DIAGNOSTIC TECHNIQUES AND SURGICAL MANAGEMENT OF BRAIN TUMORS

Edited by **Ana Lucia Abujamra**

Diagnostic Techniques and Surgical Management of Brain Tumors
Edited by Ana Lucia Abujamra

Published by InTech

Janeza Trdine 9, 51000 Rijeka, Croatia

Publishing Process Manager Iva Simcic

Technical Editor Teodora Smiljanic

Cover Designer InTech Design Team

Additional hard copies can be obtained from orders@intechopen.com

Diagnostic Techniques and Surgical Management of Brain Tumors,
Edited by Ana Lucia Abujamra
p. cm.
ISBN 978-953-307-589-1

For EU product safety concerns:
IN TECH d.o.o., Prolaz Marije Krucifikse Kozulić 3, 51000 Rijeka, Croatia, info@intechopen.com or visit our website at intechopen.com.

Meet the editor

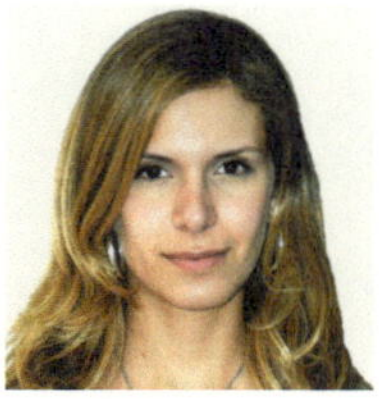

Ana Lucia Abujamra received her training at Boston University School of Medicine, where she was awarded her doctorate degree. Later she worked at Beth Israel Deaconess Medical Center and at Boston Medical Center, Boston, Massachusetts, USA. She currently lives in Porto Alegre, Brazil, working as translational research coordinator at the Children's Cancer Institute and principal investigator of the Cancer Research Laboratory, University Hospital, Federal University of Rio Grande do Sul. She holds a teaching position at the Department of Medical Sciences, Federal University of Rio Grande do Sul, and is partner and co-founder of Ziel Biosciences, a biotech start-up focusing on individualized therapy for cancer patients.

Contents

Preface

Because of their location alone, central nervous system tumors may be the hardest tumors to diagnose and manage. Numerous imaging techniques and diagnostic tools have been developed over time, in order to stage the tumor correctly and determine its precise location - events that determine the initial tumor staging and grading and that aid the surgeon in performing a thorough tumor resection while preserving this noble organ as best as possible.

Within this spectrum, the book is divided into two sections: In the first section, the principle neuroimaging techniques are described, along with other diagnostic methods. These chapters present an extensive review of the current clinical practice and evaluate the new methodologies that may aid in early detection and more precise diagnosis of tumor extent and margins. The second section reviews the neurosurgical practices commonly used for tumor resection, and present new techniques for advanced surgical management.

The main focus of this book is the gliomas, given their incidence and dismal prognosis, but other brain tumors, including brain metastases, are also discussed. Written by experts in the field, this book provides the most up-to-date information regarding the diagnostic and surgical techniques available, and each chapter is extensively referenced, providing a comprehensive bibliographical guide on the subjects discussed.

The aim of the chapters here presented is in contributing to the understanding of how better diagnosis and surgical management of brain tumors may impact on patient overall survival and quality of their life. I believe you will find that they have met this goal – it is now our duty, as healthcare professionals, to put them to practice.

Dr. Ana Lucia Abujamra
Hospital de Clínicas de Porto Alegre
Oncologia Pediátrica- Terceiro Leste, Porto Alegre
Brasil

Part 1

Neuroimaging Tools and Other Diagnostic Methods

1

Patient-Reported Outcome Monitoring in Brain Tumour Patients: Benefits and Requirements

Lisa M. Wintner, Johannes M. Giesinger and Bernhard Holzner
Innsbruck Medical University
Austria

1. Introduction

In 2008 within the European Union brain cancer and cancer of the nervous system ranked number 15 within the 20 most diagnosed cancer types (Ferlay et al., 2010). Compared to the five most frequent cancer types brain cancer seems to have a small-sized incidence-rate, but the mortality rate for this type of cancer is much higher than those of most high-incidence-cancers (except lung cancer). Though brain cancer is only seldom diagnosed, its negative impact on patients health status and well-being should not be disregarded, as survival prognosis is poor and deteriorated health-related quality of life (QOL) is common (Taphoorn et al., 2010). Treatment options comprise surgery, radiation, chemotherapy and supplementary medical therapies. Brain cancer is characterised by a large variety of tumour types and a distinction is made between primary tumours arising directly from brain tissue and secondary tumours, which are brain metastases from other malignant diseases. This differentiation is often difficult to make, though, it is of special importance since the best possible treatment e.g. for glioblastoma strongly differs from those for brain metastases (Campos et al., 2009) and inadequate intervention jeopardises patients' QOL.

Survival expectancy is strongly related to the WHO grade of the tumour and varies vigorously. Grade I tumours may not shorten life expectancy, grade II tumours are associated with a survival time of 2-10 years, grade III tumours with a survival time of 2-3 years and grade IV tumours with a survival time of only 9-12 months (Reardon & Wen, 2006). Not only the tumour itself, but also treatment-related side effects and adverse events caused by supportive medication (e.g. steroids and antiepileptic drugs (Sizoo et al., 2010)), confront the patient with a high level of physical and psychosocial burden. Brain tumour patients are affected by a diversity of tumour symptoms, which might be caused by increased intracranial pressure (e.g. headache, anorexia, seizures, nausea, vomiting, sleeping longer at night, drowsiness, napping during the day). Further physical impairments may occur due to focal neurological deficits (e.g. motor deficit, aphasia, visual field defects) and even more burdensome both for patients and care-givers might be symptoms like personality changes, decrease in mental capacity and concentration, mood disturbances, cognitive dysfunction, fatigue and anxiety (Heimans & Taphoorn, 2002; Sizoo et al., 2010). These symptoms were found to have a negative impact on both patients' and their carers' overall QOL if compared to general population (Janda et al., 2007). As brain tumour patients cannot be cured in most cases, the treatment has to focus on maintaining QOL, to make the patient's remaining life time as enjoyable as possible.

2. Patient-reported outcomes

A short and concise definition of patient-reported outcomes (PROs) is presented by the Food and Drug Administration: "A PRO is a measurement of any aspect of a patient's health status that comes directly from the patient (i.e., without the interpretation of the patient's responses by a physician or anyone else)."(U.S. Food and drug administration (FDA), 2006). Therefore, PROs allow the comprehensive evaluation of patients' perception of aspects of functioning and well-being in regard to their health status, disease, and its treatment. They comprise a variety of directly reported health-related issues: disease-related symptoms, treatment-related adverse events, functioning, well-being, health-related quality of life (QOL), perceptions about treatment, satisfaction with care and professional communication (Rothman et al., 2007). Commonly assessed PROs are e.g. QOL, depression, anxiety, pain, fatigue, gastrointestinal symptoms, social functioning, or perceived cognitive dysfunction. Thus, PROs are characterised by versatility in possible application, as they may be used for QOL evaluation both in clinical research and routine, for adverse event detection in drug-safety reports and medical product development, and for guidance in medical decision making.

Many studies already illustrate that PRO-data provides additional information, which is useful for medical decision-making and treatment choices. Two papers report the results from a study with newly diagnosed glioblastoma patients (Stupp et al., 2005; Taphoorn et al., 2005). Intensive treatment comprising radiotherapy and chemotherapy with temozolomide was compared to standard treatment in regard to survival and QOL. The combined treatment option was generally refused by clinicians, since they supposed the potential side-effects to outweigh the possible benefit of longer survival. PRO-assessment at baseline, during and after treatment showed that patients with combined radio- and temozolomide chemotherapy survived longer than patients with radiotherapy alone, without additional impairments of self-reported QOL.

Marino et al. (2008) investigated QOL and overall survival in breast cancer patients receiving conventional chemotherapy or high-dose chemotherapy. PRO-data revealed that high-dose chemotherapy caused severe impairments in functioning scales and considerably high ailments due to nausea, fatigue and pain during active treatment. Furthermore patients' QOL recovered more slowly when high-dose treatment was administered and QOL remained stable at a lower level than QOL of patients with standard treatment. This additional QOL impairment due to high-dose therapy was not associated with longer overall survival.

A study conducted by Press et al. (2001) and Ganz et al. (2003) compared treatment options for patients with early Hodgkin's disease. The patient group who received chemotherapy before standard treatment (subtotal lymphoid irradiation, SLI) did not suffer from higher toxicity, had a higher failure-free survival and fewer relapses or deaths than patients receiving only SLI. Though, these benefits in respect to clinical outcomes were associated to a greater severity of symptoms, more fatigue and poorer QOL six months after baseline. Nevertheless, it must be kept in mind that treatment with chemotherapy lasted twice as long as standard treatment and therefore time for recovery was longer in SLI patients. At the one year follow-up QOL-scores returned to baseline levels in both treatment groups.

Individual patients as well as health care providers can benefit from PROs, as these may not only support patients in selecting an available treatment, but also enhance the general understanding of the disease and improve its treatment and the management of treatment-related side-effects. Additionally, PROs may alleviate the decisional hierarchy between clinicians and patients by involving both sides into the formulation of important health and QOL domains, which are considered to need clinical attention (Snyder et al., 2010). In this way, medical issues do not longer suppress QOL domains. Besides, by giving patients' the possibility to contribute to the choice of medical treatment, their anxiety and depression can be reduced and their QOL improved (Arora, 2003).

A high percentage of clinicians support the assessment of PRO-data, but only one third of them has knowledge about PRO-instruments and procedures for data collection (Bossola et al., 2010). This lack of understanding, of what PROs exactly are and what they can contribute in daily routine, could be one reason that clinicians see their authority questioned and refuse to work with PROs. However, PROs do not intent to compete with direct physician-patient communication or to replace clinicians' expert opinion. PROs rather want to improve the ability to identify and detect specific impairments and symptoms including psychological problems. The integration of patients' individual perspective may also improve multi-professional cooperation and the combination of different medical and psychological treatment options to a patient-tailored and comprehensive therapeutic concept. Many clinicians argue that the use of PROs would take too much time, but it is reported that follow-up appointments did not or only 0.5 to 2.7 minutes prolong due to PRO-assessment (Frost et al., 2007).

The additional value of PRO-data in clinical routine was shown in some randomised-controlled trials. The prescription of pain medication in a mixed sample of cancer patients differed significantly between patients who completed a pain-self-rating and patients who did not. Prescriptions for patients who provided a self-report changed more often, both with increase and decrease. In patients without self-reports prescriptions changed less frequently and only with an increase (Trowbridge et al., 1997). In another study, clinical staff responsible for lung cancer patients was demonstrated how to read PRO-data and they were encouraged to use reports of these data to detect domains, which could guide the discussion about QOL with the patient. Patients whose clinicians used PRO-data reported more domains discussed in regard to QOL within the consultation (Taenzer et al., 2000). In patients with various cancer diagnoses undergoing palliative chemotherapy, the use of PRO-data before the follow-up visits prior to each chemotherapy cycle had a number of significant effects: communication about QOL issues improved, unobvious domains like social functioning and fatigue were more often discussed and patients' felt to a larger extent emotionally supported. Clinicians showed a tendency to be more responsive to problems in unobvious QOL-domains. The duration of the follow-up visit was not prolonged by the use of PRO-data (Detmar et al., 2002a). Another population of cancer patients with different diagnoses receiving chemotherapy gave evidence that the explicit use of PRO-data can have a positive impact on patients' QOL and emotional well-being (Velikova et al., 2004). Of these patients whose PRO-data was explicitly used, the vast majority rated the questionnaire to be useful to communicate personal feelings to the clinician (Velikova et al., 2010).

Although studies have shown that PROs can be useful for enhancing communication in clinical routine, there are also studies that do not report a beneficial impact of PROs. Some studies did not find any effect of the usage of PRO-data on global QOL of patients (Drury et al., 2000; McLachlan et al., 2001; Detmar et al., 2002a). A randomized-controlled trial conducted by Rosenbloom et al. (2007) provided PRO-data and results of structured interviews of advanced cancer patients undergoing chemotherapy to their nursing staff. No effect of the mere provision of PRO-data on clinical management strategies, satisfaction or QOL was found. The authors suggest that the communication of PRO-data is only useful, if oncology staff is also provided with concrete information about treatment and care strategies for certain QOL-impairments. This criticism concerns all of the above mentioned studies investigating PROs in clinical routine, as none of them gives any specific treatment advice to clinicians (Taenzer et al., 2000; McLachlan et al., 2001; Detmar et al., 2002a; Velikova et al., 2004; Velikova et al., 2010).

Osoba (2007) emphasizes that PROs can be useful at several stages of patient-management, especially when they are conducted in parallel to conventional medical procedures. Besides gathering information about patients' medical history, physical exams, laboratory and imaging tests, treatment and follow-up, PROs may be used to support differential diagnosis and to monitor patients' progress. Similar to these steps, which are associated with several courses of action, also PRO-data has to be associated with guidelines for clinicians, which interventions can be set, if impaired QOL-domains are detected. Clinicians have to be trained in PRO-data interpretation and in possibilities for QOL-focused support. By analogy, it would seem bizarre to argue that blood level analysis is useless, because clinicians do not adjust treatment in regard to these characteristic values due to insufficient knowledge about how to use them. Exactly this is a problem with PRO-data: most studies do not evaluate specific interventions imposed after PRO-data analysis, but only the collection of PROs. Some studies tell clinicians to use PRO-data within patient-clinician communication, but do not guide them *how* to use this data. Therefore the study results might depend on the open-mindedness, prior experience and the expertise about PRO-use of the clinician. Furthermore, some patients might already benefit from the mere collection of PRO-data and others might need focused intervention.

Regarding the studies that did not find any positive effect of PRO-data, some further limitations have to be taken into account. There was only a low compliance of clinicians' to pay attention to PRO-data and to use them regularly. Just a third of all possible offered interventions were used by patients and physical procedures were more often accepted than psychological consulting (McLachlan et al., 2001). Furthermore, ceiling effects may have disguised existing effects of PRO-data usage on patients' satisfaction (Taenzer et al., 2000; Detmar et al., 2002a).

Even if the results of randomized-controlled trials concerning the usage of PRO-data are mixed, there is evidence that PROs can enrich patient-clinician communication and in this way also influence patients' QOL. PRO-completion seems not to impose an intolerable burden to patients and many studies report high acceptance of PROs - conducted as paper-pencil or more sophisticated via a software program - even in sick patients (Mullen et al., 2004; Bush et al., 2005).

The acceptance of PROs by patients is usually very good, as they are capable to bridge the gap between favoured discussions on QOL-domains with their clinician and patients' hesitation to initiate these discussions themselves. Detmar et al. (2000) reported that QOL domains differ in regard to how often patients wish their clinician to start a conversation on a certain issue. Approximately 25-29% of patients wish their clinician to ask them about their emotional functioning, daily activities and familial issues. About 37% of patients expect their clinician to address the topic of social functioning. Hereby PROs can successfully contribute to satisfaction of clinicians and patients, as clinicians attain a deeper insight in patient's needs and may properly address relevant topics and patients do not need to answer a variety of possibly irrelevant questions during the face-to-face consultation. PROs may also sharpen clinicians' awareness for psychological, social and spiritual functioning and diminish the domination of physical functioning in patient-doctor conversation (Rodriguez et al., 2010).

2.1 PRO instruments

For PRO-assessment in cancer patients, an extendable generic cancer core-questionnaire can be administered, which might be supplemented by disease-specific questionnaire-modules. Widely used, validated and reliable cancer-targeted instruments for instance are the European Organization for Research and Treatment of Cancer core questionnaire (EORTC QLQ-C30) and the Functional Assessment of Cancer Therapy general version (FACT-G). To both of these instruments a brain cancer-specific module can be added (QLQ-BN20 for the EORTC QLQ-C30 and FACT-Br and the FACT-Br Symptom Index (FBrSI) for the FACT-G). Table 1 gives an overview of the questionnaire characteristics.

2.1.1 EORTC QLQ-C30 and QLQ-BN20

The EORTC QLQ-C30 was originally developed to evaluate QOL in cancer patients participating in clinical trials (Aaronson et al., 1993) and is a nowadays widely used and internationally validated cancer-targeted PRO-instrument. The core questionnaire consists of thirty questions and is the basic part of the QOL-instrument, which can be expanded by additional elements. These supplementary modules focus on diagnosis-specific symptoms and impairments. Altogether, the QLQ-C30 comprises nine scales and six single item symptoms. Five scales concern various functioning domains (physical, role, social, emotional and cognitive functioning), one is a scale for global QOL, and three are symptom scales (pain, fatigue, nausea/vomiting). Except for the two questions about general QOL every question needs to be rated on a likert scale from "not at all", "a little", "quite a bit" to "very much". The overall QOL scale asks the patients to grade how they experienced their general QOL and physical condition between 0 "very poor" and 6 "excellent". With the exception of the physical functioning scale, all questions use a time frame of one week before the examination date.
The EORTC Brain Cancer Module (QLQ-BN20) contains 20 items and focuses on symptoms that particularly concern brain cancer patients undergoing chemotherapy or radiotherapy. In this way, both disease symptoms and treatment toxicities are included in the item list (Sprangers et al., 1998). The QLQ-BN20 is divided into four scales (future uncertainty, visual disorder, communication deficit, motor dysfunction) and seven single items (headache, seizure, drowsiness, hair loss, itching, weakness of both legs, difficulty controlling bladder function) (Osoba et al., 2000).

2.1.2 FACT-G and FACT-Br/FBrSI

The Functional Assessment of Chronic Illness Therapy (FACIT) measurement system provides questionnaires concerning a variety of chronic illnesses and their conditions, for instance cancer, HIV/AIDS, and multiple sclerosis. Within the FACIT the FACT-G questionnaire is a cancer-specific instrument for PRO-assessment (Webster et al., 2003). Nowadays the fourth version of the FACT-G is widely used and comprises 27 items grouped into four primary QOL domains (physical well-being, social/family well-being, emotional well-being, and functional well-being). The patient has to rate each item on a five-point Likert-scale between "not at all", "a little bit", "somewhat", "quite a bit" and "very much" in relation to symptom severity during the last week. The FACT-G was examined concerning its ease of administration, brevity, reliability, validity and responsiveness to clinical change and was found to fit all the stipulated requirements (Cella et al., 1993). The questionnaire's validity was also tested for a variety of language versions (Sanchez et al., 2011).

The brain cancer-specific FACT-Br module consists of 23 items and explores how patients perceive their cognitive, neurological, sensory and psychological functioning and the impact of changes in these domains on their daily living. Additionally, the FACT-Br Symptom Index (FBrSI) is available for symptom rating of brain tumour patients. Both the FACT-Br and FBrSI proved to be reliable, valid and responsive to change (Nickolov et al., 2005).

instrument	**scales**	**items**
FACT-G Functional Assessment of Cancer Therapy-General	- physical well-being - social/family well-being - emotional well-being - functional well-being	27
FACT-Br Functional Assessment of Cancer Therapy-Brain Module	- cognitive functioning - neurological functioning - sensory functioning - psychological functioning - impact of changes in functioning on daily living.	23
FBrSI FACT-Br Symptom Index	- brain tumour specific symptom list	15
EORTC QLQ-C30 European Organisation for Research and Treatment of Cancer Quality of Life Questionnaire Core 30	- functioning (physical, role, social, emotional and cognitive) - global QOL - pain, fatigue, nausea/vomiting - dyspnoea, sleeping disturbances, appetite loss, constipation, diarrhoea and financial impact	30
EORTC QLQ-BN20 European Organisation for Research and Treatment of Cancer Quality of Life Brain Module	- future uncertainty - visual disorder - communication deficit - motor dysfunction) - headache, seizure, drowsiness, hair loss, itching, weakness of both legs, difficulty controlling bladder function	20

All instruments have been extensively validated.
All instruments use a recall period of one week.

Table 1.Commonly used PRO-instruments for cancer patients with brain modules available

2.2 The value of proxy-reported outcomes

A common symptom burden in brain cancer patients are cognitive impairments, which may be caused by the disease itself or anti-cancer treatment. Although PROs are the method of choice for QOL-assessment, this method is not suitable for patients who suffer from deteriorated cognitive function. A large amount of patients is not able to complete PRO-instruments due to serious malfunction in cognition, speech, vision, concentration or language. Even if these symptoms are perceived at a low level, PRO-assessment can be too burdensome for these patients and cause additional distress. This implies that the needs of a certain subgroup of patients are possibly not adequately met, because they are excluded from QOL-assessment and therefore also from intervention. Furthermore, the exclusion of these patients from longitudinal studies sugarcoat data and may produce compromising and misleading results (Sneeuw et al., 1997). Especially the subgroup of patients, who are not able to give information about their QOL themselves, might particularly be in need for intervention concerning impaired QOL-domains.

A complementary source of information about patients' QOL are therefore ratings from clinicians, nurses or significant others (spouses, children, family members or close friends). Normally, the usefulness of information provided by others on patients' QOL is investigated by analysing the agreement of outsiders' and patients' ratings. Therefore, proxies or health care providers have to complete the same PRO-instrument as the patient. The degree of agreement or correlation of patients' and others' answers reflects the reliability of this approach for QOL-data collection. Generally, proxy ratings tend to overestimate patients' symptom burden and underestimate their QOL, because proxies are in their ratings influenced by their own feelings and experiences of care-giving activities. Nevertheless, care-giving significant others are supposed to be a valuable source for information about patients' QOL, especially for concrete and observable domains (Addington-Hall & Kalra, 2001). In brain cancer patients there was exact agreement between proxies and patients found in 60% of the questions of the EORTC QLQ-C30 and the module BN20. If one category of difference in either direction was allowed, even over 90% of approximate agreement was obtained. There were only low correlations between ratings of social functioning, nausea/vomiting, and pain. Over time, agreement worsened significantly for patients whose condition deteriorated since the baseline assessment. Additionally, disagreements in answers were more likely if patients were more physically and neurologically impaired or mentally confused (Sneeuw et al., 1997).

In brain cancer patients a moderate-to-high patient-proxy agreement for the Linear Analogue Self-Assessment (comprises questions concerning physical condition, social interactions, psychological effects of disease and personal relationships), for hope, confusion and sadness was reported (Hahn & Dunn, 2003). Brown et al. (2008) report for patients with newly diagnosed high-grade glioma a moderate-to-high patient-proxy agreement at the FACT-Br questionnaire. They also indicate that agreement was influenced by patients' cognitive status. Low scores at the Folstein Mini-Mental State Examination were associated with a poorer agreement between proxies and patients in their rating of mood states. Giesinger et al. (2009a) report not only high discrepancies of patient-proxy rating for social functioning, dyspnoea and seizures, but also good agreement for the scales physical functioning, sleeping disturbances, appetite loss, constipation, financial impact and taste alterations (EORTC QLQ-C30 and BN20). They support the use of proxy-ratings for QOL-assessment in brain cancer patients, but also critically note that general agreement is higher for physical symptoms than for psychosocial issues.

All in all, patients and proxies exactly agreed in their answers to a high extent and variations mostly did not exceed more than one answer category (Sneeuw et al., 1997). Cognitive impairments seem to worsen agreement between patients and proxies (Sneeuw et al., 1997; Brown et al., 2008). More obvious physical symptoms show better agreement rates than psychosocial issues (Giesinger et al., 2009b). Although proxy-patient agreement deteriorates over time if patient's health and/or mental condition get worse, it still is reasonable to collect proxy-reported QOL-data for incorporating also the most ill patients in data-collection for intervention and research purposes.

3. Electronic PRO-data capture

Even though PRO assessments gain more and more importance in scientific research, e.g. concerning drug evaluation studies and label claim issues, they are not yet completely accepted as measurement method for adverse event detection, QOL-measurement and primary outcome in randomized controlled trials. Currently, many clinicians still consider clinician ratings' as being sufficient for adequate evaluation of patients' well-being and symptom burden (Basch, 2010). Patrick (2007) emphasizes the usefulness of PRO instruments, as they allow the capture of advantages and disadvantages of known or newly developed treatment options, which is valuable for choosing between therapies and for reasoning already chosen disease management strategies. One third of palliative cancer patients received adjusted treatment in respect to QOL improvement, but clinicians only focused on overall QOL instead of a variety of subscales and eclipsed QOL issues if patients showed tumour progression or increased treatment toxicity (Detmar et al., 2002b). This illustrates that specialized training for physicians is necessary to ladle the potential benefit of PRO-data in clinical routine.

Walker et al. (2003) report administrative failure as most important reason for missing data (72.2 percent) in PRO-data collection in patients suffering from malignant glioma. About 21.7 percent of patients did not fill out the PRO-instruments due to their very bad health condition and only 6.1 percent of patients refused to participate in PRO-assessments. The major problem of administrative failures in the study of Walker et al. (2003) can be traced to irregular administration time points of QOL PROs, too little explanation of instrument completion and missing specialized staff for QOL research who checks questionnaires for completeness. Such barriers can easily be overcome with the routine usage of electronic ePROs, which avoid a high percentage of missing data, as a standardized questionnaire explanation is integrated in the procedure and further questions are only displayed after all preceding questions have been answered.

3.1 Requirements for ePRO and its implementation

The implementation of ePRO in clinical routine requires some underlying circumstances, which enable effective QOL-evaluation. Firstly, there is a need for a comprehensive IT infrastructure that includes technical devices for data collection, software solutions for calculation and graphical illustration of results and network facilities for data-transmission, storage and backup. For data collection personal computers (PCs), laptops or personal digital assistants (PDAs) can be used. These devices differ in their feasibility according to patient-groups.

For outpatients a fixed PC-workstation can be useful, since these patients are supposed to be in a relatively good health condition and able to see the PC by themselves. Portable devices like laptops and PDAs seem to be more useful for inpatients, who are approached directly at the hospital bed. The IT infrastructure also should include a database for data storage and backup. A central database allows that clinicians from different wards have access to patients prior and latest QOL-assessments. A database connection can be established via a local area network (LAN) or Wifi (wireless fidelity, also WLAN, wireless local area network). Connection via LAN is more laborious as the study nurse needs to connect the tablet PC to the LAN with the purpose of preparing the patient list to who the questionnaire shall be administered. The tablet PC has to be disconnected, handed over to patients for bed-side assessment and again connected to the LAN for uploading the collected information into the database.

A connection provided by WiFi is much more comfortable, as the database can be updated anytime without special constraints. Wifi is nowadays a common and inexpensive technology that is also practicable in a hospital setting. Connection via WiFi eases work for both data collectors and clinicians, as data is transferred instantly and the immediate access to patients' data is possible. Especially for home monitoring some additional requirements are added. If home monitoring is conducted via web-access, a feasible and user-friendly website with special security features is needed. Privacy of health information, data security and patients' safety need special attention when developing an online PRO-platform (Basch et al., 2007).

Secondly, clinicians and nurses need to be trained in two ways: on the one hand in device and software handling and on the other hand in choosing interventions according to PRO-data. Acquaintance with technical equipment allows to answer most of patients' questions and to solve minor problems directly on site. Training in result interpretation is also necessary, as PRO-data is supposed to give information about patients' QOL and initiate thereby medical and/or psychosocial intervention. Although there are software solutions that offer easily interpretable graphs, precise instructions for interventions are still of crucial importance. Interpreting QOL-scores correctly is only the first step of successful ePRO-data use. The second step is to choose appropriate intervention strategies for QOL-management. Furthermore, a positive attitude of health care providers towards PRO-assessment is strongly necessary. Clinicians and nurses exert influence on patients and therefore also affect their compliance, since patients often orientate themselves by clinicians' suggestions. The vivid contribution of clinicians and nurses to assess and use PRO-data may also carry patients along and support the whole PRO-procedure in all stages.

3.2 Feasibility

Velikova et al. (1999) report a high acceptance of ePRO in a mixed sample of cancer patients. Patients were asked to complete a paper-pencil as well as an electronic version of the EORTC QLQ-C30, with an interval of three hours between the two assessments. More than half of the patients preferred the ePRO version to the traditional paper-pencil questionnaire, whilst each 24% of patients preferred the paper-pencil questionnaire or had no preference. Overall, the ePRO version was slightly quicker completed by patients, whereas older patients in general needed more time to complete the PRO-instruments, independent of the type of administration. The quality of collected QOL-data was excellent if electronic assessment was used, as no missing data occurred. Although Velikova et al. (1999) hypothesized that patients would rather refuse to take part in a study, which demands them to use a computer for data-collection, compliance rates were similar to those in traditional therapeutic clinical trials.

The assessment of QOL by means of ePROs is also feasible in a clinical routine setting with a large number of mixed cancer patients attending the ward of an oncology clinic. Wright et al. (2003) conducted two feasibility studies, whose results underline that in comparison to a separate prospective patient sample (study 1), routine ePRO-assessment (study 2) reached higher compliance rates and therefore a better data-base for the description of changes over time. In both studies the majority of patients did not feel that the ePROs made their visit more difficult or temporally longer and only few patients said that they would refuse to complete ePROs as part of clinical routine. Most patients reported that the electronic equipment was easy to use and general feedback on ePROs was positive.

Carlson et al. (2001) used a computerized version of the EORTC QLQ-C30 that was already successfully utilized by Taenzer et al. (2000) for investigating the ePRO-based changes in lung cancer outpatient care. Already in this previous study (Taenzer et al., 2000) the QOL-tool was shown to be feasible and effective in sensitizing clinicians for QOL-issues. In the study of Carlson et al. (2001), the effectiveness of ePROs was examined with a group of patients with extensive symptom burden, who attended a cancer pain and symptom control clinic. The majority of patients rated the computerized EORTC QLQ-C30 version to be easy in use and well understandable. Their satisfaction with the ePRO was high and with repeated use of ePRO they judged the use of computers more favourably. Clinical staff felt that the ePRO was appropriate for QOL-assessment and useful for guiding the interaction with the patient. All in all, both highly impaired patients and health care providers support the use of ePRO and confirmed their feasibility and usefulness.

3.3 Symptom monitoring and screening

Brain cancer patients are affected by a variety of severe clinical symptoms. Since the survival time in most brain cancer patients is rigorously limited, early and symptom-focused intervention is of paramount importance. PRO-data works in two ways concerning symptom management. On the one hand, QOL-evaluation reveals impaired domains, which need targeted intervention. On the other hand, regularly assessed PRO-data allows achieving a deeper understanding of the impact of symptom management on a variety of symptoms besides the aimed symptom (Ganz & Goodwin, 2007). By way of example, there was the intention to improve physical functioning by pain reduction and PRO-data might show that other QOL-domains changed as well. PRO-assessments also capture unexpected developments and may illustrate interrelationships among QOL-domains (Ganz & Goodwin, 2007).

Next to treatment-related symptoms, cancer patients have also to deal with psychosocial distress triggered by the disease itself and anti-cancer therapy. Since the inadequate or missing treatment of psychosocial distress may confront the patient with further impairments, as they might develop chronic mental disorders, early detection of psychosocial distress is necessary (Meraner et al., 2009). Effective screening for psychosocial distress can be performed by means of PRO-instruments like the Hospital Anxiety and Depression Scale (HADS) (Zigmond & Snaith, 1983) or the General Health Questionnaire (GHQ-12) (Goldberg, 1972). Approximately 20-40 percent of cancer patients suffer from psychosocial distress and are therefore in need for referral to psychooncological treatment (Meraner et al., 2009). A study of Zabora et al. (2001) identified brain cancer patients to be highly endangered to perceive extensive psychosocial distress. Nearly 43 percent of brain cancer patients were tested positive with a distress screening by means of the Brief Symptom Inventory and ranked second after lung cancer with only tiny difference. For these patients, PROs contribute in the detection of needs for psychooncological treatment and therefore prevent further ailments.

As a screening tool is supposed to offer a quick possibility to check for impairments that require treatment, cut-off scores are of major importance. Additionally, the comparison to norm or reference values from general population or other cancer cohorts plays an essential role for the definition of impaired or normal QOL. For the interpretation of changes in PRO-scores it is necessary to know, which score-deviations reflect clinical meaningful changes. Statistically significant effects are easily to find if a high number of patients contributed in PRO-data collection, but not every significant effect also must be a subjectively meaningful difference (Cella & Nowinski, 2002). To correctly interpret changes in PRO-scores, minimal important differences (MID) can be used. Jaeschke et al. (1989) described MID as the „smallest difference in score in the domain of interest which patients perceive as beneficial and which would mandate, in the absence of troublesome side effects and excessive cost, a change in patient's management" (as cited in Dubois et al., 2006, p 977). MIDs are diverse for PRO-instruments and may also differ between diagnoses and disease stages (Revicki et al., 2008). Furthermore, they vary in dependence on how good baseline scores were and if QOL increased or deteriorated (Farivar et al., 2004). In addition, it is necessary to know if a change in the QOL-score is associated to the patients' experience with a small, medium or large effect (Guyatt et al., 2002).

There are considerable differences in the MIDs, depending on whether individual or group scores are used for analysis. For the EORTC QLQ-C30 and the FACIT system MIDs for group levels have been established but these MIDs should not be used in the same way for individual score interpretation (Giesinger et al., 2009a). On average unchanged QOL-scores of a group may also contain individual scores that meaningfully changed (Crosby et al., 2003; Kemmler et al., 2010). Small changes on group level may be clinical significant, whereas on an individual level these changes do not reach clinical significance (Guyatt et al., 2002), since small score differences in individuals may be due to measurement errors if they do not exceed the range of variation. Moreover, not every single patient experiences the average score change of the group, but a stronger or weaker score-deviation. Thus, group comparisons are used for the evaluation of various treatments and health policy decisions, while for actual clinical decision making conclusions derived from the individual level should be used (Crosby et al., 2003). These methodological considerations illustrate how important it is to train clinicians and nursing staff in PRO-data interpretation, since a correct understanding of the data is the basis for adequate intervention.

3.4 ePRO software example

For obtaining the highest grade of feasibility and utility of PRO-assessments, the use of specialized software that fits perfectly the needs of both patients and clinicians is obligatory. In recent years some effort has been undertaken to develop and implement software solutions for QOL-assessment in clinical routine, for instance by Joerg Sigle (AnyQuest) and Galina Velikova and Irma Verdonck (OncoQuest). These tools use touch screens and have shown to be feasible in clinical practice. Implementation studies suggest that routine patient-monitoring using a software solution for assessment is beneficial for clinicians, patients and medical care in general (Wright et al., 2003; Velikova et al., 2004; Rogausch et al., 2009).

A further example for such a specific software solution is the computer-based health evaluation system (CHES). CHES has been especially been developed for electronic PRO-data capture and offers a variety of useful features for clinical routine and research purposes. Any required paper-pencil questionnaire can be implemented into the CHES program to facilitate all steps from data collection to result calculation, interpretation and statistical data analysis as well. CHES provides a database (e.g. MySQL or Oracle) for supplementary medical and psychosocial data. This database is particularly useful for research purposes, as it improves study logistics, reduces human resources and increases data quality. A so-called flag system enriches and facilitates the interpretation of QOL-data, since the implementation of reference values makes it possible to mark clinically relevant changes and problems. PRO-data can be accessed as a single assessment summary or as longitudinal graphical charts. The last one allows the immediate detection of changes and deficits in every single scale and gives an overview of the course of symptoms even if the clinician only takes a quick look at the graphs (Holzner et al., 2004). The availability of user-friendly and well-tested software for PRO-assessments is the key for successful routine implementation of PROs. CHES already offers a variety of beneficial features for PRO-application in clinical routine. A research project in cooperation with the EORCT Quality of Life Group (QLG) aims at the further development and distribution of CHES within the QLG for electronic QOL-assessment by means of the EORTC QLQ-C30 and its modules. The project comprises several steps of software development, multilingual software releases, a comprehensive manual and the work on additional features like computer-adaptive testing (CAT), telemonitoring and a web-forum for users and researchers.

Holzner et al. (2011) implemented CHES for routine QOL monitoring at a neuro-oncological outpatient unit and reported it to be feasible, as routinely conducted ePRO-assessments could be easily integrated into the schedule of the ward. The integration of QOL-data profiles into interdisciplinary team meetings offered the benefit that possible problem domains can be detected at an early stage and patient-centred care can be improved. The use of CHES for PRO-collection was also well accepted by another population of brain tumour patients (Erharter et al., 2010). On average patients needed only ten minutes to complete the EORTC QLQ-30 and the QLQ-BN20. Furthermore, repeated instrument administration was associated with a decrease of the average completion time. Clinicians reported the ePRO to be beneficial, as e.g. loss of bladder controlling would not have been detected adequately without ePRO.

3.4.1 Patient example for PRO-profile

To give an example for patient-reported symptom trajectories Figure 1 shows the PRO-profiles of the male patient D.K. born in 1953. He attended the hospital due to first occurence of epileptic seizures in December 2009 where diagnostic procedures revealed an astrocytoma (WHO grade III, right side, parietotemporal). After confirmation through stereotactic biopsy chemotherapy with temozolomide started in January 2010. In March 2010, the patient was included in routine ePRO monitoring with EORTC QLQ-C30 and QLQ-BN20 at the neurooncological unit using the software CHES (see Figure 1).

From April 2010 until May 2010 the patient received additional whole-brain radiotherapy. After end of therapy, the patient was seen monthly at the outpatient unit for follow-up. Figure 1 shows the course of self-reported physical functioning and motor dysfunction from March 2010 until October 2010. During this period, the initially high symptom level decreased considerably, reaching average scores. Horizontal lines in the charts in Figure 1 show the 10th percentile (red), the 25th percentile (orange), and the 50th percentile (green) from a reference group of neurooncological outpatients. Colouring of bars corresponds to these score ranges. Below each bar assessment date and abbreviation of treatment phase (chemotherapy (CT) and aftercare (AC)) is noted. Abbreviations on top of bars indicate specific interventions (pain intervention (PI) and psychooncological treatment (PO)).

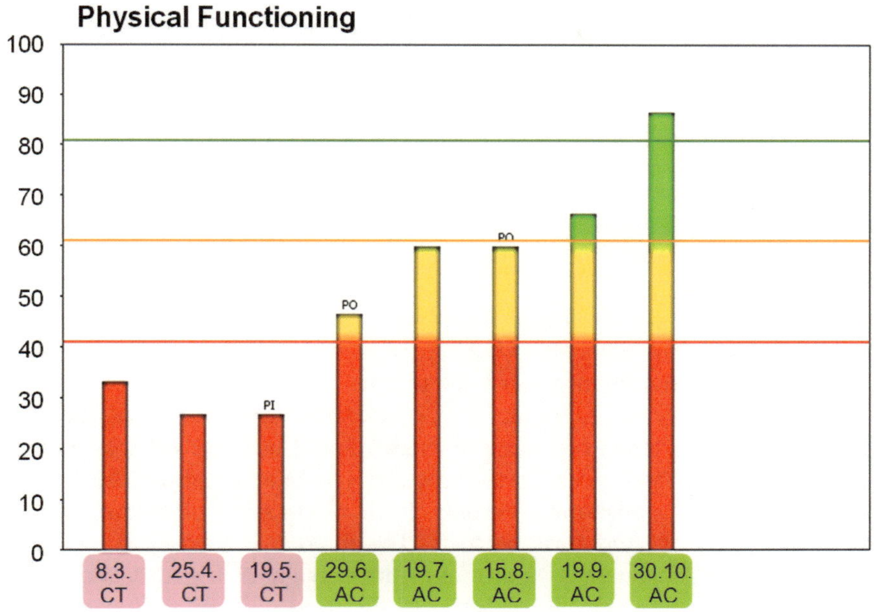

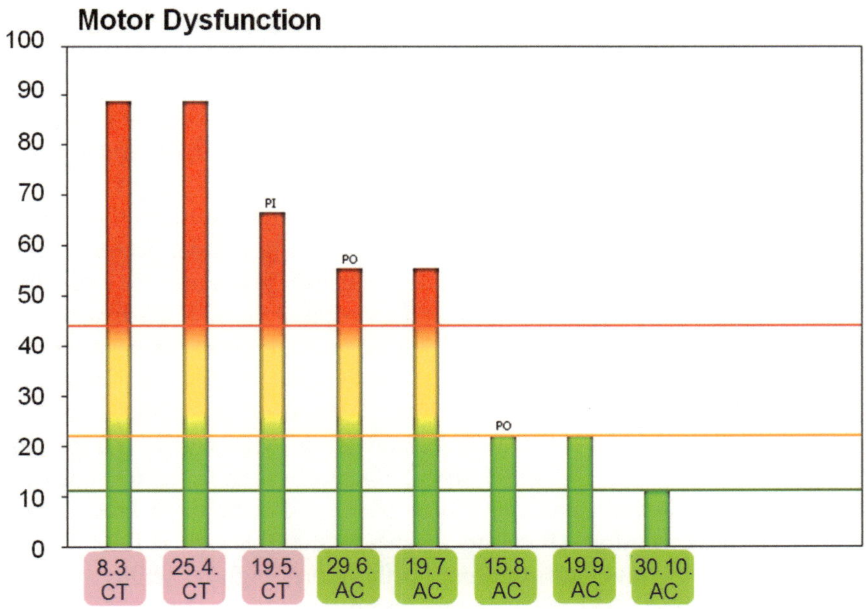

Fig. 1. Course of Physical Functioning (QLQ-C30) and Motor Dysfunction (QLQ-BN20) in a patient diagnosed with astrocytoma during chemotherapy and aftercare.

3.5 Home monitoring

Even if QOL is regularly assessed within the hospital time schedule, information about patients' well-being is still incomplete, as their PRO-monitoring ends with hospital discharge. ePRO makes it possible to follow patients' in their home environment and to accompany them also during a phase, when hospital visits are not scheduled. Especially concerning chemotherapy, side-effects and treatment-related symptom burden are known to be most severe a few days after cytostatic drug application (Hawkins & Grunberg, 2009). At that time, patients mostly are already back at home and are therefore left alone with their management of occurring adverse events. Perceived symptoms during times spent at home may be underestimated due to missing patient-monitoring. This gap may be overcome by ePROs conducted via phone or web-based assessments (telemonitoring). Telemonitoring in combination with alert systems enable clinicians to contact patients suffering from severe symptom burden and intervene appropriately even when he/she is not hospitalized (Balducci & Stanta, 2000).

PRO-data from assessments in clinical routine can be merged with data from home monitoring and provide a database, which potentially enable clinicians to get a deeper insight in disease and treatment-related symptoms in general and to identify signs of adverse events at an early stage. In this way, prospective intervention can be provided to minimize complications. However, comprehensive and close-meshed tele monotoring of patients' QOL during their home stays requires additional administrative resources. Traditional paper-pencil questionnaires only have a low rate of return and are more expensive due to printing and postage costs. The internet provides an inexpensive and nowadays widespread technology that makes an easy, user friendly and reliable data collection possible. Though web-PROM imposes the need of a minimal computer literacy and internet use of patients, there is statistical data for Europe (Seybert & Lööf, 2010) that supports the assumption that web-PROM may be feasible in a considerable percentage of cancer patients. In 2010, 70% of European households had an internet connection and 69% of internet-users across all age groups used the internet regularly. The average rate of European internet-users who obtained health-related information via online sources doubled within the last six years (from 17% in 2004 to 34% in 2010) and is supposed to increase further.

Although telemonitoring yet only reached an early stage of development, there are already a few studies available that document its use within oncological care. The most remarkable study was conducted by Bush et al. (2005) and collected QOL-data via web-PROM from patients who received hematopoietic stem cell transplantation. PRO-data was collected whether on a daily or monthly basis. Daily assessments consisted of only four out of 38 items, which varied according to a quasi-random frequency, and a global QOL item. Monthly assessments included all 38 items at once and needed to be completed within two successive days. Patients had to visit a website and log in with a private user name and a password to enter the online QOL-assessment. Overall compliance for both daily and monthly assessments was good and only three patients discontinued study participation due to their bad health condition. Therefore, data show that this way of PRO-data collection does not only include the less sick patients. Furthermore, high feasibility of web-PROM, high patient acceptance and user satisfaction war reported.

Telemonitoring takes patients' QOL outside the hospital setting into account and contributes to its integration into symptom estimation, monitoring and treatment. Especially for brain cancer patients, telemonitoring could be of particular benefit, as it may increase their feeling of security when they spend time at home. Eventually occurring symptoms are recognized by health care providers in real time despite the geographic distance between patient and medical services.

3.6 Benefits from ePRO

The traditional way of collecting PROs by means of paper-pencil questionnaires imposes several burdens to the patient, to clinical staff and financiers. Firstly missing data is more common in paper-pencil data collection as patients often may overlook an item and clinical staff is too busy to precisely control every single questionnaire. In addition, more human and time resources are needed, as questionnaires have to be printed in a sufficient number, tacked together, an stored so they can be handed over to patients, when needed. Subscales need to be calculated, put into an interpretable characteristic value and made accessible to clinicians. This procedure does not only gulp working time, costs for printing and staff, but is also vulnerable to missing data and errors in data transfer and calculation. ePRO-assessment by means of electronic devices like laptops and tablet PCs prevent these error sources and save time as well as costs. Admittedly, ePROs need some seed money to acquire technical equipment and software, but with regular use these devices amortize soon as printing of multi-paged questionnaires is no longer necessary and staff costs are reduced.

The implementation of PRO assessments of QOL or adverse events in clinical drug evaluation studies facilitates and accelerates data flow because intricate and defective data collection is cut short. Without PRO instruments clinicians ask patients about their symptoms and write a construed summary of these symptoms down in patients' charts, from which research assistants collect information and consign them into research data bases (Trotti et al., 2007). This process is highly endangered to lose and/or alter information given by patients' and needs much more human and time resources than the use of ePRO-assessments. By means of touch screen equipped tablet PCs patients can easily complete the PRO-assessment themselves. The possibility to fit font and button sizes to the needs of different patients groups allows that readability and handling of the assessment is practicable for e.g. elderly people as well (Giesinger et al., 2009a). As no computer literacy of patients is needed for PRO-completion, in principle all patients are able to participate in ePROs. They were shown to be well accepted by patients (Mullen et al., 2004; Velikova et al., 2010), valid (Abernethy et al., 2010) and equivalent to paper-pencil versions (Coons et al., 2009).

The advantage of time saving can also be applied to clinical routine. Admittedly, at the beginning of PRO implementation some time burden may be set on clinicians and nurses, as they need to be trained in software handling and result interpretation, but after a phase of familiarization PRO instruments contribute in time saving. Firstly, the completion of a PRO instrument encourages the patient to reflect more detailed on his/her health status and symptom burden and facilitates in that way the communication between patient and clinician/nurse about relevant problem areas. Secondly, via WiFi or LAN, patient's ePRO-data is immediately accessible for the clinician, whose attention can be called to clinically relevant deteriorations or improvements. In fact, such an alert system helps clinicians to focus on issues important for the patient without long-winded enquiry of possible difficulties. Queue times of patients might meaningfully be padded by PRO-completion.

Furthermore, ePROs reduce staff costs, because score calculation, graphical illustration, alert systems and data storage are performed automatically. Time-saving aspects do not only concern data collection, but also identifying impaired QOL-domains. The implementation of reference levels simplifies the comparison between patient-groups or patients and normal population and in this way the detection of problems in QOL. Automatically generated reports may comprise only affected scales, the complete assessment or trajectories over time, depending on which information the user is interested in. Due to the instantly performed data calculation, clinicians directly can be informed after PRO completion about clinically remarkable PRO data that need adequate intervention. Clinicians may therefore pick these notable domains and address them to the patient without the need to undertake a long-winded exploration. In doing so, time can more effectively be spent on treatment and patient management, than on preliminary inquiry. The illustration of results by means of eye-catching and meaningful coloured graphs makes interpretation comfortable for both clinician and patient. Software solutions that include a storage database also simplify long-term data storage and backup. ePROs enhance data quality, since missing data is prevented by forwarding only to the remaining questions when all prior items were answered.

One common criticism to PROs is that patients are forced to answer annoying questions, which might be irrelevant to them. The development of CAT eradicates this flaw and makes ePRO-assessments for patients even more comfortable. CAT generates a patient-tailored question set and chooses appropriate items based on preceding answers. Information about diagnosis, progress of disease and treatment can also be considered for question compilation (Snyder et al., 2010).

Although many advantages of PRO assessments can be communicated, there are still popular counter-arguments rampant. Even if PRO-data is available many clinicians do not pay attention to them because of lack of time, human resources and an adequate PRO-instrument and the assumption that directly from patients obtained information does not add any additional value (Luckett et al., 2009). Furthermore some clinicians argue that information on QOL are not of same importance as treatment decisions (Morris et al., 1998), equality of PRO instruments is doubtful (Barlesi et al., 2006) and the methodology of PRO measurement seems to be dubious. These objections can be devitalised, though. Meanwhile a broad variety of internationally validated and widely used PRO instruments is available (especially for cancer populations the forgoing mentioned EORTC QLQ-C30 and the FACT-G with their supplemental modules). The use of PRO-instruments does usually not or only a few minutes prolong the clinical appointment (Frost et al., 2007). Particularly the implementation of ePROs solves the problem of time constraints as data is directly entered by patients, scores are calculated automatically and immediate information processing is possible. Electronic data capture was shown to need less time for instrument completion than paper-pencil versions (Drummond et al., 1995; Velikova et al., 1999; Taenzer et al., 2000). Table 2 summarizes pros and cons of PRO-assessments and illustrates, which benefits might outweigh commonly cited disadvantages of PRO-assessments.

Some studies illustrate that in clinical routine the usage of PROs offers further benefits than only time and cost saving. Based on PRO-data clinicians adjusted the dosage of analgesics in a more sophisticated way than without PRO-data (Trowbridge et al., 1997). The patient-clinician communication was improved (Taenzer et al., 2000; Detmar et al., 2002a) and enhanced concerning discussed domains (Detmar et al., 2002a), if clinicians took advantage of provided QOL-data. Furthermore patients felt higher emotional support, clinicians became more sensitive for normally underestimated QOL-domains (Detmar et al., 2002a), patients were more satisfied with care and the building of a relationship to the clinician (Velikova et al., 2010) and reported a better QOL (Velikova et al., 2004).

advantages of PROs	disadvantages of PROs
direct assessment of patients' perspective without intermediary (e.g. clinicians, proxies) individually tailored therapy approaches in regard to PRO-data, targeted intervention (medical, psychological) improvement of patient-clinician communication detection of unobvious problem domains (e.g. social domains, fatigue, sexual issues) heightened awareness of clinicians for unobvious problem areas patients' support in clinical decision making longitudinal PRO-data capture allows to track the impact of medical intervention	additional burden for patients
ePRO: provide automated results calculation and graphical presentation time-saving assessment of relevant problem domains that need special attention	additional resources necessary (time, human and financial resources)
large variety of validated PRO-instruments (generic and specified)	dubious comparability of PRO-instruments
CAT (computer adaptive testing) makes it possible to fit PROs to the patients' needs	current, static PRO-instruments include also items irrelevant to a patients' current health status

Table 2. Advantages and disadvantages of PRO-assessments

4. Conclusion

The raising recognition of the patients' perspective in clinical research, drug evaluation and label claim issues demonstrate the importance of PRO-assessments. However, PROs could be used in more clinical settings than they are now implemented. Especially in clinical routine PRO-data have a variety of benefits to offer, since already their mere administration potentially has positive effects on patients and clinicians.

Recapitulating, the practical implications of this chapter are the following: The use of PROs within clinical routine is easily realizable since validated and reliable instruments are available. The conduction of PRO-assessments is further facilitated by effortlessly manageable software solutions. The participation in PROs encourages the patient to reflect detailed on different domains of their QOL even before the appointment with the clinician. Immediately transferred PRO-data enables the clinician to purposefully guide the conversation towards issues the patients reported to be important. In this way, time resources are optimal utilized: Queuing time is reasonably spent, because the patient gets prepared for the visit and within the appointment the clinician can spend more time on intervention and treatment. PROs allow therefore a targeted patient-clinician communication and a comprehensive as well as systematically performed screening for symptoms and impairments.

Concerning the feasibility of PRO-assessments within the schedule of a busy oncology clinic, ePROs and constantly ongoing software development support the regular use of these measures also with neurooncological patients. It is of crucial importance to fit available PRO-instruments and their electronic administration to the needs of health care providers' daily procedures. The smooth and effective implementation of PROs in clinical routine makes it more likely that they are accepted and supported by clinicians and nurses. Although the acceptance of PROs by patients is of major importance, the health care providers' attitude towards QOL-measurement should not be disregarded. Clinicians' contribution to PRO-assessment and PRO-data use influences substantially the success and effectiveness of PROs. The way how clinicians introduce PROs to patients may influence their feelings about them as well as their willingness to contribute. If patients are approached with a positive attitude they might experience PROs as an additional benefit instead of a further burden. Therefore, health care providers need to be directly approached to actively participate in QOL-measurement in the neurooncological setting. Even if patients are no longer able to provide self-reports, as it might especially occur in neurooncological patients, it is useful to ask significant others to substitutionally rate patients' QOL to continue the assessment of the patients' perception for symptom management.

Especially in neurooncological patients, whose median survival expectancy is rather low, it is of particular importance to assess QOL in order to be able to quickly intervene if impairments occur. The routine use of PRO-instruments allows a constant patient monitoring with little effort, which nevertheless makes individualized treatment possible. That patient-centred care is highly needed is demonstrated by study results of Bosma et al. (2009). They report that glioma patients differ in their QOL-patterns in regard to their survival time. Patients with a shorter survival (death within one year from diagnosis) were reported to have more general health problems during the course of disease and an increase of weakness of legs until four months after baseline. On the other hand, long-term survivors (still alive two years after diagnosis) had fewer general health problems, showed improvements of physical, social and emotional functioning and had stable or even decreasing brain specific symptom levels. The limited survival of most brain cancer patients requires a special focus on QOL, since curative treatment is unlikely and other aspects of life become more important.

Methodologically, there is still the need to establish reference scores for brain cancer patients with different diagnoses undergoing diverse therapies. Furthermore, there is a lack of randomized-controlled trials that investigate the effect of ePRO-based, targeted interventions in clinical routine. Future studies should put a focus on the evaluation of the precise impact of ePROs on medical care. A comprehensive knowledge about the impact of ePROs on the patient-clinician communication and on the provision of medical and psychosocial interventions would facilitate the patient-centred care and could therefore contribute to QOL improvement.

5. Acknowledgement

The work of Lisa M. Wintner was financially supported by a scholarship of the Leopold-Franzens-University Innsbruck, Austria.

6. References

Aaronson, N.K. Ahmedzai, S. Bergman, B. Bullinger, M. Cull, A. Duez, N.J. Filiberti, A. Flechtner, H. Fleishman, S.B. & de Haes, J.C. (1993). The European Organization for Research and Treatment of Cancer QLQ-C30: a quality-of-life instrument for use in international clinical trials in oncology. *J Natl Cancer Inst,* Vol. 85, No. 5, pp. 365-76

Abernethy, A.P. Zafar, S.Y. Uronis, H. Wheeler, J.L. Coan, A. Rowe, K. Shelby, R.A. Fowler, R. & Herndon, J.E., 2nd. (2010). Validation of the Patient Care Monitor (Version 2.0): a review of system assessment instrument for cancer patients. *J Pain Symptom Manage,* Vol. 40, No. 4, (Oct), pp. 545-58

Addington-Hall, J. & Kalra, L. (2001). Who should measure quality of life? *BMJ,* Vol. 322, No. 7299, (Jun 9), pp. 1417-20

Arora, N.K. (2003). Interacting with cancer patients: the significance of physicians' communication behavior. *Soc Sci Med,* Vol. 57, No. 5, (Sep), pp. 791-806

Balducci, L. & Stanta, G. (2000). Cancer in the frail patient. A coming epidemic. *Hematol Oncol Clin North Am,* Vol. 14, No. 1, (Feb), pp. 235-50, xi

Barlesi, F. Tchouhadjian, C. Doddoli, C. Astoul, P. Thomas, P. & Auquier, P. (2006). [Quality of life: attitudes and perspectives of doctors in a thoracic oncology regional care network]. *Sante Publique,* Vol. 18, No. 3, (Sep), pp. 429-42

Basch, E. (2010). The missing voice of patients in drug-safety reporting. *N Engl J Med,* Vol. 362, No. 10, (Mar 11), pp. 865-9

Basch, E. Iasonos, A. Barz, A. Culkin, A. Kris, M.G. Artz, D. Fearn, P. Speakman, J. Farquhar, R. Scher, H.I. McCabe, M. & Schrag, D. (2007). Long-term toxicity monitoring via electronic patient-reported outcomes in patients receiving chemotherapy. *J Clin Oncol,* Vol. 25, No. 34, (Dec 1), pp. 5374-80

Bosma, I. Reijneveld, J.C. Douw, L. Vos, M.J. Postma, T.J. Aaronson, N.K. Muller, M. Vandertop, W.P. Slotman, B.J. Taphoorn, M.J. Heimans, J.J. & Klein, M. (2009). Health-related quality of life of long-term high-grade glioma survivors. *Neuro Oncol,* Vol. 11, No. 1, (Feb), pp. 51-8

Bossola, M. Murri, R. Onder, G. Turriziani, A. Fantoni, M. & Padua, L. (2010). Physicians' knowledge of health-related quality of life and perception of its importance in daily clinical practice. *Health Qual Life Outcomes,* Vol. 8, No. pp. 43

Brown, P. Decker, P. Rummans, T. Clark, M. Frost, M. Ballman, K. Arusell, R. & Buckner, J. (2008). A prospective study of quality of life in adults with newly diagnosed high-grade gliomas: comparison of patient and caregiver ratings of quality of life. *Am J Clin Oncol*, Vol. 31, No. 2, pp. 163-168

Bush, -.N. Donaldson, -.G. Moinpour, -.C. Haberman, -.M. Milliken, -.D. Markle, -.V. & Lauson, -.J. (2005). Development, feasibility and compliance of a web-based system for very frequent QOL and symptom home self-assessment after hematopoietic stem cell transplantation. *Qual Life Res*, Vol. 14, No. 7, pp. 77-93

Campos, S. Davey, P. Hird, A. Pressnail, B. Bilbao, J. Aviv, R.I. Symons, S. Pirouzmand, F. Sinclair, E. Culleton, S. Desa, E. Goh, P. & Chow, E. (2009). Brain metastasis from an unknown primary, or primary brain tumour? A diagnostic dilemma. *Curr Oncol*, Vol. 16, No. 1, (Jan), pp. 62-6

Carlson, L.E. Speca, M. Hagen, N. & Taenzer, P. (2001). Computerized quality-of-life screening in a cancer pain clinic. *J Palliat Care*, Vol. 17, No. 1, pp. 46-52

Cella, D. & Nowinski, C., J. (2002). Measuring quality of life in chronic illness: the functional assessment of chronic illness therapy measurement system. *Arch Phys Med Rehabil*, Vol. 83, No. 12 Suppl 2, pp. S10-7

Cella, D.F. Tulsky, D.S. Gray, G. Sarafian, B. Linn, E. Bonomi, A. Silberman, M. Yellen, S.B. Winicour, P. Brannon, J. & et al. (1993). The Functional Assessment of Cancer Therapy scale: development and validation of the general measure. *J Clin Oncol*, Vol. 11, No. 3, (Mar), pp. 570-9

Coons, S. Gwaltney, C. Hays, R. Lundy, J. Sloan, J. Revicki, D. Lenderking, W. Cella, D. Basch, E. & Force, I.e.T. (2009). Recommendations on evidence needed to support measurement equivalence between electronic and paper-based patient-reported outcome (PRO) measures: ISPOR ePRO Good Research Practices Task Force report. *Value Health*, Vol. 12, No. 4, pp. 419-429

Crosby, R.D. Kolotkin, R.L. & Williams, G.R. (2003). Defining clinically meaningful change in health-related quality of life. *J Clin Epidemiol*, Vol. 56, No. 5, (May), pp. 395-407

Detmar, S.B. Aaronson, N.K. Wever, L.D. Muller, M. & Schornagel, J.H. (2000). How are you feeling? Who wants to know? Patients' and oncologists' preferences for discussing health-related quality-of-life issues. *J Clin Oncol*, Vol. 18, No. 18, (Sep 15), pp. 3295-301

Detmar, S.B. Muller, M.J. Schornagel, J.H. Wever, L.D.V. & Aaronson, N.K. (2002a). Health-related quality-of-life assessments and patient-physician communication: a randomized controlled trial. *JAMA*, Vol. 288, No. 23, pp. 3027-34

Detmar, S.B. Muller, M.J. Schornagel, J.H. Wever, L.D.V. & Aaronson, N.K. (2002b). Role of health-related quality of life in palliative chemotherapy treatment decisions. *J Clin Oncol*, Vol. 20, No. 4, pp. 1056-62

Drummond, H.E. Ghosh, S. Ferguson, A. Brackenridge, D. & Tiplady, B. (1995). Electronic quality of life questionnaires: a comparison of pen-based electronic questionnaires with conventional paper in a gastrointestinal study. *Qual Life Res*, Vol. 4, No. 1, (Feb), pp. 21-6

Drury, M. Yudkin, P. Harcourt, J. Fitzpatrick, R. Jones, L. Alcock, C. & Minton, M. (2000). Patients with cancer holding their own records: a randomised controlled trial. *Br J Gen Pract*, Vol. 50, No. 451, pp. 105-10

Dubois, D. Dhawan, R. van de Velde, H. Esseltine, D. Gupta, S. Viala, M. & de la Loge, C. (2006). Descriptive and prognostic value of patient-reported outcomes: the bortezomib experience in relapsed and refractory multiple myeloma. *J Clin Oncol*, Vol. 24, No. 6, pp. 976-82

Farivar, S.S. Liu, H. & Hays, R.D. (2004). Half standard deviation estimate of the minimally important difference in HRQOL scores? *Expert Rev Pharmacoecon Outcomes Res*, Vol. 4, No. 5, (Oct), pp. 515-23

Ferlay J, Shin HR, Bray F, Forman D, Mathers C and Parkin DM. GLOBOCAN 2008, Cancer Incidence and Mortality Worldwide: IARC CancerBase No. 10 [Internet]. Lyon, France: International Agency for Research on Cancer; 2010. Available from: http://globocan.iarc.fr

Frost, M. Bonomi, A. Cappelleri, J. Schunemann, H. Moynihan, T. & Aaronson, N. (2007). Applying quality-of-life data formally and systematically into clinical practice. *Mayo Clin Proc*, Vol. 82, No. 10, pp. 1214-28

Ganz, P.A. & Goodwin, P.J. (2007). Health-related quality of life measurement in symptom management trials. *J Natl Cancer Inst Monogr*, Vol. No. 37, pp. 47-52

Ganz, P.A. Moinpour, C.M. Pauler, D.K. Kornblith, A.B. Gaynor, E.R. Balcerzak, S.P. Gatti, G.S. Erba, H.P. McCoy, S. Press, O.W. & Fisher, R.I. (2003). Health status and quality of life in patients with early-stage Hodgkin's disease treated on Southwest Oncology Group Study 9133. *J Clin Oncol*, Vol. 21, No. 18, (Sep 15), pp. 3512-9

Giesinger, J. Kemmler, G. Meraner, V. Gamper, E.M. Oberguggenberger, A. Sperner-Unterweger, B. & Holzner, B. (2009a). Towards the Implementation of Quality of Life Monitoring in Daily Clinical Routine: Methodological Issues and Clinical Implication. *Breast Care (Basel)*, Vol. 4, No. 3, pp. 148-154

Giesinger, J.M. Golser, M. Erharter, A. Kemmler, G. Schauer-Maurer, G. Stockhammer, G. Muigg, A. Hutterer, M. Rumpold, G. & Holzner, B. (2009b). Do neurooncological patients and their significant others agree on quality of life ratings? *Health Qual Life Outcomes*, Vol. 7, No. pp. 87

Guyatt, G.H. Osoba, D. Wu, A.W. Wyrwich, K.W. & Norman, G.R. (2002). Methods to explain the clinical significance of health status measures. *Mayo Clin Proc*, Vol. 77, No. 4, (Apr), pp. 371-83

Hahn, C. & Dunn, R. (2003). Prospective study of neuropsychologic testing and quality of life assessment of adults with primary malignant brain tumors. *International Journal of Radiation, Oncology, Biology, Physica*, Vol. 55, No. 4, pp. 992-999

Hawkins, R. & Grunberg, S. (2009). Chemotherapy-induced nausea and vomiting: challenges and opportunities for improved patient outcomes. *Clin J Oncol Nurs*, Vol. 13, No. 1, (Feb), pp. 54-64

Heimans, J. & Taphoorn, M.J. (2002). Impact of brain tumour treatment on quality of life. *J Neurol*, Vol. 249, No. 8, pp. 955-60

Holzner, B. Schauer-Maurer, G. Stockhammer, G. Muigg, A. Hutterer, M. & J., G. (2011). Computergestütztes Patient-reported Outcome Monitoring in der Neuroonkologie: Lebensqualität und Rezidiv beim Glioblastom. *Wien Med Wochenschr*, Vol. 161, No. 1-2, pp. 13-19

Holzner, B. Zabernigg, A. Kemmler, G. Baier, S. Kopp, M. & Sperner Unterweger, B. (2004). Computerized assessment of quality of life in patients undergoing chemotherapy. *Qual Life Res*, Vol. 13, No. 9, pp. 1523

Janda, M. Steginga, S. Langbecker, D. Dunn, J. Walker, D. & Eakin, E. (2007). Quality of life among patients with a brain tumor and their carers. *J Psychosom Res*, Vol. 63, No. 6, (Dec), pp. 617-23

Kemmler, G. Zabernigg, A. Gattringer, K. Rumpold, G. Giesinger, J. Sperner-Unterweger, B. & Holzner, B. (2010). A new approach to combining clinical relevance and statistical significance for evaluation of quality of life changes in the individual patient. *J Clin Epidemiol*, Vol. 63, No. 2, (Feb), pp. 171-9

Luckett, T. Butow, P.N. & King, M.T. (2009). Improving patient outcomes through the routine use of patient-reported data in cancer clinics: future directions. *Psychooncology*, Vol. 18, No. 11, (Nov), pp. 1129-38

Marino, P. Roche, H. Biron, P. Janvier, M. Spaeth, D. Fabbro, M. Linassier, C. Delozier, T. Martin, A.L. Santin, G. & Moatti, J.P. (2008). Deterioration of quality of life of high-risk breast cancer patients treated with high-dose chemotherapy: the PEGASE 01 Quality of Life Study. *Value Health*, Vol. 11, No. 4, (Jul-Aug), pp. 709-18

McLachlan, S.A. Allenby, A. Matthews, J. Wirth, A. Kissane, D. Bishop, M. Beresford, J. & Zalcberg, J. (2001). Randomized trial of coordinated psychosocial interventions based on patient self-assessments versus standard care to improve the psychosocial functioning of patients with cancer. *J Clin Oncol*, Vol. 19, No. 21, pp. 4117 - 25

Meraner, V. Giesinger, J. Kemmler, G. Taucher, S. Hubalek, M. Weber, B. Rumpold, G. Sperner-Unterweger, B. & Holzner, B. (2009). Development of a screening tool for the identification of psychooncological treatment needs in breast cancer patients. *Psychooncology*, Vol. epub 13 Jan 2009, No. pp.

Morris, J. Perez, D. & McNoe, B. (1998). The use of quality of life data in clinical practice. *Qual Life Res*, Vol. 7, No. 1, pp. 85 - 91

Mullen, K.H. Berry, D.L. & Zierler, B.K. (2004). Computerized symptom and quality-of-life assessment for patients with cancer part II: acceptability and usability. *Oncol Nurs Forum*, Vol. 31, No. 5, (Sep), pp. E84-9

Nickolov, A. Beumont, J. Victorson, D. Peterman, A. Cella, D. Liepa, A. & HA, F. (2005). Validation of functional assessment of cancer therapy: brain (FACT-Br) questionnaire and FACT-Br symptom index (FBrSI) in patients with recurrent high-grade glioma. . *Paper presented at: Chicago Supportive Oncology Conference , 2005, ; Chicago, IL.*, Vol. No. (October 6-8), pp.

Osoba, D. (2007). Translating the science of patient-reported outcomes assessment into clinical practice. *J Natl Cancer Inst Monogr*, Vol. No. 37, pp. 5-11

Osoba, D. Brada, M. Prados, M.D. & Yung, W.K. (2000). Effect of disease burden on health-related quality of life in patients with malignant gliomas. *Neuro Oncol*, Vol. 2, No. 4, pp. 221-8

Patrick, D.L. Burke, L.B. Powers, J.H. Scott, J.A. Rock, E.P. Dawisha, S. O'Neill, R. & Kennedy, D.L. (2007). Patient-reported outcomes to support medical product labeling claims: FDA perspective. *Value Health*, Vol. 10 Suppl 2, No. (Nov-Dec), pp. S125-37

Press, O.W. LeBlanc, M. Lichter, A.S. Grogan, T.M. Unger, J.M. Wasserman, T.H. Gaynor, E.R. Peterson, B.A. Miller, T.P. & Fisher, R.I. (2001). Phase III randomized intergroup trial of subtotal lymphoid irradiation versus doxorubicin, vinblastine, and subtotal lymphoid irradiation for stage IA to IIA Hodgkin's disease. *J Clin Oncol*, Vol. 19, No. 22, (Nov 15), pp. 4238-44

Reardon, D.A. & Wen, P.Y. (2006). Therapeutic advances in the treatment of glioblastoma: rationale and potential role of targeted agents. *Oncologist*, Vol. 11, No. 2, (Feb), pp. 152-64

Revicki, D. Hays, R. Cella, D. & Sloan, J. (2008). Recommended methods for determining responsiveness and minimally important differences for patient-reported outcomes. *J Clin Epidemiol*, Vol. 61, No. 2, pp. 102-109

Rodriguez, K.L. Bayliss, N. Alexander, S.C. Jeffreys, A.S. Olsen, M.K. Pollak, K.I. Kennifer, S.L. Tulsky, J.A. & Arnold, R.M. (2010). How oncologists and their patients with advanced cancer communicate about health-related quality of life. *Psychooncology*, Vol. 19, No. 5, (May), pp. 490-9

Rogausch, A. Sigle, J. Seibert, A. Thuring, S. Kochen, M.M. & Himmel, W. (2009). Feasibility and acceptance of electronic quality of life assessment in general practice: an implementation study. *Health Qual Life Outcomes*, Vol. 7, No. pp. 51

Rosenbloom, S.K. Victorson, D.E. Hahn, E.A. Peterman, A.H. & Cella, D. (2007). Assessment is not enough: a randomized controlled trial of the effects of HRQL assessment on quality of life and satisfaction in oncology clinical practice. *Psychooncology*, Vol. 16, No. 12, (Dec), pp. 1069-79

Rothman, M.L. Beltran, P. Cappelleri, J.C. Lipscomb, J. & Teschendorf, B. (2007). Patient-reported outcomes: conceptual issues. *Value Health*, Vol. 10 Suppl 2, No. (Nov-Dec), pp. S66-75

Sanchez, R. Ballesteros, M. & Arnold, B.J. (2011). Validation of the FACT-G scale for evaluating quality of life in cancer patients in Colombia. *Qual Life Res*, Vol. 20, No. 1, (Feb), pp. 19-29

Seybert, H. & Lööf, A.(2010). Internet usage in 2010 – Households and Individuals, Availble from: http://epp.eurostat.ec.europa.eu/cache/ITY_OFFPUB/KS-QA-10-050/EN/KS-QA-10-050-EN.PDF

Sizoo, E.M. Braam, L. Postma, T.J. Pasman, H.R. Heimans, J.J. Klein, M. Reijneveld, J.C. & Taphoorn, M.J. (2010). Symptoms and problems in the end-of-life phase of high-grade glioma patients. *Neuro Oncol*, Vol. 12, No. 11, (Nov), pp. 1162-6

Sneeuw, K.C. Aaronson, N.K. Osoba, D. Muller, M.J. Hsu, M.A. Yung, W.K. Brada, M. & Newlands, E.S. (1997). The use of significant others as proxy raters of the quality of life of patients with brain cancer. *Med Care*, Vol. 35, No. 5, pp. 490-506

Snyder, C.F. Jensen, R.E. Geller, G. Carducci, M.A. & Wu, A.W. (2010). Relevant content for a patient-reported outcomes questionnaire for use in oncology clinical practice: Putting doctors and patients on the same page. *Qual Life Res*, Vol. 19, No. 7, (Sep), pp. 1045-55

Sprangers, M.A. Cull, A. Groenvold, M. Bjordal, K. Blazeby, J. & Aaronson, N.K. (1998). The European Organization for Research and Treatment of Cancer approach to developing questionnaire modules: an update and overview. EORTC Quality of Life Study Group. *Qual Life Res*, Vol. 7, No. 4, pp. 291-300

Stupp, R. Mason, W. van den Bent, M. Weller, M. Fisher, B. Taphoorn, M. Belanger, K. Brandes, A. Marosi, C. Bogdahn, U. Curschmann, J. Janzer, R. Ludwin, S. Gorlia, T. Allgeier, A. Lacombe, D. Cairncross, J. Eisenhauer, E. Mirimanoff, R. European Organisation for Research and Treatment of Cancer Brain Tumor and Radiotherapy Groups & National Cancer Institute of Canada Clinical Trials Group. (2005). Radiotherapy plus concomitant and adjuvant temozolomide for glioblastoma. *N Engl J Med*, Vol. 352, No. 10, pp. 987-996

Taenzer, P. Bultz, B.D. Carlson, L.E. Speca, M. DeGagne, T. Olson, K. Doll, R. & Rosberger, Z. (2000). Impact of computerized quality of life screening on physician behaviour and patient satisfaction in lung cancer outpatients. *Psychooncology*, Vol. 9, No. 3, pp. 203-13

Taphoorn, M. Stupp, R. Coens, C. Osoba, D. Kortmann, R. van den Bent, M. Mason, W. Mirimanoff, R. Baumert, B. Eisenhauer, E. Forsyth, P. & Bottomley, A. (2005).

Health-related quality of life in patients with glioblastoma: a randomised controlled trial. *Lancet Oncol*, Vol. 6, No. 12, pp. 937-944

Taphoorn, M.J. Sizoo, E.M. & Bottomley, A. (2010). Review on quality of life issues in patients with primary brain tumors. *Oncologist*, Vol. 15, No. 6, pp. 618-26

Trotti, A. Colevas, A.D. Setser, A. & Basch, E. (2007). Patient-reported outcomes and the evolution of adverse event reporting in oncology. *J Clin Oncol*, Vol. 25, No. 32, (Nov 10), pp. 5121-7

Trowbridge, R. Dugan, W. Jay, S.J. Littrell, D. Casebeer, L.L. Edgerton, S. Anderson, J. & O'Toole, J.B. (1997). Determining the effectiveness of a clinical-practice intervention in improving the control of pain in outpatients with cancer. *Acad Med*, Vol. 72, No. 9, (Sep), pp. 798-800

U.S. Food and drug administration (FDA). (2006). Guidance for Industry. Patient-Reported Outcome Measures: Use in Medical Product Development to Support Labeling Claims. *Federal Register*, Vol. 74, No. 35, pp. 65132-133

Velikova, G. Booth, L. Smith, A.B. Brown, P.M. Lynch, P. Brown, J.M. & Selby, P.J. (2004). Measuring quality of life in routine oncology practice improves communication and patient well-being: a randomized controlled trial. *J Clin Oncol*, Vol. 22, No. 4, (Feb 15), pp. 714-24

Velikova, G. Keding, A. Harley, C. Cocks, K. Booth, L. Smith, A.B. Wright, P. Selby, P.J. & Brown, J.M. (2010). Patients report improvements in continuity of care when quality of life assessments are used routinely in oncology practice: secondary outcomes of a randomised controlled trial. *Eur J Cancer*, Vol. 46, No. 13, (Sep), pp. 2381-8

Velikova, G. Wright, E.P. Smith, A.B. Cull, A. Gould, A. Forman, D. Perren, T. Stead, M. Brown, J. & Selby, P.J. (1999). Automated collection of quality-of-life data: a comparison of paper and computer touch-screen questionnaires. *J Clin Oncol*, Vol. 17, No. 3, pp. 998-1007

Walker, M. Brown, J. Brown, K. Gregor, A. Whittle, I. & Grant, R. (2003). Practical problems with the collection and interpretation of serial quality of life assessment in patients with malignant glioma. *J Neurooncol*, Vol. 63, No. 2, pp. 179-186

Webster, K. Cella, D. & Yost, K. (2003). The Functional Assessment of Chronic Illness Therapy (FACIT) Measurement System: properties, applications, and interpretation. *Health Qual Life Outcomes*, Vol. 1, No. pp. 79

Wright, E.P. Selby, P.J. Crawford, M. Gillibrand, A. Johnston, C. Perren, T.J. Rush, R. Smith, A. Velikova, G. Watson, K. Gould, A. & Cull, A. (2003). Feasibility and compliance of automated measurement of quality of life in oncology practice. *J Clin Oncol*, Vol. 21, No. 2, (Jan 15), pp. 374-82

Zabora, J. Brintzenhofeszoc, K. Curbow, B. Hooker, C. & Piantadosi, S. (2001). The prevalence of psychological distress by cancer site. *Psychooncology*, Vol. 10, No. 1, (Jan-Feb), pp. 19-28

Zigmond, A. & Snaith, R. (1983). The hospital anxiety and depression scale. *Acta Psychiatr Scand*, Vol. 67, No. 6, pp. 361-370

2

Brain Tumour Imaging

Amit Mehndiratta and Frederik L Giesel
University Hospital Heidelberg,
Department of Nuclear Medicine
Germany

1. Introduction

There is now a plethora of different imaging techniques used for diagnosing and treating brain tumours. Different contrast agents in magnetic resonance imaging - coupled with amino acid tracers used in positron emission tomography - are the new weapons in radiologists' armoury which allow them to target and measure tumours more accurately.
Brain tumours are among the top causes of tumour-related deaths, with ten to 15 out of every 100,000 people diagnosed in Europe and USA every year.
The evaluation of tumours with medical imaging modalities is now one of the primary concerns of radiology departments. Computed tomography (CT), magnetic resonance imaging (MRI) and various advanced MRI techniques like perfusion MRI and dynamic susceptibility contrast (DSC) MRI play a vital role in brain tumour assessment.
In this chapter, we will summarize the current clinical applications of Computed Tomography, gadolinium contrast agents in neuro-imaging, including contrast-enhanced MRI, perfusion-weighted imaging and positron emission tomography (PET) for evaluation of brain tumour lesions. We will also discuss the advantages and limitation of each modality with respect to answering the specific clinical concerns.

2. Role of imaging in brain tumour assessment

In the management of patients with confirmed / suspected intracranial tumours, imaging of brain is often required at various stages and has a significant role at each level. Several stages of management may be considered although they are in practice often integrated with each other [1].

i. Detection / confirmation of a structural abnormality
ii. Localization and assessment of extent of the lesion
iii. Characterization - distinction between neoplastic and non-neoplastic lesions, if neoplastic then differentiation among malignant and benign
iv. Staging of the tumour: lymphatic spread or other organ involvement
v. Looking for involvement of any vital brain area which might be of concern for therapy planning
vi. Facilitate surgical planning or other therapeutic interventions
vii. Intraoperative control of resection procedure
viii. Monitoring prognosis and follow up

CT is often the first line of imaging study in tumour assessment because it is cheap, minimally invasive and widely available in clinical settings. It is a very good screening method in demonstration of supratentorial abnormalities but MRI is additional sequences which are mandatory for better anatomical distinction when it comes to decision of surgical interventions.
There are various structural features which are of interest to radiologist in answering the critical question in tumour assessment:

i. Signal contrast with respect to normal brain parenchyma
ii. Tumour structure, margins, extent of perifocal edema
iii. Indirect tumour signs (compression syndrome, midline shift etc.)
iv. Tumour vascularity, main vessels supplying the tumour and its course
v. Degree of contrast enhancement

The information provided by MRI in evaluating brain lesions is critical for accurate diagnosis, therapeutic intervention and prognosis. Contrast-enhanced MR neuro-imaging using gadolinium (Gd) contrast agents depicts blood-brain barrier disruption, thereby demonstrating the location and extent of the tumour by depicting the increased extracellular-extravascular space (EES) contrast concentration in these areas.
However, simple contrast-enhanced morphologic imaging is limited in accurately predicting tumour aggressiveness. Adding dynamic contrast-enhanced and perfusion-weighted imaging can solve this problem by providing physiological information - such as haemodynamic and neo-angiogenic status - in addition to pure lesion morphology. T1-w and T2* perfusion imaging in a follow-up scan can differentiate treatment success by differentiating between radiation necrosis and tumour recurrence.
Most available Gd-contrast agents have similar T1 and T2 relaxivities, and thus comparable tissue-enhancing properties. The exceptions are gadobenate, gadoxetate and gadofosveset, all of which have transient protein-binding capability that is responsible for up to twice (and more) the R1 and R2 relaxivity as compared to the other agents at all magnetic field strengths [2].
Table 1 summarizes the indication, advantages and limitation of CT and MRI before we move on to each modality in details.

3. Magnetic resonance imaging studies in brain tumour

MR imaging is an important diagnostic tool in the evaluation of intracranial tumours. Its effectiveness is due to its inherent high sensitivity to pathologic alterations of normal parenchymal water content, as demonstrated by abnormal high or low signal intensity on T2- or T1-weighted images, respectively. Compared to CT, MR imaging allows more accurate determination of lesion location, extent and better demonstrates subtle mass effects or atrophy, particularly along the cerebral convexities. MR imaging better depicts the presence of subacute or chronic haemorrhage and permits more accurate distinction between a vascular structure and adjacent parenchyma. CT is superior in depicting the presence of calcification and bone abnormalities, e.g. destruction, erosion, permeation, and hyperostosis. MR imaging is superior to CT for differentiating between tumour and perifocal edema, for defining extent of tumour, and for showing the relationship of the tumour to critical adjacent structures. Heavily T2-weighted sequences are the most sensitive for the detection of tumour and edema extent (discussed later in the chapter), but the tumour focus is not well separated from surrounding edema. T1-weighted images following contrast enhancement generally provide better localization of the tumour nidus and improved diagnostic information relating to tumour grade, blood-brain barrier breakdown, haemorrhage, edema and necrosis. Contrast-enhanced T1-weighted images also better show small focal lesions such as metastases, small areas of tumour recurrence, and ependymal or leptomengeal tumour spread because of improved signal contrast. Proton density images are useful for distinguishing tumour and edema from adjacent cerebrospinal fluid, which may have a similar appearance as high-signal areas on heavily T_2-weighted images. All this information is essential for surgical planning.

Modality	*Indications*	*Limitations*
Computed Tomography	1. Shorter imaging time 2. Low cost of scanning 3. Better spatial resolution 4. Good for extra-axial brain tumour assessment 5. Superior in detection of calcifications, skull erosion, penetration, destruction	1. Poor definition of edema 2. Only one plane acquisition and most of the time non-isotropic 3. X-ray radiation risk 4. Poor tissue characterization 5. Imaging of posterior fossa is limited due to bone artifacts
Magnetic Resonance Imaging	1. Good in demonstration of edema of parenchyma (early sign for tumour detection) 2. Accurate delectating extent of edema and compression effects 3. Better detection of mass effects and atrophy 4. High neuroanatomical definition (tissue differentiation) 5. Accurate detection of vascularity of tumour (in various planes acquisition)	1. Poor detection of calcification and bone erosions 2. Not possible in intraoperative assessment 3. Lower spatial fidelity 4. Sometime sequence are very time consuming

Table 1. Comparison of CT and MRI in assessment of Brain Tumours

As indicated in various studies, imaging findings in MR studies roughly correlate with the *histologic grading* of cerebral gliomas. Generally, masses that are sharply marginated, are homogeneous in signal intensity, and show little or no contrast enhancement tend to be low-grade gliomas. Masses that have indistinct margins, are inhomogeneous in appearance, and demonstrate intense, irregular contrast enhancement tend to be high-grade gliomas. These are generalizations and all of the imaging findings and contrast-enhancing patterns must be considered together. Additionally, individual cases may differ from the norm. Some low-grade astrocytomas that are primarily infiltrating and histologically benign demonstrate poor margination with the surrounding brain and some rapidly growing malignant gliomas may show sharp margination from the surrounding brain.

Dean *et al.* (1990) found the degree of mass effect and the presence of cyst formation or necrosis to be statistically significant positive *predictors of tumour grade.* Central nonenhancing zones within an enhanced mass suggest areas of necrosis and indicate rapid tumour growth that outstrips the blood supply. This is a manifestation of malignant behaviour and should suggest the diagnosis of glioblastoma multiforme. Similarly, areas of hemorrhage within a mass also favour a malignant lesion and are most often seen with glioblastomas or metastases.

Very large zones of edema surrounding an enhancing intra-axial tumour also favour the diagnosis of a malignant lesion and contribute to the mass effect associated with these tumours. A notable exception to this rule is meningioma, which, although a benign tumour, is often associated with large areas of adjacent edema and mass effect. However, these tumours are readily distinguished from malignant gliomas by their extra-axial location. Low-grade gliomas tend to exhibit an infiltrating pattern resembling edema on neuroimaging studies, but the lack of contrast enhancement and the absence of large mass effects that generally accompanies large zones of cerebral edema help to distinguish these entities.

Calcification within a tumour usually indicates a slowly growing neoplasm. Calcification can frequently be demonstrated in classic oligodendrogliomas and gangliogliomas and may occasionally be seen in astrocytomas and ependymomas.

Limitations to the usefulness of MR imaging to date are the following:

1. It does not provide a precise histologic diagnosis because of considerable overlap between the characteristic morphologic changes associated with various intracranial lesions necessitating surgical biopsy in virtually all cases prior to definitive therapy.
2. MR images represent computer-generated maps of a spatial representation of differences in water proton T1 and T2 relaxation characteristics. Although significant pathologic abnormalities usually alter these characteristics, in some instances they may not change detectably from normal. If, as may occur with small tumours or with infiltrative gliomas, there is no significant mass effect distorting normal anatomy, the lesion may go undetected.
3. Even when there is a well-defined enhancing tumour nidus, infiltrating tumour and isolated tumour cells can extend several centimetres beyond the enhancing region into the surrounding 'edematous' zone and, in some cases, beyond any abnormality seen on the image.
4. Bulk calcium emits no MR signal, making tumour calcification difficult or impossible to detect unless present in large amounts.
5. Artefacts can degrade image quality to nondiagnostic levels. Patient motion during image acquisition may introduce abnormal 'bright' or 'dark' areas in a normal brain that can even simulate a lesion.
6. Magnetic field inhomogeneity presents problems with spatial resolution.

4. Brain tumour imaging using gadolinium contrast agents

The most common clinical application of CE-MR neuroimaging is in the evaluation of primary and secondary brain tumours. The goals of conventional brain tumour imaging are the sensitive detection and delineation of tumour to make a correct diagnosis and accurate tumour grading to facilitate appropriate intervention.

In addition, CE-MR helps localize adjacent critical structures such as vessel or nerves to aid surgical or radiotherapeutic planning. MRIs of brain lesions also play a vital role in post-interventional monitoring by determining response to treatment – and hence prognosis – as early identification of treatment failure can help to select an alternative therapeutic approach, thus potentially improving patient outcomes.

The protocol followed by most of the clinicians includes a T1w, T2w and also T1 post-contrast image acquisition of the brain tumour prior to present perfusion maps. T1 and T2 images give a good anatomical image quality and contrast with well-demarcated tumour boundaries. We also need T1-w for selecting good region of interest (ROI) of the tumour for relevant perfusion map (Figure 1). Dynamic Susceptibility Contrast (DSC) MRI can provide information on tumour vascularity which might not be obvious by T1/T2 imaging only but will be potential in grading the tumour and management options [3].
A standard dose of gadolinium contrast agent is considered to be 0.1mmol/kg bodyweight, although many studies have been published demonstrating improved diagnostic performance with double (0.2mmol/kg) or even triple (0.3mmol/kg) doses,[4;5] and this has become routine clinical practice.
Although higher doses of contrast agent have potentially increased the cost of MR examinations and are associated with higher false-positive rates,[5;6] such doses are very sensitive when determining the extent of the disease is the primary goal. The high molarity 1% Gd contrast gadobutrol (Gadovist) is also shown to be very sensitive (Figure 1) in detecting tumour activity [7]. Essig et al. compared 0.1 and 0.2 mmol/kg body weight doses of 1 M gadobutrol and gadobenate dimeglumine at 1.5 T in healthy volunteers and found that although the peak signal fall with the double dose of both agents was larger, there were no statistical differences between agents or doses (Fig. 5) [8]. Moreover, a signal drop of approximately 40% was produced by single doses of both agents, sufficient to permit calculation of highquality CBV and CBF maps. In this case, bolus widths achieved with gadobenate dimeglumine and gadobutrol were sharp and comparable, and therefore, the reduced injection time of gadobutrol did not have a positive effect on the bolus geometry. Essig and colleagues concluded that at 1.5 T, both the 1 M gadobutrol and the higher relaxivity gadobenate dimeglumine permitted a sufficient drop in SI to afford robust and reproducible quantification of haemodynamic parameters and that the slightly lower volume of the injection of gadobutrol did not produce any major advantage in terms of bolus geometry [8].
Improving the diagnostic performance by using a higher relaxivity contrast agent is an equally good alternative to increasing gadolinium dose. Early dosing studies demonstrated that double doses of gadobenate dimeglumine are potentially beneficial, with enhanced sensitivity in brain tumour detection, although no further benefit is seen when increasing to triple dose [9;10].
The more significant evidence of improved diagnostic performance by the higher relaxivity agent, however, came from a series of intra-individual crossover studies directly comparing gadobenate dimeglumine with gadopentetate dimeglumine,[11-16] gadoterate meglumine [11;13], gadodiamide[11;17] and gadofosveset trisodium. In these crossover studies, patients underwent two otherwise identical MR examinations, one with each contrast agent, within a gap of two days to two weeks, thus enabling any differences between the two imaging sets to be directly attributed to the contrast agents being used (Figure 2-5) [2;12-14].
The first such crossover study, performed in 2001, demonstrated that in patients with metastatic central nervous system (CNS) disease, the sensitivity for lesion detection with gadobenate dimeglumine (93%-100%) was much higher than that with an equal dose of comparator (65%-73%), like gadopentetate dimeglumine (N=13), gadodiamide (N=4), or gadoterate meglumine (N=5)[11]. In addition, tissue contrast in the main lesion-to-normal

brain parenchyma was consistently greater for gadobenate dimeglumine (143%) than for an equal dose comparator (127%) as compared to unenhanced images.

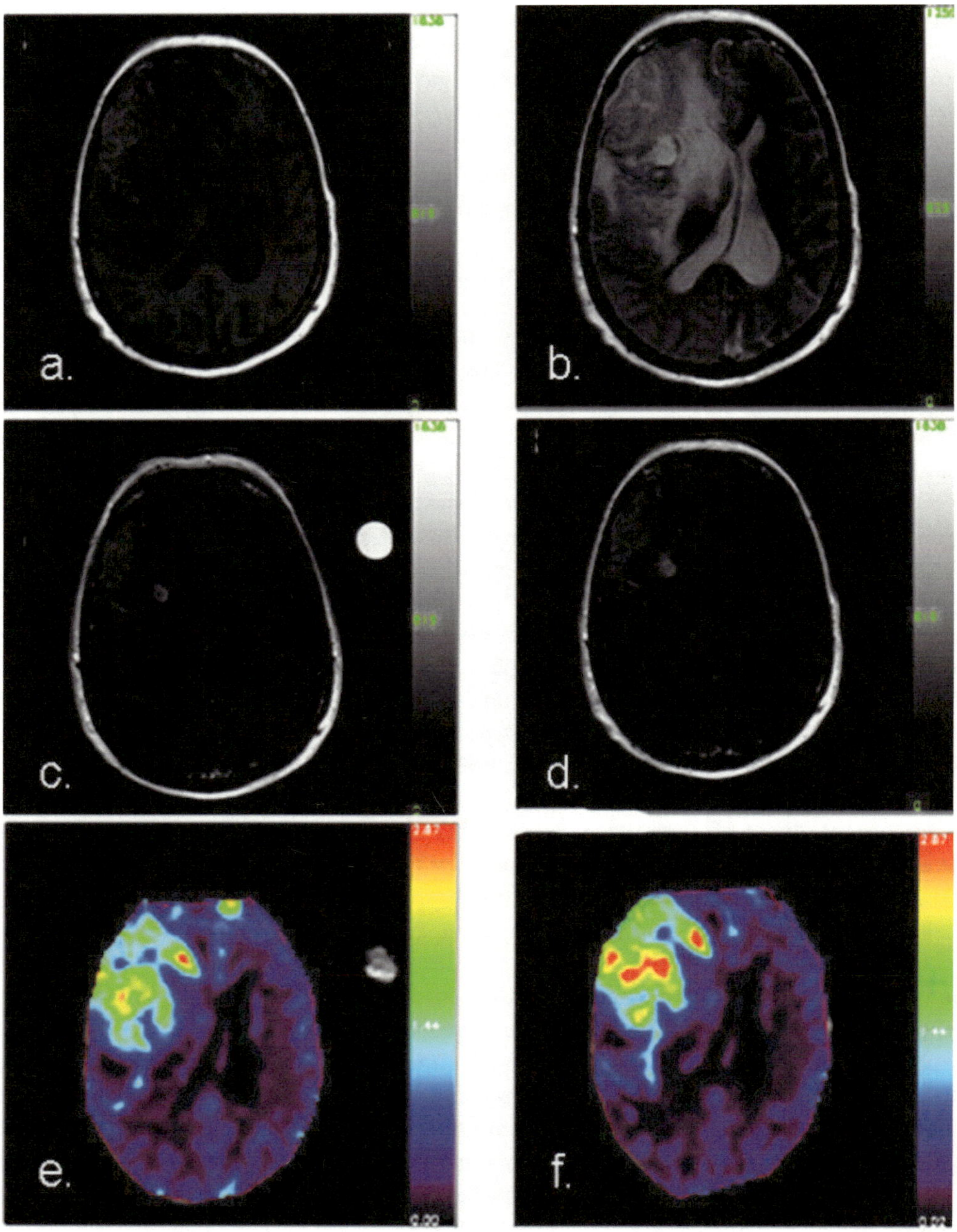

Fig. 1. a) T1-weighted; b) T2-weighted; c) T1-w post Gd-DTPA contrast; d) T1-w post Gadobutrol contrast; e) T2* weighted parametric CBV map with Gd-DTPA; f) T2* weighted parametric CBV map with Gadobutrol. Gadobutrol is shown to be more sensitive and show more number of active lesions in tumour with high blood supply.[4].

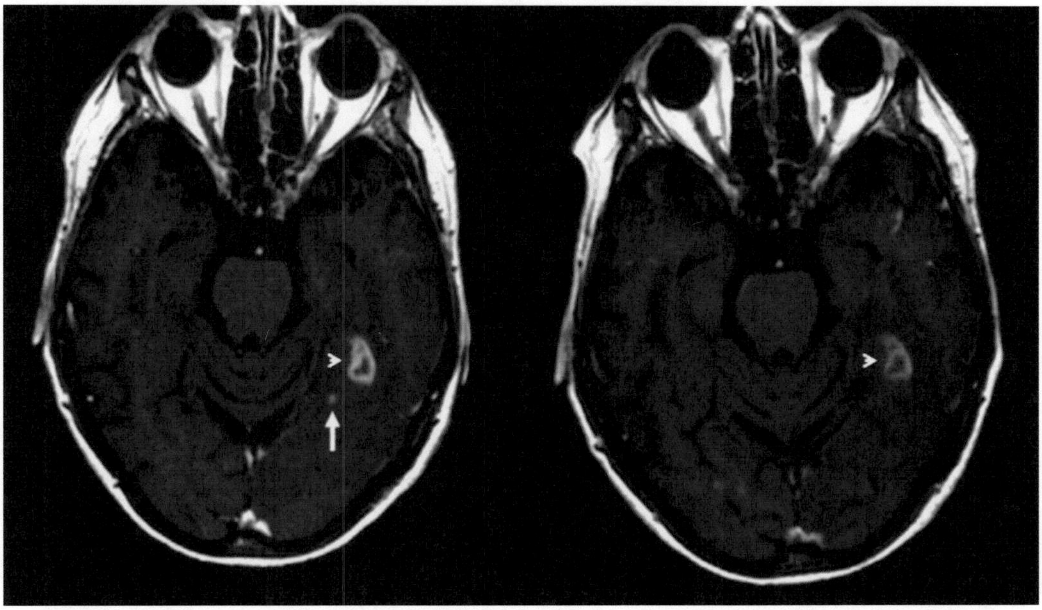

Fig. 2. Matched pairs of T1-weighted spin echo images from intraindividual comparative studies with high relaxivity enhanced images shown on the left and the comparator-enhanced image on the right. Where present, arrows highlight additional information present on gadobenate-dimeglumine-enhanced images. From Colosimo et al. [13] presenting a patient with malignant glioma (arrow head) gadobenate dimeglumine-enhanced MRI, which allows beside the stronger enhancement, the depiction of a satellite lesion (arrow) not present on the comparator image. The satellite-enhancing lesion should be integrated into the target volume for therapeutic intervention.

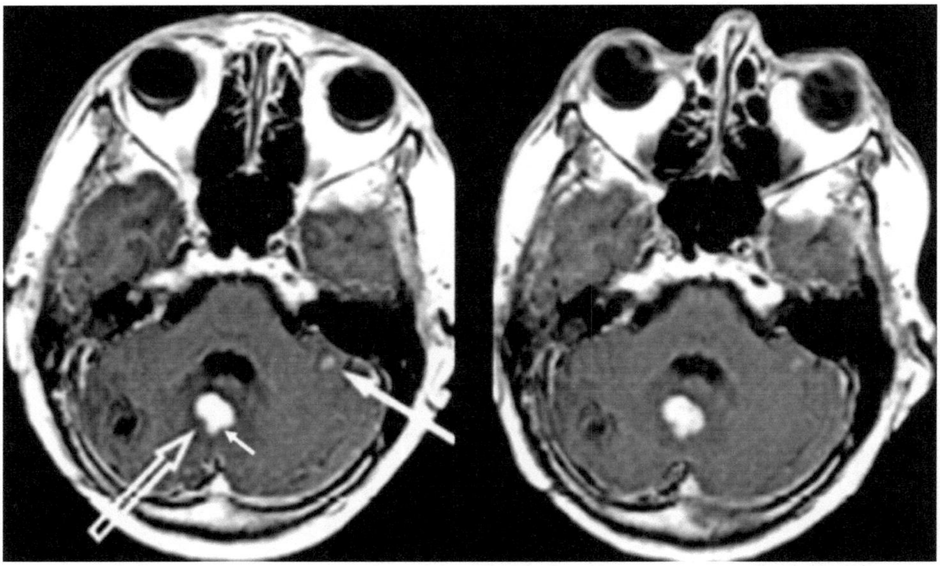

Fig. 3. A patient with multiple cerebral metastases, gadobenate dimeglumine-enhanced MRI is able to show additional metastases in the left cerebellar hemisphere (left) and a larger appearance of the lesion in projection of the midline (from Knopp et al. [12]). High relaxivity enhanced images shown on the left and the comparator-enhanced image on the right.

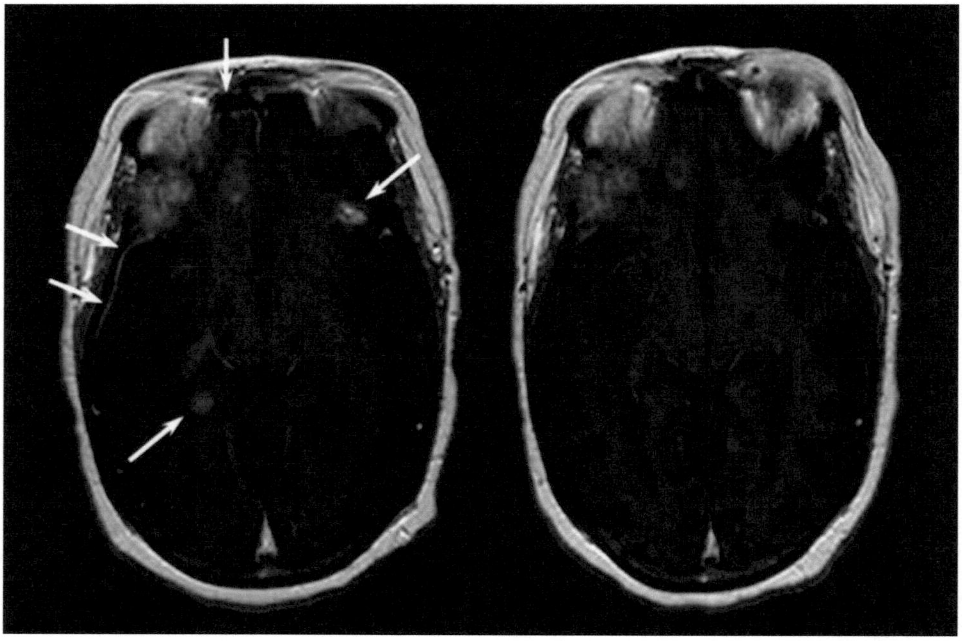

Fig. 4. A patient with multiple metastases, a high relaxivity agent allowed the detection of additional lesions and the proved the infiltration of the meninges (from Maravilla et al. [14]). High relaxivity enhanced images shown on the left and the comparator-enhanced image on the right.

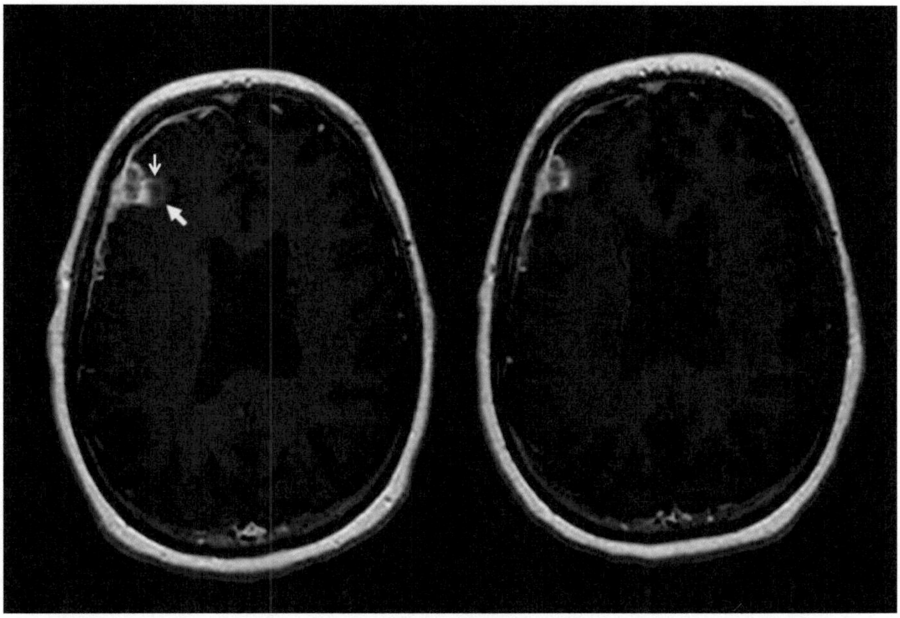

Fig. 5. The patient with an infiltration of the menigiosis carcinomatosa and a focal metastatic lesion, the enhancement is more pronounced with the use of a high relaxivity agent, and the lesion appears to be substantially larger (from Essig et al.[2]). High relaxivity enhanced images shown on the left and the comparator-enhanced image on the right.

Since then, five larger, prospective, randomised, intra-individual crossover studies have been performed with a total of 355 patients in which gadobenate dimeglumine was directly compared with an equal dose of other non-protein-binding contrast agents for MRI of primary and secondary CNS lesions[12-14;16;17].

Qualitatively blinded readers expressed global preference for images enhanced with gadobenate dimeglumine versus the other standard agents. Additionally, an independent analysis of intra-axial enhancing brain lesions (N=158) demonstrated a highly significant ($p \leq 0.0156$, all readers) improvement with gadobenate dimeglumine compared to gadopentetate dimeglumine, both qualitative and quantitatively[15].

All of the above-mentioned comparison studies between various MR contrast agents were performed using the field strength of 1.5T or less, while the recent crossover study by Rumboldt et al was performed using a 3T magnet[16]. The study demonstrated the persistent benefits of high-relaxivity agents even at higher field strengths, which will be the focus of clinical research in coming years.

An additional consideration recently is the fear of nephrogenic systemic fibrosis (NSF) developing in certain patient populations when higher doses of Gadolinium are used [18-20], NSF and other side-effects of MR contrast agents are beyond the remit of this chapter, but are worth mentioning here.

5. T1 weighted MR imaging in brain tumours

T1 weighted (T1w) MRI needs a special mention in brain tumour evaluation, because on many occasions the blood-brain barrier (BBB) is damaged in tumours, which alters the normal one-compartment physiological model used in imaging for perfusion analysis. The T1-w enhancement of contrast agent is attributed to BBB leakage associated with angiogenesis and capillary damage in regions of active tumour growth.

Angiogenesis is an important contributor to tumour growth and correlates with tumour aggressiveness. As angiogenesis increases microvascular cerebral blood volume (CBV), CBV-imaging may provide a unique insight into tumour physiology, histology and response to therapeutic agents. Different imaging modalities such as PET and MRI-CBV methods have been employed in tumour imaging for some time, but both require appropriately timed injection of contrast agents and subsequent post-processing, making them logistically difficult.

Recently, a new MRI approach called vascular-space-occupancy (VASO) imaging was developed as a non-invasive method for detecting CBV changes accompanying neuronal activation. VASO is a T1-weighted MRI approach that exploits the T1 difference between blood and tissue to null intravascular blood signal, simultaneously giving an image of extravascular tissue water, but only as it relates to parenchyma tumour.

While VASO has shown consistent sensitivity to CBV changes in functional MRI, it has not been tested extensively in the clinical setting for tumour imaging. Recently, VASO images with and without contrasts were combined to quantitatively assess absolute CBV in brain tumours, showing promise for assessing tumour grade assessment. However, this approach is confounded by the assumption that the administered contrast remains in the vasculature (single-compartment perfusion model), which may not be applicable in regions of BBB breakdown (two-compartment perfusion model).

The studies have also demonstrated that VASO and MPRAGE (magnetisation prepared rapid gradient echo) MRI provide contrast complementary to Gd-T1w and FLAIR (fluid attenuation inversion recovery) MRI for tumour imaging. Interestingly, FLAIR, VASO and MPRAGE are all inversion-based MRI sequences. However, they each offer a range of T1w contrasts, of which a collective analysis provides information not otherwise evident[21].

6. MR Spectroscopy (MRS) in tumour grading

Clinical applications of magnetic resonance spectroscopy (1H-MRS) are increasing as the techniques with (techniques and hardware have become more robust with fast processing) hardware have become more robust and fast processing. Proton MRS provides biochemical and metabolic information about tumours and normal brain [22]. The information obtained from MRS for tumour is unique and complimentary to other MR Imaging techniques.

As with other organs spectroscopy of brain tumours can be done in single- or multi- voxel forms. The two most widely used methods for volume selection are stimulated echo acquisition mode (STEAM) and point-resolved spectroscopy sequence (PRESS). In general STEAM is better as shorter echo times can be achieved with it but, it is more sensitive to motion related artefacts [23]. In theory, for the same total echo time, the signal of PRESS is twice as great as that of STEAM; also PRESS is also less sensitive to motion. With faster and better softwares PRESS is getting more commonly used method of volume selection in clinical practice.

Single voxel MRS is sometimes better as it's faster and quick to acquire but it lacks the high spatial resolution and hence regional mapping of metabolic variations. Brain tumours are heterogeneous in their tumours potentials; therefore single voxel spectroscopy might not be very reliable in tumour grading based on its metabolic activity. Poor spatial resolution also makes it vulnerable to high partial volume artefacts.

In the spectroscopy the most commonly used echo times are 144 msec and 270 msec at which the spectrum is dominated by 5 different metabolite peaks. These are the choline (Cho), creatine (Cr), N-acetylaspartate (NAA), lactate, and lipid. The choline peak reflects cell membrane turnover; Creatine is a good marker for energy synthesis, and NAA is exclusive to neuronal cells. Lactate resulting from anaerobic metabolism (which is uncommon in normal brain parenchyma) is detected in necrotic/infarcted tumour [24]. Cellular and myelin breakdown products result in prominent lipid peaks in MRS. MR Spectroscopy allows analysis of these specific metabolites within brain tissue. Tumours, especially primary brain tumours show very specific pattern in elevation of choline and loss of N-Acetyl Aspartate peaks [25;26].

Combined with MRI, MRS can aid in the evaluation of tumour type and grade. The higher-grade gliomas tend to exhibit higher Cho/Cr and Cho/NAA ratios. MR spectroscopy can help differentiate enhancing tumour from other causes of enhancement (mainly necrosis) and is more specific in differentiating nonenhancing tumour from edema and other causes of T2 prolongation. These qualities have been exploited in order to better define the true extent and morphology of gliomas. This information has the potential to significantly alter target volumes and radiation therapy doses of brain gliomas when compared with conventional radiotherapy. Although this is an attractive concept, there are no studies to show benefits, changes in failure patterns, or improved survival. MR spectroscopy is utilized more and more by different groups in assessing response to therapy in patients with primary brain tumours or metastases. MR spectroscopy can noninvasively enable the distinction between a solitary metastasis and high-grade gliomas, particularly when combined with perfusion MR imaging [27]. In their study, Law et al showed that measurements of Cho and mean rCBV in the perienhancing region are useful in differentiating solitary metastases from high-grade gliomas. In the perienhancing region, T2 prolongation is partly due to tumour infiltration (nonenhancing tumour) in patients with high-grade gliomas. Whereas in the case of metastases, the hyperintensity surrounding the region of enhancement is due to vasogenic edema or nonspecific treatment effects rather than infiltrating tumour. Therefore, elevated levels of choline and/ or rCBV surrounding a peripherally enhancing mass reflect tumour infiltration in a high-grade glioma.

Post- treatment, MRS has a much limited role in the assessment of patients. Frequently, there is a mixture of ruminant tumour and necrosis after therapy. This limits the utility of MRS in differentiating residual/recurrent tumour from radiation necrosis, as is the case with MR perfusion. As a tumour responds to treatment, the choline decreases and lactate and/or lipids may increase [28;29]. MR spectroscopy can play a useful role after treatment in assessing the therapeutic response. This is particularly important for early detection of treatment failure so that an ineffective treatment can be modified prior to a significant progression of disease.

7. Molecular imaging and PET in brain tumour imaging

PET imaging is a non-invasive diagnostic imaging tool that has an advantage over anatomical imaging in that it is a metabolic imaging tool that is able to distinguish between benign and malignant tumours. It is often used to accurately determine the stage of the brain tumour. PET images produce visual impression of detailed biochemical changes caused by brain tumours and their metabolic activities.

Despite the recognized limitations of fluorodeoxyglucose positron emission tomography (FDG-PET) in brain tumour imaging due to the high background of normal gray matter, this imaging modality provides critical information for the management of patients with cerebral parenchyma tumours by providing a:

- Global picture of the tumour and thus guiding the appropriate site for biopsy, thereby improving accuracy of the technique and reducing the number of biopsy samples
- Prediction of metabolic activity and aggressiveness of the tumour, thereby enhancing the ability to provide a prognosis.

Another area, which has been investigated extensively in tumour imaging, is differentiating between recurrent tumour and treatment-related changes - for example, radiation necrosis or postsurgical changes. The aggressive tumour responds with a bright signal because of its high uptake of FDG, but radiation necrosis will show no changes.

FDG-PET has equally demonstrated its usefulness in differentiating lymphoma from infectious toxoplasmosis in patients with acquired immune deficiency syndrome with almost 100% accuracy, and is the investigation of choice in that setting [30].

In recent years, an increasing number of brain tumour PET studies have used other tracers, such as labeled methionine, tyrosine, thymidine, choline, fluoromisonidazole, EF5 and so on, of which positron-labeled amino acid analogues, nucleotide analogues, and the hypoxia imaging tracers are of special interest [30]. The major advantage of these radiotracers over FDG is the markedly reduced background activity in gray matter, which allows detection of even smaller lesions and low-grade tumours with high precision.

The promise of the amino acid PET (Figure 6) tracers has been emphasized due to their higher sensitivity in imaging recurrent tumours (particularly the low-grade) and better accuracy for differentiating between recurrent tumours and treatment-related changes compared with FDG. O-(2-[18F]fluoroethyl)-L-tyrosine (FET) is a potential new amino acid PET tracer that has been shown to be helpful as an additional tool in few patients by allowing better differentiation of tumour tissue from inflammatory tissue. Another possible application of 18F-FET PET being considered is in the monitoring of radio- or chemo-therapy of squamous cell carcinoma (SCC), because the reaction of the tumour tissue may be specifically detected without the interfering the uptake by inflammatory or reactive tissue [31].

The newer PET tracers have also shown great potential to image important aspects of tumour activity and thereby demonstrate ability in predicting right prognosis response. The value of hypoxia imaging tracers (such as fluoromisonidazole or more recently EF5) is substantial in radiotherapy planning and predicting treatment response. In addition, they may play an important role in the future in directing and monitoring targeted hypoxic therapy for tumours with hypoxia.

8. Future trends

With the further technological advancements in imaging modalities and contract agents the brain tumour imaging is getting benefited. The high relaxivity contrast agents are able to provide vital information on tumour vascularity and higher magnetic strength scanner having higher SNR are getting more focus for clinical usage. The PET-MR is no more a research prototype but is getting validated with clinical trials which will be available for clinics very soon. Even the newly available CT technology, Multi-Energy Computed Tomography, which operates on material characterization properties by multi-energy (commonly two) CT acquisition is the promising technology for anatomical and tumour functional information accessed at the same time [32].

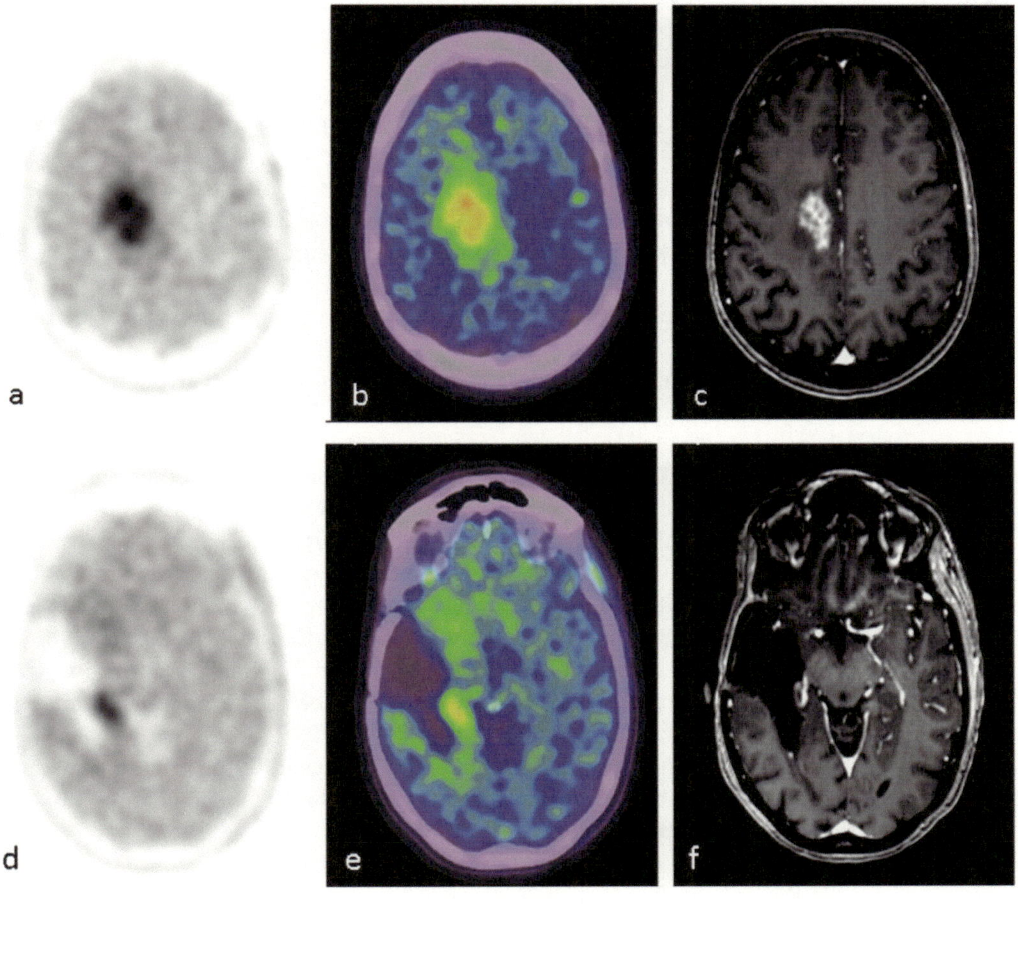

Fig. 6. Patient with a recurrent locoregional brain lesion - images show tumour before and after neurosurgery and radio-chemotherapy. a, d) FET-PET image showing intense uptake in the tumour tissue before and recurrent tumour after neurosurgery; b, e) Fused PET-CT image confirming the location of the tumour and recurrent lesion before and after surgery; c, f) post contrast MRI image in concordance to strong FET-tracer uptake shown in PET/CT. Furthermore, an additional brain lesion was identified in the right parietal lobe medial area of the brain tissue resected area, presenting a high FET-tracer uptake in PET/CT and strong contrast enhancement in MRI.

9. Conclusion

Brain tumour imaging consists of anatomical imaging with CT and perfusion MRI and functional imaging with PET. Physicians need both anatomical and functional imaging information to be assessed at the same time for appropriate treatment planning. The future of tumour imaging lies in developing optimal image registration and segmentation strategies from multimodality imaging as well as novel PET tracers. This approach is also set to play a role in the era of intensity-modulated radiotherapy, and is likely to have important clinical and research applications in radiotherapy planning in patients with brain tumours.

10. Reference

[1] Kandel EI, Schavinsky YV. Stereotaxic apparatus and operations in Russia in the 19th century. J Neurosurg 1972; 37:407-411

[2] Giesel FL, Mehndiratta A, Essig M. High-relaxivity contrast-enhanced magnetic resonance neuroimaging: a review. Eur Radiol 2010; 20:2461-2474

[3] Essig M. Clinical experience with MultiHance in CNS imaging. Eur Radiol 2003; 13 Suppl 3:N3-10

[4] Goyen M. Gadofosveset-enhanced magnetic resonance angiography. Vasc Health Risk Manag 2008; 4:1-9

[5] Sze G, Johnson C, Kawamura Y, et al. Comparison of single- and triple-dose contrast material in the MR screening of brain metastases. AJNR Am J Neuroradiol 1998; 19:821-828

[6] Schneider G, Kirchin MA, Pirovano G, et al. Gadobenate dimeglumine-enhanced magnetic resonance imaging of intracranial metastases: effect of dose on lesion detection and delineation. J Magn Reson Imaging 2001; 14:525-539

[7] Giesel FL, Mehndiratta A, Risse F, et al. Intraindividual comparison between gadopentetate dimeglumine and gadobutrol for magnetic resonance perfusion in normal brain and intracranial tumors at 3 Tesla. Acta Radiol 2009; 50:521-530

[8] Essig M, Lodemann KP, Le-Huu M, Bruning R, Kirchin M, Reith W. Intraindividual comparison of gadobenate dimeglumine and gadobutrol for cerebral magnetic resonance perfusion imaging at 1.5 T. Invest Radiol 2006; 41:256-263

[9] Schneider G, Kirchin MA, Pirovano G, et al. Gadobenate dimeglumine-enhanced magnetic resonance imaging of intracranial metastases: effect of dose on lesion detection and delineation. J Magn Reson Imaging 2001; 14:525-539

[10] Baleriaux D, Colosimo C, Ruscalleda J, et al. Magnetic resonance imaging of metastatic disease to the brain with gadobenate dimeglumine. Neuroradiology 2002; 44:191-203

[11] Colosimo C, Ruscalleda J, Korves M, et al. Detection of intracranial metastases: a multicenter, intrapatient comparison of gadobenate dimeglumine-enhanced MRI with routinely used contrast agents at equal dosage. Invest Radiol 2001; 36:72-81

[12] Knopp MV, Runge VM, Essig M, et al. Primary and secondary brain tumors at MR imaging: bicentric intraindividual crossover comparison of gadobenate dimeglumine and gadopentetate dimeglumine. Radiology 2004; 230:55-64

[13] Colosimo C, Knopp MV, Barreau X, et al. A comparison of Gd-BOPTA and Gd-DOTA for contrast-enhanced MRI of intracranial tumours. Neuroradiology 2004; 46:655-665

[14] Maravilla KR, Maldjian JA, Schmalfuss IM, et al. Contrast enhancement of central nervous system lesions: multicenter intraindividual crossover comparative study of two MR contrast agents. Radiology 2006; 240:389-400

[15] MJ, Picozzi P, Maldjian JA, et al. Evaluation of intraaxial enhancing brain tumors on magnetic resonance imaging: intraindividual crossover comparison of gadobenate dimeglumine and gadopentetate dimeglumine for visualization and assessment, and implications for surgical intervention. J Neurosurg 2007; 106:557-566

[16] Rumboldt Z, Rowley HA, Steinberg F, et al. Multicenter, double-blind, randomized, intra-individual crossover comparison of gadobenate dimeglumine and gadopentetate dimeglumine in MRI of brain tumors at 3 tesla. J Magn Reson Imaging 2009; 29:760-767

[17] Rowley HA, Scialfa G, Gao PY, et al. Contrast-enhanced MR imaging of brain lesions: a large-scale intraindividual crossover comparison of gadobenate dimeglumine versus gadodiamide. AJNR Am J Neuroradiol 2008; 29:1684-1691

[18] Broome DR, Girguis MS, Baron PW, Cottrell AC, Kjellin I, Kirk GA. Gadodiamide-associated nephrogenic systemic fibrosis: why radiologists should be concerned. AJR Am J Roentgenol 2007; 188:586-592

[19] Sadowski EA, Bennett LK, Chan MR, et al. Nephrogenic systemic fibrosis: risk factors and incidence estimation. Radiology 2007; 243:148-157

[20] Kanal E, Broome DR, Martin DR, Thomsen HS. Response to the FDA's May 23, 2007, nephrogenic systemic fibrosis update. Radiology 2008; 246:11-14

[21] Donahue MJ, Blakeley JO, Zhou J, Pomper MG, Laterra J, van Zijl PC. Evaluation of human brain tumor heterogeneity using multiple T1-based MRI signal weighting approaches. Magn Reson Med 2008; 59:336-344

[22] Howe FA, Opstad KS. 1H MR spectroscopy of brain tumours and masses. NMR Biomed 2003; 16:123-131

[23] Castillo M, Kwock L, Mukherji SK. Clinical applications of proton MR spectroscopy. AJNR Am J Neuroradiol 1996; 17:1-15

[24] Nelson SJ. Multivoxel magnetic resonance spectroscopy of brain tumors. Mol Cancer Ther 2003; 2:497-507

[25] Usenius JP, Kauppinen RA, Vainio PA, et al. Quantitative metabolite patterns of human brain tumors: detection by 1H NMR spectroscopy in vivo and in vitro. J Comput Assist Tomogr 1994; 18:705-713

[26] Usenius JP, Vainio P, Hernesniemi J, Kauppinen RA. Choline-containing compounds in human astrocytomas studied by 1H NMR spectroscopy in vivo and in vitro. J Neurochem 1994; 63:1538-1543

[27] Law M, Cha S, Knopp EA, Johnson G, Arnett J, Litt AW. High-grade gliomas and solitary metastases: differentiation by using perfusion and proton spectroscopic MR imaging. Radiology 2002; 222:715-721

[28] Shino A, Nakasu S, Matsuda M, Handa J, Morikawa S, Inubushi T. Noninvasive evaluation of the malignant potential of intracranial meningiomas performed using proton magnetic resonance spectroscopy. J Neurosurg 1999; 91:928-934

[29] Graves EE, Nelson SJ, Vigneron DB, et al. Serial proton MR spectroscopic imaging of recurrent malignant gliomas after gamma knife radiosurgery. AJNR Am J Neuroradiol 2001; 22:613-624

[30] Basu S, Alavi A. Molecular imaging (PET) of brain tumors. Neuroimaging Clin N Am 2009; 19:625-646
[31] Pauleit D, Zimmermann A, Stoffels G, et al. 18F-FET PET compared with 18F-FDG PET and CT in patients with head and neck cancer. J Nucl Med 2006; 47:256-261
[32] Mehndiratta A, Kapal JM, A P. Iodine mapping in brain tumor imaging using dual-energy computed tomography. Med Hypotheses 2011 May, 76(5):764.;

3

Imaging Techniques in Brain Tumor

Mingkun Yu, Wei Ye, Xiangqian Qi, Jun Qian,
Zhenyang Liu and Wenfeng Fang
*Department of Neurosurgery, Changzheng Hospital,
Second Military Medical University, Shanghai
China*

1. Introduction

Recent years, the emerging new imaging techniques not only show the detailed and complete aspects of brain neoplasm, but also promote clinical doctors using new techniques, such as CT three-dimensional reconstruction, magnetic resonance spectroscopy (MRS), diffusion weighted imaging (DWI), diffusion tensor imaging (DTI) to research the mechanism of those diseases in the aim of better treatment. The X-ray is the fundamental technology in clinical medicine. As CT and MRI make a great progress, the X-ray takes smaller and smaller part. When the neoplasm causes skull destruction or erosion, such as osteoma or Ewing's sarcoma of skull and pineal gland calcification, a significant X-ray can give us some useful information in diagnosis. The application of CT new technology, such as electron beam CT, dynamic CT enhancement, CT angiography and CT perfusion enhancement unfold a new boundary to neurosurgeons. Dynamic CT can not only reveal the pathophysiological change, but also make us keep an eye on local blood flow alteration. The CT angiography contains 4 methods which are threshold shaded surface display (SSD), maximum intensity projection (MIP), curved planner reformation (CPR) and volume rendering (VR). In those methods, three-dimension reconstruction takes the most important place, which gives us comprehensive observation by the complex show. On the other hand, if the blood vessels of tumor tissue need to be showed, the CT perfusion enhancement is a not bad choice, which can give clinical doctors accurate risk evaluation. The location, structure and perfusion of the neoplasm are the most important, and the answers of those significant aspects could be offered by conventional MRI. According to the distribution of the blood vessels, brain tumors can be divided into 3 types, and those provide a better differential diagnosis. Time-of-flight (TOF) and phase-contrast (PC) are the basic image formation methods. Multiple overlapping thin-slab acquisition (MOTSA) is the updated technology, which can elevate the signal overlapped vessels, display the relationships between vessels and brain. MRS can show the fineness and further, the metabolic characters of intracranial tumor. The MRS is complementary in brain neoplasm diagnosis, differential diagnosis, grading, evaluating and recurrence predicting. By determining the micro-metabolite such as N-acetyl-aspartate (NAA), creatinine (Cr), choline (Cho) etc in brain, MRS could be generally applied to the brain tumor. NAA is generally accepted as a marker in central nervous system. It decreases in almost all malignant brain tumors. The Cho extremely increases in malignant brain tumors, in the meaning that conversion function of cellular membrane is greatly accelerated. In most cases of malignant brain tumors, the Cr often lays on a lower level, compared to the normal value. With the use of MRS, the localization methods should be mentioned, which contain depth-resolved surface coil spectroscopy (DRESS), pointed- resolved surface coil spectroscopy (PRESS), spatially resolved spectroscopy (SPARS), the stimulated-echo acquisition method (STEAM), image selected in vivo spectroscopy (ISIS), fast-rotating spectroscopy (FROGS), point-resolved rotating-gradient surface-coil spectroscopy (PROGRESS) and volume-selective excitation (VSE). The MRS can be used to classify glioma, meningioma, metastatic tumor and other intracranial neoplasm by special peak and some characters. So, the MRS can tell us the characters and growth potential of a certain kind of brain tumor, and help us choose a correct and appropriate treatment strategy. Functional MRI is used to show the changes in the ratio of intravascular oxyhemoglobin to deoxyhemoglobin in response to a stimulus. It is widely used in many fields, such as vision, auditory perception, sensation, motor etc. which can be an addition to conventional MRI by discriminating neoplasm and edema. The functional MRI will be a guide in neurosurgery surgical approach to decrease the mortality in preoperative period. The diffusion of the water in central nervous system is depended on the integrity of the cell membrane and the osmotic balance. Though each brain tumor has its own special DWI, which can supply some valuable information of diagnosis and differential diagnosis, but DWI is mainly used in brain ischemic processes. The diffusion of water first decreases due to cell swelling, in the reason of decreasing the extracellular space. During the recovery stage, the loss of cell wall causes the diffusion to increase. In MRI, fiber bundles' integrity, compactability and parallelism are described by fractional anisotropy (FA). DTI is the conversion of FA value to FA figure. FA figures can distinguish grey matter and white matter, disclose the diffusion character of brain and the details as internal capsule, corpus callosum which could not be seen clearly on conventional MRI. Another echo planar imaging (EPI) is used to measure tissue perfusion. As diffusion, its effect can be easily swamped by patient's minor motion. The method of imaging tissue perfusion is to create an endogenous contrast by presaturating the blood flowing into the brain tumor in a reasonable radio frequency pulse. So, the ever developing world will provide us more and more useful image techniques, and now let's go into details of the summary we talked above.

2. X-RAY and brain tumor

Since 1895, Roentgen discovered x-ray which was used as a traditional x-ray machine till to 1970s.The x-ray machine brought about a structural change and improved its qualitative leap in performance in 1980s. In the late 1990's, CT and x-ray technology were combined to produce a new generation of digital x-ray (DR) radiographic techniques. So far, DR technology is widely used in clinic. X-ray diagnosis of brain tumors is mainly made by indirect signs. Skull destruction or hyperplasia or cranial calcification showed on x-ray, can be used for rough diagnosis of brain tumor. As X-ray technology is relatively simple and low cost, it is important in the initial diagnosis of brain lesions for the people living in some remote areas or underdeveloped regions. DR powerful quality control module of the post-processing techniques ensures the stability of image quality and avoids image distortion caused by scattering, blur and distortion. But the DR image as ordinary x-ray image, two-dimensional image is not only lack of three-dimensional effect, but also to be strict in the design requirements of the body. DR images are more sensitive to respiratory and body movements。 In the diagnosis of brain tumors, x-ray technology is far lower than CT, MR imaging technology. Plain film can sometimes show some signs which suggest the location of the intracranial space-occupying lesions according to the site of tumor calcification. Lesions could occupy some space within the cranial cavity, which are bound to cause some intracranial structural movement. Lesions near the skull may cause local bone destruction or proliferation often due to tumor oppression or erosion. These changes with positioning significance, directly or indirectly suggest the location of lesions. Tumor calcification results from tumor necrosis or hemorrhage, and often locates in the tumor and its vascular wall. Therefore, the appearance of calcification may specify the location of the tumor. Calcification ranges from a few millimeters to several centimeters, but the size of calcification can not represent the size of the tumor region. The site of tumor calcification is confined to the cranial cavity, which may be deep in the cranial cavity (such as glioma, etc.). Tumor calcification form may be irregular, nodular, patchy or small point, and wall calcification more features, which often has loop-shaped outline form cysts. If the calcification occurs and develops slowly, it mostly looks like benign calcification. The incidence of calcified craniopharyngioma ranks first in intracranial tumors in children. Most of intrasellar calcification is close to the saddle diaphragm and the minority may locate in the saddle back. The most common sign is the small number of high-density spots, or tiny piles of small pieces together. These spots or small pieces of calcified wall of the tumor spread fairly frequently so that the location can be another form of projection such as the arc form whose dense wall calcification is prone to shape and even depicts the outline of the entire tumor. The number and extent of calcification vary in size and sparsely scattered mostly from 1 to several centimeters in diameter. Large calcification is rare. Sometimes only one or two small point's calcification occurs, but the tumor is very large. Calcification of meningioma may be seen only in sand type and curing specific form. Calcification of meningioma generally occurs around 10%, sometimes up to 20% -50%. Most of calcification locates in the periphery of the cranial cavity, or the skull base close to the parietal bone surface. Differential diagnosis between Physiological intracranial calcification and calcified tumor are more difficult. CT and MRI should be further examined if there is difficult in diagnosis. The existence and the site of intracranial lesions could be inferred according to the displacement of the normal physiological intracranial calcification such as pineal calcification. Pineal calcification locates in the midline of cranial cavity. Cerebral hemisphere lesions can easily lead to its opposite displacement. Local bone changes include decreased density, bone destruction and bone hyperplasia due to the long-term oppression and erosion of the brain tumor. Lesions beside the sella may cause deformation, destruction or resorption of the ipsilateral sella bone structure. Invasive skull base tumor in the sella can cause destruction or resorption of cranial bone. Lesions near the skull base, can cause the expansion and deformation of the local canals. The pore size of the normal skull base is individually different, and both sides of them can also be slightly asymmetric, so diagnosis must be carefully considered. The expansion of the internal auditory canal is common in acoustic neuroma.

3. The computer tomography of brain neoplasm

As the popularity of the computer tomography (CT), it has been the first choice in diagnosing intracranial neoplasm. The X-ray getting through the collimator forms lots of electronic beam, and there is a detector bar in appropriate position in the aim of receiving the information of electron beam. After signal enhancement and analog/digital converter, the information will be processed by MATRIX, and the CT picture could be got. The highlighted character of CT is the discriminating ability such as showing brain structure. Therefore CT can not only show the white matter and grey matter, but also disclose internal capsule and basal ganglion. And the less loss of information can provide us more useful message to diagnose and evaluate prognosis. However, completely relying on CT in diagnosis and differential diagnosis, is not a good idea. Because the same tumor may present different picture and different neoplasm can show the same character, the application of different imaging method should be put in the first place, and this can give us clinical doctor lots of useful messages. Before CT scanning, some points should be talked about. First one is CT value and partial volume effect. The X-ray absorption in certain area can be evaluated by CT value which presents the density of normal and abnormal tissue in human. The partial volume effect will affect the result of CT picture. In case of neoplasm not displayed in all scanning pictures, CT value will show different density around the same tissue. The adjustment of window width can show the fine difference between normal tissue and neoplasm, and this is the second point should be noticed. The choice of window width and window center depends on the requirement of clinical doctor. Large window width leads to more structures presenting and less details showing. So the correct window width and window center is very important in CT scanning. And the third point is the enhancement. The picture will be enhanced when the neoplasm contains rich blood supply. This can give doctors better judgment in diagnosing and treatment. The last point is the artifact which come from different additional reasons, and in this situation, a re-examining should be in consideration. CT perfusion imaging is a new technology. Through this method, some parameter as blood flow, blood volume, mean transit time and time to peak could be acquired to evaluate the brain neoplasm. It is simple and feasible, and could be used in lots of area. After contrast enhancement, a time density curve could be got through multi-scanning to a certain area, and reconstructure of the data could provide us the perfusion situation of the organ. The growth period of brain tumor can be divided into two parts: first one without vessel and the second with vessel. In first period, the slow growth of tumor is in the short of nutrition supply, and then the formed vessels supply tumor rich nutrition so that the tumor grows at a higher speed. Pathologist Weidner N analyzed the tumor vessels and formed notion of microvascular density, which can give us information of the neoplasm to make appropriate treatment schedule. At present, microvascular density has become the "golden standard" in evaluation the growth of tumor vessels. But in the clinical process, the use of the criteria needs re-evaluating because of dynamic change reasons. Because different tumor has its own perfusion parameter (Wintermark et al; 2001), CT perfusion imaging could be used for diagnosis of brain tumor. The CBV of high grade glioma is quite different from that of the low one. And the more blood supply, the higher the CBV and CBF value will be detected. Recent research shows that the CBF value increase significantly in glioma and meningioma. Conventional CT and MRI cannot outline the tumor for infiltration, the reason of which lies in the integrity of blood vessel. While perfusion CT can give us the message of different parameter we want （Cenic et a1; 2000）. In guiding biopsy, our clinical doctor could take the tissue from the higher perfusion area, and elevate the successful chance of biopsy, promote us make the very suitable plan for patient treatment. The perfusion parameter has close relationship with the blood supply of neoplasm (Natbavi et a1; 2001). Use this technology, the necrosis after radiology and recurrence can be distinguished. If CBF ratio of the enhanced area to the normal brain higher than 2.6, the tumor recurrence is in consideration, while the ratio lower than 0.6, a tendency to be necrosis should be thought over.

The principle of dynamic CT is that time density curve will be obtained through processing a series of scanning after enhancement. Different tumor has different time density curve. The curve could be divide into five kinds: first, fast perfusion and diminishing with high peak, which can be seen in vascular disease; second, slow perfusion and diminishing with no so high peak, whose curve is mostly seen in meningioma, pituitary adenoma and metastasis tumor; third, slow perfusion and diminishing with low peak, which can be seen in glioma; fourth, slow perfusion and fast diminishing with low peak and the 5th one, a linear form. As the dynamic CT can show the brain vessels very clearly, so it not only can distinguish brain tumor from the vascular disease, but also have some meanings in differential diagnosis of brain tumor. Dynamic CT can help us understand the enhancement process in a convenient way. Before the peak, the data mean the perfusion of tumor and after the peak, the data show the resident of enhancer. There are four stages in dynamic CT time-density curve, slow increase of density, fast increase of density, fast decrease of density and slow decrease of density. The average time should be from 12 to 19 seconds. The peak can distinguish tumors rich or short of blood supply.

4. MRI and brain tumors

Magnetic resonance imaging has been an important component in the medical imaging diagnostic field. The research showed that MRI for intracranial tumor is better than CT, whose accuracy reaches 98% in positioning diagnosis and 70% - 85% in qualitative diagnosis. MRI has the following advantages: First, MRI has better soft tissue contrast; Second, 3-D imaging is more advantageous to accurate orientation of the lesions by multiple parameters and directions of the organs; Third, MRI can show intracranial vascular structure without contrast; Forth, No radiation damage, which is safe and reliable. In recent years, new technology of magnetic resonance imaging including DWI, DTI, PWI, fMRI and MRS, which have been in clinical research and application, is developing quickly. It not only reflects the information of the anatomy changes, but also provides the information of pathology, physiological function and biochemistry. So more accurate positioning of brain tumor and more reasonable design of surgery have been made in pre-operation or operation, which can reduce the damage of brain function and neural networks effectively. The advanced technology of MRI has been widely applied.

4.1 Conventional MRI and brain tumor

At present, the 1.5 to 3.0 tesla MRI have been used in most hospitals. The usual screening MRI of the brain begins with a sagittal localizer of the brain. The other includes T1 and T2 weighted axial images and FLAIR sequence. In some centers, gadolinium is routinely injected for a contrast enhancement picture so as to have a better diagnosis.

Gliomas are the most common primary brain tumors in both adult and children, taking approximate 1/2 to 2/3 parts of all brain tumors. Gliomas are usually divided into four distinct histologic subgroups: astrocytomas, oligodendrogliomas, ependymomas and choroid plexus tumors. The appearances of gliomas in MRI can be quite different. In some cases, the neoplasms have a distinct location and performance, which lead into correct diagnosis. While in other cases, the MRI image is not specific, and the clinical diagnosis should be made after pathologic diagnosis. MRI appearances are also depended on the histological grade of the neoplasm. In other words, the low-grade tumors usually exhibiting minimal or no peritumoral vasogenic edema, and high-grade tumors show prominent vasogenic edema. However, the sensitivity and specificity of MRI are limited in assessing the degree of anaplasia neoplasm. Astrocytoma accounts for 20% to 30%of all gliomas. The histological subtypes such as fibrillary, protoplasmic and gemistocytic varieties, are hardly distinguished by MRI. Some other types, such as cystic pilocytic astrocytomas, are typically found in the cerebellum in children, and subependymal giant cell astrocytomas with tuberous sclerosis can be distinguished by MRI based on their typical appearance, location and clinical manifestation. On MRI T1-weighted images, astrocytomas usually present hypointense to normal, while on T2-weighted and FLAIR images, astrocytomas present hyperintense to normal. Sometimes the MRI pictures cannot completely reliable, but the general rules should be noted. Low-grade astrocytoma shows slight peritumoral edema and homogeneous in signal characters on both T1 and T2-weighted images, while high-grade astrocytomas are usually more infiltrative without defined borders, associated with significant surrounding edema and more likely to be heterogeneous with the cystic and necrotic changes typically found in those tumors. Enhancement of astrocytomas on postgadolinium T1-weighted images can be quite variable. Although high grade tumors generally demonstrate more prominent enhancement than low grade tumors do, exceptions often occur. So the presence or absence of significant enhancement should not be used to estimate the degree of tumor which might be certificated by pathology. Post-contrast T1-weighted images can improve the sensitivity of MRI in the preoperative diagnosis and postoperative recurrence of those neoplasms. This sensitivity can be further improved by MR spectroscopy, which shows significantly elevated choline amplitude rated to creatine would suggest a recurrent form. The absence of elevated choline in a background of mobile lipids and lactate would favor radiation necrosis or post-surgical changes. New MRI techniques such as perfusion MRI and functional MRI are now more and more used. The MRI of oligodendroglioma shows more calcification, and usually hypointense on T1 and T2-weighted image, but microcalcifications can present hyperintense on T1-weighted images. So it is not very reliable by MRI to differentiate those tumors. The ependymomas have a protean MRI appearance and variable signal intensities on T1 and T2-weighted images, which are consistent with the variable cellularity and histologic composition of tumors. They are typically hypointense on T1-weighted images and hyperintense on T2-weighted images. However, calcification and cystic or hemorrhagic components often result in a variable, heterogeneous MR signal and enhancement.

Meningiomas are the second most common primary brain tumors. They are usually found in middle-aged to older women. As to pathology, they arise from the arachnoid cap cells and are commonly found over the parasagittal cerebral convexity, sphenoid wing, parasellar, tuberculum sella, olfactory groove, and cerebellopontine angle regions. They are usually isointense to grey matter on both T1 and T2-weighted images and therefore can be overlooked on screening MRI studies without contrast. They are often associated with an enhanced, thickened dura along the lateral margins of the tumor, which is known as a "dural tail". Meningiomas sometimes have areas of necrosis, calcification, hemorrhage and cystic changes, which generally lead to relatively small amount of edema.

Pituitary adenoma is one of the more common neoplasms encountered in adult neurosurgical patients. The tumor may be functional or non-functional adenoma. The functional adenoma can secrete prolactin, adrenocorticotropic hormone, growth hormone and so on. But MRI can not distinguish those subtypes. However, MRI is valuable in identifying a microadenoma. In case of macroadenoma, MRI can accurately identify the sellar, suprasellar, and parasellar extension of the tumor and the relationship between tumor and surrounding structures such as optic chiasm, optic nerves, hypothalamus, and cavernous sinus and supraclinoid segments of internal carotid arteries. The most important imaging sequence is the T1-weighted images with gadolinium contrast, which should include thin coronal images through sella turcica with a small field of view and filmed with magnification. In microadenomas, dynamic images should be done with a series of thin (3 to 4 mm) coronal images rapidly obtained over 2 to 3 minutes during bolus intravenous injection of gadolinium. It can identify a relatively slow enhancing microadenoma, within a rapidly and homogeneously enhancing normal pituitary parenchyma. Some other image findings include a deviation of the infundibulum away from the centre of the gland containing the adenoma, asymmetrical convexity of the superior border of the gland, and abnormal contour of the floor of the sella turcica. In the evaluation of macroadenomas, additional imaging sequence including T1-weighted sagittal images with contrast and T2-weighted coronal images, are valuable in defining tumor extension and associated parenchymal changes.
MRI with gadolinium contrast is the most sensitive imaging technique for the evaluation of the central nervous system metastasis. For the reason of multiplanar evaluation and no CT artifacts, MRI is superior to CT in tissue contrast. The appearance of metastasis tumor depends on the original tissue. The lesions are typically localized at grey matter-white matter junction of the supratentorial brain and occur more commonly in the anterior circulation. On T1-weighted images, the lesion often show iso- to hypo- intense, while on T2-weighted images, the lesion often present iso- to hyper- intense with prominent surrounding vasogenic edema.

4.2 Contrast-enhanced MRI and brain tumor

The MRI of enhanced T1-weighted images has great values of orientation, qualitative assay and curative effect evaluation in intracranial neoplasm (Zimmerman et al., 1999). It also exists some certain limitations, such as the difficulty for showing lesions in ventricle side or cortex area, not accurately reflecting the blood, the actual size and the scope by strengthening region and not offering the information of function in tumor. Currently the new technologies of MRI including contrast enhanced FLAIR MRI, dynamic contrast enhanced MRI, perfusion weighted MRI can provide more information for clinical treatment, which compensated for the shortage of conventional enhanced MRI. FLAIR is a stronger T2-weighted image by extremely long TR, TE and TI around 2000ms. The characteristic of image is that free water signal is zero and the contrast of brain grey matter is low. But the contrast between the lesion and the background is significantly increased in T2-weighted images. So the lesion is showed more clearly due to eliminating the influence of cerebrospinal fluid in ventricle side or brain ditch (Husstedt et al., 2000; Singh et a1., 2000). The research (Mathews et al., 2000) showed that enhanced FLAIR not only can express enhanced T1-weighted images but also can better detect the lesions of superficial parts compared with it. Enhanced FLAIR images which can observe the strengthened lesions and the edema area, makes up for the shortage of T1-weighted and T2-weighted images in some degree (Fig.4-1). Some scholars (Ercan et a1. , 2004) suggest that enhanced FLAIR images should be used as conventional scan and then the T1-weighted and T2-weighted images abolished, especially in detection of brain metastases and following-up for treatment of brain tumor.

The basic principle of dynamic enhanced MRI is the T1-weighted relaxation effect and magnetic sensitive effect of organizations caused by paramagnetic contrast agents through vein injection. Smaller doses of contrast agents can obtain higher resolution images. After several scans continuously, the change of strengthening degree in organization can be observed dynamically, and the hemodynamic quantitative material also can be obtained (Wong et al. , 1998). Through observing and analyzing the parameters of the interesting area such as SI-T curve, SImax, Tmax, Va and MCER, the information of differential diagnosis, the type and the grade of tumor can be obtained. Because it has the characteristics of no magnetic sensitive artifact and little effect by the surrounding edema, the basal ganglia lesions can be displayed obviously. PWI is the images of using dynamic contrast through magnetic sensitivity. It can obtain hemodynamic materials that MRI and MRA can't get such as rCBV, rCBF, and rMTT. It also can get the information of neural function and cerebrovascular state. So PWI can be used to identify primary or metastatic tumor, benign or malignant tumor, recurrence or the necrosis after radiation therapy (Wetzel et al. , 2002). Because it has obvious magnetic sensitive border artifact in the bone-brain or gas-brain interface, PWI currently only applies to hemisphere lesions which is still have some limitations in skull base or raised-face lesions.

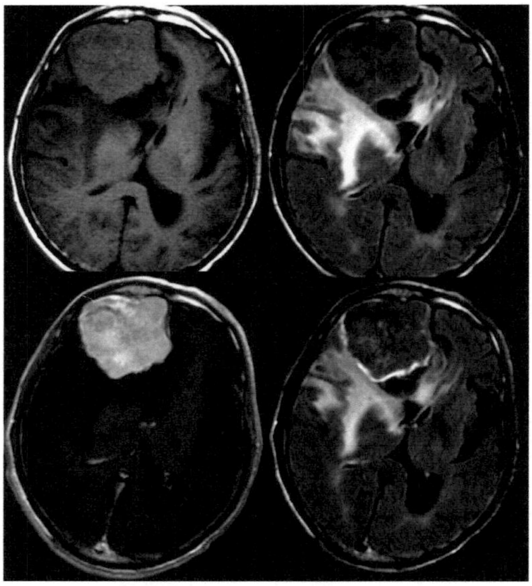

Fig. 4-1. T1WI (upper left), FLAIR (upper right), enhanced T1WI (lower left); contrast enhanced FLAIR (lower right).

4.3 DWI and brain tumor

DWI reflects the Brownian motion of tissue water. The diffusion of water molecules is faster, the signal is lower. The slower part of diffusion shows high signal. In ADC images, the organization with faster diffusion has high ADC values, and ADC value is low in the organization with lower diffusion. It can be used to diagnosis or differential diagnosis in intracranial neoplasm. It also not only can provide the clinical basis of rational operation plan, but also can be a method for monitoring the results after healing, which makes up for the shortage of conventional MRI.

4.3.1 DWI in diagnosis and differential diagnosis

Intracranial cystic lesions mainly include epidermoid cyst, dermoid cyst and arachnoid cysts. In SE sequences, there are long T1, T2 signal and no strengthening with enhancement. In DWI, epidermoid cyst and dermoid cyst are showed high signal and low ADC values, but arachnoid cyst is expressed low signal and high ADC values (Reddy et al., 2006). Common intracranial lesions including cerebral abscess, glioma and metastasis with hoop strengthening in MRI traditional sequence, have the same performance whose diagnosis is difficult. There are a variety of inflammatory cells, bacteria, necrotic tissue and sticky liquid secretion in the brain abscess in which the diffusion speed of water molecules is significantly limited. So the ADC values drop obviously, and DWI has high signal. But the cystic changes or necrotic area of brain tumor only include necrotic cells, bits of inflammatory cells and serums. Its ADC values and DWI signal are similar to CSF (Mishra et al., 2004).

In conventional MRI images, it is difficult to distinguish between the central nervous system lymphoma and gliomas before the operation. Because lymphoma cells density is higher, the ADC value is often lower than that of gliomas (Guo et al., 2002) (Fig.4-2).

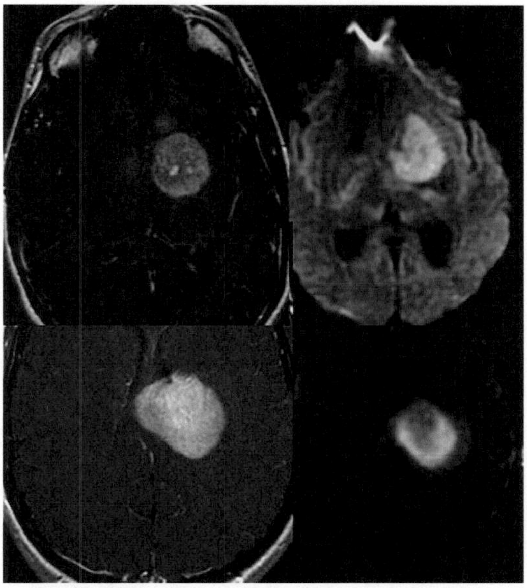

Fig. 4-2. T1 with contrast (left), DWI (right), primary central nervous system lymphoma (top row), GBM (bottom row).

4.3.2 Preoperative assessment of surgical resection range

DWI has certain effect in judging the low grade glioma with no strengthening and the malignant tumor boundaries which invade surrounding tissues. The edema area around glioma can be found not only the capillaries and edema, but also the invasive growth of tumor cells scattering along the new blood vessels or expand blood vessels especially in high grade glioma. Because of the inverse relationship between ADC values and cell density (Hayashida et al. , 2006), the ADC value of edema area around malignant glioma is relatively lower. It is very important to determine the range of surgical resection in preoperation.

4.3.3 Monitoring the effect of therapeutic response

ADC images which have potential value for evaluating the efficacy of fixed-point treatment such as radiation and local intracerebral injection of chemotherapy drug can be used to reflect the local treatment response quantitatively. The research (Hamstra et al., 2004) showed that ADC value before treatment is negatively correlated with extinctive degree of tumor after treatment. ADC level of tumor has been regarded as a imaging indicator of forecasting therapeutic effect. Another research (Morat et al. , 2005) also confirmed fDM in the treatment period can predict the response to treatment correctly in the 20 patients which was calculated the correlation between tumor diffusion value and clinical response by DWI imaging before radiotherapy or chemotherapy and after three weeks, and regarded the dispersion value of water molecules in tumor as an early markers before tumor volume change.

4.4 DTI and brain tumor

In recent years, DTI has been rapidly developed a new MRI imaging technology based on weighted imaging. It is currently the only alive, noninvasive and individualized 3D imaging technique which can display the fiber structure of cerebral white matter (Poupon et al. , 2000) (Fig. 4-3). DTI is similar to DWI but involves the collection of additional data

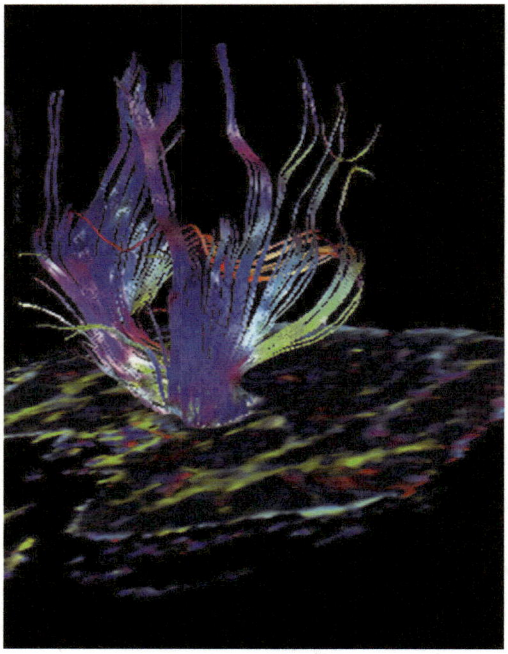

Fig. 4-3. Tractogram from a third subject illustrates the standard technique for displaying DTI data for surgical planning. (tractogram images courtesy of Kelvin Wong, PhD, using Philips Pride Software at Jockey Club MRI Center, University of Hong Kong.)

necessary to define the tensor describing the preferential direction and magnitude of water diffusion. The degree to which water diffusion in tissue is facilitated in one direction and hindered in another-referred to as diffusion anisotropy is often characterized by a scalar value derived from the diffusion tensor: fractional anisotropy.

4.4.1 DTI in diagnosis and differential diagnosis

Compared with metastases, the FA value is significantly lower in glioblastoma (Wang et al., 2009). However, the FA value is higher and the MD value is lower around glioblastoma (Lu et al., 2004). The FA, ADC value and the ratio of them in lymphoma is obviously lower than in glioblastoma (Toh et al., 2008). Compared with meningioma, the FA value around the area of tumor is lower in glioma (Provenzale et al., 2004). The average FA value of edema surrounding metastatic and its ratio is lower than in meningioma, but the MD values and its ratio are higher (Toh et al., 2007). The FA value in DTI is controversial in classifying the gliomas (Inoue et al., 2005; Goebell et al., 2006; Lee et al., 2008). The main reason of inconsistent results is hard to limit interested standard regions for effective data analysis.

4.4.2 DTI in treatment

Because DTI can clearly show the relationship between white matter fibers and brain tumor, it has great clinical value for guiding surgery including preoperative plan, intraoperative navigation and postoperative evaluation. The relationship between nerve fibers and brain tumor can be divided into three kinds: damage, shift and infiltration. The results showed that meningioma, glioblastoma and astrocytomas make the fiber bundles shifted, destroyed and infiltrated respectively (Wei et al., 2007). As a result, we can formulate operation plan and decide to surgical approach through confirming the relationship between white matter fiber bundles and brain tumor in preoperation. Through combined intraoperative DTI with fMRI and navigation technology to locate the positions of fiber bundles, brain function and brain tumor, it can be used as guiding tumor resection in intraoperation. At the same time, the maximum range of tumor is resected with the result that the important functional areas and fiber bundles are preserved greatly (Talos et al., 2006). DTI can also be applied to observe the therapeutic effect of drugs on tumor by dynamic tracking display in addition to the comparison of integrity and position of fiber bundles in postoperative evaluation (Wu et al., 2007; Gerstner et al., 2008). Meanwhile, the FA value is also a useful biological index of nerve damage caused by the treatment (Khong et al., 2006).

4.5 Bold-fMRI and brain tumor

BOLD-fMRI image is got by using endogenous hemoglobin as contrast agents through blood oxygen saturation alteration which reflects the changes of blood flow, blood volume and hemoglobin oxygen cooperation at neural activity . The different signal changes of cerebral blood oxygen consumption between activated area and not activated area are statistically analyzed to identify functional area.

4.5.1 The application of fMRI in surgery

The relationship and changes between lesions and functional areas in patients with brain tumor inspected by fMRI in preoperation contribute to design operation plan precisely. It can significantly reduce the risk of postoperative dysfunction. So fMRI should be the routine preoperative inspection in patients with brain tumor (Tomczak et al., 2000; Haberg et al.,

2004). There may be an adapted response of functional areas after injury because of mass effect by tumor which makes the cortex functional area deformation, shift and restructuring. Combined with intraoperative behavior evaluation, fMRI can protect the patients' cognitive function in intraoperation (Amiez et al., 2008). Understanding the relationship between cortical activated area and tumor in preoperation, it may help us predict the dysfunction risk degree and the possibility of tumor recurrence after tumor resection (Wildfőrster et al., 1998).

4.5.2 The combined application of fMRI and other methods

4.5.2.1 The combined application of fMRI and neural navigation

Intraoperative navigation which is conducted through the anatomical and functional orientation logged in stereotactic neurosurgery navigators by fMRl in preoperation can effectively remedy the defects of intraoperative orientation, avoid intraoperative injury of cortical functional areas, reduce postoperative complications and lower the recurrence rate after surgery (Hall et al., 2009).

4.5.2.2 The combined application of fMRI and DTI

The combined images of fMRI and DTI in preoperation can show not only the cerebral cortex function, but also the brain white matter fiber bundles. Its value is higher than fMRI alone which make less postoperative complications and help to improve the prognosis because of the good assessment of function in language, movement and vision (Ulmer et al., 2004) (Fig.4-4).

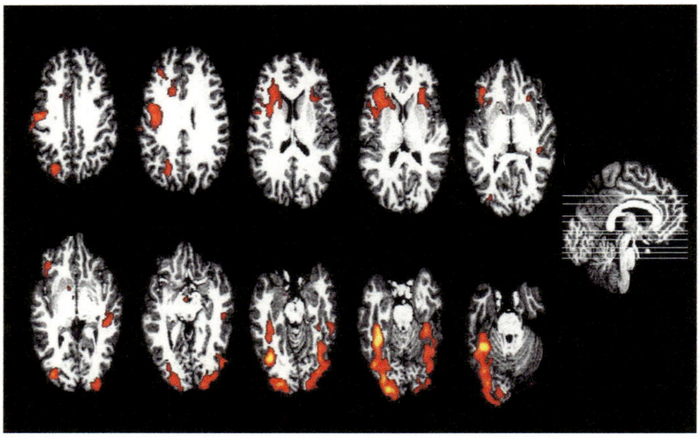

Fig. 4-4. fMRI results to word reading.

4.5.2.3 The combined application of fMRI and 3D-ultrasound

The data of fMRI and DTI can be integrated into 3D-ultrasound in order to correct the deviation caused by brain shift (Rasmussen et al., 2007).

4.6 MRS and brain tumor

As the MRS was admitted to the clinical application in 1995, neuroradiology has step into a brand new world. Being a non-invasive examination method, MRS can provide us the metabolic information which the conventional MRI and CT cannot tell us, and the one more important aspect, the MRS can not only find some abnormal earlier than conventional MRI, but also provide the prognosis information. Each compound in brain obtains its own picture in different frequency, and so it can be detected for several reasons: made of hydrogen, concentration more than 0.5mmol/L, own different frequency on chemical shift. As to the atoms used in the MRS, all of us will place the hydrogen in the first place. MRS can provide a "biopsy on line" without any invasive operation (Buascher et al., 2000), and can evaluate metabolic information on brain tumor (Fountas et al., 2000). Middle-time-echo (144ms) shows the elevation of choline ideally, which is the major presentation in brain tumor. Short-time-echo (30ms or 35ms) can detect mI to grade the neoplasm. The peak of NAA decreases because of the death of neuron, and the peak of Cr decreases in the reason of tumor metabolism. Cho is the most important chemical compound in evaluating the neoplasm, the increase of which often tells us the reproduction of the membrane. When the neoplasm present alike in the cMRI, MRS could be used for differential diagnosis. Cho is recognized as the special marker in brain tumor (Gruber et al., 2005). In high-grade (grade Ⅱ and Ⅲ) glioma (Negendan et al., 1996), MRS can show the high level of choline, but when the collecting of images in the necrosis area, the choline could diminish. So, trying to avoid necrosis area, is very important to presenting the Cho in glioma. In adult MRS, Lac peak could be detected and the high grade tumor often links with higher peak of Lac. And in meningiomas, increase of Glx can be detected(McKnight，2004).

The accuracy of grading malignant brain tumor by MRS is higher than aimless biopsy. For two reasons: one is that MRS can analyze the relatively big amount tissue, and the other is when biopsy taken the part not in the active area could not provide the accurate grading of the tumor. The sensitivity, accuracy and specificity of discriminating high-grade tumor or low-grade tumor are 100%, 96% and 86% respectively. In assurance of tumor grading, the Cho, Lac, Lip, NAA, Cr and mI can provide us lots of useful information (Murphy et al., 2004). Within the high-grade tumors, the higher Cho, Lac, Lip and mI can be detected, but NAA and Cr often show a decreasing form. In the malignant brain tumors, because cMRI cannot show the exact boundary, MRS or PWI should be considered. MRS can also provide useful message on tumor progressing, the Cho increasing more than 45% often shows the progress of tumor. The cMRI and MRS has been used in neurosurgery operation in the aim of resecting the neoplasm in a great and safe way, which take more and more important part in neurosurgery (Hemfinghaus et al., 2002).

5. Digital subtraction angiography

Digital subtraction angiography (DSA) is a type of fluoroscopy technique used in interventional radiology to clearly visualize blood vessels in a bony or dense soft tissue environment. DSA eliminates the unnecessary organization image, leaving only the vascular image through digital processing. Its distinct image and high resolution provide a real three-dimensional image for the position measurement, diagnosis and interventional treatment of vascular disease. DSA is mainly used for examination and treatment of systemic vascular diseases and cancer. Before the application of CT and MR, angiography was one of the most important methods for brain tumor imaging which display the displacement, stenosis and occlusion of normal blood vessels caused by tumor and determine the tumor size and location combined with tumor angiogenesis (tumor stain), then make a diagnosis. It is generally considered that the characteristics of a benign tumor are of uniform thickness, more radial of vascular morphology, homogeneous dense tumor staining and clear outline (Fig.5-1.). The developing time is similar with cerebral circulation because of more mature blood vessels. Contrarily, the characteristics of a malignant tumor are of different thickness, inhomogeneous distribution of rough edges of vascular and unclear light profile of tumor stain. Because of the immature vascular structures, veins often develop early as a result of the direct intersection of arteriovenous. With the development and wide application of CT and MR, angiography plays a declining role in the diagnosis of brain tumor. Now angiography is mainly used for the identification of cancer and vascular disease, preoperative evaluation and embolization of the intracranial tumors.

DSA can help us understand the blood supply and scope of brain tumors which is useful for interventional treatment and followed-up. For hypervascular intracranial tumors, especially meningioma and glomus jugulare tumor, preoprative angiography is mainly used for displaying tumors' blood supply and impact of important veins. Taking the meningioma for example, its blood supply is often divided into the following categories (Manelfe et al, 1973). ECA alone, ECA and ICA mainly by ECA, ECA and ICA mainly by ICA, ICA alone. For meningioma supplied both by ECA and ICA, the ICA often supplies the peripheral of tumor, while the ECA for the centre, most of which come from the ECA branch such as the dura artery. It's very important in the preoperative preparation for a parasinus meningioma to make sure whether sinus was completely obliterated (Caroli et al, 2006). Completely occluded dural sinus means a considerable formation of collateral circulation. For this type of tumor and related dural venous sinuses which has been blocked, completely removing them usually doesn't cause venous thrombosis. However, the occurrence of dural venous sinus obstruction after surgery is of high risk if the tumor has accumulated in the dural venous sinus without blocking, especially in the back of the superior sagittal sinus, transverse sinus and sigmoid sinus. The goal of preoperative embolization of intracranial meningiomas is to facilitate their surgical removal by reducing tumor vascularity and decreasing blood loss during surgery (Richter & Schachenmayr, 1983; Manelfe et al., 1986; Engelhard, 2001; Hirohata et al, 2003). Preoperative embolization appeared to be very useful in large tumors with pure or predominant external carotid artery supply (convexity meningiomas), in skull-base meningiomas, and in middle fossa and paracavernous meningiomas. It was also useful in falx and parasagittal meningiomas receiving blood supply from the opposite side and in posterior fossa meningiomas (Manelfe et al., 1986).The external carotid artery embolization is often adopted for safety consideration. And the gelatin sponge or particles of 200-300 micron is often selected as material for embolization. The catheter should be as closer as possible to the vascularity of tumor when embolism begins (Fig.5-1). Embolization in tumor is better than that simply for feeding artery. The main complications of embolization include cerebral vasospasm, local fever and headache, skin necrosis may also occur. For there could be "dangerous anastomasis" or reflux, so the most serious complications are blindness, aphasia, and sensory-motor disorder as a result of embolization in the intracranial blood vessels. Therefore, the operation process of embolization should be slow and careful to prevent refluxing. DSA is also used for malignant brain tumor in arterial infusion chemotherapy. There has certain effect, fewer complications and less systemic adverse reactions when applying intracranial arterial infusion therapy in patients with brain metastases. For patients with brain metastases unsuitable for surgical treatment, arterial infusion chemotherapy is effective in improving the quality of life and prolonging the life.

Despite of the rapid development of CT and MRI, DSA technology is still the "gold standard" of diagnosis and treatment for vascular disease. Following the development of the computer technology, imaging equipment and contrast agents in the future, DSA technology will play an important role in diagnosis and treatment for brain tumor.

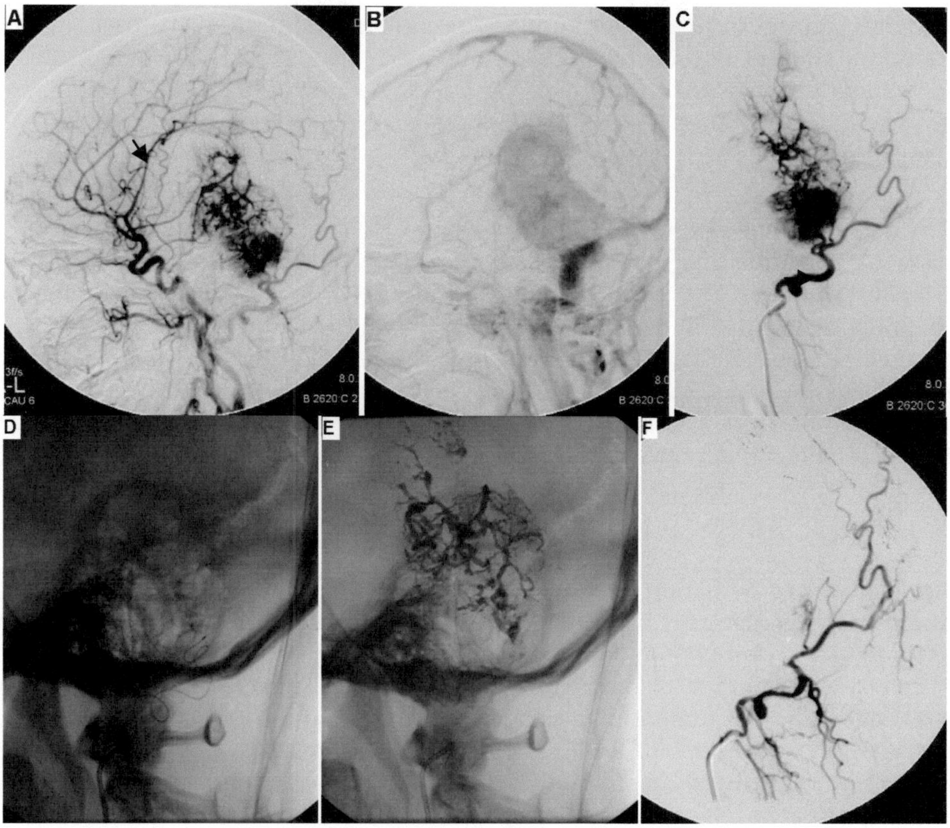

Fig. 5-1. Preoperative embolization for a meningioma. A, B, DSA displays the displacement of MCA (black arrow) and stain of the tumor. C, A super-selected angiography of the occipital artery shows the feeding artery (black arrow). D, Microcatheter in occipital artery arrived at the feeding artery. E, The emboliaztion agents in the tumor. F, Angiography of the occipital artery post-embolization.

6. Perfusion imaging

Perfusion imaging with CT or MRI is an exciting new radiological technique for noninvasive evaluation of cerebral hemodynamics in brain tumor. Cerebral perfusion imaging describes the passage of blood through the brain's vascular network. In this part, we will focus on the role of perfusion MR imaging in improving accurate diagnosis and monitoring brain tumors during therapy.

6.1 The basic principle of CT perfusion imaging

The theory foundation of CT perfusion imaging is nuclear medicine radioactive tracer dilution and center volume principles. The radioactive tracer is quickly injected into people's vein, which go to the target organ through the left ventricular. By the dynamic CT scanning for the selected slices, we can get the time-density curve (TDC) for each pixel in these slices. According to time-density curve, blood flow (BF), mean transit time (MTT) and blood volume (BV) could be calculated by using different mathematical models. This method can be used for evaluation of blood perfusion conditions in the tissue. Common perfusion parameters include reginal cerebral blood volume (rCBV) which means total blood volume in the specific brain area, and reginal cerebral blood flow (rCBF) which means blood volume that flows through particular brain regions in unit time. Their mathematical relationship is rCBF=rCBV／MTT.

6.2 The basic principle of MR perfusion imaging

MR cerebral perfusion imaging shows blood condition of brain in the capillaries level by application of markers. The common parameters are blood flow, perfusion, and time and so on of brain tissue in unit volume. The main parameters include cerebral blood flow (CBF),cerebral blood volume (CBV), mean transit time(MTT) that the contrast agents go through the tissue, and time to peak (TTP) of contrast agents concentration, etc. Gd-DT-PA is commonly used as external markers. Arterial water molecules are often used as endogenous markers. Arterial spin labeling is a new perfusion technique that does not require exogenous contrast; instead it exploits the spins of endogenous water protons that perfuse the imaging plane.

6.3 Applications of perfusion Imaging

Perfusion imaging, especially with MRI has become an integral component of the complete radiological assessment of brain tumors. Perfusion imaging may reflect angiogenesis status and hemodynamic change of brain tumor. There are two kinds of tumor blood vessels sources, one kind is tumorous neoangiogenesis of the host, and another kind is neovascularization of tumour itself. There is obvious relationship between biological behaviour and vascularization of brain tumor, whose characteristics are the damage of the blood brain barrier so as to increase vascular permeability. Therefore perfusion imaging can be used for the diagnosis and differential diagnosis of brain tumors. Because the flow of blood to the tumor increased significantly, regional cerebral blood volume (rCBV) value can reflect how much there are functional capillary quantity. The increase of rCBV, quickly leaking into the surrounding tissue (contrast agents quickly enter extracellular clearance), can reflect tumorous biological activities. The more active tumor grows, the higher the malignant degree of tumor will be, and the greater rCBV value is, also the faster the risk of leakage. The new vessels are more tortuous than the native cerebral vessels, leading to increased mean transit times (MTT). Therefor, perfusion imaging is often useful to establish the diagnosis of tumor and to distinguish tumor from tumor mimics, for example, infective granulomas or tumefactive demyelination, which are hypoperfused with low values of CBV, CBF, and MTT. Perfusion computed tomography (PCT) allows to reliably classify gliomas and lymphomas based on quantitative measurements of CBV and KTrans (Schramm, et al. 2010）. In comparison with normal parenchyma, low grade gliomas showed no significant difference of perfusion parameters, whereas high-grade gliomas demonstrated significantly higher values for KTrans, CBV and CBF. Lymphomas displayed significantly increased mean KTrans values compared with unaffected cerebral parenchyma but no elevation of CBV. High-grade gliomas show significant higher CBV values than lymphomas (Figure 6-1 and 6-2). MR cerebral perfusion imaging can also identify the benign or malignant brain tumors. In addition, rCBV of the brain tumor will significantly reduce after the chemotherapy, embolization or radiation therapy. MR perfusion imaging can also be used to identify with tumor recurrence or focal necrotic after treatment and evaluate prognosis or monitor the efficacy of treatment. Furthermore, numerous studies (Park et al., 2009; Schramm et al., 2010; Ludemann et al., 2009; Park et al., 2009) have shown that perfusion imaging have special superiority in noninvasively grading tumor histology preoperatively. Low-grade astrocytomas are hypoperfused as compared to grade III and IV lesions (Figure 6-3). Up to one-third of the high-grade tumors do not enhance on post contrast T1 weighted images, which may lead to a false radiological impression of low grade; unless a perfusion study is performed, which demonstrates hyperperfusion due to neoangiogenesis, which is associated with higher grade (Figure 6-4). Some authors (Law et al., 2002) have suggested that MR perfusion along with spectroscopy may aid in differentiating a high-grade primary tumor from solitary cerebral metastasis. Primary high-grade tumors are infiltrative by nature; hence the peritumoral edema shows elevated CBV values. In contrast, metastases are well encapsulated and noninfiltrative by nature and therefor the perilesional edema being purely vasogenic shows low CBV values. MR perfusion may also be used as a guide to direct stereotactic biopsies from the most aggressive component of a heterogeneous tumor. Up to one-third of high-grade tumors are under-reported at stereotactic biopsy and this may be because the biopsy has not been acquired from the most aggressive portion of the lesion.

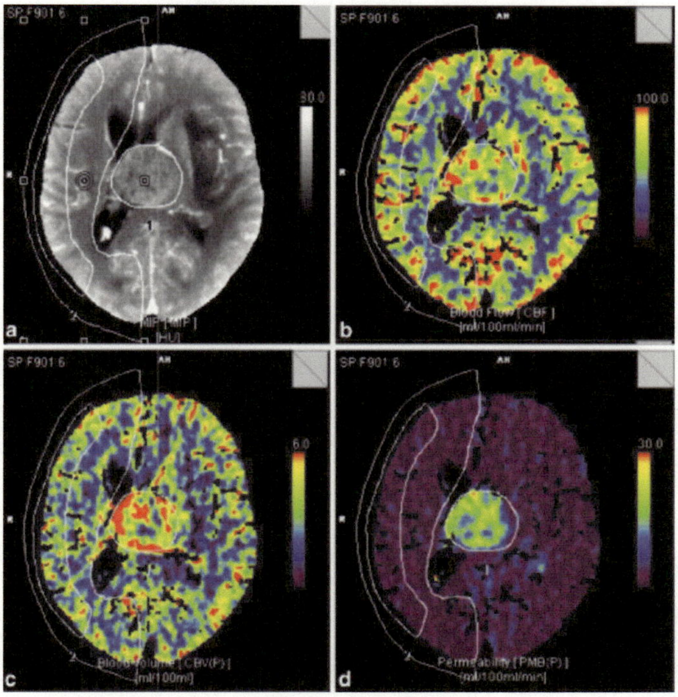

Fig. 6-1. A 58-year-old man with histopathological diagnosis of glioblastoma multiforme WHO IV. Axial contrast-enhanced MIP reconstruction image (a) shows a contrast-enhanced mass, which demonstrates intensely elevated blood flow (b) and volume (c) as well as strongly increased regional Ktrans (d) in comparison with the normal cortical and subcortical cerebral parenchyma (Schramm, et al. 2010).

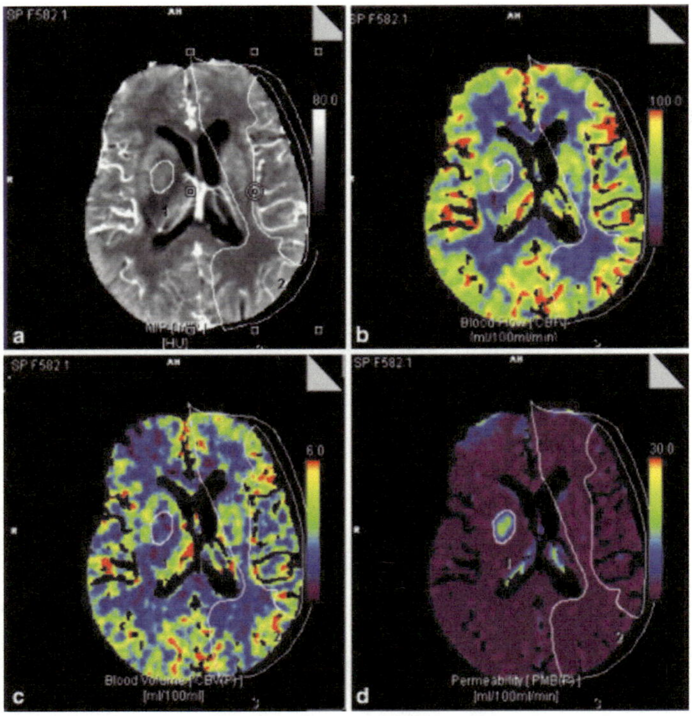

Fig. 6-2. A 72-year-old woman with histopathological diagnosis of primary cerebral lymphoma. In comparison with the contralateral normal cerebral parenchyma, the lesion depicted in the right lentiform nucleus demonstrates the typical perfusion characteristics of lymphoma: enhancement (a), no significant increase in CBF (b) or CBV values (c), though intensely increased regional permeability (KTrans, d), indicating a massive disturbance of the blood-brain barrier (Schramm, et al., 2010).

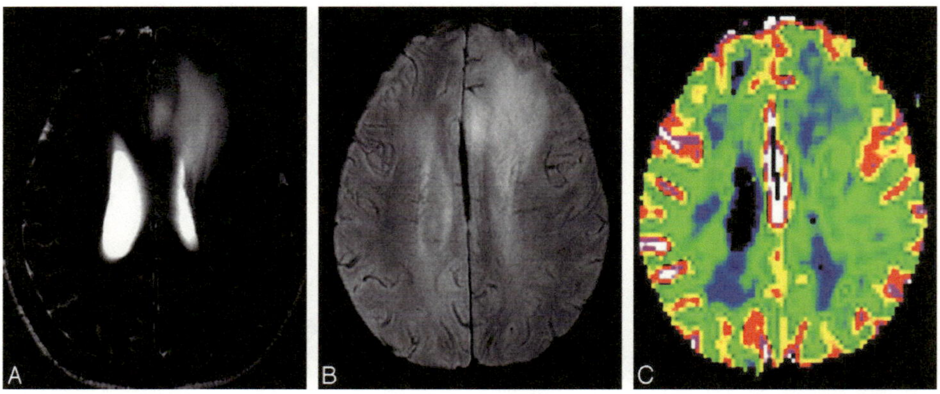

Fig. 6-3. MR images of a 39-year-old woman with left frontal low-grade astrocytoma (WHO grade II). A, The axial T2-weighted image shows an ill-defined mass with high signal intensity in the left frontal lobe. B, High-resolution susceptibility-weighted imaging (HR-SWI) demonstrates no evidence of the intratumoral susceptibility signal intensity (ITSS). C, Corresponding rCBV map shows relatively low rCBVmax values of 1.31. (Park et al., 2009).

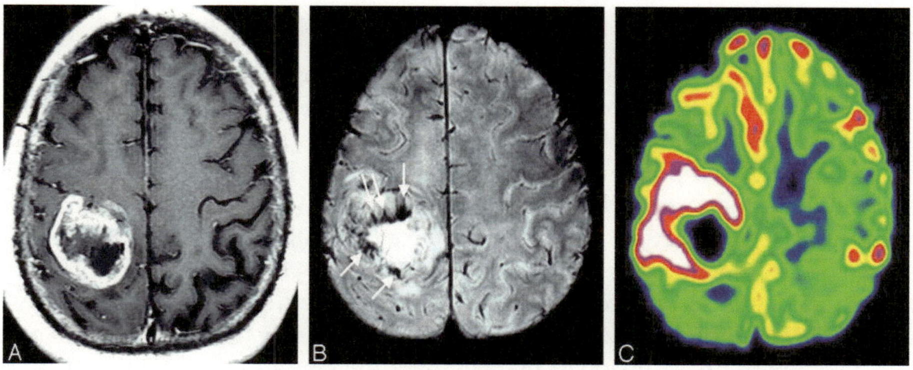

Fig. 6-4. MR images of a 55-year-old man with a glioblastoma multiforme. A, The contrast-enhanced axial T1-weighted image shows a mass with irregular peripheral rim enhancement in the right parietal lobe. B, HR-SWI reveals conglomerated fine linear ITSSs just in the inner portion of the enhancing rim on the contrast-enhanced T1-weighted image (White arrows show tumor vessels). C, Corresponding rCBV map shows high rCBVmax values (4.71) in the tumor segment, including a maximum degree of ITSS. (Park et al., 2009).

MR perfusion can help distinguish gliomas from nonglial lesions like lymphoma and metastases or extra-axial tumors like meningioma. rCBV maps demonstrate increased blood volume in the enhancing high-grade glioma and decreased blood volume in lymphoma and metastases or extra-axial tumors, which are more significant in the area of peritumoral edema. This is because extra-axial tumors and nonglial lesions lack a blood brain barrier (BBB), hence, a very large fraction of the bolus leaks into the extravascular space during the first pass (Young G.S. & Setayesh K., 2009; Sasao et al., 2010; Hartmann et al., 2003; Noguchi et al., 2008). On the other hand, gliomas have a BBB that is impaired but not absent and this could be reflected in the perfusion data. The difference between these perfusion patterns can contribute significantly to the discrimination of tumor types in cases of peripherally located enhancing tumors when the differential diagnosis includes meningioma and peripheral GBM, and in periventricular enhancing lesions when the differential diagnosis includes choroid plexus papillocarcinoma and GBM (Kaur et al., 2004). It has been reported that MR perfusion is more accurate in determining the true anatomical extent of a lesion as compared to conventional imaging. This is because the perilesional edema often contains microscopic tumors, which manifest on perfusion studies as areas of increased CBV. So perfusion maps may show true tumor margins beyond what is visible on conventional MR imaging. The demonstration of the true anatomical extent of a tumor aids in proper surgical and radiation therapy planning. Perfusion imaging is excellent in the differentiation of tumor recurrence from radiation necrosis, which can be confusing on conventional MR imaging (Hu et al., 2009). On conventional imaging, both recurrent high-grade tumor and radiation necrosis appear as space occupative lesions with post contrast enhancement, perilesional edema, mass effect, and intralesional hemorrhage. Furthermore, for reason not well understood, radiation necrosis most commonly occurs in the tumor bed, even in cases of whole brain irradiation. However, radiation therapy leads to endarteritis and therefore the lesions of radiation necrosis are hypoperfused, whereas, recurrent tumor being most often high-grade, is hyperperfused. Finally, it is expected, that in the future, perfusion imaging may be a surrogate marker to study response in clinical trials of newer antiangiogenic pharmaceuticals.

7. Conclusion

Recent Neuroimaging technology has developed from a purely morphology-based discipline to the complete anatomy, physiology, pathophysiology, hemodynamics and biochemical assessment of a brain tumor. These techniques have important implications in planning therapy and in prognostication. Imaging diagnosis has come from general level deeply into the cellular, molecular, and genetic level. With the advent of the new contrast agents (including organization, organ specific contrast agents, specific gene expression, specific metabolic process, special physiological function contrast agents, etc.), diagnosis and differential diagnosis of specificity will be stronger. Neurosurgeons can design surgery scheme and decide approach for surgical total resection of the tumor during the operation by using a variety of image fusion technology with the application of computer simulation technology and digital image navigation system, which will make the scope of operation more precise and effective, and maximally reserve postoperative neurological function. Recent advances in imaging methods will help us to better assess treatment response, more accurately determine tumor activity during therapy, and differentiate recurrent tumor and treatment related complications.

8. References

Amiez C, Kostopoulos P, Champed AS, et al. (2008). Preoperative functional magnetic resonance imaging assessment of higher-order cognitive function in patients undergoing surgery for brain tumors. J Neurosurg, Vol.108, No.2, pp.258-268.

Buascher IM, Skagerberg G, Geijer B, et a1. (2000). Proton MR spectroscopy and preoperative diagnostic accuracy: an evaluation of intracranial mass lesions characterized by stereotactic biopsy findings.Am J Neuroradiol, Vol.21, No.1, pp.84-93.

Caroli E, Orlando ER & Mastronardi L, et al (2006). Meningiomas infiltrating the superior sagittal sinus: surgical considerations of 328 cases. Neurosurg Rev, Vol. 29, No. 3, pp. 236-41.

Craen R.A., et a1. (2000). A CT method to measure hemodynamics In braintumors: validation and application of cerebral blood flow maps. Am J Neuroradiol, Vol.1, No.3, pp.462-470.

Engelhard HH(2001). Progress in the diagnosis and treatment of patients with meningiomas. Part I: diagnostic imaging, preoperative embolization. Surg Neurol, Vol.55, No.2, pp.89-101.

Ercan N, Guhekin S, Celik H, et a1. (2004). Diagnostic value of contrast-enhanced fluid-attenuated inversion recovery MR imaging of intracranial metastases. American Journal of Neuroradiology, Vol.25, No.5, pp.761-765.

Fountas KN, Kapsalaki EZ, Gotsis SD, et a1.In vivo proton magnetic resonance spectroscopy of brain tumors. Stereotact Funct Neurosurg, Vol.74, No.1, (2000), pp.83-94.

Gerstner ER, Sorensen AG, Jain RK, et al. (2008). Advances in neuroimaging techniques for the evaluation of tumor growth, vascular permeability, and angiogenesis in gliomas. Curr Opin Neurol, Vol.21, No.6, pp.728-735.

Goebell E, Paustenbach S, Vaeterlein O, et al. (2006). Low-grade and anaplastic gliomas: differences in architecture evaluated with diffusion-tensor MR imaging. Radiology, Vol.239, No.1, pp.217-222.

Gruber S, Stadlbauer A, Mlynarik V, et a1. Proton magnetic resonance spectroscopic imaging in brain tumor diagnosis. Neurosurg Clin N Am, Vol.16, No.1, (2005), pp.101-104.

Guo AC,Cummings TJ, Dash RC, et al. (2002). Lymphomas and high-grade astrocytomas: comparison of water diffusibility and histologic characteristics. Radiology, Vol.224, No.7, pp.177-183.

Haberg A, Kvistad KA, Unsgard G, et al. (2004). Preoperative blood oxygen level-dependent functional magnetic resonance imaging in patients with primary brain tumors: clinical application and outcome. Neurosurgery, Vol.54, No.7, pp.902-914.

Hall WA, Kim P, Truwit CL. (2009). Functional magnetic resonance imaging guided brain tumor resection. Top Magn Reson Imaging, Vol.19, No.4, pp.205-212.

Hamstra DA, Lee KC, Tychewicz JM, et al. (2004).The use of 19F spectroscopy and diffusion weighted MRI to evaluate difference in gene dependent enzyme prodrug therapies. Mol Ther, Vol.10, No.5, pp.916-928.

Hartmann M., Heiland S., Harting I., et al. (2003). Distinguishing of primary cerebral lymphoma from high-grade gliomas with perfusion-weighted magnetic resonance imaging. Neurosci Lett, Vol.338, No.2, pp. 119-122.

Hayashida Y, Hirai T, Morishita S, et al. (2006). Diffusion-weighted imaging of metastatic brain tumors: comparison with histologic type and tumor cellularity. Am J Neuroradiol Vol.27, No.7, pp.1419-1425.

Hemfinghaus S, Pilatus U, Moiler-Hartman W, et a1. Increased choline levels coincide wil1 enhanced proliferative activity of human neuroepithelial brain tumors. NMR Biomed, Vol.15, No.3, (2002), pp.385.

Hirohata M, Abe T, Morimitsu H, et al(2003). Preoperative selective internal carotid artery dural branch embolisation for petroclival meningiomas. Neuroradiology, Vol.45, No.9, pp.656-60.

Hu L.S., Baxter L.C., Smith K.A., et al. (2009). Relative Cerebral Blood Volume Values to Differentiate High-Grade Glioma Recurrence from Posttreatment Radiation Effect: Direct Correlation between Image-Guided Tissue Histopathology and Localized Dynamic Susceptibility-Weighted Contrast-Enhanced Perfusion MR Imaging Measurements. Am J Neuroradiol, Vol.30, No.3, pp.552–58.

Husstedt HW, Sickert M, Kstler H, et al. (2000). Diagnostic value of the fast-FIAIR sequence in MR imaging of intracranial tumors. Eur Radiol, Vol.10, No.5, pp.745-752 ·

Inoue T, Ogasawara K, Beppu T, et al. (2005). Diffusion tensor imaging for preoperative evaluation of tumor grade in gliomas · Clin Neurol Neurosurg, Vol.107, No.3, pp.174-180.

Kaur B., Tan C., Brat D.J., et al. (2004). Genetic and hypoxic regulation of angiogenesis in gliomas. J Neurooncol, Vol.70, No.2, pp.229-43.

Khong PL, Leung LH, Fung AS, et al. (2006). White matter anisotropy in post-treatment childhood cancer survivors: preliminary evidence of association with neurocognitive function. J Clin Oncol, Vol.24, No.6, pp.884-890.

Law M., Cha S., Knopp E.A., et al. (2002). High grade gliomas and solitary metastases: Differentiation by using perfusion and proton spectroscopic MR imaging. Radiology, Vol.222, No.3, pp.715-21.

Lee HY, Na DG, Song IC, et al. (2008). Diffusion-tensor imaging for glioma grading at 3-T magnetic resonance imaging: analysis of fractional anisotropy and mean diffusivity. J Comput Assist Tomogr, Vol.32, No.2, pp.298-303.

Lu S, Ahn D, Johnson G, et al. (2004). Diffusion-tensor MR imaging of intracranial neoplasia and associated peritumoral edema: introduction of the tumor infiltration index. Radiology, Vol.232, No.1, pp.221-228.

Ludemann L., Warmuth C., Plotkin M., et al. (2009). Brain tumor perfusion: comparison of dynamic contrast enhanced magnetic resonance imaging using T1, T2, and T2* contrast, pulsed arterial spin labeling, and H2O positron emission tomography. Eur J Radiol, Vol.70, No.3, pp. 465-74.

Manelfe C, Guiraud B & David J, et al (1973). Embolization by catheterization of intracranial meningiomas. Rev Neurol (Paris), Vol.128, pp. 339–351.

Manelfe C, Lasjaunias P & Ruscalleda J(1986). Preoperative embolization of intracranial meningiomas. Am J Neuroradiol, Vol.7, No.5, pp.963-72.

Mathews VP, Caldemeyer KS, Lowe MJ, et al. (2000). Brain: gadolinium-enhanced fast fluid-attenuated inversion-recovery MR imaging. Radiology, Vol.211, No.1, pp.257-263.

McKnight TR. Proton magnetic resonance spectroscopic evaluation of brain tumor metabolism. Semin Oncol, Vol.31, No.5, (2004), pp.605-617.

Mishra AM, Gupta RK, Jaggi RS, et al. (2004). Role of diffusion-weighted imaging and in vivo proton magnetic resonance spectroscopy in the differential diagnosis of ring-enhancing intracranial cystic mass lesions. J Comput Assist Tomogr, Vol.28, No.4, pp.540-547.

Morat BA, Chenevert TL, Lawrence TS, et al. (2005). Functional diffusion map: A noninvasion MRI biomarker for early stratification of clinical brain tumor response. PNAS, Vol.102, No.15, pp.5524-5529.

Murphy PS, Viviers L, Abson C, et a1. Monitoring temozolomide treatment of low -grade glioma with proton magnetic resonance spectroscopy. Br J Cancer, Vol.90, No.6, (2004), pp.781.

Natbavi D.G., Cenic A., Henderson S., et a1. (2001). Perfusion mapping using computed tomography allows accurate prediction of cerebral infarction in experimential brain ischemia. Stroke, Vol.32, No.1, pp. 175-183.

Negendan k W, Sauter R. Proton magnetic resonance spectroscopy in patients with glial tumors：a multicenter study. J Neurosurg, Vol.84, No.3, (1996), pp.449-458.

Noguchi T., Yoshiura T., Hiwatashi A., et al. (2008). Perfusion imaging of brain tumors using arterial spin-labeling: correlation with histopathologic vascular density. Am J Neuroradiol, Vol.29, No.4, pp. 688-93.

Park M.J., Kim H.S., Jahng G.H., et al. (2009). Semiquantitative assessment of intratumoral susceptibility signals using non-contrast-enhanced high-field high-resolution susceptibility-weighted imaging in patients with gliomas: comparison with MR perfusion imaging. Am J Neuroradiol, Vol.30, No.7, pp. 1402-8.

Poupon C, Clark CA, Frouin V, et al. (2000).Regularization of diffusion-based direction maps for the tracking of brain white matter fascicles. Neuroimage, Vol.12, No.8, pp.184-195.

Provenzale JM, McGraw P, Mhatre P, et al. (2004). Peritumoral brain regions in gliomas and meningiomas: investigation with isotropic diffusion weighted MR imaging and diffusion-tensor MR imaging. Neuroradiology, Vol.232, No.6, pp.451-460 ·

Rasmussen IA, Lindseth F, Rygh OM, et al. (2007). Functional neuronavigation combined with intra-operative 3D ultrasound: initial experiences during surgical resections close to eloquent brain areas and future directions in automatic brain shift compensation of preoperative data. Acta Neurochir, Vol.149, No.4, pp.365-378.

Reddy JS, Mishra AM, Behari S, et al. (2006).The role of diffusion-weighted imaging in the differential diagnosis of intracranial cystic mass lesions: a report of 147 lesions. Surg Neurol, Vol.66, No.9, pp.246-250.

Richter HP & Schachenmayr W(1983). Preoperative embolization of intracranial meningiomas. Neurosurgery, Vol.13, No.3, pp.261-8.

Sasao A. Hirai T. Nishimura S. et al. (2010). Assessment of Vascular Supply of Hypervascular Extra-Axial Brain Tumors with 3T MR Regional Perfusion Imaging. Am J Neuroradiol, Vol.31, No.3, pp.554–58.

Schramm P., Xyda A., Klotz E., et al. (2010). Dynamic CT perfusion imaging of intra-axial brain tumours: differentiation of high-grade gliomas from primary CNS lymphomas. Eur Radiol, Vol.20, No.10, pp.2482-90.

Singh SK, Agris JM, Leeds NE, et a1. (2000). Intracranial leptomeningeal metastases: comparison of depiction at FLAIR and contrast-enhanced MR imaging. Radiology, Vol.217, No.1, pp.50-53

Talos IF, Mian AZ, Zou KH, et al. (2006). Magnetic resonance and the human brain: anatomy, function and metabolism. Cell Mol Life Sci, Vol. 63, No.10, pp.1106-1124.

Toh CH, Castillo M, Wong AM, et al. (2008). Primary cerebral lymphoma and glioblastoma muhiforme: differences in diffusion characteristics evaluated with diffusion tensor imaging. Am J Neuroradiol, Vol.29, No.4, pp.471-475.

Toh CH, Wong AM, Wei KC, et al. (2007). Peritumoral edema of meningiomas and metastatic brain tumors: differences in diffusion characteristics evaluated with diffusion-tensor MR imaging. Neuroradiology, Vol.49, No.6, pp.489-494.

Tomczak RJ, Wunderlich AP, Wang Y, et al. (2000). fMRI for preoperative neurosurgical mapping of motor cortex and language in a clinical setting. J Compur Assist Tomogr, Vol.24, No.6, pp.927-934.

Ulmer JL, Salvan CV, Mueller WM, et al. (2004). The role of diffusion tensor imaging in establishing the proximity of tumor borders to functional brain systems: implications for preoperative risk assessments and postoperative outcomes. Technol Cancer Res Treat, Vol.3, No.6, pp.567-576.

Wang W, Steward CE, Desmond PM. (2009). Difusion tensor imaging in glioblastoma multiforme and brain metastases: the role of p, q, L, and fractional anisotropy · Am J Neuroradiol, Vol.30, No.1, pp.203-208.

Wei CW, Guo G, Mikulis DJ. (2007). Tumor effects on cerebral white matter as characterized by diffusion tensor tractography. Can J Neurol Sci, Vol.34, No.1, pp.62-68.

Wetzel SG, Cha S, Law M, et al. (2002). Preoperative assessment of intracranial tumors with perfusion MR and a volumetric interpolated examination: a comparative study with DSA. Am J Neuroradiol, Vol.23, No.11, pp.1767-1774.

Wildfőrster U, Falk A, Harders A. (1998). Operative approach due to results of functional magnetic resonance imaging in central brain tumors. Comput Aided Surg, Vol.3, No.4, pp.162-165.

Wintermark M., Philippe J. & Nabavi T.(2001). Simultaneous Measurement of Regional Cerebral Blod Flow by Perfusion and Stable Xenon CT: A Validation Study. Am J Neuroradiol, Vol.22, No.5, pp.905-914.

Wong ET, Jackson EF, Hess KR, et al. (1998). Correlation between dynamic MRI and outcome in patients with malignant gliomas. Neurology, Vol.50, No.3, pp.777-781.

Wu JS, Zhou LF, Tang WJ, et al. (2007). Clinical evaluation and follow-up outcome of diffusion tensor imaging-based functional neuronavigation: a prospective, controlled study in patients with gliomas involving pyramidal tracts. Neurosurgery, Vol.61, No.5, pp.935-948.

Young G.S. & Setayesh K. (2009). Spin-Echo Echo-Planar Perfusion MR Imaging in the Differential Diagnosis of Solitary Enhancing Brain Lesions: Distinguishing Solitary Metastases from Primary Glioma. Am J Neuroradiol, Vol.30, No.3, pp.575–7.

Zimmerman RA, Gibby WA, Carmody RF. (1999). Neuroimaging: clinical and physical principles. Springer, ISBN 0387949631, New York ·

4

Brain Tumors: How Can Images and Segmentation Techniques Help?

Alejandro Veloz, Antonio Orellana, Juan Vielma,
Rodrigo Salas and Stéren Chabert
Universidad de Valparaíso, Biomedical Engineering Department
Serivicios de Imagenología y Neurocirugía, Hospital Carlos Van Buren, Valparaíso
Chile

1. Introduction

These days, cancer is one of the diseases that scares people the most. Brain cancer may be considered among the most difficult cancers to treat, as it involves the organ which is not only in control of the body, but is also responsible for the self-definition of the person. During surgery or any kind of treatment, eloquent areas must not be affected in order to minimize iatrogenic risks. Therefore good diagnosis and planning of treatment choices is essential. This is why images are now of paramount importance in the evaluation of brain tumors: oncologists, neurosurgeons and the entire medical team need to know how to understand them and how to use the current tools provided by computational techniques to take advantage of the information retrieved from them. A wide variety of images is available to support the physician's actions at different levels, including diagnosis, treatment election, interventional support, and follow-up. Investigation in this area is very active; attempts are being made to go beyond the current pixel resolution, and to gain information with "molecular images"; not only in nuclear medicine but also in magnetic resonance images.

Everybody agrees that images are now an invaluable service in the practice of medicine. However, the present and future use of images is intrinsically associated with larger numbers of images, which are not easily manageable by either radiologists or surgeons. Neuroradiology is conceived as a discipline in which the health status of a patient is inferred according to the visual inspection of images taken from different modalities. This implies that the success of the clinical diagnosis depends on the physician's particular skills, and also on the information that the clinical team can handle. In addition, numerous image modalities are used frequently at different time points; therefore there is also a need for integration of the features reflected by these different sources of images. In order to provide support for this integration, automatic processing methods have been developed. Many Computer Aided Diagnostic (CAD) software packages have been developed, in particular to provide second readings in mammography, lung or brain cancer (Doi, 2007). These developments have motivated several clinical applications.

Regarding brain tumor image processing, what is usually expected is to detect the localization and extension of the tumor, in other words to segment the tumor in the image.

However, the inherent aggressive behavior of brain tumors causes uncertainty in the definition of neoplastic borders, limiting an accurate diagnosis at the macroscopic level and a proper definition of treatment. Further analysis of image segmentation results may also provide an objective quantification of the relevant properties of tumors, such as information related to size or shape, metabolic-related information, and analysis of the molecular changes associating a pathologic behavior to a therapy outcome. Consider for example the work of (Drabycz et al., 2010), in which the response of Glioblastoma Multiforme to chemotherapy was analyzed by segmenting the tumor. Another group emphasized that determination of the growth rates of low-grade gliomas based on image analysis was helpful to assess the risk of transformation of this tumor state to a malignant one (Rees et al., 2009). Heterogeneity-related features of brain tumors have shown a strong relationship with the differentiation of a low-grade glioma from a malignant tumor (Kaye et al., 2001). On the other hand, the edema of white matter has been related to the aggressiveness of the tumor (Gaensler, 1998); separation from edema sometimes can be accomplished by the practiced eye of the specialist, but is difficult to define automatically. The situations mentioned above, namely high heterogeneity and edema, can be handled by computational-based methods, providing support to improve patient management.

Segmentation of brain tumors is a difficult task, due to the complex anatomy and several problems that are inherent to the nature of the image. The heterogeneous and diffuse manifestation of this pathology in medical images complicates the implementation of computational techniques able to deal with this great variability of patterns. Also, all image modalities present limitations and artifacts that must be addressed by segmentation methods. For instance, Magnetic Resonance (MR) images are often corrupted with a smooth-varying intensity inhomogeneity, known as the bias field. This is a non-uniform intensity pattern, for a given tissue, over an image which is invisible to the human eye but highly perceptible by an automatic process on a computer, which makes segmentation more complicated. Because of the complex shape of the brain and the finite resolution of medical images, some voxels may lie on the border between two or more tissue types, in other words the same voxel intensity reflects the contributions from different tissue types at the same time. This phenomenon is usually known as partial volume effect (Bankman, 2009).

The purpose of this chapter is to give the reader a survey of the key aspects to understand and manipulate efficiently brain tumor images (section 2) and their segmentation techniques (section 3). Emphasis will be placed on the fundamental concepts to understand what it is possible to do nowadays, and what are the challenges in this area.

2. Neuroimaging of brain tumors: interpretation and limits

Neuroimaging is an essential part of planning and performing surgical interventions and treatment of brain tumors. In this section some definitions and explanations will be given in order to show the relevant aspects of the three main image modalities currently used for characterizing brain tumors; Nuclear Medicine (NM) imaging techniques such as Single Photon Emission Computed Tomography (SPECT) and Positron Emission Tomography (PET), Computed Tomography (CT) and Magnetic Resonance Imaging (MRI). MRI and CT are comparable methods in the sense that they provide high spatial resolution anatomical images, while NM techniques offer functional but not anatomical information. The purpose of this section is to give the reader the keys to understanding the basics of image and contrast formation in the context of brain tumors; a detailed explanation of the imaging techniques may be found in (Oppelt, 2006) and (Drevelegas, 2011) presents visualization of brain tumors in a more exhaustive manner.

2.1 Nuclear medicine

Nuclear Medicine images are based on the intake by patient of a radiolabeled substance, a radiopharmaceutical, which continuously emits electromagnetic radiation. The radiation emitted can have different energies, according to the radioelement used, all in the γ-ray range. γ-ray detection is performed by a γ-camera, rotating around the patient in case of SPECT, fixed in case of PET, and specifically by scintillation crystals that will scintillate, in other words that will create a certain amount of visible light depending on the amount of energy captured from γ-rays. This light is then detected and amplified by optoelectronics, and fitted by a computer program to create an image from the detected signals. Images obtained usually present spatial resolutions of the order of 5 - 10 mm in case of SPECT, and of 3 - 7 mm in case of PET.

The basic principle behind PET and SPECT is identical, yet there are some important differences worth mentioning. First and foremost, the radioelements used are different; in case of SPECT γ-emitting elements are used, such as ^{99m}Tc, ^{131}I or ^{201}Tl for instance, while PET is based on positron-emitting elements, such as ^{18}F, ^{11}C, ^{13}N, ^{15}O, elements that are usually closer to natural organic substances. The emitted positron is shortly annihilated by its anti-particle, an electron, and two γ-rays of 511 keV are emitted, parallel and in opposite directions. These are the γ-rays that are detected to form the final PET image. This point is important because it implies two main differences on a technical level: first, PET looks for the detection of two γ-rays coming from a same event, which is called coincidence detection, and the event detected is not the emission of the positron but its annihilation, which may be a millimeter away from its initial emission. An entire ring of scintillation crystals is needed around the patient to be able to undertake coincidence detection. This is the reason why images from PET show higher spatial resolution and Signal-to-Noise Ratio (SNR) than SPECT images. Second, the energy of γ-rays in PET studies is fixed and greater than the energy of the γ-rays in SPECT studies, frequently around 140 keV. The crystals used for detection must be adequate for each type of electromagnetic radiation emitted. Last but not least, full-ring detectors and the frequent necessity of producing radiopharmaceuticals on site, using a cyclotron, make PET imaging much more expensive than SPECT imaging.

What is shown in nuclear medicine images is the distribution of the radiopharmaceutical inside the body, which may include abnormal accumulation in pathological tissues due to increased metabolism for instance, or on the contrary, abnormal lack of substance in a pathological tissue, due to necrosis for example. Visualization of the pharmaceutical is what makes these images interesting, being a reflection of a specific and functional interaction with a drug at the cellular level. Even though NM spatial resolution may be poor, the contrast is obtained from a phenomenon occurring at a much smaller scale. As pathological changes usually occur at this level before inducing any anatomical modification, nuclear medicine images offer a way of access to this type of modification.

Various pharmaceuticals in SPECT provide images with marked contrast between parenchyma and tumor and can be used as markers for tumor cell proliferation, such as ^{201}Tl, a potassium analogue, or ^{99m}Tc-Sestamibi (MIBI), which concentrates in mitochondria

(Drevelegas, 2011). These tumor imaging pharmaceuticals accumulate in tumors through leaks in the Blood-Brain Barriers (BBB), and are particularly useful to differentiate low grade from high grade gliomas (Drevelegas, 2011). Radiolabeled amino acids may also be used as tumor markers, since many tumors present enhanced protein synthesis. The large number of radiopharmaceuticals available permits obtaining high specificity information, using for instance radiolabeled receptor ligand analogs. Perfusion studies can be done in SPECT using ^{99m}Tc, or agents giving information proportional to regional cerebral blood flow such as the amphetamine analogue ^{123}IMP, or diamine H ^{123}IPDM. These images offer a way of quantifying tumor aggressiveness.

Most pharmaceuticals used in PET usually cross the BBB and accumulate in the entire brain. Their distribution depends on the functionality of the pharmaceutical in use, and provides metabolic images. Of particular interest is ^{18}F-Fluoro-deoxy-glucose (FDG); it accumulates in cells and reflects their glucose uptake. It has been shown that FDG uptake is an indicator to differentiate tumor grades (Drevelegas, 2011). Uptake of FDG has also been shown to be a determinant parameter for predicting survival and time to tumor progression (Douglas et al., 2006). This is an advantage of NM images; they provide valuable information at the moment of establishing prognosis. Many radiopharmaceuticals are used in PET; it is worth mentioning ^{18}F or ^{11}C labeled amino acids which are used in the same way as FDG, such as ^{18}F dihydroxyphenylalanine (FDOPA), or ^{11}C-methionine (^{11}C MET), that reflects cell membrane transport of amino acids.

Nuclear medicine offers versatility of use in imaging applications, according to the chosen radiomarker. Functional brain mapping may be done in NM through FDG or ^{15}O labeled water, and therefore supports neurosurgery preparation. NM has proven useful to differentiate low grade from high grade tumors, especially in lesions not revealed by other imaging means. This is particularly the case for patients who already have been treated once and for whom it is not always easy to separate necrosis induced by radiotherapy or stereotactic surgery from tumor recurrence. NM also offers support when CT and MR cannot differentiate tumor from infection or from abscess (Drevelegas, 2011). The advantage and limitation of NM is that it provides functional information; additional anatomical images are needed. Combined PET-CT and whole body MR-PET equipment (Judenhofer et al., 2008) are currently available.

2.2 Computed tomography

Interest in Computed Tomography comes from the fact that, contrary to nuclear medicine methods, it is widely available and offers high spatial resolution images with fast acquisition modes: a slice can be acquired in less than a second, with common spatial resolution of about 1 mm. Most CT equipment is composed of an X-ray tube and a certain number of detecting elements rotating together around the patient, at the same time as the patient table advances though the detection ring, which provides a "spiral" or "helicoidal" acquisition.

Contrast in CT images arises from interactions of X-rays with tissues. There are different types of interaction, the principal one being the photoelectric effect. Photoelectric effects result in total absorption of the incident X-rays, and therefore induce the maximum possible contrast: no X-ray reaches the detector (no signal, the photosensitive film stays white), but when the incident X-ray reaches the detector with little if any modification or full signal, the film blackens. The probability of the photoelectric effect depends essentially on the atomic number (Z) of the elements of the tissue to be exposed. This is what explains the high contrast in X-ray or CT images of soft tissues, composed mainly of carbohydrate elements with low Z, and mineralized hard tissue such as bone, with important concentration of high Z calcium (^{20}Ca). As the atomic number of iodine is quite high (^{53}I) most CT contrast media contain this element and provide marked contrast in the organ or system to be visualized, such as the vascular system in case of intravenous medium injection. On the other hand, the occurrence probability of the photoelectric effect depends inversely on the third power of the incident X-ray energy; this energy is equivalent to the X-ray tube kilo-voltage selected by the user. This implies that the greater the X-ray energy, the lower the image contrast. However, the lower the X-ray energy, the lower is the penetration capacity of thick body elements by X-rays. The tube voltage is a crucial parameter for the user to choose according to what is desired from the image, along with the number of X-ray photons to be produced, which is directly related to the tube filament current intensity. An interesting point of CT is the quantification available through Hounsfield Units (HU): pixel values reflect the X-ray linear attenuation coefficient, normalized to the water coefficient.

In terms of contrast production there is no flexibility in CT as there is in NM or MRI. Current developments are focused upon improving signal detection; looking for better and faster signal collection (changes in hardware), and better reconstruction techniques (image improvements and radiation dose decreases). Recent improvements have decreased considerably the time needed for each acquisition (cardiac, abdominal and some kinetic studies).

Application of CT images in brain tumor detection is based essentially on two types of images; low-contrast images and iodine-based Contrast-Enhanced (CE) studies, as shown in Figure 1. Low-contrast images present soft tissue contrast and visualization of parenchyma, edema, hemorrhage, timorous tissues and Cerebro-Spinal Fluid (CSF), among others. In the case of calcified tumors, CT images show good contrast, while conventional MR images do not always present variation of signal. CE images provide high contrast between tumor and parenchyma due to BBB disruption; the contrast medium accumulates in the tumor extracellular space and causes a greater X-ray attenuation. Perfusion studies allow assessment of cerebral blood volume and cerebral blood flow, offering a way of characterizing how aggressive the tumor is. However, there has been recently some debate about the adequate use of this type of acquisition and consequent radiation overdoses to patients in several sites (Food and Drug Administration [FDA], 2010a).

The advantages of CT are numerous; availability and good quality images made this method a "must have" in most radiology units. However, the concern over patients and workers exposed to ionizing radiation is increasing. Recent technical advances, such as spiral, or multi-slice CT, are accompanied by higher doses to patients. The concern is even greater for child and infant imaging, due to their young age at exposure and probability of developing some cancer due to this exposure, while all radiology units do not have adequate protocols (The Alliance for Radiation Safety in Pediatric Imaging). The compromise between risk and benefit must always be carefully balanced.

2.3 Magnetic resonance imaging

Magnetic resonance images (MRI) combine a common advantage with CT - high spatial resolution images - but with no ionizing radiation exposure, which makes it a safer technique. MRI holds a very specific place among imaging modalities as it is highly flexible from various points of view; it provides a wide variety of contrast types with the same equipment, accessible through a unique imaging session, and it offers flexibility of slice positioning at any angle in the three dimensional space, added to a naturally good soft

tissue contrast. These advantages make MRI one of the main imaging tools for neurological studies, even though total examination time is usually longer than with other types.
Image formation is based on manipulation of the magnetic properties of the nucleus of water hydrogen, and consequent manipulation of "tissue magnetization", made possible in the context of a very high magnetic field. The interesting thing is that, as each tissue has a unique chemical composition and microstructure, each tissue will have different global magnetic properties that can be taken advantage of. This is usually referred to as each tissue having different *longitudinal* and *transversal relaxation times*, T_1 and T_2 respectively. The longitudinal relaxation time, T_1, expresses how much time the magnetization needs to recover its initial state; a shorter T_1 means faster magnetization recovery and higher signal. The transversal relaxation time T_2 reflects the rate of signal decay; a shorter T_2 implies faster signal decay and lower signal. T_1 and T_2 arise from disconnected causes and present different and separate tissue characteristics.
There are various ways of manipulating tissue magnetization, creating and acquiring a MR signal. This is what allows obtaining T_1- or T_2-weighted images, which are the basic contrast types accessible in MRI. As the signal originates in the water hydrogen nucleus, net signal quantity depends on tissue water concentration, and gives rise to the last of the three main types of contrasts available; proton density (PD) weighted images. The selection of which contrast type to obtain is made through the adequate selection of an imaging *sequence* and of its parameters; the MR signal is created and manipulated through chronological application of a few elements, namely radiofrequency pulse (RF pulse), and magnetic field gradient, along the three spatial axes. The different and convenient temporal application of these elements is called the MR sequence. A typical MR imaging protocol consists of acquiring images with different types of sequences, chosen according to what is looked for.

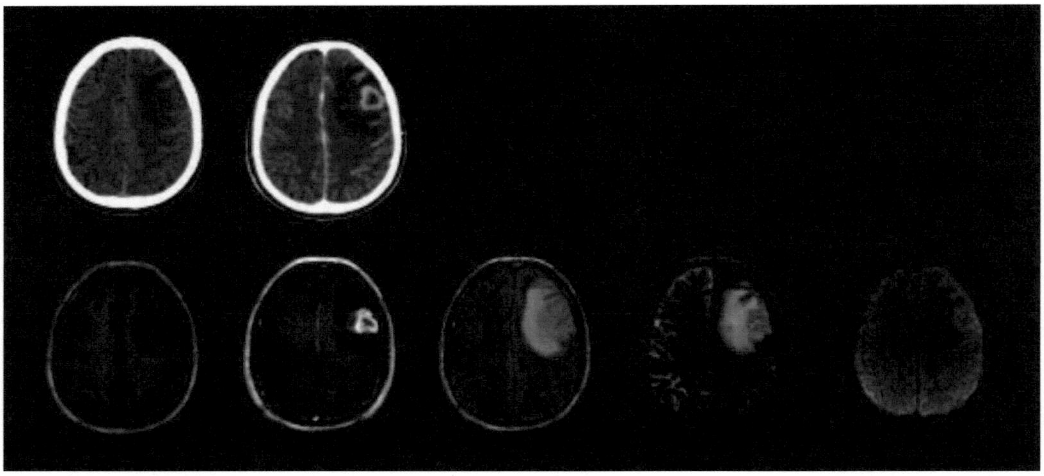

Fig. 1. Glioblastoma Multiforme. Top row: CT images, without CE (left), and with CE (right). Bottom row: MR images. From left to right: T_1-weighted, Contrast-Enhanced T_1-weighted, FLAIR, T_2-weighted, diffusion-weighted.

Most brain tumors have longer relaxation times than healthy tissues, which implies that on T_2-weighted images tumors appear hyperintense while on T_1-weighted images they appear hypointense. On PD-weighted images tumors show intermediate signals. The tumor itself frequently presents different levels of cellular density and different types of abnormalities appear around the tumors, such as hemorrhage, necrosis, calcification, additional fat content, etc.; many brain tumors have a heterogeneous appearance in MR images, such as the Glioblastoma Multiforme shown in Figure 1. From an automatic segmentation point of view this is one of the challenges to address, to be able to delimitate the tumor the same way an expert would.

Inversion Recovery (IR) sequences are commonly used in neurological applications. IR consists of sequences that permit suppression of the signal from certain specific tissues based on the knowledge of their longitudinal relaxation time, and thus provide very good gray matter - white matter contrast. The best known IR sequence is FLuid Attenuated Inversion Recovery (FLAIR), which suppresses the CSF signal and offers images with good definition between edema and tumor. FLAIR sequences are frequently combined with contrast agent injection, presenting images with high contrast between tumors and background tissues.

Contrast enhanced images in MRI are obtained using media containing gadolinium (Gd) chelate: the latter shortens T_1 and causes hypersignal in the organ or system where it lies. Gd chelates accumulate in the tumor extracellular space, in the same way as iodine contrast agents do in CT studies, since the BBB breaks down, thus offering images with better tumor visualization and with higher specificity. Common MR protocols include contrast media injection and image acquisition post injection. Figure 1 presents a typical ring-like enhancement around the tumor area. High doses of gadolinium can improve the quality of enhancement in case of gliomas or metastasis. It has been shown that cell tumors are found beyond the area defined by the contrast enhancement (Drevelegas, 2011). Recently, health problems have been related to the use of gadolinium-based contrast media, particularly in patients reporting kidney dysfunction (FDA, 2010b). Other techniques besides gadolinium-based contrast are needed, especially to assess tumor aggressiveness, as Gd enhancement relies strongly on BBB breakdown. It has been shown that there is a significant fraction of non-enhancing gliomas that are malignant, and that there are enhancing gliomas which are benign (Arvinda et al., 2009). Various techniques are available for MR angiography and perfusion measurements, such as "black blood" acquisition, "Time of Flight" (TOF), or based on contrast agent injection and consequent repetitive acquisitions, among others. Signal variations can be quantified in time and volume. Information on tumor microvasculature may be obtained and allows the determination of its degree of aggressiveness and potential proliferation (Aromen et al., 1994).

Magnetic resonance is characterized by being a very active area of investigation, and many different applications are now available besides the common T_1-, T_2-, and PD-weighted images. The elastic modulus of tissues can be assessed *in vivo* through MR elastography, also feasible in brain imaging (Sack et al., 2008); pH measurements can be made (Gillies et al., 2004). Development of new contrast media and techniques are being undertaken; magnetic nanoparticles are being used, such as super paramagnetic iron oxide SPIO, which tries to detect angiogenesis and amid proton transfer, aiming at imaging at the protein and peptide leven. It is worth mentioning functional MRI (fMRI), used since the mid-1990s to localize cortical areas activated during the realization of a specific task. In the context of brain tumor management, fMRI has been useful to detect patient eloquent areas, offering helpful information to support neurosurgery preparation (Stippich, 2007).

Proton magnetic resonance spectroscopy (MRS) (Horská & Barker, 2010) was first reported more than 20 years ago and is now used for evaluation of brain tumors. There are two techniques; single voxel, either PRESS or STEAM sequences, and multivoxel, MRSI, each with its own advantages and disadvantages. Almost all brain tumors have decreased N-acetyl aspartate (NAA) and increased choline (Cho), producing increased Cho/NAA ratios (Bruhn et al., 1989). Lactate, lipid and other metabolic changes have also been studied (Castillo et al., 2000). Cho has been found to correlate with the degree of tumor infiltration (Croteau et al., 2001), and therefore is able to define tumor boundaries. Nevertheless, MRS has not been widely accepted as a routine clinical tool. Carefully designed Multicenter trials are lacking. For this reason this technique is only being used in major academic medical centers.

Last but not least, about 15 years ago a new MR imaging technique attracted attention as a way of practicing "non-invasive biopsy through images", Diffusion Weighted Images (DWI). DWI consists of weighting signal magnitude according to how many water molecule translations, from natural diffusion phenomena, occur within the voxel during a defined diffusion time (Le Bihan, 1995). The more motion in the voxel, the less signal is measured. Motion is quantified using the Apparent Diffusion Coefficient (ADC). DWI refers to the images directly acquired from the magnet, however, it is not possible to distinguish ADC variations from T_2 variations with DWI. It is thus common to compute ADC maps in order to get rid of this so-called "T_2-shine through" effect (Le Bihan, 1995). DWI focuses on measuring motion; this measurement can be made in three dimensions and give information about the diffusion anisotropy, called Fractional Anisotropy (FA), and the Mean Diffusivity (MD). These 3D measures are obtained acquiring Diffusion Tensor Images (DTI), over a longer acquisition time than regular DWI acquisitions.

Although all mechanisms are not fully understood, it has been shown that in biological tissues the diffusion coefficient value may be affected by cell density, intra- and extra-cellular volumes and viscosity, and by the presence of numerous semi-permeable membranes restricting motion (Chabert & Scifo, 2007). It has been reported that ADC reflects tissue microstructure, organization and integrity. Diffusion coefficient variations have been shown to vary in correlation with tumor cellularity and tumor grade (Murakami et al., 2009), in particular in combination with perfusion images (Arvinda et al., 2009); tumor tissue tends to present higher cell density, that may be related to lower ADC and appear hyperintense in DWI, while necrotic tissues have higher ADC ("freer water") and appear hypointense in DWI. FA has been shown to be greater in high-grade tumors (Drevelegas et al., 2011). Diffusion coefficients in tumors are heterogeneous, for intrinsic reasons of microstructure heterogeneity. Various current investigations are looking for finer indices, for instance characterizing non-Gaussian diffusion using a kurtosis index, as a potential marker of higher structural complexity in high grade tumors (Raab et al., 2010).

On the other hand, since water motion is less in the direction perpendicular to the main axis of white matter fibers than in the direction parallel to the fibers, measuring diffusion anisotropy gives a good indication of white matter integrity (Mori, 2007). This is particularly relevant not only to detect pathologies such as multiple sclerosis; it is now also possible to track white matter fibers *in vivo* based on DT images, extracting information from the main direction of the white matter fibers on a pixel basis, and then connecting them (Mori, 2007). In the presence of tumors, DTI fiber tracking can assess displacement and deformation of fiber bundles, as a consequence modifying the surgical intervention (Bello et al., 2008).

In summary, MRI is considered to be safe and non-invasive. It provides information with high contrast and high spatial resolution, and can provide different visualizations at the same time. Investigation is very active in this field; new sequences and applications are available every day. Magnetic resonance is now considered a main tool for neurological studies. Even though it is not accessible to patients with ferro-magnetic implants or pacemakers, recent technical developments are aiming at improving compatibility.

3. Review of computational techniques for image segmentation

Several computational approaches have been proposed for brain tumor segmentation. Since Magnetic Resonance Imaging gives functional and anatomic information with high resolution and several types of contrast at the same time, most methods for segmenting brain tumors have been proposed based on this kind of image. These situations enable both simultaneous analysis of different contrasts produced and monitoring of the disease over time. However, in order to extract information from the damaged tissue on the basis of these large numbers of images, advanced computational techniques must be applied. Depending on how the information from the image is used, there are two prominent approaches for image segmentation: intensity-based and region-based methods (Bankman, 2009).

Intensity-based techniques have been extensively applied in medical image segmentation. The most important constraints for segmenting brain tumors such as partial volume effect, fuzzy definition of pathological boundaries, brain tumor heterogeneity, MRI artifacts, etc., have been addressed using this formulation. These techniques are constructed based on the information contained in the voxel intensity to estimate the region to which this voxel belongs. In other words, the image is partitioned into a specific number of regions, each region representing one tissue type, and a label is attached to each voxel to characterize its membership within one of the image regions. The most important intensity-based methods used for medical image segmentation will be presented below in section 3.1.

Similarly, the region-based approach constitutes an important family of methods that operate in a spatial context and exploit information based on global shape, intensity, texture or edge-related features of the object to be segmented. Pathology-related difficulties and MRI artifacts affect the performance of this family of techniques, although this influence is diminished because the approach integrates more information (shape, edges of objects, intensity, etc.) to segment a region. The most relevant techniques in this category will be treated below in section 3.2.

3.1 Intensity-based techniques

The aim of intensity-based techniques is to classify the set of voxels $\{x_1, x_2,\ldots, x_n\}$ of an image to each tissue type present in the image. Each voxel is represented by a p-dimensional feature vector, i.e., $x_i \in R^p$, $i = 1,\ldots, n$, whose elements are related to anatomical or functional features of tissues at this image location. For instance, each voxel could be composed of p intensity values from T_1-weighted, T_2-weighted, proton density MR images, CT, PET, local texture measures on a neighborhood (such as average or standard deviation), metabolic behavior from MRS, or any other information provided by a neuroimage method. If voxels are represented by scalar values, a monospectral formulation of the segmentation problem is given, however if vector-valued voxels are considered, the formulation of the segmentation problem is known as multispectral.

The assignment of each voxel to the corresponding tissue type is accomplished by building a mathematical model that assigns a label from the set $\{y_1, y_2, \ldots, y_c\}$ used to represent each of the c tissue types present on the image. As the tissue types from a pathological or normal brain image are known *a priori*, the set of possible labels are restricted to those regions that compose the image (one particular label represents one specific region of the image). To segment brain tumors on MRI using intensity-based methods, studies commonly consider five classes; white matter, gray matter, CSF, edema and tumor.

A fundamental issue that should be addressed with intensity-based approaches is related to overlapping intensities of different tissue types that have similar behavior in terms of intensity values. For example, some domains of a brain tumor on MRI may have a similar behavior with respect to surrounding healthy tissues of the brain, in this case the discrimination between two voxels, one corresponding to healthy tissue and other that belongs to the tumor region, is a difficult task when voxels are considered as isolated entities without a global context such as the shapes of the objects that are being segmented. Another important problem is related to the bias field that may cause misclassification of tissues when segmentation techniques are applied, especially when only intensity-based methods are used.

Two fundamental approaches have been proposed to develop a model that assigns a label to a voxel. The first consists of estimating the relation from a large number of voxels whose labels are known *a priori*. The model is estimated, or trained, from this set of labeled voxels; this is commonly known as a training set and usually corresponds to labels provided by experts. This strategy is called supervised methods for voxel classification; models constructed under this paradigm are estimated in order to emulate the labeling process made by experts. Due to the inherent variability of the intensity patterns of brain pathological structures, the construction of the training data set can be a difficult task. Also, for a proper establishment of voxel labels, a variety of pathological behaviors need to be captured by the training data set for a proper estimation of the segmentation model. This is another aspect that makes its construction difficult.

If a training data set is not available, there are several additional methods that assign voxels labels according to a similarity measure. This has lead to the development of many unsupervised methods for voxel classification. The lack of information is compensated by including other sources of information, such as *a priori* information provided by a user or by a digital atlas of the brain. In the following subsections, the more well known supervised and unsupervised methods for brain tumor segmentations are described.

3.1.1 Histogram-based thresholding

Image histograms are the basis for numerous image processing techniques. The histogram of a digital image is a discrete function that quantifies the number of voxels that lie in a certain range of the gray scale. Defining a threshold based on the histogram is the simplest approach for image segmentation, due to its simplicity and low computational demand. The basic idea behind this approach is that voxels of the image can be separated into two regions whose intensities are as similar as possible for the same region and as different as possible for different regions. There are two main approaches for image thresholding. The first corresponds to the application of a single threshold calculated for the entire image; this threshold is called global thresholding. The other approach is based on defining a threshold taking into account only a restricted neighborhood of voxels; this method is called local thresholding and the computation of this threshold commonly depends on local features across the image, such as statistical properties of a neighborhood (how smooth, how heterogeneous, etc.). Several methods for automatic selection of a proper threshold have been proposed. These techniques work by seeking a numerical value that separates the

intensities of an image to obtain nearly uniform regions as a result. A popular approach was proposed by (Otsu, 1979) that derives a discriminant function that maximizes between-class variance.
Due to the simplicity of Otsu's method, it cannot deal with the complex behavior of brain tumors and their MR images properties. Although bias field estimation and correction may be applied as a previous step to the segmentation process, thresholding techniques are not able to deal with the overlapping intensities of healthy and pathological tissues. In (Gibbs et al., 1996) a global threshold was manually selected from samples of enhanced tumor and surrounding tissues, and afterwards region-based methods combined with edge information were used to refine the final segmentation. Local thresholds may be especially useful when a single threshold is not able to segment the image in a global context. The values of local thresholds may be estimated by considering partial volume artifacts of each region to determine the threshold for segmenting each component on an MR image (see Sung et al. 2000).

3.1.2 Supervised techniques for voxel classification

As stated earlier, a model for voxel classification is estimated from training data where the latter consists of a set of voxels with multispectral features labeled by an expert. The distributions of different tissue types must be represented by capturing the particularities of each. This constitutes the most important and difficult issue to be satisfied using this paradigm. Once this training set is available, a training algorithm is applied to estimate a model which emulates the labeling process. This model is known as classifier and it is used to predict labels from unseen data, i.e., new features of voxels are presented to the model that assigns a label according to what was previously learned.
There is a large list of models that follow the principle mentioned above. One of the most important supervised techniques for voxel classification is called the Multilayer Perceptron (MLP). MLPs are computational models used to model complex relationships between inputs and outputs (Bishop, 2006). In spite of the performance degradation of the resulting segmentation obtained using this supervised technique, that is affected by overlapping intensities between tissue types, the complex non-linear relationships that this model establishes as a decision function tend to minimize its effect. Therefore, the discriminant function that allows distinguishing between two similar voxels from different tissue types may be very abrupt, whether or not the training data set reflects this situation consistently. This is an important aspect that allows dealing with the segmentation of heterogeneous brain tumors. The pioneering studies related to the application of MLP to brain tumor segmentation were those of (Clarke, 1991) and (Ozkan et al., 1993). These studies were based on a training procedure that initially uses a single slice from a specific patient. With a training data set generated from this first slice, a MLP model was constructed and was used to segment the adjacent slice of this patient image set. The labels obtained from the adjacent slice were used to generate a second training data set, which was then used to segment the adjacent slice. This process continued until the entire available image data set was segmented. A different approach was proposed by (Dickson et al., 1997) in which a set of non-patient-specific hand-labeled MR slices was used for training an MLP model for classifying acoustic neuromas. In addition to the intensities of the voxels, the intensities of neighboring voxels and their locations were used. In order to avoid some difficulties related to the complexity of the MLP model for segmenting brain tumors, (Tayel et al., 2006)

proposed some compression-based methods to deal with the size of the model itself, the size of the training data set and the training time.
A different method was proposed by (Villalta et al., 2006) in which a neural network was used to obtain the spatial distribution of brain tumors using information coming from Magnetic Resonance Spectroscopy and Relaxometry (T_2-weighted MR image), and with an appropriate spatial resolution, the segmentation accurately determined the Gross Tumor Volume. The decay patterns were classified according to different states of the tissue (normal, pathologic, necrotic or edema) in comparison to Chemical Shift Imaging (CSI) data.

3.1.3 Unsupervised techniques for voxel classification

Techniques proposed for unsupervised classification, or clustering, of voxels for image segmentation seek to group a data set according to their similarity. The data set is composed of p-dimensional feature vectors that represent voxel intensities, as for instance in T_1- or T_2-weighted MR images, or also using local texture measures. Let us consider the set of voxels $\{x_1, x_2, \ldots, x_n\}$ forming a multispectral image. The i-th voxel of the image is denoted by $x_i \in R^p$, whose elements are the corresponding features used for segmentation. The best discriminative ability will be achieved by the clustering method if the most representative information about the structure of the pathology to be segmented is included in the feature vectors.
A very popular unsupervised method for medical image segmentation is fuzzy c-means (FCM) clustering algorithm, which was first suggested by (Dunn, 1973) and later improved by (Bezdek et al., 1999). Unlike k-means clustering, in which each observation has a hard binary membership in the set of clusters, the FCM method proposes a fuzzy partition that assigns a degree of membership between 0 and 1 to each voxel in each group. Given an observed feature vector, a membership degree equal to 0 expresses non-membership while 1 means full membership of this observation to the class. An important constraint in the assignment of membership degrees for a given observation is that the sum of the membership degrees must be equal to 1. Instead, in the possibilistic fuzzy c-means (PFCM) method proposed by (Krishnapuram & Keller, 1996), this constraint is relaxed and the membership degrees between 0 and 1 are assigned for each observation according to their proximity to the cluster centers.

Fuzzy c-means and possibilistic fuzzy c-means methods

FCM has motivated a significant amount of research in the context of MRI brain tumor segmentation. An important aspect for the application of the FCM-like method is related to the specification of the number of clusters by the user. This is not a trivial task, since the tumor presents a heterogeneous intensity pattern that overlaps with healthy brain tissues. This determines that in different clusters that represent different healthy tissues, e.g., white matter, gray matter, etc., the tumor domain is expressed with a high degree of membership (see Figure 2). Several studies dealt with this problem by incorporating knowledge-based criteria to include constraints (e.g., information about shapes) in the membership degree assignments. (Clark et al., 1998) performed multispectral segmentation (using T_1, T_2-weighted and proton density images) of Glioblastoma Multiforme using the FCM algorithm, multispectral histogram analysis and knowledge-based criteria to improve the final tumor segmentation. Also, (Fletcher-heath et al., 2001) proposed a knowledge-based fuzzy clustering approach for multispectral segmentation of non-enhancing brain tumors. An initial segmentation is computed using an unsupervised fuzzy clustering algorithm and the domain knowledge, and 3D connected components (across slices of the MR volume) are evaluated to build the tumor segmentation. A solution to address the problem of determination of cluster number has been given by developing some cluster validity indices in order to determine automatically the number of clusters. Consider (Saha et al., 2007) as an example based on the Genetic Algorithm applied to MRI segmentation.

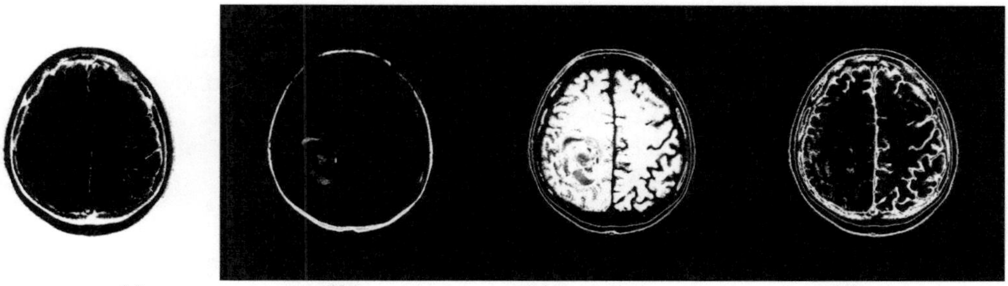

(*a*) (*b*) (*c*) (*d*)

Fig. 2. (a)(b)(c)(d) Different clusters obtained with the multispectral Fuzzy C-Means technique (T_1 + contrast enhancement, T_1 FLAIR, T_2). The tumor is presented with a high membership degree in (b), but in (c) is also presented significantly.

Another important aspect of the FCM algorithm is concerned with the spatial or contextual information considered for the generation of tissue classes. Originally, voxels were considered as isolated entities by clustering algorithms, which failed to deal with the strong correlations between neighboring voxels. To overcome this problem several methods have been proposed using local spatial information to compute membership degrees to a given cluster (see, for instance, Cai et al., 2009).

Mixture modeling

Mixture models try to take advantage of the knowledge of the image characteristics to determine the best image partition, specifically the knowledge of the probability distribution of the intensity that each tissue type should follow; the most frequently used distribution being the normal distribution. It is a way of expressing how the voxel intensities will disperse around the average value associated with their tissue type, as is illustrated in the histogram of Figure 3. Let us consider again the set of voxels $\{x_1, x_2,\ldots, x_n\}$, with $x_i \in R^p$ that compose an image as a realization of a random variable X, whose density function is determined by the weighted sum of K components (distributions). Each of these components represents the intensity behavior of a region that composes the image, e.g., white matter, gray matter, CSF, tumor or edema. The k-th component of the mixture model expresses the probability that voxel x_i belongs to the tissue type represented by this component. The entire set of parameters φ (the weighting factors and the parameters of the probability distributions) will be estimated from the available data by the maximization of the (log) likelihood function. When an estimate of the model parameters φ is available, each voxel can be assigned to the tissue type (mixture component) that best explains its intensity. In Figure 3, a mixture model for segmenting normal structures of the brain is illustrated.

In the context of medical image segmentation, (Van Leemput et al., 2001) proposed an approach for segmenting normal and pathologic tissues from MRI. An initial estimate of the unknown parameters is obtained using a digital brain atlas that contains spatially varying prior probability maps for the location of white matter, gray matter, and CSF. A mixture model is used to explain healthy tissues and the pathology is detected as voxels that are not well explained by the statistical model constructed for the normal brain. Also, bias field estimation is performed by including an extra term in all the mixture components that depends on the spatial positions of the voxels. Based on these ideas, (Moon et al., 2002) further extended the mixture modeling approach for segmenting brain tumors. These authors introduced a fully automatic method for segmenting MR images presenting tumor and edema, both mass-effect and infiltrating structures. The prior probabilities for the normal tissue classes were defined by a digital atlas and the spatial tumor prior was calculated from the T_1 pre- and post-contrast difference image. Also, (Menze et al., 2010) presented a tumor appearance model for multispectral images. The method uses information about the spatial location of the lesion for each voxel and the probability of observing tumor in each one is computed.

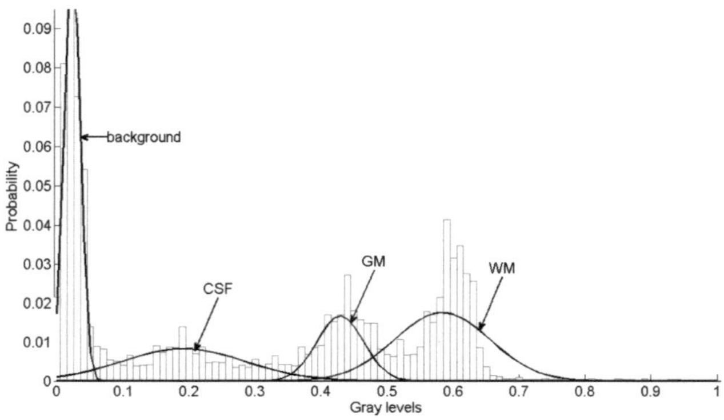

(a)

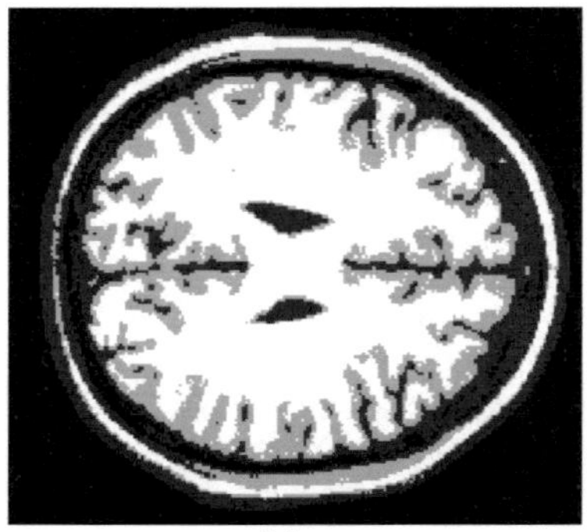

(b)

Fig. 3. (a) Histogram of a typical MR image and Mixture Model Components fitted to each tissue class. (b) Label map obtained according the Mixture Model of (a)

Markov Random Fields image segmentation

Markov Random Fields (MRFs) are stochastic processes that have been used in a wide range of medical image processing applications (Zhang et al., 2001) to represent spatial dependences between neighboring voxels to group them in a specific class, i.e., it is probable that if a voxel belongs to a certain group, its neighbors also belong to this group. This method was first presented by (Besag, 1986). In many cases, this method reduces both the possible problem of clusters overlapping, which is essential in the context of tumor segmentation, and the effect of noise on the clustering results.

The classification of a voxel as a part of a region considering the labels of neighboring voxels is the basic idea of this approach for image segmentation. MRFs typically use a generative approach, modeling the joint probability of the features (e.g., multispectral intensities, texture measures, etc.) of the set of voxels $x = \{x_1,\ldots, x_n\}$ and their corresponding set of labels y, i.e., $p(x,y) = p(x \mid y)p(y)$. Traditionally, to solve this problem it is assumed that the distributions $p(x \mid y)$ are independent of each other, in order to make the calculation of the joint probability $p(x,y)$ tractable. This is a limiting factor for representing complex spatial relationships between feature vectors and their corresponding labels. To define spatial dependences, a neighborhood system over the image and a clique configuration must be defined. A clique is a subset of voxels that are all neighbors and allows the incorporation of spatial dependences between labels. The specific shape of cliques is user-defined. The term $p(y)$ will be considered as an MRF if it follows a Gibbs distribution (see Li, 2008) that defines a spatial dependence between neighboring labels.

In general, an initial estimate of the set of labels is needed to apply MRF-based strategies, making the subsequent estimation process highly dependent on the quality of this initial estimate. For instance, (Capelle et al., 2000) presented an unsupervised MRF-based approach for brain tumor segmentation using a Gaussian mixture model to represent gray matter, white matter, CSF, tumor and edema. The MRF model was estimated using the Iterated Conditional Modes (ICM) algorithm. An important disadvantage of MRF-based segmentation is that some of the parameters involved, such as the size and shape of the clique, may be very difficult to specify. The consequence may be that the definition of labels in borders of the structures of the image may fail. This is prohibitive for brain tumor segmentation applications and several authors have proposed MRF-based strategies to deal with this disadvantage by integrating information about edges or region properties. (Gering et al., 2003) proposed a framework for brain tumor segmentation, extending EM-based segmentation with region-level properties and deriving a multi-level MRF. Another iterative MRF-based segmentation method was proposed by (Chen et al., 2003) in which a Gibbs Prior model and a deformable model are combined. The Gibbs Prior model provides binary region estimations which the deformable model uses for fitting. The deformable model can refine the segmentation result and update the parameters of the Gibbs Prior model for the next iteration. (Solomon et al., 2006) proposed an automated method using probabilistic reasoning over both space and time to segment brain tumors from 4D spatio-temporal MRI data. The 3D expectation-maximization method is extended using Hidden Markov models to infer tumor classification based on previous and subsequent segmentation results. (Capelle et al., 2004) proposed a segmentation method based on evidence theory for brain tumors on MRI. This method takes into account the spatial dependency between the voxels through an evidential spatial merging process.

3.2 Region-based techniques

The above mentioned approaches based on voxel classification often rely on the properties of single or nearby voxels and do not consider global shape and boundary information of the region that must be segmented. Applied to brain tumor segmentation, intensity-based approaches may have only limited success if overlapping intensity distributions of healthy tissue, tumor, and surrounding edema are not considered. In this context, region-based approaches constitute an important family of methods that operate in a spatial context and exploit information based on global shape, intensity, texture or edge-related features of the object to be segmented, to generate an accurate result. An important problem that needs to be addressed by this approach is related to the partial volume effect that limits the success in defining the boundary of the segmented region. The most important region-based methods used for brain tumor segmentation will be explained below.

Region Growing

The region growing algorithm is a classical region-based approach used for medical image segmentation. The basic idea is to start with a set of seed points of voxels manually selected that are located inside of the region(s) to be segmented. The selection of seed points is typically made by a trained user, however automatic approaches have been proposed. Starting from these seed points, regions grow by adding to each seed its neighboring voxels that have similar properties based on predefined similarity criteria. The establishment of the similarity criterion and the selection of seed points are crucial to obtain an accurate segmentation. Evidently, it is necessary to provide an efficient mechanism to represent the inherent complexities of the region to be segmented. The selection of seed points in the context of brain tumor segmentation will depend directly on the histopathological behavior of the pathology and on the user capacity to identify the several tumor domains that are present (necrosis, high cellular activity area and other biological features characteristic of each class of brain tumor; see Salman et al., 2005; Chong et al., 2004). The idea is to select seed points to construct homogeneous domains of the tumor and merge them afterwards. Some authors developed a way of defining seed points automatically in an efficient way. (Veloz et al., 2007) addressed this problem by the method known as Fuzzy Spatial Growing that was specifically proposed for the segmentation of Glioblastoma Multiforme (GBM) from T_1-weighted MR images with contrast enhancement agent. Different GBM domains on MRI are captured as the initial step by using the FCM algorithm and mathematical morphology-based methods, whereby intensity patterns are established that reflect specific tumor behavior. With these intensity patterns, a membership function is defined to assign for each voxel a membership degree to define the tumor class. In Figure 4, the original image and the tumor class obtained with this method is presented. In Figure 5 the resulting membership functions are shown together with the image and tumor class histogram. With the defined tumor class a growing process is performed in the tumor class, applying fuzzy operations to include neighboring voxels to the starting points; then the tumor is segmented according a stopping criterion defined by the user. Another fuzzy-based representation of brain tumor MR image was proposed by (Gordillo et al., 2010) in which, in addition to using patterns derived from the intensities of the image, expert knowledge was also incorporated. (Sato et al., 2000) proposed a modified region growing method to deal with the partial volume effect problem. This method implements a boundary-based homogeneity criterion that takes into account the gradient magnitude to establish the segmented region. (Dubey et al., 2010) extended this approach for brain tumor segmentation. In (Salman, 2009) a further analysis of this method was performed efficiently in the context of 3D brain tumor segmentation.

Many approaches often use region-growing-based algorithms as an intermediate step of a more sophisticated segmentation method. For instance, (Dou et al., 2007) proposed a framework of fuzzy information fusion to segment brain tumor areas from multispectral MRI. *A priori* knowledge of tumors, described by radiologists, is modeled by fuzzy models whose information is fused using fuzzy operators. An adjustment is performed afterwards, applying a region-growing-based approach. (Kaus et al., 2001) proposed a classification based scheme which involves iteration of a statistical classification to assign labels to tissue types, and nonlinear registration to align a digital anatomic atlas to the patient data. This registration process is applied in order to include additional information about the spatial location of anatomic structures. Finally, objects of interest are identified on the classified images with local segmentation operations, specifically, using mathematical morphology and region growing methods. (Rexilius et al., 2007) proposed an efficient multispectral segmentation of brain tumors based on a probabilistic intensity model, followed by an iterative refinement of the initial segmentation. A progressive region growing that combines probability and distance information is applied. (Gibbs et al., (1996) used region growing for brain tumor segmentation after applying a threshold to the original image to compute statistical properties of the pathologic region (average and variance) and to obtain the edge map using gradient magnitude. With these two information sources the similarity criterion to delineate the tumor was derived. In (Stadlbauer et al., 2004), a biochemical map of gliomas obtained from MR spectroscopic imaging was segmented via thresholding and was compared with region growing segmentation from T_2-weighted MR images.

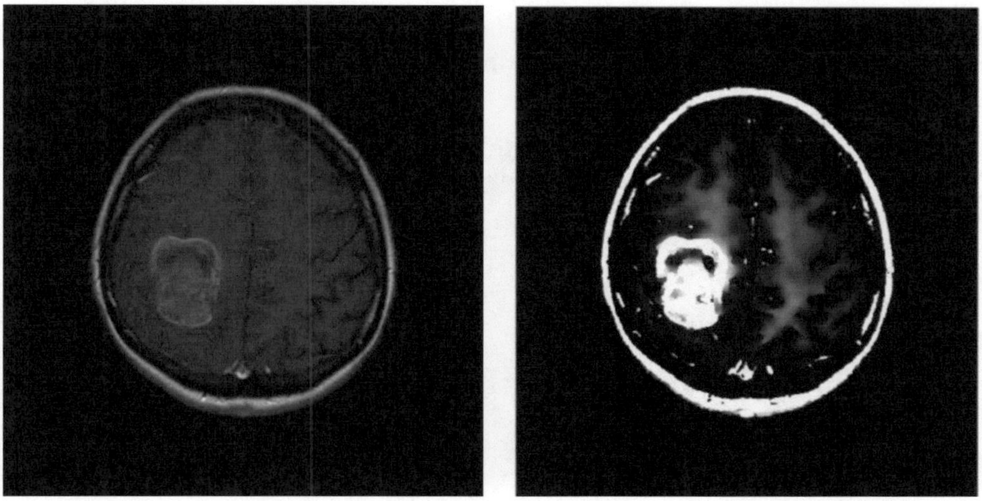

(a) (b)

Fig. 4. (a) Original GBM T_1-weighted MR image and (b) fuzzy definition of the tumor class.

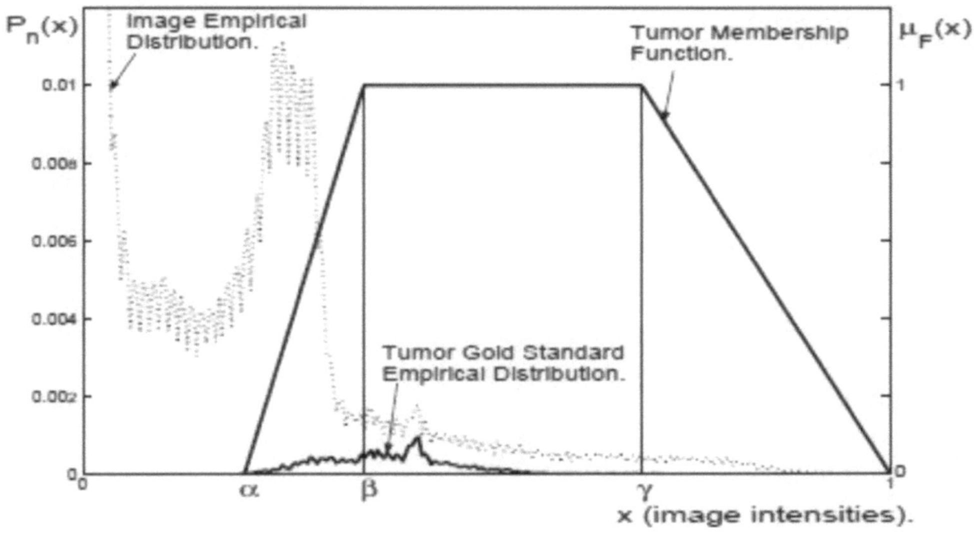

Fig. 5. Membership function constructed according to tumor intensity patterns extracted by the Fuzzy Spatial Growing method. Also shown are the normalized histogram of the entire image (estimate of the empirical distribution of intensities) and the normalized histogram of the tumor, obtained according to the manual segmentation performed by a radiologist (gold standard).

Deformable models

Deformable models establish a connected and continuous contour model for a specific anatomic structure; this contour evolves over the image (see Figure 6) according to some high-level information about the object shape and is fit to extract smooth and closed boundaries. Deformable models are also known as active contours, active surfaces, deformable templates or snakes. The existing active contour models may be broadly classified as either parametric or geometric active contour models, according to their representation and the evolution strategy.

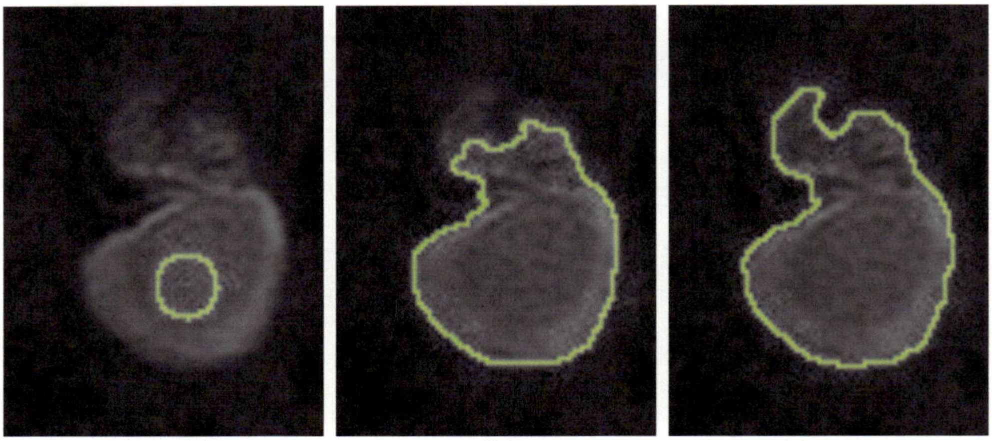

(a) (b) (c)

Fig. 6. (a) Initial contour defined inside the tumor region (b) that will evolve iteratively toward the boundary of this region. (c) Final region obtained with a classical geometric deformable model.

Parametric deformable models were first introduced by (Kass et al., 1987). The deformation of the dynamic curve is best explained from an energy minimization perspective. The contour that minimizes the total energy $E=E_{int}+E_{ext}$ provides the final solution for the segmentation problem, which is determined by starting from an initial seed contour placed by the operator or by an automatic procedure. The external energy (E_{ext}) of the system is defined by local image features and user-defined constraints, which is analogous to kinetic energy deforming the contour and attracting toward the image features such as edges. The magnitude of the gradient of an image is the most popular choice for describing external energy because of its computational simplicity. On the other hand, shape-related constraints are restricted to an internal energy (E_{int}) term, which acts in a way similar to potential energy that aims to prevent the contour from losing its shape-related properties, e.g., smoothness and curvature. It is necessary to calculate the contribution of the continuity and curvature terms to define these shape-related properties.

(Khotanlou et al., 2009) proposed an automatic method for brain tumor segmentation. Initially, the brain tumor is roughly segmented using two alternative approaches: fuzzy clustering based on the possibilistic fuzzy c-means (PFCM) algorithm or symmetry analysis of the brain. Symmetry analysis of the brain consists of analyzing the differences in histograms obtained from the healthy hemisphere and from the hemisphere where the tumor is present. Comparison of these two histograms provides useful information about the intensity classes induced by the tumor. Even though symmetry analysis may fail in the case of a symmetrical tumor across the mid-sagittal plane, it is usually preferred over PFCM, because with fuzzy clustering it is difficult to obtain a good performance for any type of tumor when heterogeneous neoplasic domains are present. Afterwards, a segmentation refinement is performed using a deformable model.

Geometric deformable models are based on the level set method introduced by (Osher et al., 1988) and were proposed by (Caselles et al., 1993) and (Malladi et al., 1995). The basic idea is to represent the curve in a higher dimension as a zero level set, usually referred to as the level set function. This function evolves according a partial differential equation (PDE). The main advantage of this approach with respect to parametric deformable models is that complex topological changes can be handled by the contour and it is able to merge the curve during the evolution process. This becomes very useful for three dimensional segmentation frameworks that are inherently more complex for parametric representations.

According to (Li et al., 2005), there are two formulations of the segmentation problem based on the level set method. The first is the Lagrangian formulation and corresponds to the early geometric active contour models (Caselles et al., 1993; Malladi et al., 1995). An initial contour evolves iteratively according to the PDE of a parametrized curve, taking into account information related to the gradient of the image; the deformation is stopped in high gradient locations, locating the curve in the boundary of an object. This approach may become very expensive in three dimensions (Xu et al., 2003). Also, if boundaries are poorly defined the curve may pass through them (see, for instance, Caselles et al., 1993), because the edge-related information becomes insufficient as a stopping criterion for the curve evolution. This is especially true in medical image segmentation where complex behavior of biological structures is observed. An alternative approach for the evolution of the contour is related to the variational formulation, where no edge-stopping functions based on the gradient of the image are defined. The evolution PDE is directly derived by minimizing certain energy functions defined on the level set function (see Li et al., 2005).

(Ho et al., 2002) introduced an improved approach in which brain tumors are automatically segmented, modulating the propagation of the curve with a local statistical force to avoid the need for careful initialization of snakes with constant propagation. This method starts with an intensity-based fuzzy classification of voxels into tumor and background classes. The initial fuzzy classification is used to guide locally the propagation direction and speed of a level-set-based contour, and is also used for automatically initializing the contour. (Prastawa et al., 2004) extended the approach described in (Moon et al., 2002). First, the detection of abnormal tissues was performed using a registered brain atlas (as a model of a normal brain) and a robust estimate for the location and dispersion of the normal brain tissues was calculated. From the T_2-weighted MR images, it was determined whether edema appears together with tumor in the abnormal regions, described as outliers (voxels that are not explained by the normal brain model estimated as a first step). Finally, the geometric level set method was applied with the same evolution strategy used in (Ho et al., 2002) and also prior knowledge was included to refine the segmentation of tumor and edema. Similar approaches were proposed by (Cobzas et al., 2007) and (Popuri et al., 2009), but instead of using a level set for refinement in a final step as done by (Prastawa et al., 2004), a feature set of specific anatomical priors was fully integrated into the region-based variational formulation. (Xie et al., 2005) presented a hybrid approach, i.e., the evolution of the curve is governed simultaneously by region and boundary information that serves as propagation force and stopping function, respectively.

4. Concluding remarks

Brain Tumor Segmentation methods are an active research area with increasing interest to improve treatment and diagnosis of patients. Currently, a large amount of information is generated by several image modalities and computational techniques are required to support decisions in tasks related to diagnosis, surgical planning and evaluation of treatments.

Fundamental issues related to the improvements of acquisition methods and image processing techniques are the main focus of the current research efforts in the field of brain tumor segmentation. Image modalities are evolving quickly, and are providing more and better information about the pathology. Magnetic Resonance Imaging plays a remarkable role in providing good spatial resolution and several contrasts that reflect anatomical and functional properties of tumoral and healthy tissues in very precise ways.

In general, intensity-based and region-based approaches for brain tumor segmentation take into account the histological heterogeneity and the diffuse infiltration that characterize the pathology. Drawbacks related to image modalities, such as the bias field, partial volume effect, overlapping intensity distributions of tumor/healthy tissues, etc., are also addressed by most methods proposed to segment brain tumors. Intensity-based approaches and multispectral analysis are essential tools in order to integrate different sources of information on anatomy and functionality provided by the available image modalities. Furthermore, region-based techniques are useful in dealing with overlapping intensity distributions. A large number of studies have been devoted to integrate approaches to improve the outcomes of segmentation approaches and to take advantage of each methodology.

It is important to take advantage of the information retrieved by image modalities, either anatomical or functional, to represent in a more informative way the specific complexities of the pathology. The computational representations of brain tumor features that guide the segmentation process may be limited; they are usually not able to capture the inherent anatomical complexities made manifest with image modalities. On the other hand, the validation of medical image segmentation methods has been an important problem from the beginning. Usually, this is done by using gold standards constructed from manual delineation of tumor boundaries conducted by experts. Evidently, this is very time-consuming approach, and subject to high variability. Another approach is related to the use of simulated images that may be helpful for characterizing the performance of a proposed segmentation method.

In the scientific community there is no consensus about which segmentation approach best fits brain tumor segmentation. The most promising schemes for brain tumor segmentation are those in which the information from several image modalities is combined and where the information on regions and multispectral intensities are also considered simultaneously.

5. References

Aromen, J.H.; Gazit, I.E.; Louis, D.N., Buchbinder, B.R.; Pardo, F.S.; Weisskoff, R.M.; Harsh, G.R.; Cosgrove, G.R.; Halpern, E.F. & Hochberg, F.H. (1994). Cerebral blood volume maps of gliomas: comparison with tumor grade and histologic findings. *Radiology*, Vol.191, No.1, (April 1994), pp. 41-51, ISSN 0033-8419

Arvinda, R.; Kesavadas, C.; Sarma, P.S.; Thomas, B.; Radhakrishnan, V.; Gupta, A.; Kapilamoorthy, T. & Nair, S. (2009). Glioma grading: sensitivity, specificity, positive and negative predictive values of diffusion and perfusion imaging. *Journal of Neurooncology*, Vol.94, No.1, (August 2009), pp. 87-96, ISSN 0167-594X

Bankman, I. (2009). *Handbook of Medical Image Processing and Analysis*, Elsevier, ISBN 978-0-12-373904-9, USA

Bello, A.; Gambini, A.; Castellano, G.; Carrabba, F.; Acerbi, E.; Fava, C.; Giussani, M.; Cadioli, V.; Blasi, A.; Casarotti, C.; Papagno, A.K.; Gupta, S.; Gaini, G.; Scotti, A. & Falini (2008). Motor and language DTI Fiber Tracking combined with intraoperative subcortical mapping for surgical removal of gliomas. *NeuroImage*, Vol. 39, No.1 (January 2008), pp. 369–382. ISSN 1053-8119

Besag, J. (1986). On the Statistical Analysis of Dirty Pictures. *Journal of the Royal Statistical Society - B*, Vol.48, No.3, (May 1986), pp. 259-302, ISSN 00359246

Beyer, T.; Townsend, D.W.; Brun, T.; Kinahan, P.E.; Charron, M.; Roddy, R.; Jerin, J.; Young, J.; Byars, L. & Nutt, R. (2000). A combined PET/CT scanner for clinical oncology. *Journal of Nuclear Medicine*, Vol.41, No.8, (August 2000), pp. 1369-1379, ISSN 0161-5505

Bezdek, J.; Pal, M.; Keller, J. & Krishnapuram, R. (1999). *Fuzzy Models and Algorithms for Pattern Recognition and Image Processing*, Kluwer Academic Publishers Norwell, ISBN 0792385217, MA, USA

Bishop, C. (2006). *Pattern Recognition and Machine Learning*, Springer, ISBN 0387-31073-8, NY-USA

Bruhn, H. ; Frahm, J. ; Gyngell, M.L. ; Merboldt, K.D. ; Hänicke, W. ; Sauter, R. & Hamburger, C. (1989). Noninvasive differentiation of tumors with use of localized H-1 MR spectroscopy in vivo: initial experience in patients with cerebral tumors. *Radiology*, Vol 172, No.2, (August 1989), pp. 541-548, ISSN 0033-8419

Cai, W.; Chen, S. & Lei, L. (2009). A Fuzzy Clustering Algorithm for Image Segmentation Using Dependable Neighbor Pixels, *Chinese Conference on Pattern Recognition*, ISBN 978-1-4244-4199-0, Nanjing-China, November 4-6, 2009

Capelle, A.; Alata, O.; Fernandez, C.; Lefevre, S. & Ferrie, J. (2000). Unsupervised segmentation for automatic detection of brain tumors in MRI, *Proceedings of IEEE the International Conference on Image Processing*, ISBN 0-7803-6297-7, Canada, September 10-13, 2000

Capelle, A.; Colot, O. & Fernandez, C. (2004). Evidential segmentation scheme of multi-echo MR images for the detection of brain tumors using neighborhood information. *Information Fusion*, Vol.5, No.3, (September 2004), pp. 203-216, ISSN 1566-2535

Caselles, V.; Catte, F.; Coll, T. & Dibos, F. (1993). A geometric model for active contours in image processing. *Numerische Mathematik*, Vol.66, No.1, (October 1993), pp. 1-31, ISSN 0029-599X

Castillo, M.; Smith, J.K. & Kwock, L. (2000) Correlatio of myo-inositol levels and grading of cerebral astrocytomas. *Am. J Neuroradiol*, Vol.21, No.9, (October 2000), pp.1645-1649, ISSN 0195-6108

Chabert, S. & Scifo, P. (2007). Diffusion Signal in Magnetic Resonance Imaging: Origin and Interpretation in Neurosciences. *Biological Research*, Vol.40, No.4, (December 2010), pp. 385-400, ISSN 0716-9760

Chen, T. & Metaxas, D. (2003). Gibbs prior models, marching cubes, and deformable models: A hybrid framework for 3d medical image segmentation, *Proceedings of 6th International Conference of MICCAI*, ISBN 3-540-20462-8, Canada, November 15-18, 2003

Chong, V.; Zhou, J.; Khoo, J.; Huang, J. & Lim, T. (2004). Tongue carcinoma: tumor volume measurement. *International Journal of Radiation Oncology - Biology - Physics*, Vol.59, No.1, (May 2004), pp. 59-66, ISSN 0360-3016

Clark, M.; Hall, L.; Goldgof, D.; Velthuizen, R.; Murtaugh, R. & Silbiger, M. (1998). Automatic tumor segmentation using knowledge-based techniques. *IEEE Transactions on Medical Imaging*, Vol.17, No.2, (April 1998), pp. 187-201, ISSN 0278-0062

Clarke, M. (1991). MR Image Segmentation Using MLM and Artificial Neural Nets. *Medical Physics*, Vol.18, No.3, (1991), pp. 673-, ISSN 0094-2405

Cobzas, D.; Birkbeck, N.; Schmidt, M.; Jagersand, M. & Murtha, A. (2007). 3D Variational Brain Tumor Segmentation using a High Dimensional Feature Set, *IEEE Computer Society Workshop on Mathematical Methods in Biomedical Image Analysis* (*MMBIA*), ISBN 978-1-4244-1631-8, Rio de Janeiro-Brasil, October 14-15, 2007

Croteau, D. ; Scarpace, L. ; Hearshen, D. ; Gutierrez, J. ; Fischer, J.L. ; Rock, J.P. & Mikkelsen, T. (2001) Correlation between magnetic resonance spectroscopy imaging and image-guided biopsies: semiquantitative and qualitative histopathological analyses of patients with untreated glioma. *Neurosurgery*, Vol.49, No.4, (October 2001), pp.823-829, ISSN 0148-396X

Dickson, S. & Thomas, B. (1997). Using Neural Networks to Automatically Detect Brain Tumours in MR Images. *International Journal of Neural Systems*, Vol.8, No.1, (February 1997), pp. 91-99, ISSN 0129-0657

Doi, K. (2007). Computer-aided diagnosis in medical imaging: Historical review, current status and future potential. *Computerized Medical Imaging and Graphics*, Vol.31, No.4-5, (June-July 2007), pp. 198-211, ISSN 0895-6111

Dou, W.; Ruan, S.; Chen, Y.; Bloyet, D. & Constans, J. (2007). A framework of fuzzy information fusion for the segmentation of brain tumor tissues on MR images. *Image and Vision Computing*, Vol.25, No.2, (February 2007), pp. 164-171, ISSN 0262-8856

Douglas, J.G.; Stelzer, K.K.; Mankoff, D.A.; Tralins, K.S.; Krohn, K.A.; Muzi, M.; Silbergeld, D.L.; Rostomily, R.C.; Scharnhorst, J. & Spence, A.M. (2006). [F-18]-fluorodeoxyglucose positron emission tomography for targeting radiation dose escalation for patients with glioblastoma multiforme: clinical outcomes and patterns of failure. *Int J Radiat Oncol Biol Phys*, Vol.64, No.3, (Mar 2006), pp. 886-891, ISSN 0360-3016

Drabycz, S.; Roldán, G.; de Robles, P.; Adler, D.; McIntyre, J.; Magliocco, A.; Cairncross, J. & Mitchell, J. (2010). An analysis of image texture, tumor location, and MGMT promoter methylation in glioblastoma using magnetic resonance imaging. *NeuroImage*, Vol.49, No.2, (January 2010), pp. 1398–1405, ISSN 10538119

Drevelegas, A. (2011). *Imaging of Brain Tumors with Histological Correlations*. Springer-Verlag, ISBN 978-3-540-87648-9, Berlin, Germany

Dubey, R.; Hanmandlu, M.; Gupta, S. & Gupta, S. (2010). An Advanced Technique for Volumetric Analysis. *International Journal of Computer Applications*, Vol.1, No.1, (February 2010), pp. 91-98, ISSN 1206-212X

Dunn, J. (1973). A fuzzy relative of the ISODATA process and its use in detecting compact well-separated clusters. *Cybernetics and Systems*, Vol.3, No.3, (1973), pp. 32-57, ISSN 0196-9722

Fletcher-heath, L.; Hall. L.; Goldgof, D. & Murtagh, F. (2001). Automatic Segmentation of Non-enhancing Brain Tumors in Magnetic Resonance Images. *Artificial Intelligence in Medicine*, Vol.21, No.1, (January 2001), pp. 43-63, ISSN 0933-3657

Food and Drug Administration (November 9, 2010). FDA working to prevent radiation overdoses during CT scans. 4.02.2011. Available from http://www.fda.gov/NewsEvents/Newsroom/PressAnnouncements/ucm233245.htm

Food and Drug Administration (December 2010). FDA Drug Safety Communication: New warnings for using gadolinium-based contrast agents in patients with kidney dysfunction. 4.02.2011. Available from http://www.fda.gov/Drugs/DrugSafety/ucm223966.htm

Gaensler, E. (1998). *Neurorradiología Fundamental*, Madrid: Marbán, ISBN 8471012480, Madrid-España

Gering, D. (2003). *Recognizing Deviations from Normalcy for Brain Tumor Segmentation*, MIT, PhD thesis, retrieved from http://people.csail.mit.edu/gering/.

Gibbs, P.; Buckley, D.; Blackband, S. & Horsman, A. (1996). Tumour volume determination from MR images by morphological segmentation. *Physics in Medicine and Biology*, Vol.41, No.11, June 1996, pp. 2437-2446, ISSN 0031-9155

Gillies, R.; Raghunand, N.; Garcia-Martin M. & Gatenby, R. (2004). pH imaging. *IEEE Engineering in Medicine and Biology Magazine*, Vol.23, No.5, (September/October 2004), pp. 57-64, ISSN 0739-5175

Gordillo, N.; Montseny, E. & Sobrevilla, P. (2010). A new fuzzy approach to brain tumor segmentation, *Proceedings of the IEEE International Conference on Fuzzy Systems*, ISBN 978-1-4244-6919-2, Barcelona-España, July 18-23, 2010

Ho, S.; Bullitt, E. & Gerig, G. (2002). Level-Set Evolution with Region Competition: Automatic 3-D Segmentation of Brain Tumors, *Proceedings of the 16th International Conference on Pattern Recognition*, ISBN 0-7695-1695-X, QC-Canada, August 11-15, 2002

Horská, A. & Barker, P.B. (2010). Imaging of brain tumors: MR spectroscopy and Metabolic Imaging. *Neuroimag Clin N Am*, Vol.20, No.3, (August 2010), pp.293-310, ISSN 0022-510X

Judenhofer, M.; Wehrl, H.; Newport, D.; Catana, C.; Siegel, S.; Becker, M.; Thielscher, A.; Kneilling, M.; Lichy, M.; Eichner, M.; Klingel, K.; Reischl, G.; Widmaier, S.; Rocken, M; Nutt, R.; Machulla, H.; Uludag, K.; Cherry, S; Claussen, C. & Pichler, B. (2008). Simultaneous PET-MRI: a new approach for functional and morphological imaging. *Nature Medicine*, Vol.14, No.4, (April 2008), pp. 459-465, ISSN 1078-8956

Kass, K.; Witkin, A. & Terzopolous, D. (1987). Snakes: Active Contour Models. *International Journal of Computer Vision*, Vol.1, No.4, (January 1987), pp. 321-331, ISSN 0920-5691

Kaus, M.; Warfield, S.; Nabavi, A.; Black, P.; Jolesz, F. & Kikinis, R. (2001). Automated segmentation of MR images of brain tumors. *Radiology*, Vol.218, No.2, (February 2001), pp. 586-591, ISSN 0033-8419

Kaye, A. & Laws Jr., E. (2001). *Brain Tumors* (2nd edition), Churchill Livingstone, ISBN 0443064261, NY-USA

Khotanlou, H.; Colliot, O.; Atif, J. & Bloch, I. (2009). 3D brain tumor segmentation in MRI using fuzzy classification, symmetry analysis and spatially constrained deformable models. *Fuzzy Sets and Systems*, Vol.160, No.10, (May 2009), pp. 1457-1473, ISSN 0165-0114

Krishnapuram, R. & Keller, J. (1996). The possibilistic c-means algorithm: insights and recommendations. *IEEE Transactions on Fuzzy Systems*, Vol.4, No.3, (August 1996), pp. 385-393, ISSN 1063-6706

Le Bihan, D. (1995). *Diffusion and Perfusion Magnetic Resonance Imaging: Applications to Functional MRI*. Raven Press, ISBN 978-0781702447, New York, USA

Li, S. (2008). *Markov Random Field Modeling in Image Analysis* (3rd edition), Elsevier, ISBN 9781848002784, London-UK

Li, C.; Xu, C.; Gui, C. & Fox, M. (2005). Level Set Evolution Without Re-initialization: A New Variational Formulation, *Proceedings of the IEEE Computer Society Conference on Computer Vision and Pattern Recognition*, ISBN 0-7695-2372-2, CA-USA, June 20-26, 2005

Malladi, R.; Sethian, J. & Vemuri, B. (1995). Shape modeling with front propagation: a level set approach. *IEEE Transactions on Pattern Analysis and Machine Intelligence*, Vol.17, No.2, (February 1995), pp. 158-175, ISSN 0162-8828

Menze, B.; Van Leemput, K.; Lashkari, D.; Weber, M.; Ayache, N. & Golland, P. (2010). A Generative Model for Brain Tumor Segmentation in Multi-Modal Images, *Proceedings of the International MICCAI Workshop on Medical Computer Vision. Recognition Techniques and Applications in Medical Imaging*, ISBN 978-3-642-18420-8, China, September 20-24, 2010

Moon, N.; Bullitt, E.; Van Leemput, K. & Gerig, G. (2002). Model-Based Brain and Tumor Segmentation, *Proceeding of the International Conference on Pattern Recognition*, ISBN 0-7695-1695-X, Canada, August 11-15, 2002

Mori, S. (2007). *Introduction to Diffusion Tensor Imaging*. Elsevier Science, ISBN 9780444528285, Oxford, UK.

Murakami, R.; Hirai, T.; Sugahara, T.; Fukuoka, H.; Toya, R.; Nishimura, S.; Kitajima, M.; Okuda, T.; Nakamura, H.; Oya, N.; Kuratsu, J. & Yamashita, Y. (2009) Grading Astrocytic Tumors by Using Apparent Diffusion Coefficient Parameters: Superiority of a One-versus Two-Parameter Pilot Method. *Radiology*, Vol.251, No.3, (June 2009), pp. 838-845, ISSN 0033-8419

Oppelt, A. (2006). Imaging Systems for Medical Diagnostics: Fundamentals, Technical Solutions and Applications for Systems Applying Ionizing Radiation, Nuclear Magnetic Resonance *and Ultrasound*. Publicis Corporate Publishing, ISBN 3-89578-226-2, Erlangen, Germany

Osher, S. & Sethian, J. (1988). Fronts Propagating with Curvature Dependent Speed: Algorithms based on Hamilton-Jacobi formulations. *Journal of Computational Physics*, Vol.79, No.1, (November 1988), pp. 12-49, ISSN 0021-9991

Otsu, N. (1979). A threshold selection method from gray-level histogram. *IEEE Transactions on Systems, Man and Cybernetics,* Vol.8, No.1, (January 1979), pp. 62-66, ISSN 0018-9472

Ozkan, M.; Dawant, B. & Maciunas, R. (1993). Neural-Network-Based Segmentation of Multi-Modal Medical Images: A Comparative and Prospective Study. *IEEE Transactions on Medical Imaging,* Vol.12, No.3, (September 1993), pp. 534-544, ISSN 0278-0062

Popuri, K.; Cobzas, D.; Jagersand, M.; Shah, S. & Murtha, A. (2009). 3D variational brain tumor segmentation on a clustered feature set, *Proceedings of SPIE Medical Imaging,* ISBN 9780819475107, Florida-USA, February 7-12, 2009

Prastawa, M.; Bullitt, E.; Ho, S. & Gerig, G. (2004). A brain tumor segmentation framework based on outlier detection. *Medical Image Analysis,* Vol.8, No.3, (September 2004), pp. 275–283, ISSN 1361-8415

Raab, P.; Hattingen, E.; Franz, K.; Zanella, F. & Lanfermann, H. (2010). Cerebral gliomas: diffusional kurtosis imaging analysis of microstructural differences. *Radiology,* Vol.254, No.3, (March 2010), pp. 876-881, ISSN 0033-8419

Rees, J.; Watt, H.; Jäger, H.; Benton, C.; Tozer, D.; Tofts, P. & Waldman, A. (2009). Volumes and growth rates of untreated adult low-grade gliomas indicate risk of early malignant transformation. *European Journal of Radiology,* Vol.72, No.1, (October 2009), pp. 54-64, ISSN 0720-048X

Rexilius, J.; Hahn, H.; Klein, J.; Lentschig, M. & Peitgen, H. (2007). Multispectral brain tumor segmentation based on histogram model adaption, *Proceedings of the SPIE conference on Medical Image computing,* ISBN 9780819466303, CA-USA, February 17-22, 2007

Sack, I.; Beierbach, B.; Hamhaber, U. Klatt, D. & Braun, A. (2008). Non invasive measurment of brain viscoelasticity using magnetic resonance elastrography. *NMR in Biomedicine,* Vol.21, No.3, (March 2008), pp. 265-271, ISSN 0952-3480

Saha, S. & Bandyopadhyay, S. (2007). MRI brain image segmentation by fuzzy symmetry based genetic clustering technique, *IEEE Congress on Evolutionary Computation,* ISBN 978-1-4244-1339-3, Singapore, September 25-28, 2007

Salman, Y. (2009). Modified technique for volumetric brain tumor measurements. *Journal of Biomedical Science and Engineering,* Vol.2, No.1, (February 2009), pp. 16-19, ISSN 1937-6871

Salman, Y. & Badawi, A. (2005). Validation Techniques for Quantitative Brain Tumor Measurements, *Proceedings of the 27th Annual International Conference of the IEEE Engineering in Medicine and Biology Society,* ISBN 0-7803-8741-4, Shanghai-China, September 1-4, 2005

Sato, M.; Lakare, S.; Wan, M; Kaufman, A. & Nakajima, M. (2000). A gradient magnitude based region growing algorithm for accurate segmentation, *Proceedings of the IEEE International Conference on Image Processing,* ISBN 0-7803-6297-7, Canada, September 10-13, 2000

Solomon, J.; Butman, J. & Sood, A. (2006). Segmentation of brain tumors in 4D MR images using the hidden Markov. *Computer Methods and Programs in Biomedicine,* Vol.84, No.2, (December 2006), pp. 76-85, ISSN 0169-2607

Stadlbauer, A.; Moser, E.; Gruber, S.; Buslei, R.; Nimsky, C.; Fahlbusch, R. & Ganslandt, O. (2004). Improved delineation of brain tumors: an automated method for segmentation based on pathologic changes of 1H-MRSI metabolites in gliomas. *NeuroImage*, Vol.23, No.2, (October 2004), pp. 454-461, ISSN 10538119

Stippich, C. (2007). *Clinical Functional MRI. Presurgical Functional Neuroimaging*. Springer, ISBN 978-3-540-24469-1, Berlin, Germany

Sung, Y.C.; Han, K.S.; JunSong C.; Noh, S.M. & Park, J.W. (2000). Threshold estimation for region segmentation on MR image of brain having the partial volume artifact, *Proceedings of 5th International Conference on Signal Processing*, ISBN 0-7803-5747-7, China, August 21-25, 2000

Tayel, M. & Abodou, M. (2006). A Neuro-Difference Fuzzy Technique for Automatic Segmentation of Region of Interest in Medical Imaging, *Proceedings of the 23rd National Radio Science Conference*, ISBN 9775031842, Egypt, March 14-16, 2006

The Alliance for Radiation Safety in Pediatric Imaging (n.d.). Image gently. 4.02.2011. Available in
www.imagegently.org

Van Leemput, K.; Maes, F.; Vandermeulen, D.; Colchester, A. & Suetens, P. (2001). Automated Segmentation of Multiple Sclerosis Lesions by Model Outlier Detection. *IEEE Transactions on Medical Imaging*, Vol.20, No.8, (August 2001), pp. 677-688, ISSN ISSN 0278-0062

Veloz, A.; Chabert, S.; Salas. R.; Orellana, A. & Vielma, J. (2007). Fuzzy Spatial Growing for Glioblastoma Multiforme Segmentation on Brain Magnetic Resonance Imaging, *Proceedings of the 12th Iberoamerican conference on Progress in pattern recognition, image analysis and applications*, ISBN 3-540-76724-X, Viña del Mar-Chile, November 13-16, 2007

Villalta, R. & Martín-Landrove, M. (2006). Brain Tumor Image Segmentation Using Neural Networks, *Proceedings 14th Scientific Meeting International Society for Magnetic Resonance in Medicine*, ISBN 1522-2594, Seattle-Washington-USA, May 6-12, 2006

Xie,K.; Yang, J.; Zhang, Z. & Zhu, Y. (2005). Semi-automated brain tumor and edema segmentation using MRI. *European Journal of Radiology*, Vol.56, No.1, (October 2005), pp. 12-19, ISSN 0720-048X

Xu, J. & Zhao, H. (2003). An Eulerian Formulation for Solving Partial Differential Equations along a Moving Interface. *Journal of Scientific Computing*, Vol.19, No.1-3, (December 2003), pp. 573-594, ISSN 0885-7474

Zhang, Y.; Brady, M. & Smith S. (2001). Segmentation of brain MR images through a hidden Markov random field model and the expectation-maximization algorithm. *IEEE Transactions on Medical Imaging*, Vol.20, No.1, (January 2001), pp. 45-57, ISSN 0278-0062

5

Glial Tumors: Quantification and Segmentation from MRI and MRS

Weibei Dou[1] and Jean-Marc Constans[2]
[1]*Tsinghua University,*
[2]*CHU de Caen*
[1]*China*
[2]*France*

1. Introduction

Brain tumor segmentation is an important technique in computer-assisted diagnosis. To improve brain tumor diagnosis, it is necessary to use biochemical information provided by magnetic resonance spectroscopy (MRS). Some of the challenges involved are determining how to combine multimodal signals such as proton MRS and morphological or structural images, then knowing how to use the combined information to make a decision. In this paper, we propose using a data fusion method to perform an automatic segmentation of the brain tumor areas.

To diagnose brain tissue abnormalities such as tumors, we need to use multispectral magnetic resonance images (MRIs), e.g. T1-weighted, T2-weighted, gadolinium, or FLAIR to determine some properties of the tumor, including size, position, sort, and relationship with other tissues. However, the tumor type and grade are usually diagnosed from histopathological examination of a surgical specimen. Proton (^{1}H) magnetic resonance spectroscopy (MRS) is a non invasive MR technique that provides biochemical information about metabolites. The major biochemical characteristics can provide useful information about brain tumor type and grade (Howe et al., 2003a; 2003b). In many studies, the use of in vivo ^{1}H-MRS has been described for determining tumor type and grade (Howe et al., 2003a; Howe et al., 2003b; Preul et al., 1996; Majós et al., 2009).

Since analysis of in vivo MRS measurements are dependent on acquisition techniques that could compromise the spatial resolution and accuracy of resulting metabolite values (Maudsley et al., 2009), metabolic changes associated with disease are frequently small and diffuse. Furthermore, using the chemical-shift imaging (CSI) technique, metabolite images, known as MR spectroscopic imaging (MRSI) images, can be created using multivoxel MRS information, but it is not as visually interpretable as in a structural MRI (Maudsley et al., 2009). So, for tumor tissue classification, it is important that MRSI be combined with MRI to make a more accurate estimation of variations in metabolites, support hypotheses of metabolite variation causes, and to yield sufficient information about the tissue.

For over a decade, scientists have been developing automated brain-tumor classification methods using MRS (Garcia-Gomez et al., 2009), but a more clear definition of brain tumor type and grade may be obtained by combining MRS or MRSI and MRI (Garcia-Gomez et al., 2009). A technique used to differentiate glioblastoma from metastatic lesions using MRI and

MRS data has been published (Luts et al., 2009). Wang et al. described a classification of brain tumors using feature selection and fuzzy connectedness (Wang et al., 2007). These features are extracted from MRI and MRS data.

There are 2 difficulties for combining MRSI data and MRI data. Firstly, these data are presented in different modalities, so they do not have the same spatial resolution. There is very low spatial resolution per voxel for MRSI, and high spatial resolution per pixel for MRI. Secondly, one MR image corresponds to the distribution of many tissues, or many tissue structures. But one MRS image is an image which corresponds to 1 metabolite or a ratio between several metabolites. So, the different metabolite values cause variation in MRS images, as in the mapping of metabolite distributions by MRSI presented in a previous study (Maudsley et al., 2009). One of the main questions for application is how to combine these MRS images and MR images to give a good automated tissue classification result. The key point of the combination is how to model the metabolite distribution from MRS, which is coherent with information from MR images.

For an automated description of a brain tumor type and grade, we propose a modelization method of glioma tissues by combining the information from MR images and mulitivoxel MRS data. It can create an MRS-weighted MR image automatically, which retains the high spatial resolution of an MR image and the grey levels corresponding to biochemical abnormalities of pathological processes in brain tissues. The combined data of MRS and T2-weighted images should be enhanced by an operation of exponential companding. It consists of 5 steps: multi-voxel MRS (or CSI) data processing, localization and volume of interest (VOI) extraction, data combination, exponential companding, and region growing as the last step of segmentation. Data from 2 glioma patients, provided by Tiantan hospital in China, have been used to evaluate our method. Two "ground truth", tumors with edema and tumor only, used for result comparison are with manual labels made by neuroradiologists at Tiantan and Nanfang hospitals in China. The segmentation result represents MRS-weighted T2 structure image in the tumor region. As a performance assessment, we obtain 99% correct detection for tumor only and 98% for tumor with potential edema, and a false detection rate of 9% and 6% inside VOI, respectively. The proposed method is also a simple information fusion strategy.

2. Quantitative analysis of glial tumor metabolism

Conventional magnetic resonance imaging (MRI) provides information about tumor anatomy, its extent, and pathology; however, the specificity of diagnosis used to distinguish between benign and malignant disease and the grade severity is still not optimal. Furthermore, MRI does not provide information on the underlying biochemical processes associated with tumor progression and potential regression under therapies. Thus, the biochemical information from tissues may be useful for specific diagnosis, accurate prognosis and follow-up of therapeutic response when used as an adjunct to anatomical details obtained from MR images. This can be achieved through in vivo proton Magnetic Resonance Spectroscopy (MRS) that provides unique metabolic information, at the molecular level, of diagnostic and prognostic importance for tumor typing and grading (Galanaud et al., 2007). The tissues contain several biologically important metabolites (biochemicals) in addition to water and fat hydrogen atoms that could be followed by MRS. It also provides information on the alterations in metabolic pathways during disease processes by detection and quantification of metabolites and their temporal variation. MRS is also a useful tool in the planning and evaluation of treatments and in predicting tumor progression and treatment response. It is known that tumor growth is not a simple regulated phenomenon. There are variations in metabolism and cell density, and in the presence of cystic and necrotic regions (particularly in heterogeneous malignant tumors and under therapies). Thus, the MR spectrum obtained from tumor tissue can be a mixture of different tissue types, including those of different grades, which complicates the spectral interpretation. Most MRS measurements are based on the use of proton (^{1}H) nuclei, due to its great sensitivity. The integration of ^{1}H MRS with clinical MRI investigation is relatively straightforward and easy to implement. Addition of in vivo ^{1}H MRS protocol increases the overall acquisition time by approximately 10 to 20 minutes but it drastically improves the diagnostic, prognostic accuracy and the follow-up of therapeutic response. This method has generated considerable interest in recent years and the added value of the vivo ^{1}H MRS is in the process of evaluation in clinical application. In particular it would allow quantification of metabolites from a well-defined region of interest (ROI) or volume element (voxel). Moreover, the heterogeneous nature of tumors could be understood and detected, which would be of great interest for biopsy guidance in time and space (with CSI) and planning, monitoring, and evaluation of treatments (Soffietti et al. 2010) such as surgery, radiotherapy, and chemotherapy (Hart et al. 2008). Therefore, the possibility of obtaining in vivo quantitative biochemical information has revolutionized the field of clinical neurooncology. In the present work on gliomas, metabolic information obtained in quantitative single voxel MRS measurements, associated with anatomic and perfusion data, allows us to establish an accurate prognosis based on a spectral and metabolic classification system and start to evaluate therapies. In addition, in longitudinal follow-up studies, multimodality (with perfusion and with Positon Emission Tomography (PET) especially in glioblastomas) allow us to study the relationship between MRS, MRI segmentation and perfusion, together with some biologic parameters (eg, proliferation, infiltration, glycolysis metabolism, necrosis) thus helping to characterize sensitive biomarkers and to detect early changes in order to assess costly and heavy (for the patient) therapies rapidly and more accurately. Moreover, MRS data to be evaluated have to be related to data such as the response to therapy, histology, and genetic prognostic mutations (Isocitrate Dehydrogenase 1 IDH1, 1p19q, Methyle guanine methyl transferase MGMT).

Numerous studies reported in the literature have shown that ^{1}H MRS contributes significantly to the management of brain tumors. The major metabolites seen at long, intermediate, and short echo times are N-Acetyl-aspartate (NAA; 2.02 ppm), total creatine (tCr; 3.03 ppm), and choline-containing compounds (tCho; 3.2 ppm). NAA is found predominantly in neurons. The tCr level is reduced in astrocytomas and is nearly absent in meningiomas and schwannomas, indicating changes in energy metabolism. Gliomatosis cerebri is an uncommon and infiltrative type of glioma which is difficult to diagnose but has higher levels of tCr, thus distinguishing it from low grade gliomas (Galanaud et al., 2003). The tCho/tCr ratio increases with the grade of the glioma (Gill et al., 1990) but the large overlap of ratios between grades prevents its individual use as a reliable grading index. The level of tCho increases from grade II to grade III in astrocytomas, but grade IV tumors show wide variation due to the heterogeneity in cell density and necrosis. It is even more variable in gliomatosis. The ratio tCho/NAA was shown to correlate with long-term survival independent of tumor type (Nelson et al., 2002). In addition to the above predominant metabolites observed at long echo times, additional metabolites such as Glx (glutamate

(Glu) and glutamine (Gln), at 3.6-3.9 ppm and 2.1- 2.6 ppm) and myo-inositol (mI, at 3.56 ppm) are seen at shorter echo times and these also have diagnostic and prognostic potential. Lactate (a doublet at 1.33 ppm) is observed in tumors resulting from glycolysis (Stubbs et al., 1995), and lipids (1.3 and 0.9 ppm) are seen in high grade tumors (Howe et al., 2003a; Auer et al.,2001; Kuesel et al., 1994).

For evaluating therapies, one of the purpose is to better understand glial tumor metabolism and post chemotherapy, radiotherapy, and antiangiogenic variations. To determine cerebral variation in MRS area, amplitude, and ratios of metabolites and spectral profiles during a 6-year longitudinal follow-up in 26 patients with low grade gliomas (oligodendroglial tumors (n=12) or gliomatosis (n=14)) without initial hyperperfusion and treated with Temodal and to detect differences in infiltration (NAA), proliferation (Cho/Cr), necrosis (lipids), glycolytic metabolism (lactate) or energetic metabolism (glucose and glutamine) at different tumoral stages and after therapies. Gliomatosis Cerebri (GC) is a challenging tumor, considered to have a poor prognosis and poor response to treatment.

2.1 Materials, methods and measures

2.1.1 Patient population

The World Health Organization (WHO) classification of gliomas is based on the presumed cell origin, and distinguishes between astrocytic, oligodendrocytic, and mixed gliomas. A grading system is based on the presence of the following criteria: increased cellular density, nuclear atypia, mitosis, vascular proliferation, and necrosis. The main histological subtype of grade I gliomas is pilocytic astrocytoma, which is benign. Diffuse astrocytomas, oligodendrogliomas, and oligoastrocytomas are low grade (II) or high grade (III and IV) tumors. Glioblastomas correspond to grade IV astrocytomas.

We studied glioblastomas and mainly low grade gliomas (oligodendrogliomas and gliomatosis).

2.1.2 MRI acquisition and segmentation

Measurements of Sagittal T1, axial proton density, T2, FLAIR, diffusion, perfusion, 3D T1 and 3D T1 planes after gadolinium were acquired (Fig. 1c). Total tumoral volume, volume of FLAIR and T2 hypersignal, contrast enhancement, hyperperfusion, and necrosis volumes are available on the MRI. A late enhancement should be taken into account. Segmentation allows a more quantitative multispectral MRI analysis to estimate tumor volumes, edema and necrosis (Fig. 1a and 1b, (Dou et al., 2007a; Dou et al., 2006; Constans, 2006)). These data allow us to show that treated tumor volumes, observed on MRI, change little between 2 measurements, while spectroscopic profiles and Cho/Cr or mI/Cr ratios decrease (see in Results of spectroscopy).

2.1.3 Perfusion

This NMR technique allows us to study cerebral microcirculation with very fast slice acquisition after gadolinium injection (first past perfusion). In glial tumor, the map of relative CBV ratio is proportional to area under the curves to evaluate tumoral vascularization after intravenous gadolinium injection and showing hyperperfusion.

The data show some tumoral angiogenesis with severe lesions of the BBB (blood-brain barrier). The extravasation of radiocontrast agents induces suceptibility changes, an increase in the curve area of first passing above the baseline. Only a few low grade gliomas

(gliomatosis and oligodendrogliomas) have shown hyperperfusion (without contrast enhancement) at the beginning. Then, more hyperperfusion and small amounts of contrast enhancement appear during the progression.
The relative Cerebral Blood Volume (rCBV) in low grade gliomas is not often elevated, between 1 and 3, showing relative hyperperfusion compared to the contralateral side.
This technique has high temporal resolution and low S/N, and relatively low spatial resolution. For this reason, there is interest in the fusion of perfusion data with MRI data (T1, gadolinium T1, FLAIR and T2).

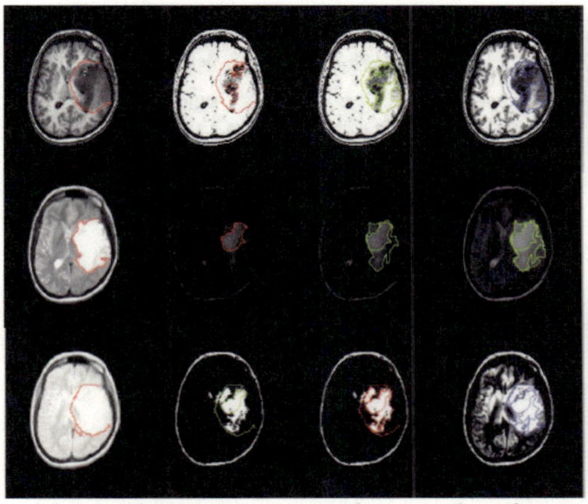

a) Manual segmentation and tissue classification of the different compartments from different weighted (T1, T2 and proton density) images from an oligodendroglioma that became gliomatosis

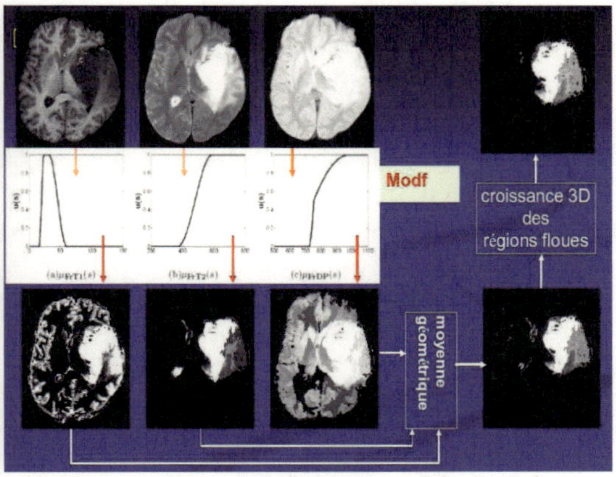

b) Segmentation, classification, and fusion of an oligodendroglioma that became gliomatosis

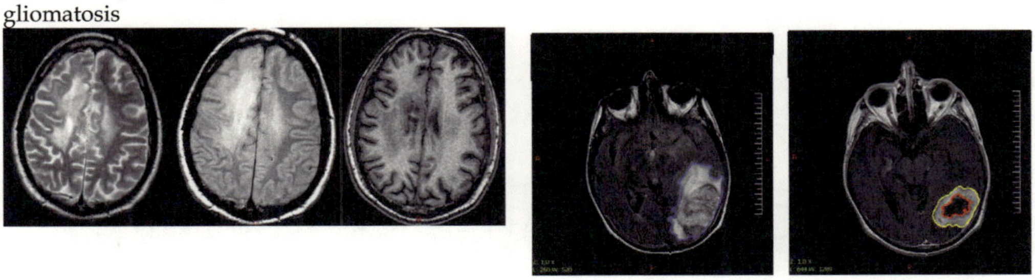

c) Gliomatosis and glioblastoma after segmentation

Fig. 1. MRI acquisition and segmentation of different types of gliomas,

2.1.4 MRS Acquisition and data processing

Single voxels (6 to 12 cm^3) from a 1,5 T machine were done on the most aggressive area (Fig. 2b and 2c) and in the contralateral side (Fig. 2a) using PRESS MRS sequence and with multiple TEs (35, 144, 288, 432ms).
MRS acquisition is sensitive to some parameters and some instrumental problems: localization quality, saturation bands, and homogeneity (Constans, 2006). This is even more evident in large volumes like CSI. SA/GE software (Fig. 3a) and a home-written SCI-MRS-LAB (Delcroix, 2000; Chechin, 2001) (Fig. 3b) (at CHU and Caen University and in Scilab INRIA-ENPC open source code) automated processing software packages yield amplitudes,

areas, ratios, and relative concentrations. Quantification based on amplitude and area (proportional to concentration and relaxation) estimation in spectral domain needs solvent resonance(s) suppression and presents some difficulties such as unknown resonances and molecule metabolization. This process requires normalization with a relative scale with a ratio to another metabolite such as water, NAA, Cr, or absolute metabolite concentration (absolute scale).

Data Processing

There are few quantification methods (SA/GE, JMRUI, SCI-MRS-LAB, THU-MRS0.5 (Dou et al., 2009), THU-MRS1.0 (Chi et al., 2011), sparse representation (Guo et al., 2010), which include different processing steps, e.g. water suppression, baseline estimation, fitting and analysis (Provencher et al., 1982; Nelson, 1989; Nelson, 2001; Hossu, 2009). Fig. 3 shows an example of a quantification methods comparison between Vendors such as SAGE (Spectroscopy Analysis by General Electric) (Fig. 3a) and SCI-MRS-LAB (Fig. 3b).

Usually, we can obtain much better water signal suppression and baseline estimation with SCI-MRS-LAB than with SAGE, especially for overlapped coupled spins, eg, glutamate and glutamine, citrate, or unusual additional resonance to fit.

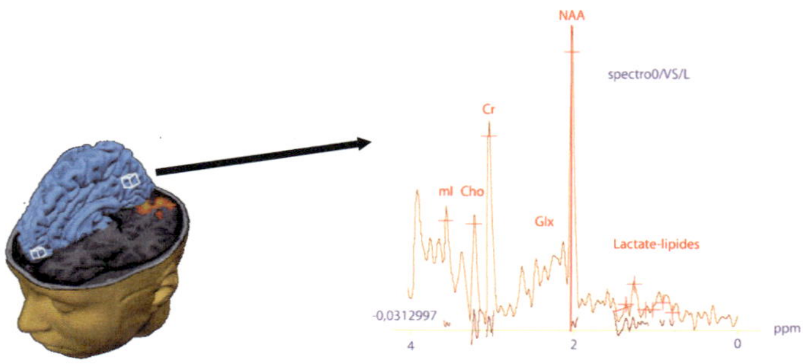

a) Magnetic resonance spectroscopy single voxel short TE 35 ms spectrum from white matter contralateral side similar to a normal spectrum

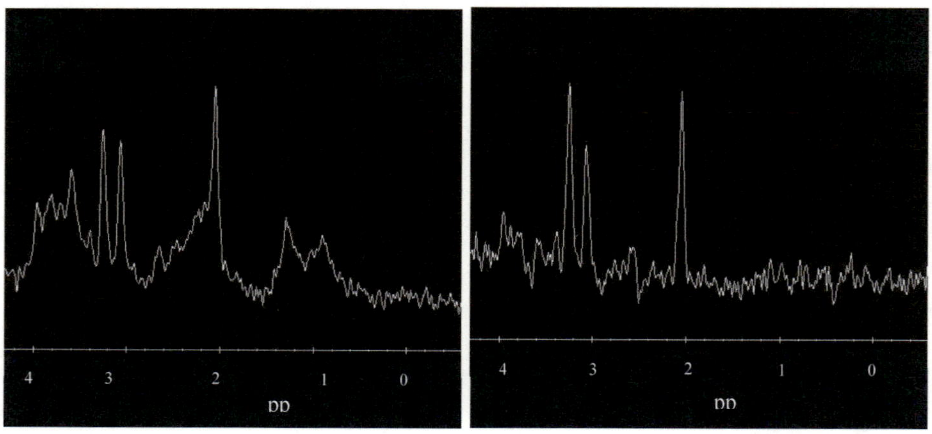

b) Example of spectra from gliomatosis tumor onset at 1.5 Tesla in PRESS sequences at different TE: 35 ms (left) and 144 ms (right) and showing infiltration (NAA/Cr decrease), gliotic activity (slight increase of mI and Cr) with some lactate and demyelination compared to onset ,

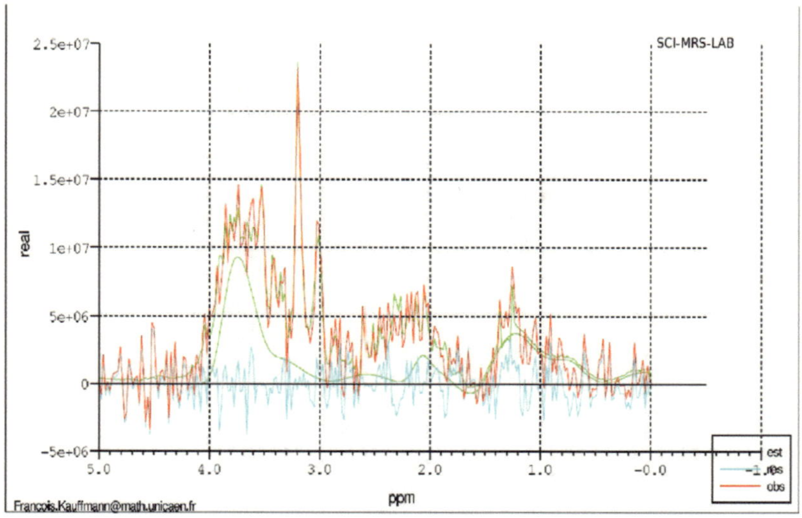

c) Example of spectral variations in glioma modelized by SCI-MRS-LAB processing software:

Cho (containing mainly the metabolites glycerophosphocholine (GPC) and elevated phosphocholine (PC) at 3.22 ppm): proliferation
Lactate (at 1.33 ppm): glycolysis
Decreased NAA/Cr (NAA at 2.02 ppm and Cr at 3.03 ppm): infiltration

The raw signal is in red, modelization by SCI-MRS-LAB, in green, baseline in green, and residuals in blue.In this example, Cho/Cr and ml/ Cr decrease under chemotherapy (Temozolomide [Temodal ®]). NAA/Cr ratios are variable and have a tendency to improve under Temozolomide in gliomatosis.

Fig. 2. MRS acquisition and modelization from a health volintier 2a), and giloma tumors 2b) and 2c)

After therapy, a study of the contralateral side is very important to assess effects of these therapies on the remaining non tumoral neuronal tissues.

Statistical Analysis

In segmentation, tissular classification, and FLAIR hypersignal extension volume the largest variation between n+1 and n exams was retained. Statistical analyses of longitudinal spectroscopic data with z_{test} were done (every 3 months over 60 months).
The longitudinal evolution of Cr concentration was calculated and, because of its low concentration variation in time, this metabolite was used as the reference for the different metabolite ratios. Then, Cho/Cr, NAA/Cr, Myoinositol/Creatine (ml/Cr) and Choline/N-Acetyl-Aspartate (Cho/NAA) were used; their longitudinal variations were studied and analysed.

2.2 Results

2.2.1 Segmentation

The segmentation of gliomas is easier to measure than the segmentation of gliomatosis, especially when assessing contrast enhancement, necrosis and total volumes. In these glioma cases, methods of mathematical morphology or classifications, e.g. Support vector machine (SVM) can be used. The segmentation of glioblastomas and oligodendrogliomas is also easier than gliomatosis because in this type of glioma with more infiltration, it is difficult to separate the different tumoral compartments and to accurately judge the extent of the infiltration, especially when there is little edema and small contrast differences.

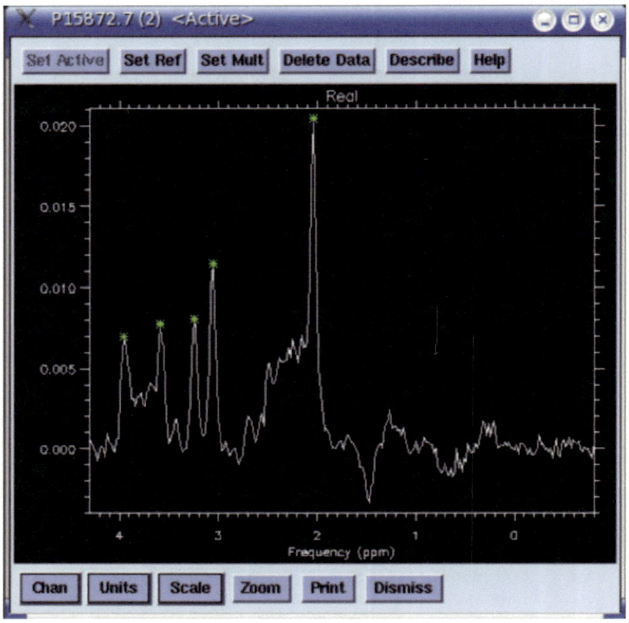

a) Spectral analysis software from General Electric (SA/GE)

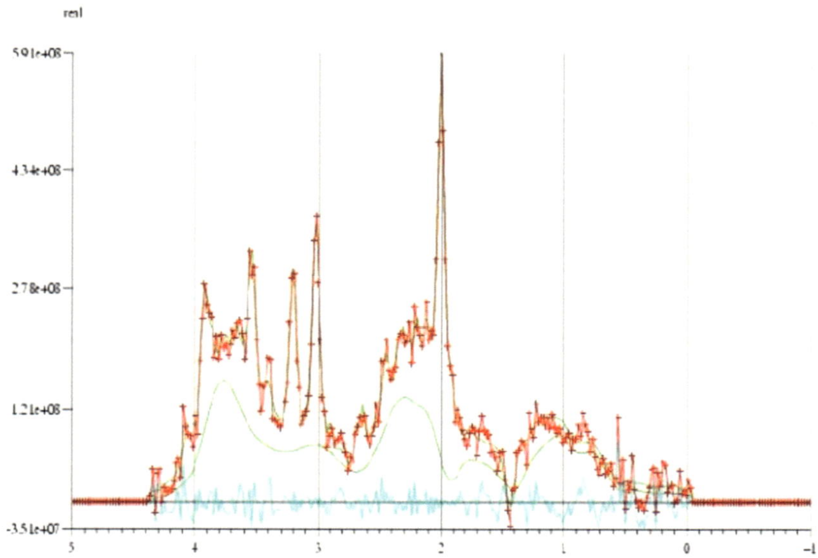

b) The raw signal (in red), modelization by SCI-MRS-LAB (in green the signal), base line (in green) and residuals (in blue)

Fig. 3. Example and comparison of SAGE (Figure 3a) and SCI-MRS-LAB (Figure 3b) processing for short TE spectra from a normal healthy volunteer, ,

2.2.2 Spectroscopy results

Treated (with chemotherapy or radiotherapy) tumoral volumes in MRI, change little (< 20 %) in low-grade gliomas between 2 exams, while spectroscopic profiles and ratios do change (> 60 %) with increases in NAA/Cr and decreases in cho/Cr or ml/Cr ratios, sometimes with a tendency to return to more normal values (even in some gliomatosis lesions).
Without chemotherapy, spectroscopic profiles worsen, with increases in Cho/NAA, Cho/Cr and ml/Cr ratios, decreases in NAA/Cr and sometimes with increases in lactate.
After chemotherapy, treated tumoral volumes in MRI change little between 2 exams, while spectroscopic profiles and ratios do change. MRS could, in fact, be more sensitive than MRI and could, in some cases, be predictive of worsening.

2.2.3 Results of longitudinal follow-up

Some patients with low grade gliomas are still alive 10 years after diagnosis, whereas for glioblastoma, we only obtained a few measures because the patients died within 2 years, on average. Therefore, we will present longitudinal follow-up studies of low grade gliomas (oligodendroglioma and gliomatosis) (Fig. 4).
Water and creatine are quite stable, which could justify using them for some other ratios to quickly detect spectroscopic variations. Cho concentration was predictive in 12 of 26 cases and more sensitive than ratios (8/26). Cho concentration increased in 5 patients with subsequent aggravation.

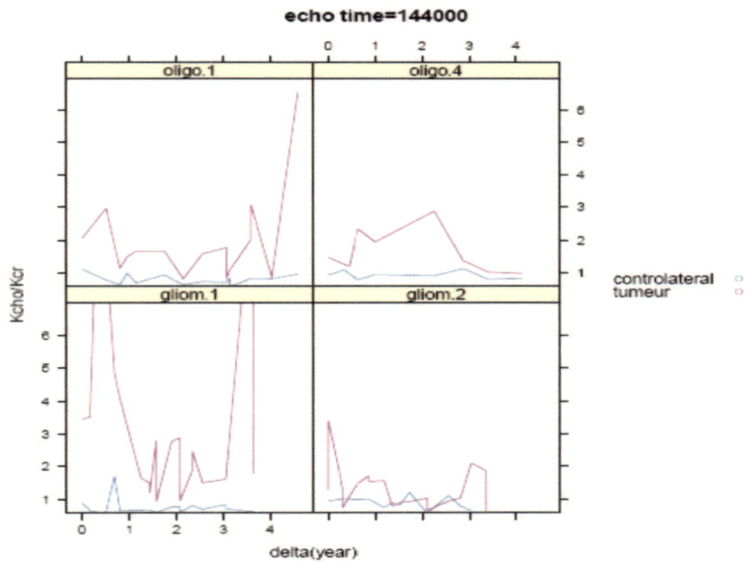

Fig. 4. Progression with time of a metabolite ratio under treatment: Cho/Cr in oligodendroglioma (above) and in gliomatosis (below).

Cho/Cr seems to decrease more rapidly and more frequently between exams in gliomatosis than in oligodendrogliomas. There is sometimes a decrease in the Cho/Cr ratio, but also an increase in the ml/Cr ratio (as in Fig 5).
Concentration of NAA has a tendency to increase with time under Temozolomide, more in contralateral, but sometimes in the tumor as well. NAA/Cr ratios are variable and seem to

improve with treatment in gliomatosis, but sometimes they show a decrease that precedes increased atrophy with FLAIR and T2. Effect of TE on measurements: concentration of NAA always shows a higher estimation on the short TE , while lactate shows a higher estimation on long TE.

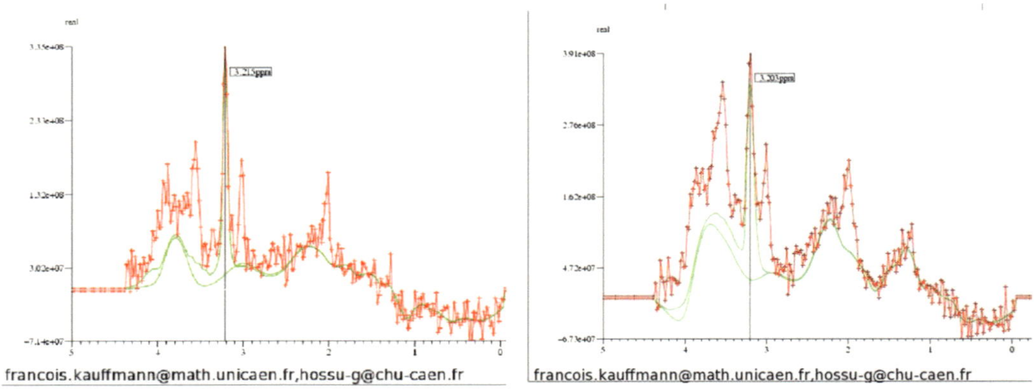

Fig. 5. Example of Cho/Cr ratio decrease under Temodal, but increase in mI/Cr ratio.

2.2.4 Example of perfusion and spectroscopy cases under antiangiogenic therapy

Later in the progression in 4 patients with hyperperfusion which disappeared with antiangiogenic therapy, but proliferation, infiltration, and glycolytic metabolism remained at a high level or worsened. (Fig. 6)

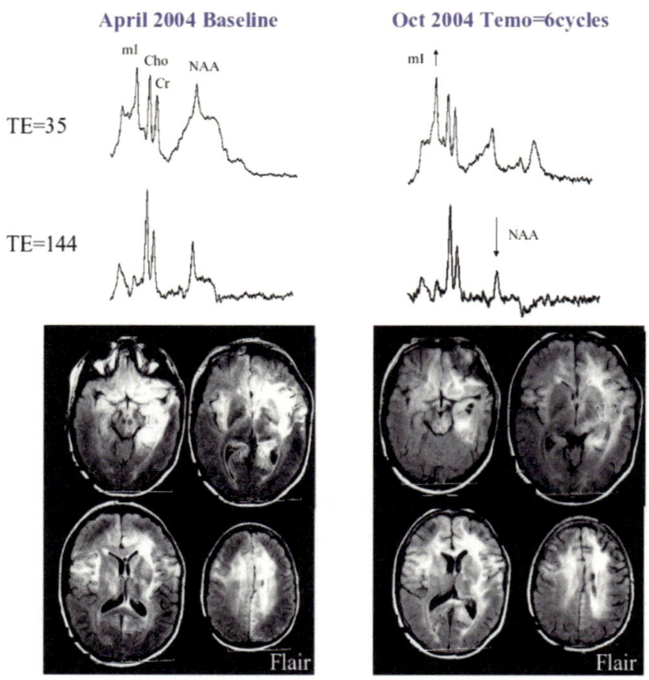

a) Example of MRI and MRS follow-up of a patient with gliomatosis

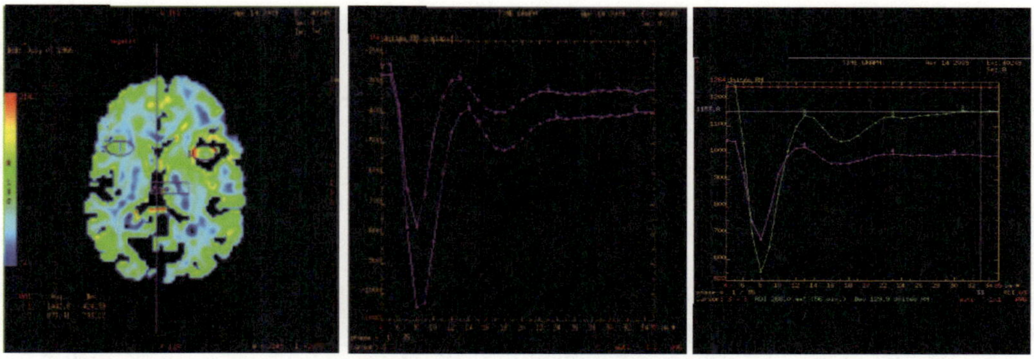

b) Example of MR Perfusion in another gliomatosis patient with decreased hyperperfusion that normalizes

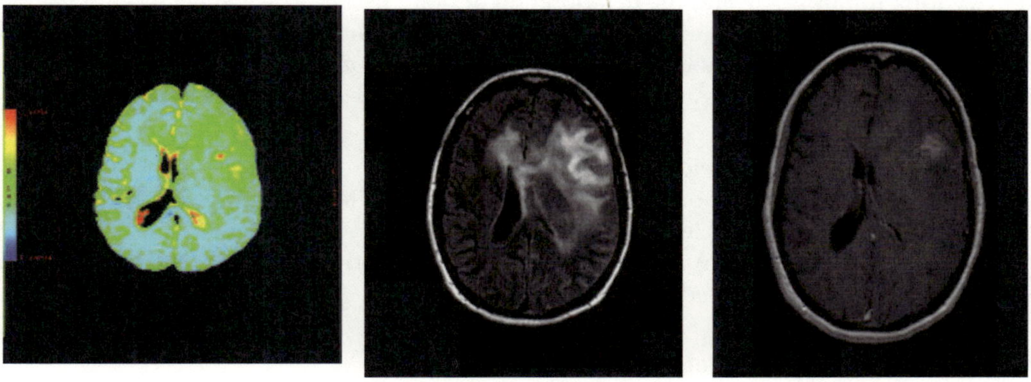

c) Diffusion, FLAIR, contrast enhancement: stability in diffusion and ADC, with FLAIR, and persistent contrast enhancement

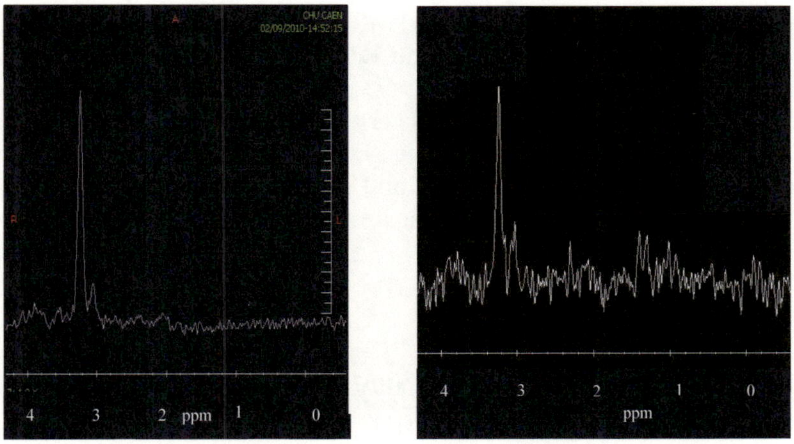

d) MRS: Increased proliferation (Cho at 3,22 ppm), glycolytic metabolism (lactate at 1,27-1,33 ppm), and infiltration (NAA at 2,02 ppm) at TE 144 and TE 288 ms

Fig. 6. Patient with good perfusion response to antiangiogenic treatment (Fig. 6b), but with a small amount of persistent contrast enhancement (Fig. 6c), intense increased proliferation, glycolytic metabolism, and infiltration (Fig. 6d)

3. Segmentation of brain tumor tissues using information fusion of MRI and MRS

For automated segmentation of brain tumor area, we have proposed a fuzzy information fusion based method (Dou, 2006; Dou et al., 2007a; Dou et al., 2007b), using T1-, T2-weighted and proton-density images. It is a feature fusion system, but it misses important biochemical information. The major biochemical characteristics can non invasively provide useful information on brain tumor type and grade (Howe et al., 2003b). Therefore, we propose a data-fusion strategy to segment brain tumors. This is an exponential companding method for enhancing the combination data from T2-weighted image and CSI signal. It automatically creates an MRS-weighted T2 structure image, which retains the high spatial resolution and brain structure information of the MR image while its grey levels correspond to the deterioration of brain tissues. The biochemical information is coherent for representing tumor grade and the deterioration of brain tissues. It is the key step in feature fusion for creating the feature models of glioma tissues, both for MRS values and for MR images. The combination modeling of these 2 types of information should separate the glioma tissues and normal tissues.

3.1 Features in models of glioma tissues

According to research done on brain tumor diagnosis by MR imaging and MRS, we can summarize 2 types of characteristics of glioma: one is the signal intensity of T1-weighted (with or without gadolinium) and T2-weighted images, and the other is the chemical-shift values of metabolites presented in MRS data.

3.1.1 Signal intensity characteristics of MR images

We have proposed some fuzzy modeling methods of different tumoral cerebral tissues on MR images based on fusion of tissue features (Dou et al. 2005a; 2005b; Dou, 2006; Dou et al., 2007a). Table 1 describes the characteristics of brain tissues by creating a gradation of signal intensity as a function of different tissues and MRI sequences (Dou et al., 2005a), where CSF is cerebral spinal fluid, GM is gray matter, and WM is white matter. In Table 1, the "Seqs" is used for "Sequences of MRI". The symbol "+" represents a hyper-signal; it means that the signal intensity is very high and the image is very bright. The symbol "-" represents a hypo-signal; the intensity is very low and the image is very dark. The symbol "-+" means that the signal intensity is higher than hypo-signal, and "+-" means that it is darker than hyper-signal. "- -" means that the signal intensity is lower than the hypo-signal, and "++" means that it is brighter than the hyper-signal.

Examples of T1-weighted image noted as T1, and T2-weighted image noted as T2 are shown in Fig. 7.

Sequences	Graduality of signal intensity					
	CSF	*GM*	*WM*	*Glioma*	*Edema*	*Necrosis*
T1	----	-	+++	---	--+	----
T2	++++	+	--	++	+++	++-

Table 1. Signal intensity characteristics of brain tissues on MR images.

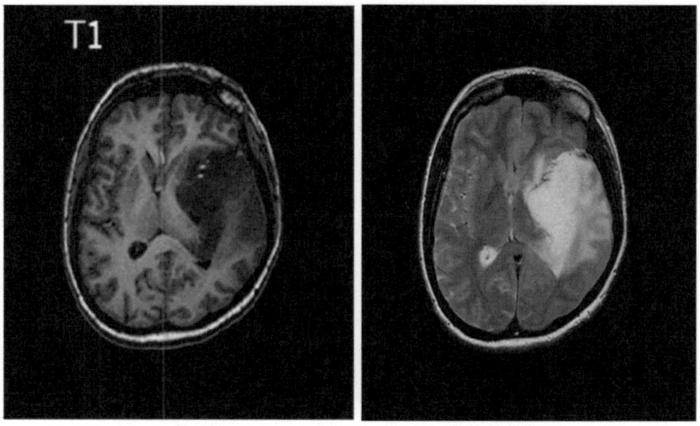

a) b)

Fig. 7. Original MRI images (a) T1 image, (b) T2 image

3.1.2 Features of metabolite changes in MRS

Among the large number of metabolites in the human body, there are only some that correspond to glioma. These include N-acetyl-asparate (NAA), creatine (Cr), choline (Cho), myo-inositol (mI), lactate (Lac), and free lipids (Lip). The variation in these metabolites can be ordered in a scalar form, as shown in Table 2, where the scalar order is: absent, very low, low, moderately (mod.) low, medium, moderately (mod.) high, high, or very high, which correspond to metabolite values from 0 to maximum. The metabolic changes with brain tissues are shown in Table 3. Data was obtained from previous studies (Brandao et al., 2003; Constans, 2006; Hoa, 2009; Dou et al., 2009).

Metabolite level	absent	very low	mod. low	low	medium	mod. high	high	very high
abbreviation	A	VL	LL	L	M	LH	H	VH

Table 2. Scalar description of metabolite values

Metabolite	**variation of metabolites corresponding with brain tissues**					
	CSF	***GM***	***WM***	***Glioma***	***Edema***	***Necrosis***
NAA	VL	VH	H	L/VL	M	A
Cho	A	M	LH	H/VH	LH	A
Cr	L	H	H	M/L	LL	A
mI	L	M	LH	H	LH/M	A
Lip	A	VL	L	H	L	VH
Lac	LH	VL	A	VH/H/LH	LH	H

Table 3. Metabolite change features in brain tissues on MRS

The metabolite-ratio characteristics of brain tissues, noted as *MetaR* and shown in Table 4, representing the *MetaR* characteristics of glioma, edema, and necrosis, are enhanced and the normal tissues are reduced. They correspond to signal intensity characteristics of the T2-weighted image described in Table 1.

Metabolite	**variation of metabolites corresponding with brain tissues**					
	CSF	***GM***	***WM***	***Glioma***	***Edema***	***Necrosis***
Cho/NAA	A	VL	L	VH	H	A
Cho/Cr	A	L	L	H	H	A
mI/Cr	M	L	M	H	H	A
Lip/Cr	A	VL	VL	H	M	VH
Lac/Cr	LH	VL	A	H	H	H

Table 4. Metabolite ratio characteristics of brain tissues

3.2 Data combination

There are 2 steps in the stage of data combination. The first, an important operation, is data localization, similar to data registration, used to adjust different data into a common coordination space. The second step is the actual combination.

3.2.1 Data localization

The operation of data localization is used to locate the MRS data to the CSI data, similar to a registration process. As their position vectors, recorded in the header of raw data, are under the same space coordinate, the volume of interest (VOI) field of MRS could be aligned to the image with the help of voxel spacings and position vectors. As shown in Fig. 8, the green grid represents the planar position of the voxels of a CSI on its reference image.

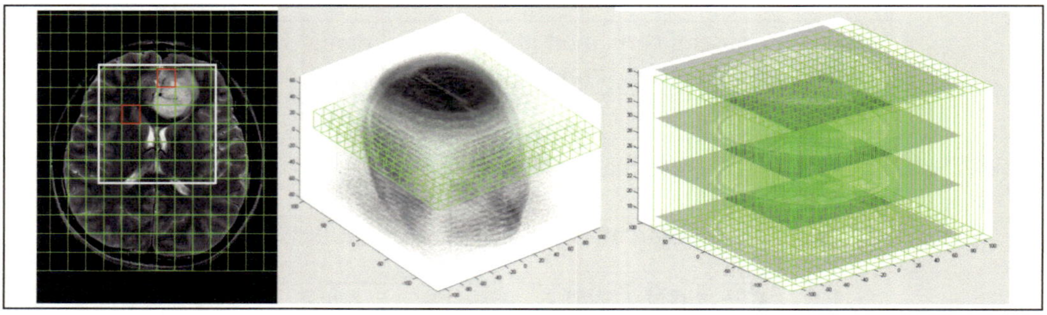

Fig. 8. An example of data location of MRS and T2 (left), the localization results are shown in 3D coordinate space (middle and right)

3.2.2 Data combination

Data combination is done as a multiplication operation as in (1). The MRS ratio is noted as *MetaR(i,v)*, where "*i*" is the metabolite index and "*v*" is the voxel index of CSI. The MR image is noted as *MRIm(p, g)*, where "*p*" is the pixel index, and "*g*" is the grey level of the MR image. Normally, *MetaR* is a function of the voxel determined by the CSI slice shown in Fig. 9. So, it is a 2-dimensional function noted as *MetaR(i,v)*. For the same reason, *ComIm* can be created as a 3-dimensional function, noted as *ComIm(v, p, g)*, where "*p*" is the pixel index corresponding to *MRIm*, and "*g*" is the grey level of a selected MR image and corresponds to "*p*". In fact, *MRIm* is a 2- dimensional function noted as *MRIm(p, g)*, where

$$g \in \mathbf{G},\ \text{and}\ \mathbf{G} = \{T1, T2, PD, FLAIR, Gado, Diffusion, Perfusion...\}$$

Consider 2 variables: *MRIm* and *Comlm*. *MRIm* is a given image like T2 and *Comlm* is an estimated image. The correlation model *MetaR* can be considered as some relationship between them. So, the regression-like model for estimating Gliolm from *MRIm* can be created as in equation (1).

$$ComIm(v, p, g) = MetaR(i, v)\Theta MRIm(p, g) \tag{1}$$

where "Θ" denotes a necessary operator and "*p*" corresponds to "*v*". If a linear regression is necessary, equation (1) can be rewritten as (2):

$$Glio\,\text{Im}(v, p, g) = MetaR(i, v) \times MR\,\text{Im}(p, g) + MetaR(j, v) \tag{2}$$

where "*i*" and "*j*" indicate different metabolites.

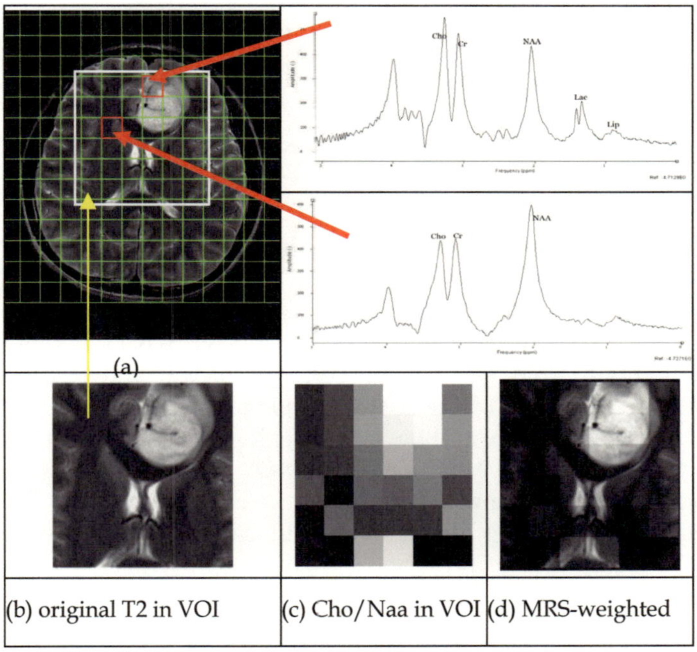

Fig. 9. Example of data combination of MRS and T2-weighted image. (a) is location image of CSI with VOI label (white line) on T2. The original image inside the region of VOI is enlarged and shown at (b). Two processed MRS resulting from step 1 are shown in the top right, corresponding to the voxels of CSI at the position of (1,4) and (3,2) of VOI, respectively. MRS ratio in (c) and combined image in (d).

T2 with localization information of CSI data is shown in Fig. 9 (a). Because MRS is available inside a VOI, marked with 6×6 white squares in Fig. 9(a), the combination of T2 and MRS should be done inside the VOI. Since the VOI contains multiple image slices, 1 MRS voxel corresponds to multi-pixel and multi-slices of an image.

Two examples of MRS are shown in Fig. 9 on the upper right. The top figure is MRS of a tumor voxel with coordinates (1, 4) in the VOI, and the bottom figure is that of normal tissue located in (3,2) of the VOI. The ratio of Cho/Naa for each voxel is shown in Fig.9(c). The data combination of MRS and MR image produces an MRS-weighted image shown in Fig.9 (d).

3.3 Exponential companding segmentation

To avoid mosaic effects, we propose a nonlinear regression-like model with spatial resolution registration in (3).

$$ComIm(v,p,g) = \exp\left[\frac{MRIm(p,g)}{T} \times MetaR(i,v)\right] + MetaR(j.v) \quad (3)$$

where "*T*" is a time constant corresponding to *MRIm* (*p*,*g*).
According to the correlation model of Table 4, the Lip/Cr and Lac/Cr are specific features w dependent on the tumor grade. So, in the model of equation (2), we have:

$$i \in \mathbf{I}, j \in \mathbf{J}, \quad MetaR = \mathbf{I} \cup \mathbf{J}$$
$$\mathbf{I} = \{Cho/Naa, Cho/Cr, mI/Cr\}$$
$$\mathbf{J} = \{Lip/Cr, Lac/Cr\}$$

Because the **J** of *MetaR* is the grade marker, it takes an interceptive role to make a different grey level from other voxels and indicates a variable grade.

3.3.1 Example of exponential companding segmentation

The segmentation method consists of 5 steps:

Step 1. Processing CSI data to get the relative quantitation of MRS, a ratio of peak amplitude or area between 2 metabolites, such as Cho/Naa, as shown in Fig. 9 (c).

Step 2. Extracting brain from original T2-weighted image, and selecting image slices contained in the volume of CSI as shown in Fig.10 (I).

Step 3. Combining the MRS ratio and the grey level information of selected image slices by multiplying the ratio of MRS, e.g. Cho/NAA, to attain MRS-weighted images as mentioned in 3.2, and shown in Fig.10 (II).

Step 4. Exponential companding to extend the difference of grey levels between normal tissue and tumor, is done as (2), and shown in Fig.10 (III).

$$ExpIm(v,p,g) = \exp(ComIm(v,p,g)/T) \quad (2)$$

where "*T*" is a time constant corresponding to *ComIm* and it is determined by the first peak of *ComIm* 's histogram.

Step 5: Tumor area segmentation by region growing, with the brightest pixel selected automatically as seed. The results are shown in Fig.10 (IV).

3.3.2 Material

The test data consists of CSI raw data and T2-weighted image. These data were acquired with STEAM sequence at the Beijing Tiantan hospital (China), with Siemens MR TrioTim (3T) and syngo MR B15. The MRS raw data are measured by csi_st/90 protocol with TR3000/TE72/TM6. T2-weighted images are measured by t2_tse_tra protocol with TR4500/TE80. An example of original test data is shown in the first row of Fig. 7.

The resolution of T2 is 0.57×0.57mm² pixel size and 5mm slice thickness. It can be noted as an image voxel of 0.57×0.57×5 mm³. The CSI location image shows that the MRS voxel size is 14×14×20mm³. According to the header information of CSI raw data, we can locate 3 ordinal slices of T2, as shown in Fig. 10(I).

3.3.3 Segmentation results

The first step is to process the CSI data to obtain the metabolite ratio. We use THU-MRS1.0, a software tool developed by our research group (Dou et al., 2009; Chi et al., 2011) for automated processing and quantitative analysis of MRS data, to calculate Cho/Naa voxel-by-voxel. An example is shown in Fig.9.

The segmentation result is shown in the fourth row of Fig.10. The output of each step of our method can be observed in Fig.10. The first row shows the result from step 2: 3 slices of original T2 contained in the volume of CSI. The second row shows the results of step 3: the product of the T2 intensity value and the ratio of MRS. The output of step 4, the exponential companding result, is shown in the third row.

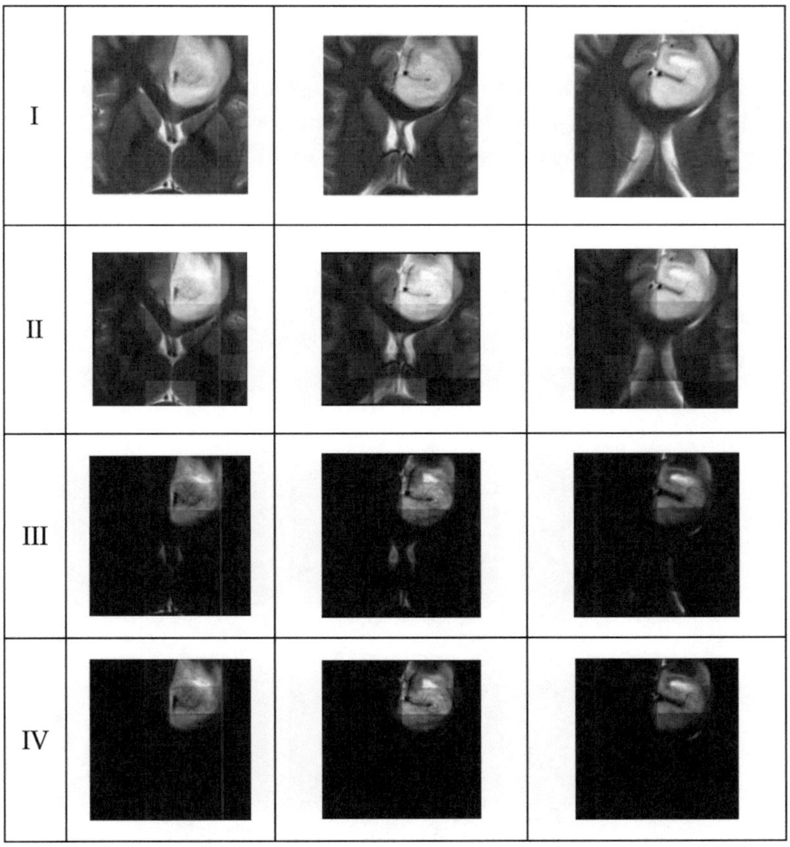

Fig. 10. Experiment results inside VOI of CSI. The first row shows 3 slices of original T2, which are contained in the volume of CSI, and resulting from step 2 of the proposed method; the second row presents the results of step 3, the third row resulted from step 4; and the last row represents the segmentation result from step 5.

3.3.4 Result evaluation

To evaluate the efficiency of our proposed method, we define the ratio of correct detection P_c and false detection P_f as (3) and (4), respectively.

$$p_c = \frac{N_{TruePositive}}{N_{RTumor}} \times 100\% \tag{3}$$

and

$$p_f = \frac{N_{FalsePositive}}{N_{RNormal}} \times 100\% \tag{4}$$

where $N_{RNormal}$ is the number of voxels in the region of normal brain tissues, and N_{RTumor} is that in the region of tumor tissues, as shown inside the red line in Fig.11. So, the total voxel number inside the VOI (white square in Fig.11) is the sum of $N_{RNormal}$ and N_{RTumor}. $N_{TruePositive}$ is the number of voxels which are detected as true positives and $N_{FalsePositive}$ is that of false positives.

A true or false positive is related to a standard model, called "ground truth". In our experiment, the ground truth is determined by manual labeling by 2 neuroradiologists, shown as a red circle in Fig.11. the first row is the "ground truth" of tumor plus potential edema area, called G1, and the second row is that of tumor only, called G2.

Comparing the segmentation result and the "ground truth", we obtain the evaluation results presented in Table 5. The correct detection rate is 98.89% for tumors with edema, and 99% for tumor only. The false detection rate in VOI is 6.48% for tumor with edema and 9.34% for tumor only.

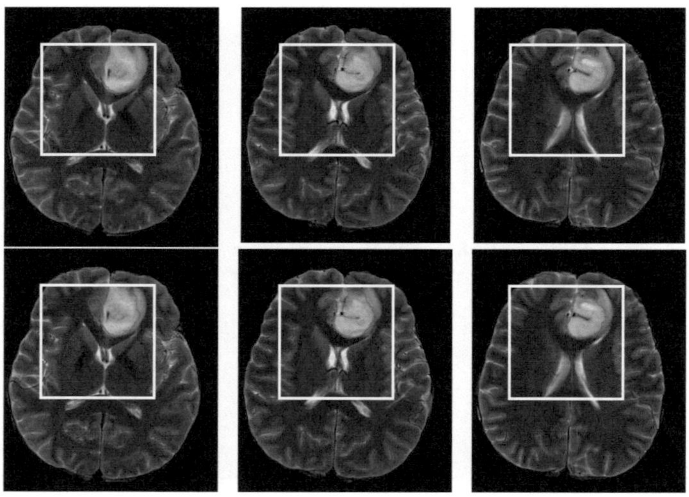

Fig. 11. The manual label results with potential edema, G1 (the first row), and without edema or tumor only, G2 (the second row).

4. Discussion

MRI remained stable for all patients, except for 2 late partial responses. MRS showed variable ratios of mI/Cr, Cho/Cr and NAA/Cr at baseline. We observed a decrease in Cho/Cr ratio and mI/Cr (to a lesser extent) and an increase in NAA/Cr ratio for patients whose clinical conditions improved and the reverse results for those whose conditions deteriorated.

Chemotherapy, radiation, and antiangiogenic therapies are widely used in the treatment of malignant brain tumors (Stupp et al., 2009; Tuettenberg et al., 2006), especially in gliomatosis that is inoperable, often leading to a mass effect in the progression, motor or language deficits or seizures and and development into high grade gliomas. Temozolomide was well tolerated. Patients had initial clinical and MRS improvement and stable MRIs. After 18 cycles, MRS showed an increase in the Cho/Cr ratio (proliferation). However, later in progression in 4 patients with hyperperfusion, this disappeared but proliferation (Cho/Cr), infiltration (NAA), and glycolytic metabolism (lactate) remained at a high level.

The glial tumor segmentation method using data fusion and exponential companding, is sensitive to the results of CSI processing and the quantitative analysis of MRS. The area ratio of metabolites is widely used in clinics when using single voxel spectroscopy (SVS). However, when using CSI data, the partial volume effects will affect neighboring voxels. It is then difficult to get a perfect MRS. In our experiment, the amplitude ratio of metabolites is better than area ratio because it is not as sensitive to processing results as the area ratio.

We used only one metabolite ratio, Cho/Naa, in our experiment, but for tumor grade definition the Lac and Lip are useful. An improved study will focus on CSI processing, data combination among other metabolites and other MR images, eg, T1-weighted, FLAIR, and gadolinium.

Ground truth	Segmentation validation in VOI	
	correct detection P_c (%)	*false detection* P_f (%) in VOI
G1	98.89	6.48
G2 (tumor only)	99	9.34

Table 5. Result evaluation of tumor segmentation in VOI

5. Conclusion

The spectroscopic and metabolic changes mentioned here, in addition to improve prognostic assessment (Law et al., 2003), occurred well before clinical deterioration and just before improvement. MRS allows non invasive follow-up of treated cerebral tumors. Therefore, MRS could be more sensitive and could detect changes earlier than MRI and is sometimes predictive.

There is a large amount of variability, but repetition and modelization of spectroscopic measurements during longitudinal follow-up could allow us to diminish it and to improve prognostic evaluation, especially in cases being treated with antiangiogenic therapy.

MRI, spectroscopy (MRS), and perfusion could be useful for monitoring energy (glutamine and glucose), glycolytic metabolism (lactate), necrosis (lipid metabolism), cell proliferation (Cho/Cr), and infiltration (NAA/Cr), and for classifying disease as stable or progressive. (Bendszus et al., 2000). These changes, as was shown, can be studied longitudinally and non invasively in humans with glial brain tumors after therapies (Callot et al., 2008). These repeated measures could give us more insight into the evolution at different times of the pathological processes, stages, tumor progression and response to therapies.

It will be important to follow gliomas to see if they become high grade glioma and even glioblastoma (Kannuki et al., 1998) in which we can study anatomical FLAIR, metabolism and proliferation with parameters from other modalities like MR, PET (11C-MET and 18F-FLT (Valable et al., 2011) and MRS. Studying the relationship between quantitative MRS measures, PET, MRI segmentation, and perfusion parameters could lead to a better understanding of tumoral pathological processes and therapeutic response, especially with regard to chemotherapy and antiangiogenic molecules, and in the future, hypoxia modulators and antioxidant molecules. These relationships could serve as a priori knowledge or constraints to improve fusion between CSI and MRI.

The segmentation method using data fusion of MRI and MRS is only a simple information fusion strategy, but it is effective for image segmentation. There are 2 important steps in this method: data combination and exponential companding; here, they act as image enhancement. It is a good example of image segmentation using data fusion of multimodal signals.

6. Acknowledgment

We would like to extend our thanks to Shaowu Li, professor of the Neuroimaging Center of Tiantan Hospital, Capital Medical University, Beijing, China, for his hard work on data scanning and his diagnostic experience; thanks to Yanping Chen, professor of Imaging Diagnostic Center of Nanfang Hospital, Guangzhou, China, for her hard work on manual labeling; thanks to François Kauffmann, assistant professor in the mathematics department of Caen University, for his hard work on data and signal processing; thanks to our excellent students Solène Collet, Gabriela Hossu, Aoyan Dong, Ping Chi and Shuai Wang for their hard work on some experiments. Also special thanks to Tsinghua National Laboratory for Information Science and Technology (TNList) Cross-discipline Foundation.

7. References

Auer DP, Gössl C, Schirmer T, et al. (2001) Improved analysis of 1H-MR spectra in the presence of mobile lipids. *Magn Reson Med.* 46: 615-8.

Bendszus M, Warmuth-Metz M, Klein R et al. (2000) MR Spectroscopy in Gliomatosis Cerebri, *American Journal of Neuroradiology* 21:375-380

Brandao, L. A. Domingues, R. C., (2003). MR spectroscopy of the brain, *Livraria e Editora Revinter Ltda.* 2003

Callot V, Galanaud D, Le Fur Y, et al. (2008) 1H MR spectroscopy of human brain tumours: a practical approach, *European Journal of Radiology* 67(2):268-274

Chi, P. Dou, W. Constans, J-M.,(2011). A Post-processing Approach of HLSVD Used for Automatic Quantitative Analysis of Multi-voxel Magnetic Resonance Spectra, *Proceedings of The 5th international conference on bioinformatics and biomedical engineering (iCBBE2011)*, May 10-12, 2011, Wuhan, China.

Chechin D, (2001) Méthode de traitement et de filtrage de signaux de SRM cérébrale proton simple volume, PhD Thesis.

Constans J.M., (2006) Sources de variabilité en SRM proton simple volume quantitative court TE STEAM chez des volontaires sains, PhD.thesis, 2006.

Delcroix N., (2000) Construction d'un système à base de connaissances pour le traitement du signal en spectroscopie 1H simple volume, PhD Thesis, Caen University, France.

Dou, W. Ren, Y. Chen, Y. Ruan, S. Bloyet, D. and Constans, J-M., (2005a). Histogram-based Generation Method of Membership Function for Extracting Features of Brain Tissues on MRI Images, *LNAI*, Vol.3613, 2005, pp.189-194.

Dou, W. Wu, Q. Chen, Y. Ruan, S. & Constans, J.-M., (2005b). Fuzzy modelling of different tumorous cerebral tissues on MRI images based on fusion of feature information, *Proceedings of 27th Annual International Conference of the IEEE Engineering in Medicine and Biology Society (EMBC 2005)*, pp.1-4, Shanghai, China, September 2005.

Dou W., (2006) Segmentation d'images multispectrales basées sur la fusion d'informations:application aux images IRM, PhD. thesis, 2006, Caen University, France.

Dou, W. Ruan, S. Chen, Y. Bloyet, D. & Constans, J.-M. (2007a). A framework of fuzzy information fusion for the segmentation of brain tumor tissues on MR images, *Image and Vision Computing*, Vol.25, 2007, pp. 164–171.

Dou W, Ren Y, Constans JM et al. (2007b) Fuzzy Kappa Used for the Agreement measure of Fuzzy Classifications. *Neurocomputing* Vol.70, 2007, pp:726-734.

Dou, W. Wang, S. Li, S. Constans, J-M.,(2009). Automatic Data Processing to Relative Quantitative Analysis of 1H MR Spectroscopy of Brain, *Proceedings of The 3rd international conference on bioinformatics and biomedical engineering (iCBBE2009)*, June 11-16, 2009, Beijing, China.

Dou, W. Dong, A. Chi, P. Li, S. Constans, J-M.,(2010). Glioma Tissue Modeling by Combining the Information of MRI and in vivo Multivoxel MRS, *Proceedings of The 4th international conference on bioinformatics and biomedical engineering (iCBBE2010)*, June 18-20, 2010, Chengdu, China.

Dou, W. Dong, A. Chi, P. Li, S. Constans, J-M.,(2011). Brain Tumor Segmentation Through Data Fusion of T2-Weighted Image and MR Spectroscopy, *Proceedings of The 5th international conference on bioinformatics and biomedical engineering (iCBBE2011)*, May 10-12, 2011, Wuhan, China.

Galanaud D, Nicoli F, Confort-Gouny S, et al. (2007) Indications for cerebral MR proton spectroscopy in 2007. *Rev Neurol.*; 163(3):287-303

Galanaud D, Chinot O, Nicoli F, et al. (2003) Use of proton magnetic resonance spectroscopy of the brain to differentiate gliomatosis cerebri from low-grade glioma. *J Neurosurg.* 98: 269-76.

Garcia-Gomez, J. Luts, J. Julia-Sape, M. Krooshof, P. Tortajada, S. Vicente, J. Melssen, W. Fuster-Garcia, E. Olier, I. Postma, G. Monleon, D. Moreno-Torres, A. Pujol, J. Candiota, A.-P. Martinez-Bisbal, MC. Suykens, JAK. Buydens, L. Celda, B. Van Huffel, S. Arus, C. & Robles, M. (2009) Multiproject-multicenter evaluation of automatic brain tumor classification by magnetic resonance spectroscopy, *Magnetic Resonance Materials in Physics, Biology and Medicine,* vol. 22, (Feb. 2009), pp. 5-18.

Gill SS, Thomas DG, Van Bruggen N, et al. (1990) Proton MR Spectroscopy of intracranial tumors: in vivo and in vitro studies. *J Comput Assist Tomogr.* 14: 497-504.

Guo Y., Ruan S., Landré J., Constans J-M., (2010) A Sparse Representation Method for Magnetic Resonance Spectroscopy Quantification. *IEEE Trans Biomed Eng.* 57(7):1620-7.

Hart MG, Grant R, Garside R, Rogers G, Somerville M, Stein K, (2008) Temozolomide for high grade glioma, Cochrane Database Syst Rev. **2008** Oct 8;(4):CD007415

Hoa, D. (September 2009). Metabolites Explored in 1H-MRS, September 2009, Available from http://www.imaios.com/en/e-Courses/e-MRI/Magnetic-Resonance-Spectroscopy-MRS

Hossu G, (2009) Spectroscopie quantitative par Résonance Magnétique proton en conditions cliniques: étude de la variabilité d'un dispositif ERETIC et spectres de médicaments, PhD Thesis, France, 2009

Howe FA. Opstad KS. (2003a). 1H MR Spectroscopy of brain tumors and masses. *NMR Biomed.* 16: 123-31.

Howe, FA. Barton, SJ. Cudlip, SA. Stubbs, M. Saunders, DE. Murphy, M. Wilkins, P. Opstad, KS. Doyle, VL. McLean, MA. Bell, BA. & Griffiths JR. (2003b). Metabolic profiles of human brain tumors using quantitative in vivo 1H magnetic resonance spectroscopy. *Magn Reson Med.* Vol.49, No.2, (Feb. 2003), pp.223-32.

Kannuki S, Hirose T, Horiguchi H, et al. (1998) Gliomatosis cerebri with secondary glioblastoma formation: report of two cases, *Brain Tumor Pathol.* 15(2):111-6

Kuesel AC, Sutherland GR, Halliday W, et al. (1994) 1H MRS of high grade astrocytomas: mobile lipid accumulation in necrotic tissue. *NMR Biomed.* 7: 149-155

Law M, Yang S, Wang H et al. (2003) Glioma grading: sensitivity, specificity, and predictive values of perfusion MR imaging and proton MR spectroscopic imaging compared with conventional MR imaging. AJNR Am J Neuroradiol. 2003;24(10):1989-98

Luts, J. Laudadio, T. Martinez-Bisbal, MC., Van Cauter, S. Molla, E. Piquer, J. Suykens, JAK. Himmelreich, U. Celda, B. & Van Huffel, S. (2009). Differentiation between brain metastases and glioblastoma multiforme based on MRI, MRS and MRSI", *in Proc. of the 22nd IEEE International Symposium on Computer-Based Medical Systems (CBMS)*, pp. 1-8, Albuquerque, New Mexico, Aug. 2009.

Majós, C. Aguilera, C. Cos, M. Camins, A. Candiota, AP. Delgado-Goñi, T. Samitier, A. Castañer, S. Sánchez, JJ. Mato, D. Acebes, JJ. & Arús, C. (2009). In vivo proton magnetic resonance spectroscopy of intraventricular tumours of the brain, *Eur Radiol.* Vol.19, No.8, (Aug. 2009), pp.2049-59.

Maudsley, AA. Domenig, C. Govind, V. Darkazanli, A. Studholme, C. Arheart, K. & Bloomer, C. (2009). Mapping of brain metabolite distributions by volumetric proton MR spectroscopic imaging (MRSI), *Magnetic Resonnance in Medicin,* Vol.61, (2009), pp.548-559.

Naressi A. (2001) Parametric quantive method and simulation with cerebral metabolites knowledge from modelisations of spectroscopic signatures (jMRUI) and physical properties of molecules. *Computers in Biol. and Med* 31: 269.

Nelson SJ, Graves E, Pirzkall A, et al. (2002) In vivo molecular imaging for planning radiotherapy of gliomas: an application of 1H MRSI. *J Magn Reson Imaging*. 16: 464-476

Nelson S., (1989) Semi-parametric method. *J. Magn. Reson. Imag*. 84: 95.

Preul, MC. Caramanos, Z. Collins, DL. Villemure, J-G. Leblanc, R. Olivier, A. Pokrupa, R. & Arnold, D. (1996) Accurate, non-invasive diagnosis of human brain tumors by using proton magnetic resonance spectroscopy. *Nat Med,* Vol.2, (1996), pp.323–325.

Provencher S., (1982) Parametric method (LCModel) with cerebral metabolites knowledge from modelisations of spectroscopic signatures. *Comput. Phys. Commun* 27: 213.

Soffietti R, Baumert BG, Bello L, Von Deimling A, Duffau H, Frénay M, Grisold W, Grant R, Graus F, Hoang-Xuan K, Klein M, Melin B, Rees J, Siegal T, Smits A, Stupp R, Wick W, (2010) Guidelines on management of low-grade gliomas: report of an EFNS–EANO† Task Force, European Journal of Neurology, Vol17, Issue 9,p 1124-1133, September 2010

Stubbs M, Veech RL, Griffiths JR, (1995) Tumor metabolism: the lessons of magnetic resonance spectroscopy. *Adv Enzyme Regul.* 35: 101-115.

Stupp R, Hegi M, Mason W, et al., (2009) Effects of radiotherapy with concomitant and adjuvant temozolomide versus radiotherapy alone on survival in glioblastoma in a randomised phase III study: 5-year analysis of the EORTC-NCIC trial, *The Lancet Oncology* 10: 459 - 466,

Tuettenberg J, Friedel C, Vaikoczy P, (2006) Angiogenesis in malignant glioma - A target for antitumor therapy? *Crit Rev Oncol Hematol* 59:181-193

Valable S, Petit E, Roussel S et al Complementary information from MRI and [18F]-FMISO PET in the assessment of the response to an anti-angiogenic treatment in a rat brain tumor model, Nuclear Medicine and Biology, in press

Wang, Q. Eirini Karamani Liacouras, Erickson Miranda, Uday S. Kanamalla, and Vasileios Megalooikonomou, (2007). Classification of brain tumors using MRI and MRS data, *Proc. SPIE* 6514, (2007) pp.65140S-1~8.

6

3D Tumor Segmentation from Volumetric Brain MR Images Using Level-Sets Method

Kamel Aloui and Mohamed Saber Naceur
National Engineering School, LTSIRS Laboratory – Tunis
Tunisia

1. Introduction

1.1 Statement of the problem

Segmentation in volumetric images is a tool allowing a diagnostics automation and as well will assist experts in quantitative and qualitative analysis. It's an important step in various applications such as visualization, morphometrics and image-guided surgery. In the context of neuro-imaging, brain tumor segmentation from Magnetic Resonance Images (MRI) is extremely important for treatment planning, therapy monitoring, examining efficacy of radiation and drug treatments and studying the difference between healthy subjects and subjects with brain tumor. The task of manually segmentation of brain tumor from MR images is generally time-consuming and difficult. Anyway, the task is done by marking by hand the tumor regions slice-by-slice which generates set of jaggy images, so the practitioner is confronted with a succession of boundary which he mentally stacked up to be made a 3D shape of brain tumor. This shape is inevitably subjective and becomes infeasible when dealing with large data sets, also there is losing of information in the third dimension because is not taken into account in the segmentation process. All this, affect the quality and accuracy of clinical diagnosis. An automatic or semi-automatic segmentation method of brain tumor that takes entire information within the volumetric MR image into account is desirable as it reduces the load on the human raters and generates optimal segmented images (Wang & al., 2004), (Michael & al., 2001), (Lynn & al., 2001). Specially, automatic brain tumor segmentation presents many challenges and involves various disciplines such us pathology, MRI physics and image processing. Brain tumors are difficult to segment because they vary greatly in size and position, may be of any size, may have a variety of shapes and may have overlapping intensities with normal tissue and edema. This leads to numerous segmentation approaches of automatic brain tumor extraction. Low-level segmentation methods, such as pixel-based clustering, region growing, and filter-based edge detection, requires additional pre-processing and post-processing as well as considerable amounts of expert intervention and a priori knowledge on the regions of interest (ROI) (Sahoo & al., 1988). Recently, several attempts have been made to apply deformable models to brain image analysis (Moon & al., 2002). Indeed, deformable models refer to a large class of computer vision methods and have proved to be a successful segmentation technique for a wide range of applications. Deformable models, on the other hand, provide an explicit representation of the boundary and the ROI shape. They combine several desirable features such as inherent connectivity and smoothness, which counteract noise and boundary irregularities, as well as the ability to incorporate knowledge about the ROI. However, parametric deformable model must be re-parameterized dynamically to recover the object boundary and that has difficulty in dealing with topological adaptation such as splitting or merging model parts. A level-Sets deformable model, also referred to as a geometric deformable model, provides an elegant solution to address the primary limitations of parametric deformable models (Taheri & al., 2009), (Taheri & al., 2007), (Lefohn & al., 2003). These methods have drawn a great deal of attention since their introduction in 1988. Advantages of the contour implicit formulation of the deformable model over parametric formulation include: no parameterization of the contour, topological flexibility, good numerical stability and straightforward extension of the 2D formulation to n-D.

1.2 Outline of our method

In this work, we describe various segmentation tools for segmenting brain tumor from volumetric MR images based on Level-Sets method. Figure 1 shows a general diagram of developed segmentation tools. We develop a first technique of brain tumor segmentation by stacking a sequence of 2D tumor contours, detected by 2D level-Sets method in the parallel cross-sectional MRI images. It consists on applying to each brain MRI slice the 2D level-Sets method and to propagate the result by taking as initial data the result of the preceding slice. The first approach is similar to an expert reasoning. This approach has several advantages such as simplicity to implement; it is fast, it requires less time than manual segmentation but it has a major disadvantage : the information loss because the third dimension is not taken into account. However, an evolution was necessary to the glance of its defects. The second and third developed approaches come to improve segmentation quality, based on carry out the computation in 3D space and detect the 3D tumor surface directly using 3D level-Sets method. In the second approach the 3D level-sets model evolves according to information related to contours on IRM volume. The third proposed method is similar to the segmentation with a deformable model with two phased image. Explicitly no need for gradient information, the level-Sets model evolves according to related regions information in the volumetric MR image.
In order to evaluate the proposed segmentation tools, MRI volumetric images have been used. They can be downloaded from the well known MeDEISA database « Medical Database for the Evaluation of Image and Signal Processing Algorithms », (MeDEISA, 2010).

1.3 Structure of the chapter

This chapter is organized as follows:

- In the next section, we present the level-Sets formulation and principal steps of the segmentation algorithm.
- In Section 3, 3D brain tumor segmentation by stacking a sequence of its 2D contours is described. For this purpose, 2D level-Sets method is required to detect tumor contours in the parallel cross-sectional MRI images.
- In section 4, we present 3D brain tumor segmentation using volumetric approaches based on boundary and region information on volumetric MRI data to check the deformable surface propagation.
- Finally, a summary and discussion related to this work are given in section 5.

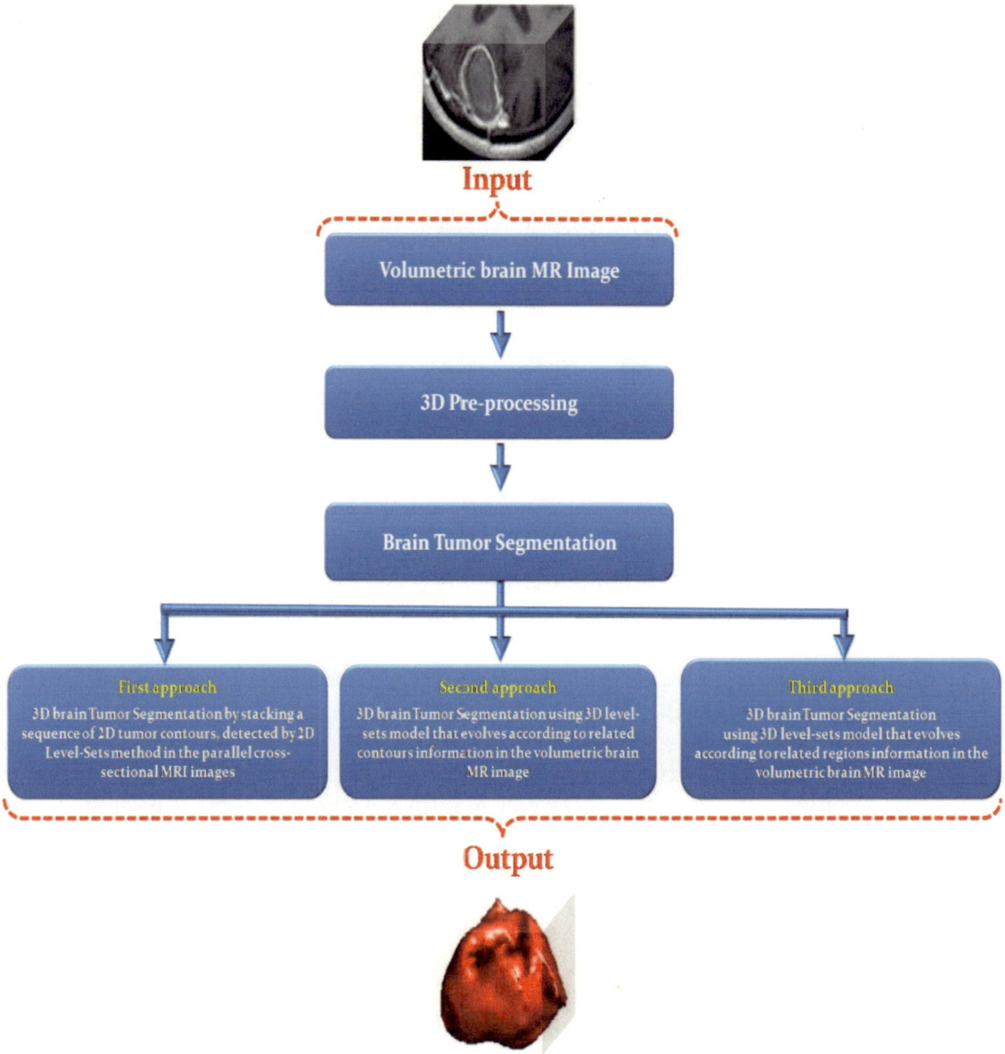

Fig. 1. General diagram of developed segmentation tools for segmenting 3D brain tumor from volumetric MR images based on Level-Sets method.

2. Level-set method: Presentation

In this Section, we describe a modeling technique based on a level-Sets approach for recovering shapes of objects in two and three dimensions. The modeling technique may be viewed as a form of active modeling such as "snakes" (Kass & al., 1988) and deformable surfaces (Terzopoulos & al. 1988). The model which consists of a moving front, until is plated on the desired shape, by externally applied stop criteria synthesized from the image data (Fig. 2.). Specially, deformable models are curves or surfaces defined in a digital image that can move under the influence of external and internal forces. External forces, which are computed from the image data, are designed to keep the model smooth during deformations. The external forces are defined from the deformable curve or surface like curvature in order to move the model to the boundary of a region of interest (ROI) in the digital image. Using these two forces, deformable models offer robustness to both image noise and boundary gaps, by constraining extracted ROI's boundaries to be smooth and incorporating other prior information about the ROI shape. Moreover, the resulting boundary representation can achieve subpixel accuracy which is considered a highly desirable property for medical imaging applications.

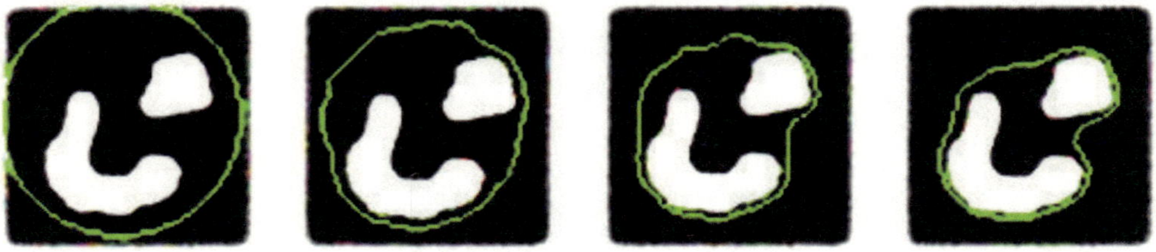

a) b) c) d)

Fig. 2. Principle of deformable curve in two space dimensions. We show curve evolution in time.

There are basically two types of deformable models:

- Parametric deformable models (Kass & al., 1988), (Amini & al., 1990), (Cohen, 1991) and (McInerney & al., 1995);
- Geometric deformable models (Caselles & al., 1993), (Milladi & al., 1995), (Caselles & al., 1995) and (Whitaker, 1994).

Parametric deformable models represent curves and surfaces explicitly in their parametric forms during deformation. This representation allows direct interaction with the model and can lead to a compact representation for fast real-time implementation. Adaptation of the model topology such as splitting or merging parts during the deformation can be difficult using parametric models. However, geometric deformable models can handle topological changes naturally. These models, based on the theory of curve evolution (Sapiro & Tannenbaum, 1993), (Kimia & al., 1995), (Kimmel & al., 1995), (Alvarez & al., 1993) and the level set method (Osher & Sethian, 1988), (Sethian, 1999) represent curves and surfaces implicitly as a level-Sets of a higher-dimensional scalar function. Their parameterizations are computed only after complete deformation, thereby allowing topological adaptively to be easily accommodated. Despite this fundamental difference, the principles of both methods are very similar. Level-Sets method as a geometric deformable model; provide an elegant solution to address the primary limitations of parametric deformable models. In particular, curves and surfaces move using only geometric measures and other prior information from the image data to recover ROI boundaries.

In this section, we first review the fundamental concepts in curve evolution theory and the level-Sets method.

2.1 Curve evolution theory

The purpose of curve evolution theory is to study the deformation of curves using only geometric measures such as the curvature and the unit normal. Let us consider a moving curve $\Gamma(t)$, where t represents the time;

The evolution of the curve along its normal direction can be characterized by the following partial differential equation (Fig. 3.):

$$\frac{\partial \Gamma}{\partial t} = F(k)\vec{N} \tag{3}$$

Where:

- N denote inward unit normal;
- k is the curvature.

Where F is called speed function, since it determines the curve evolution speed. We note that a curve moving in some arbitrary direction can always be reparameterized to have the same form as Eq. 3 (Kimia, 1990). The intuition behind this fact is that the tangent deformation affects only the curve's parameterization, not its shape and geometry.

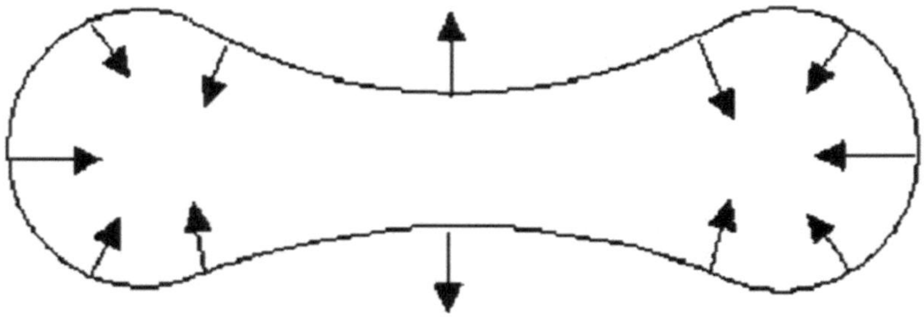

Fig. 3. Curve moving in the normal direction.

The most extensively studied curve deformations are constant deformation and curvature deformation. Constant deformation is given by:

$$\frac{\partial \Gamma}{\partial t} = V_0 \vec{N} \tag{4}$$

Where V_0 is a coefficient determining the speed and direction of deformation (shrinks or expands). Constant deformation plays the same role as the pressure force in parametric deformable models.
Curvature deformation is given by the so-called geometric heat equation (Osher & Sethian, 1988):

$$\frac{\partial \Gamma}{\partial t} = \alpha k \vec{N} \tag{5}$$

Where α is a positive constant. This equation will smooth a curve, eventually shrinking it to a circular point (Grayson, 1985). The use of the curvature deformation has an effect similar to the use of the elastic internal force in parametric deformable models.
The properties of curvature deformation and constant deformation are complementary to each other. Constant deformation can create singularities from an initially smooth curve while curvature deformation removes singularities by smoothing the curve.
The basic idea of the geometric deformable model is to couple the speed of deformation (using curvature and/or constant deformation) with the image data, so that the evolution of the curve stops at ROI's boundaries. The evolution is implemented using the level-Sets method.

2.2 Level-Sets method: Basic algorithms

We now review the level-Sets method for implementing curve evolution. The level-Sets method is used to account for automatic topology adaptation, and it also provides the basis for a numerical scheme that is used by geometric deformable models. The level-Sets method for evolving curves is due to Osher and Sethian (Osher & Sethian, 1988), (Sethian, 1985) and (Sethian, 1989). The interface Γ bounds a (possibly multiply connected) region Ω. The goal is to compute and analyze the subsequent motion of Γ under a velocity field F. This velocity can depend on position X (Where $X = (x, y)$ in tow space dimensions or $X = (x, y, z)$ in three space dimensions), time, the geometry of the interface and the external physics. The interface is captured as the zero level-Sets of a smooth function:

$$\varphi(X,t), \text{ i.e., } \Gamma(t) = \{X | \varphi(X,t) = 0\} \tag{6}$$

φ is positive inside Ω, negative outside Ω and is zero on $\Gamma(t)$, has the following properties:

$$\begin{cases} \varphi(X,t) \succ 0 & for \quad X \in \Omega \\ \varphi(X,t) \prec 0 & for \quad X \notin \Omega \\ \varphi(X,t) = 0 & for \quad X \in \partial\Omega = \Gamma(T) \end{cases} \tag{7}$$

Thus, the interface is to be captured for all later time, by merely locating the set $\Gamma(t)$ for which φ vanishes.

We note that the only purpose of the level-Sets function is to provide an implicit representation of the evolving curve and the topological merging and breaking are well defined and easily performed. Instead of tracking a curve through time, the level-Sets method evolves a curve by updating the level-Sets function at fixed coordinates through time. A useful property of this approach is that the level-Sets function remains a valid function while the embedded curve can change its topology. The motion is analyzed by convecting the φ values (levels) with the velocity field F. This elementary equation is:

$$\frac{\partial \varphi}{\partial t} + \vec{F}(k) \nabla \varphi = 0 \tag{8}$$

Where $\nabla \varphi$ denotes the gradient of φ.

Here F is the desired velocity on the interface, and is arbitrary elsewhere.

Actually, only the normal component of F is needed. The inward unit normal to the level-Sets curve is given by:

$$\vec{N} = \frac{\nabla \varphi}{|\nabla \varphi|} \tag{9}$$

Then

$$F_N(k) = \vec{F}(k) \frac{\nabla \varphi}{|\nabla \varphi|} \tag{10}$$

Accordingly, Eq. 8 becomes

$$\frac{\partial \varphi}{\partial t} + F_N(k)|\nabla \varphi| = 0 \tag{11}$$

Finally, the curvature k at the zero level-Sets is given by:

$$k = div\left(\frac{\nabla \varphi}{|\nabla \varphi|}\right) = \frac{\varphi_{xx}\varphi_y^2 - 2\varphi_x\varphi_y\varphi_{xy} + \varphi_{yy}\varphi_x^2}{\left(\varphi_x^2 + \varphi_y^2\right)^{2/3}} \tag{12}$$

2.3 Level-sets: Speed function

The geometric deformable contour formulation, proposed in (Caselles & al., 1993) and (Malladi & al., 1995), takes the following form:

$$\frac{\partial \varphi}{\partial t} + F_N(k)|\nabla \varphi| = g(I)(V_0 + \varepsilon k)|\nabla \varphi| \tag{13}$$

Where

$$g(I) = \frac{1}{1 + |\nabla \hat{I}|^p} \tag{14}$$

Positive V_0 shrinks the curve, and negative V_0 expands the curve. The curve evolution is coupled with the image data through a multiplicative stopping term $g(I)$. Where $\hat{I}$ is the image corrected by a Gaussian operator and $p = 1\ or\ 2$. This scheme can work well for objects that have good contrast. However, when the object boundary is indistinct or has gaps, the geometric deformable contour may leak out because the multiplicative term only slows down the curve near the boundary rather than completely stopping the curve. Once the curve passes the boundary, it will not be pulled back to recover the correct boundary.

2.4 Level-Sets: Numerical implementation

Various numerical implementations of deformable models have been reported in the literature. For examples, the finite difference method (Kass & al., 1988), dynamic programming (Amini & al., 1990), and greedy algorithm (Williams & Shah, 1992) have been used. In this section, we present the finite difference method implementation for level-Sets method as described in (Kass & al., 1988).

2.4.1 Initialization

An initial function $\varphi(X, t = 0)$ must be constructed such that its zero level-Sets correspond to the position of the initial contour or surface. A common choice is to set:

$$\varphi(X, t = 0) = d(x) \tag{15}$$

Where $d(x)$ is the signed distance from each grid point to the zero level-Sets.
For example, when the zero level-Sets can be described by the exterior boundary of a circle, the signed distance function can be computed as follows:

$$\varphi(x, y, t = 0) = \sqrt{(x - x_0)^2 + (y - y_0)^2} - r \tag{16}$$

Where $X_0 = (x_0, y_0)$ is the center and r is the radius of the circle.

2.4.2 Discretization of the motion equation

Since the motion equation Eq. 13 is derived for the zero level-Sets only, the speed function $F(k)$, in general, is not defined on other level-Sets. Hence, we need a method to extend the speed function $F(k)$ to all of the level-Sets. A re-initialization of the level-Sets function to a signed distance function is often required for level-Sets schemes.
The discretization of equation Eq. 13 is given as follows; noting (i, j) is a position in the tow space dimensions image data:

$$\frac{\varphi_{ij}^{n+1} - \varphi_{ij}^{n}}{\Delta t} = F_{ij} \left| \nabla_{ij} \varphi_{ij}^{n} \right| \tag{17}$$

where :

- φ_{ij}^{n} : φ values in position (i, j) at the iteration $n\Delta t$.
- $\nabla_{ij} \varphi_{ij}^{n}$: Spatial gradient approximation space of φ_{ij}^{n} with the finite difference.
- $F_{ij} = g_{ij}(I)(F_{0ij} + \varepsilon k_{ij})$.

2.4.3 Discretization of gradient

If the temporal gradient approximation does not pose a problem, it is not the same for the spatial gradient. According to the spatial gradient is a factor in the curvature or constant term, it takes a different form (Osher & Sethian, 1988), (Malladi & al., 1995) and (Sethian, 1985). Indeed, if the curve evolves in various directions (eg according to its curvature), there is no particular problem. But, if the curve evolves in a given direction (eg. Constant deformation V_0), the choice of the spatial gradient is crucial: if it is calculated on a "simple", it can lead to loops formation during the deformation. Once the corner is developed, it is not clear how to continue the deformation, since the definition of the normal direction becomes ambiguous (Fig. 4.). A natural way to continue the deformation is to impose the so-called entropy condition originally proposed in the area of interface propagation by Sethian (Sethian, 1982), (Sethian, 1994).
Since the numerical scheme of the spatial gradient in one space dimension can be written as follows:

$$|\nabla \varphi_i| = \left| \frac{\varphi_{i+1} - \varphi_{i-1}}{2\Delta x} \right| \tag{18}$$

When, there is a deformation in various directions, (when $|\nabla \varphi_i|$ is the curvature k factor);

$$|\nabla \varphi_i| = \left(\left(\max\left(D_x^- \varphi_i, 0\right)\right)^2 + \left(\min\left(D_x^+, 0\right)\right)^2 \right)^{1/2} \tag{19}$$

When, there is a constant deformation, (when $|\nabla \varphi_i|$ is constant deformation V_0 factor);

Where

- $D_x^- \varphi_i = \dfrac{\varphi_i - \varphi_{i-1}}{\Delta x}$
- $D_x^+ \varphi_i = \dfrac{\varphi_{i+1} - \varphi_i}{\Delta x}$

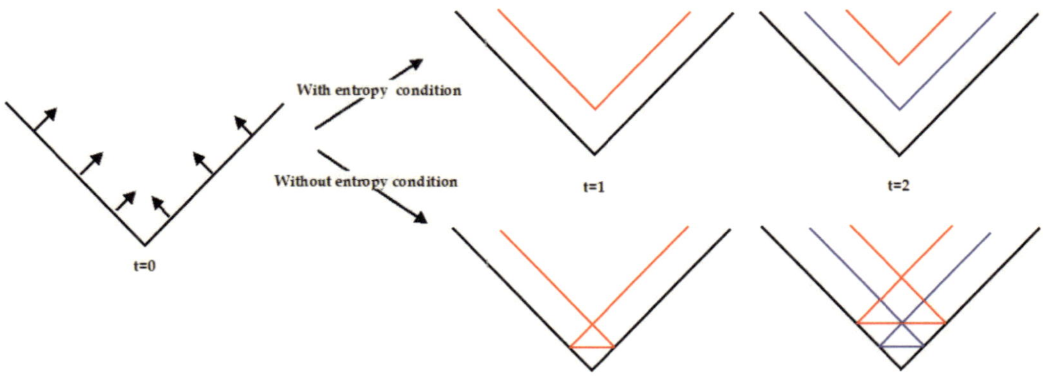

Fig. 4. Curve moving in the normal direction with the entropy condition. Deformation without entropy condition shows swallowtails and loops during the deformation.

2.5 Numerical scheme of the motion function

In this section, we provide a numerical implementation that is adapted from (Sethian, 1999) for Eq. 13, in which ε and V_0 are allowed to be functions. The spatial derivatives are implemented using a special numerical scheme that can handle the formation of sharp corners during deformation. The numerical implementation is given as follows:

$$\varphi_{ij}^{n+1} = \varphi_{ij}^{n} + \Delta t \begin{pmatrix} g_{ij}(I)\varepsilon k_{ij}^{n}\left[\left(D_{ij}^{0x}\right)^2 + \left(D_{ij}^{0y}\right)^2\right]^{1/2} + \\ \max\left(g_{ij}(I)V_{0ij}, 0\right)\nabla^{+}\varphi + \min\left(g_{ij}(I)V_{0ij}, 0\right)\nabla^{-}\varphi \end{pmatrix} \quad (20)$$

Where

$$D_{ij}^{0x} = \frac{\varphi_{i+1,j}^{n} - \varphi_{i-1,j}^{n}}{2\Delta x}, \qquad D_{ij}^{0y} = \frac{\varphi_{i,j+1}^{n} - \varphi_{i,j-1}^{n}}{2\Delta x}$$

$$D_{ij}^{+x} = \frac{\varphi_{i+1,j}^{n} - \varphi_{i,j}^{n}}{\Delta x}, \qquad D_{ij}^{+y} = \frac{\varphi_{i,j+1}^{n} - \varphi_{i,j}^{n}}{\Delta x}$$

$$D_{ij}^{-x} = \frac{\varphi_{i,j}^{n} - \varphi_{i-1,j}^{n}}{\Delta x}, \qquad D_{ij}^{+y} = \frac{\varphi_{i,j}^{n} - \varphi_{i,j-1}^{n}}{\Delta x}$$

$$\nabla^+\varphi = \begin{bmatrix} \left(\max(D_{ij}^{-x}\varphi_{ij},0)\right)^2 + \left(\min(D_{ij}^{+x}\varphi_{ij},0)\right)^2 \\ \left(\max(D_{ij}^{-y}\varphi_{ij},0)\right)^2 + \left(\min(D_{ij}^{+y}\varphi_{ij},0)\right)^2 \end{bmatrix}^{1/2}$$

$$\nabla^-\varphi = \begin{bmatrix} \left(\min(D_{ij}^{-x}\varphi_{ij},0)\right)^2 + \left(\max(D_{ij}^{+x}\varphi_{ij},0)\right)^2 \\ \left(\min(D_{ij}^{-y}\varphi_{ij},0)\right)^2 + \left(\max(D_{ij}^{+y}\varphi_{ij},0)\right)^2 \end{bmatrix}^{1/2}$$

As it has been specified previously, the level-Sets function evolves using a speed function for the zero level-Sets only and using extended speed functions. Accordingly, the level-Sets can lose its property of being a signed distance function, causing inaccuracy in curvature and normal calculations. As a result, re-initialization of the level-Sets function to a signed distance function is often required for these schemes.

Usually, the distance map is reset using the following equation (Sussman & al., 1997):

$$\frac{\partial \varphi}{\partial t} = signe\,(\varphi) \times \left(1 - |\nabla \varphi|\right) \tag{21}$$

Where

$$signe\,(\varphi) = \begin{cases} -1 & si \quad \varphi \prec -1 \\ |\varphi| & si \quad -1 \prec \varphi \prec 1 \\ +1 & si \quad \varphi \succ 1 \end{cases}$$

Since the curve or the surface of ROI is recovred from the zero level-Sets only. We must therefore detect the zero values of the function φ .We can only detect differences in sign between two consecutive points in either direction, horizontal and vertical. The detection of points $P(i,j)$ of zero level-Sets by Malladi (Malladi & al., 1995) is done according to the following algorithm:

Recovering interface algorithm:

Function $isfront\,(\varphi)$

$\forall i, j \in \varphi$

if	$\left(\max\left(\varphi(i,j), \varphi(i+1,j), \varphi(i,j+1), \varphi(i+1,j+1)\right) \succ 0\right)$ ***and***
	$\left(\min\left(\varphi(i,j), \varphi(i+1,j), \varphi(i,j+1), \varphi(i+1,j+1)\right) \prec 0\right)$ ***or***
	$\left(\max\left(\varphi(i,j)\right) = 0\right)$

then

$P(i,j) \in \Gamma(t)$

else

$P(i,j) \notin \Gamma(t)$

end

end

2.6 Level-sets: Stop function

The multiplicative stopping term of the speed function is defined as $g(I)$ given by eq. 14. It has values that are closer to zero in regions of high image gradient and values that are closer to unity in regions with relatively constant intensity. $\hat{I}$ denotes the image convolved with a Gaussian smoothing filter whose characteristic width is σ. In some image slices, the boundary feature of the tumor is not salient enough and the image gradient information is weak. It usually causes the "boundary leaking" problem when we apply the level set method to detect the 3D tumor surface. The problem of the Gaussian filtering is the smoothing of the entire image, destroys and moves edges.

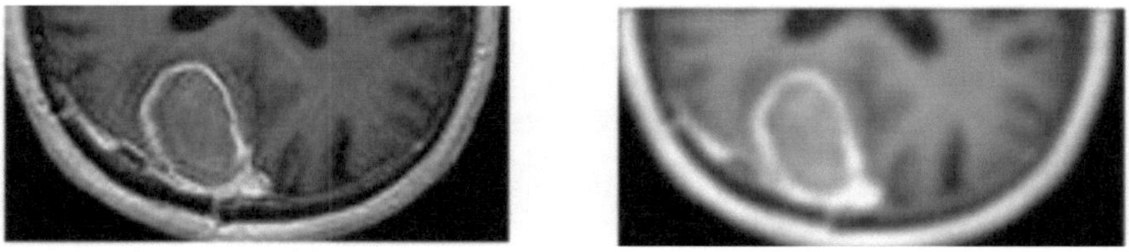

(a) (b)

Fig. 5. Gaussian filters: destroys and moves edges. (a) Original image, (b) image smoothed by a Gaussian filter.

So we need to limit or prohibit the smoothing operation of the contours in the MR images. For this, we must choose a filter aiming at reducing image noise without removing significant parts of the image content, typically edges, lines or other details of the MR image. The anisotropic diffusion filter proposed by P. Perona and J. Malik (Perona & Malik, 1990) meets our needs. The action of such filter is given by the following nonlinear equation:

$$\frac{\partial I(X,t)}{\partial t} = div\left(c(X,t).\nabla I(X,t)\right) \tag{22}$$

That preserves edges and only smooths regions with relatively constant intensity, $c(X,t)$, is called conduction coefficient. When the diffusion coefficient is chosen as an edge seeking function, the resulting equations encourage diffusion (hence smoothing) within regions with relatively constant intensity and prohibit it across strong edges. Hence, the edges can be preserved while removing noise from the image.
An illustration of the action of anisotropic diffusion filter is given by the following figure:

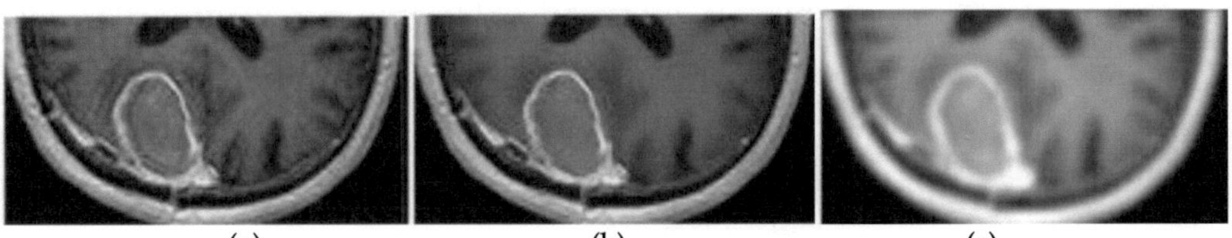

(a) (b) (c)

Fig. 6. Non linear diffusion filters: Preserves edges. (a) Original image, (b) image smoothed by a non linear diffusion filter.

The following illustrations (Fig.) show the variation of the stop function given by the equation 14, where we apply a Gaussian filter (a) and where we apply an anisotropic filtering (b).

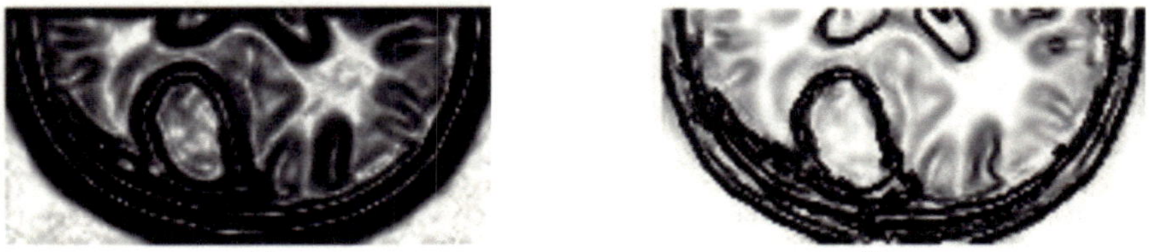

(a) (b)

Fig. 7. Stop function $g(I)$. (a) Using Gaussian filter, (b) Using an anisotropic diffusion filter.

3. 3D tumor reconstruction from its 2D contours

We develop a first technique of 3D brain tumor segmentation by stacking a sequence of 2D tumor contours, detected by 2D level-Sets method in the parallel cross-sectional MRI images (Fig. 7). It consists on applying to each brain MRI slice the level-Sets method in 2D and to propagate the result by taking as initial data the result of the preceding slice.

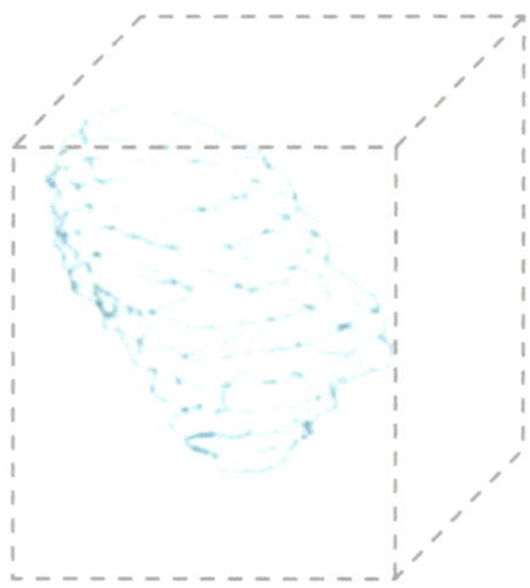

Fig. 8. 3D object reconstruction from its 2D contours.

The main stages of our algorithms are the following (Fig. 9.):

- Initialization of a curve around the tumor in the middle cross-sectional MRI images is called 'main slice' in this work.
- Run a level-Sets algorithm as it has been specified previously by the equation 20, in the main slice.
- The brain tumor boundary in the main slice is used as initial curve in its tow contiguous slices (one upper slice and one lower slice) and so forth.
- The algorithm stops when all the cross-sectional MRI images are processed. After all tumor boundaries are stacked and 3D tumor shape is reconstructed.

The following figures (Fig. 10. and Fig. 11.) show various views of the surface of the tumor obtained by 3D reconstruction of its 2D contours and some projections of 2D tumor contours related of somes cross-sectional MRI images.

This approach is similar to an expert reasoning. This approach has several advantages such as simplicity to implement, it is fast, it requires less time than manual segmentation and based on 2D level-Sets method that has shown robustness in the segmentation of MRI images.

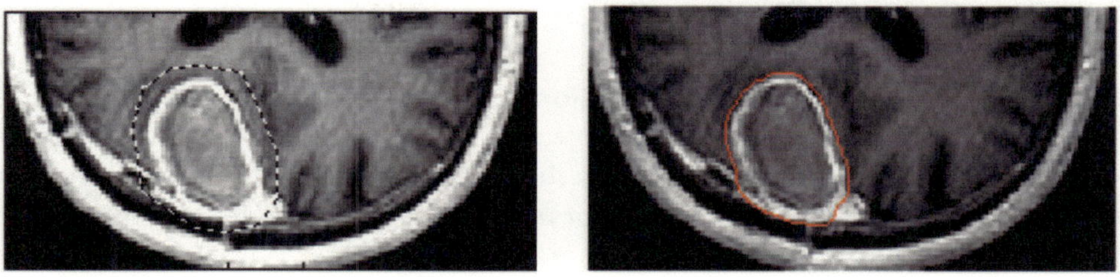

(a) (b)

Fig. 9. Result of brain tumor segmentation in the middle MRI slice. (a) Initialization or initial curve, (b) final boundary of brain tumor.

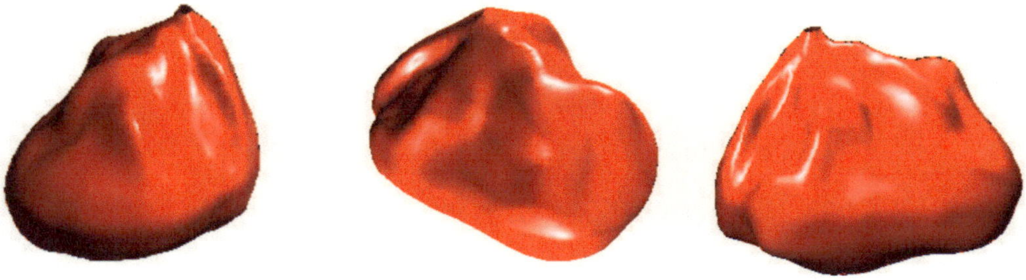

Fig. 10. 3D brain tumor surface visualization by stacking of its 2D boundaries.

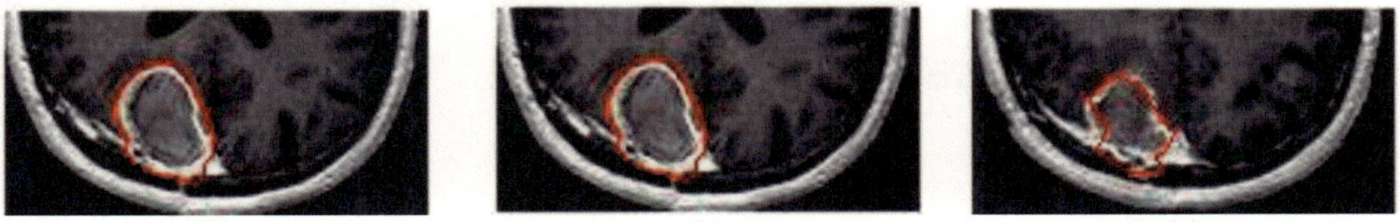

(a) (b) (c)

Fig. 11. Result of 2D segmentation: (a) slice 80, (b) slice 75, (c) slice 70.

4. Volumetric approach

Despite the advantages cited above related to segmentation based on stacking a sequence of 2D contours detected in the parallel cross-sectional images, it has many disadvantages: there is information loss because the third dimension is not taken into account, broken boundary in one slice and overlapping intensities usually lead to poor detected results. This approach supposes that the distance between the slices is very small and the reconstruction of the surface and its properties from 2D contours may lead to inaccurate results. However, an evolution was necessary to the glance of its defects. The following developed approaches come to improve segmentation quality, based on carrying out the computation in 3D space and detects the 3D tumor surface directly using 3D level-Sets method. First, the 3D level-

Sets model evolves according to information related to contours on IRM volume specifically the data gradient information. Second, the level-Sets model evolves according to related regions information in the volumetric MR image.

4.1 3D level-Sets method with contours information

The first stage of this method is to initialize a small sphere around the border of the brain tumor. Then the level-Sets model evolves according to information related to edges in the volumetric brain MR images. This movement comes to its end when the deformable surface found the actual border of the brain tumor.
3D discrete evolution equation of the level-Sets model is the following:

$$\varphi_{ijk}^{n+1} = \varphi_{ijk}^{n} + \Delta t \begin{pmatrix} g_{ijk}(I)\varepsilon k_{ijk}^{n}\left[\left(D_{ijk}^{0x}\right)^2 + \left(D_{ijk}^{0y}\right)^2 + \left(D_{ijk}^{0z}\right)^2\right]^{1/2} + \\ \max\left(g_{ijk}(I)V_{0ijk}, 0\right)\nabla^{+}\varphi + \min\left(g_{ijk}(I)V_{0ijk}, 0\right)\nabla^{-}\varphi \end{pmatrix} \tag{23}$$

Where

$$\nabla^{+}\varphi = \begin{bmatrix} \left(\max(D_{ijk}^{-x}\varphi_{ijk},0)\right)^2 + \left(\min(D_{ijk}^{+x}\varphi_{ijk},0)\right)^2 \\ \left(\max(D_{ijk}^{-y}\varphi_{ijk},0)\right)^2 + \left(\min(D_{ijk}^{+y}\varphi_{ijk},0)\right)^2 \\ \left(\max(D_{ijk}^{-z}\varphi_{ij},0)\right)^2 + \left(\min(D_{ijk}^{+z}\varphi_{ijk},0)\right)^2 \end{bmatrix}^{1/2}$$

$$\nabla^{-}\varphi = \begin{bmatrix} \left(\min(D_{ijk}^{-x}\varphi_{ijk},0)\right)^2 + \left(\max(D_{ijk}^{+x}\varphi_{ijk},0)\right)^2 \\ \left(\min(D_{ijk}^{-y}\varphi_{ijk},0)\right)^2 + \left(\max(D_{ijk}^{+y}\varphi_{ijk},0)\right)^2 \\ \left(\min(D_{ijk}^{-z}\varphi_{ij},0)\right)^2 + \left(\max(D_{ijk}^{+z}\varphi_{ijk},0)\right)^2 \end{bmatrix}^{1/2}$$

The curvature is given as follows:

$$k = \frac{2\varphi_x\varphi_y\varphi_{xy} - \varphi_x\varphi_z\varphi_{xz} + 2\varphi_y\varphi_z\varphi_{yz}}{\left(\varphi_x^2 + \varphi_y^2 + \varphi_z^2\right)^{2/3}} \tag{24}$$

To stop the evolution of 3D level-sets model in the desired boundaries we used 3D version of the anisotropic diffusion filter in order to reduce noise without removing significant parts of the brain MRI volume and without evolving the deformable surface toward the brain tumor borders.
We show in the following figure the results of the 3D brain tumor surface reconstruction using 3D level-Sets based contour's information. The following figure shows different stages of evolution of the deformable surface until reaching the final surface of the tumor and some projections in 2D slices (Fig. 12. and Fig. 13.).
Segmentation of 3D tumor in MR Images using volumetric approach based on the level-Sets as the surface detection mechanism. We note that the main problem with this approach is related to leakage or overflow of the deformable surface in regions where overlapping intensities are present and that usually leads to poor detected results.

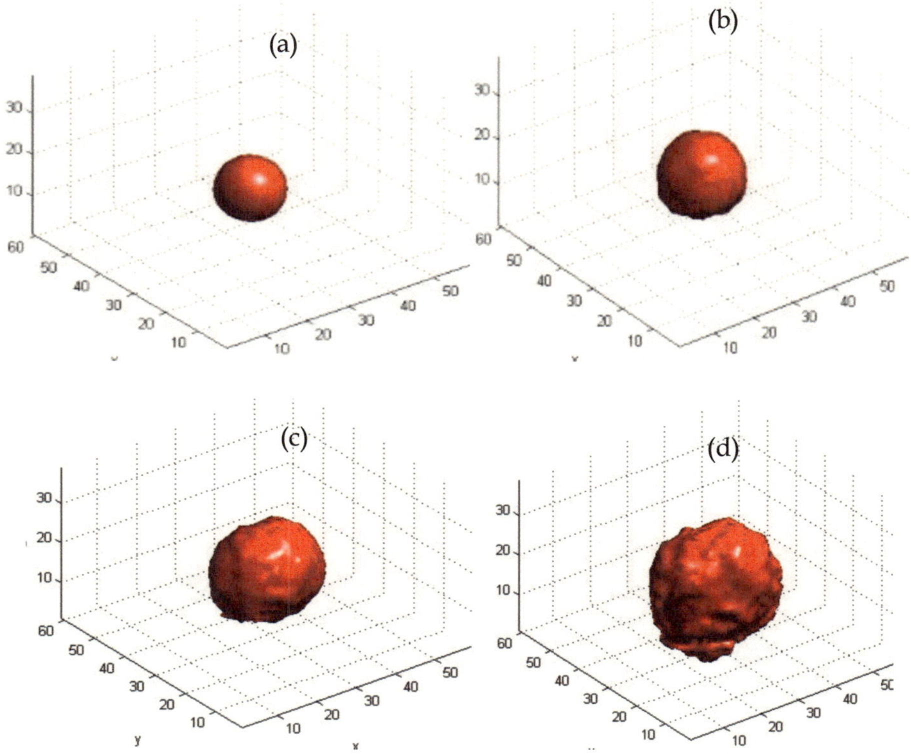

Fig. 12. 3D visualization of the surface of the brain tumor: (a) Initialization, (b) Iteration 10, (c) itiration 30, (d) iteration 50.

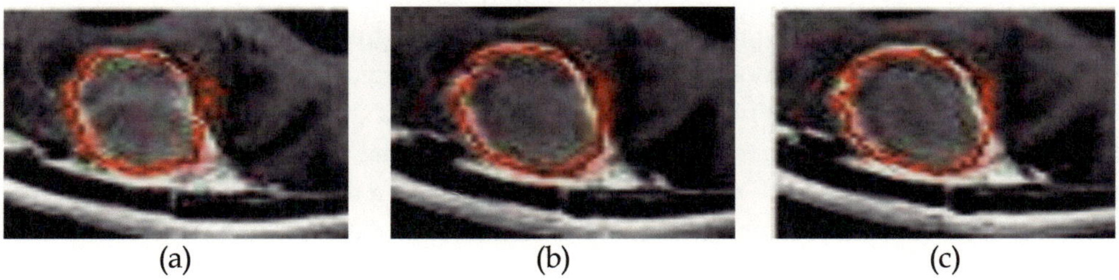

Fig. 13. 2D boundary visualization of the brain tumor: (a) slice 80, (b) slice 70, (c) slice 60.

4.2 3D level-Sets method with regions information

In the previous approach,the segmentation quality is not good, it means that the gradient information which is local information insufficient to control the evolution of the level-Sets model. An alternative is to integrate statistical information related to regions in the brain MRI volume to improve the quality of brain tumor segmentation. Technically speaking, the new proposed method is similar to the segmentation with a deformable model with a two phased image (Chan & Vese, 1999). The general principle is based on the evolution of a surface Γ which partitions the volume data into several regions of different statistical characteristics.

A single deformable surface Γ allows segmentation into two regions Ω_{in} and Ω_{out}, where Ω_{in} represents the region that circumscribed by the surface Γ and Ω_{out} the outer region (Angelini, 2005). The information that controls the evolution of the the new level-Sets model is usually based on statistical modelling of the various region in the volumetric data.

We assume that the image $I(x,y,z)$ defined on the domain Ω is composed of two homogeneous regions of distinct values I_0 and I_1 and that the tumor region to detect corresponds to the region of intensity I_0. We denote the boundary of the tumor with intensity I_0 by Γ. For a given surface Γ of the domain Ω, we consider the following energy functional $E(\Gamma)$:

$$E(\Gamma) = \mu L(\Gamma) + \nu A(\Gamma) + \lambda_0 \int_{\Omega_{in}} |I_0 - c_0|^2 d\Omega + \lambda_0 \int_{\Omega_{out}} |I_1 - c_1|^2 d\Omega \tag{25}$$

Where c_1 and c_2 are equal respectively to the average value of inside and outside of the surface Γ. $L(\Gamma)$ and $A(\Gamma)$ are the regularizing terms corresponding respectively to the length of the curve and the area of the object enclosed by the curve.

μ, ν, λ_1, λ_2 are fixed positive parameters.

Segmentation of the brain tumor from volumetric MRI image is performed via minimization of the energy functional defined in Eq. (26). Minimization of the functional is proceeded using a steepest gradient descent on a discrete spatial grid indexed with $(i,j,k) \in \Re^3$ and introduction of a temporal index (n) leads to an iterative scheme with the following equation of the level-Sets evolution model:

$$\varphi_{ijk}^{n+1} = \varphi_{ijk}^{n} + \nabla t \times \delta_\varepsilon(\varphi_{ijk}^{n})\left(-\mu k \varphi_{ijk}^{n} + \lambda_1 (I_{ijk} - c_1 \varphi_{ijk}^{n})^2 + \lambda_2 (I_{ijk} - c_2 \varphi_{ijk}^{n})^2\right) \tag{26}$$

To segment the brain tumor using this approach (Fig. 14.), we initialized an initial surface through its boundary. Then this surface evolves until reaching the actual border of the tumor. Several criteria can be incorporated to stop the process of segmentation: when the area of the deformable surface becomes constant or the volume of the region bounded by the deformable surface becomes constant or Energy function $E(\Gamma)$ reaches its minimum value. The latter criterion is sufficient but it has a problem of computational cost. The convergence of the deformable surface to the tumor border implies that the area and the volume of deformable surface becomes constant. However, area and volume computational is less. For this, we used as a stopping condition, area and volume of the deformable surface at a time.

We present above a flowchart designed in our research to isolate a brain tumor using level-Sets method based on region informations:

This method consists in initializing a small sphere through the border of the brain tumor. Then the level-Sets model evolves according to related region information in the image in order to plate itself on the surface of the tumor. We show in the following the results of the 3D reconstruction of the brain tumor surface relayed to this approach. The following figure shows different stages of evolution of the deformable surface until reaching the final surface of the tumor and some projections in 2D slices (Fig. 15. and Fig. 16.).

These results show that this approach combine the following advantages: arbitrary initialization of the object anywhere in the image, no need for gradient information, self adaptation for inward and outward local motion.

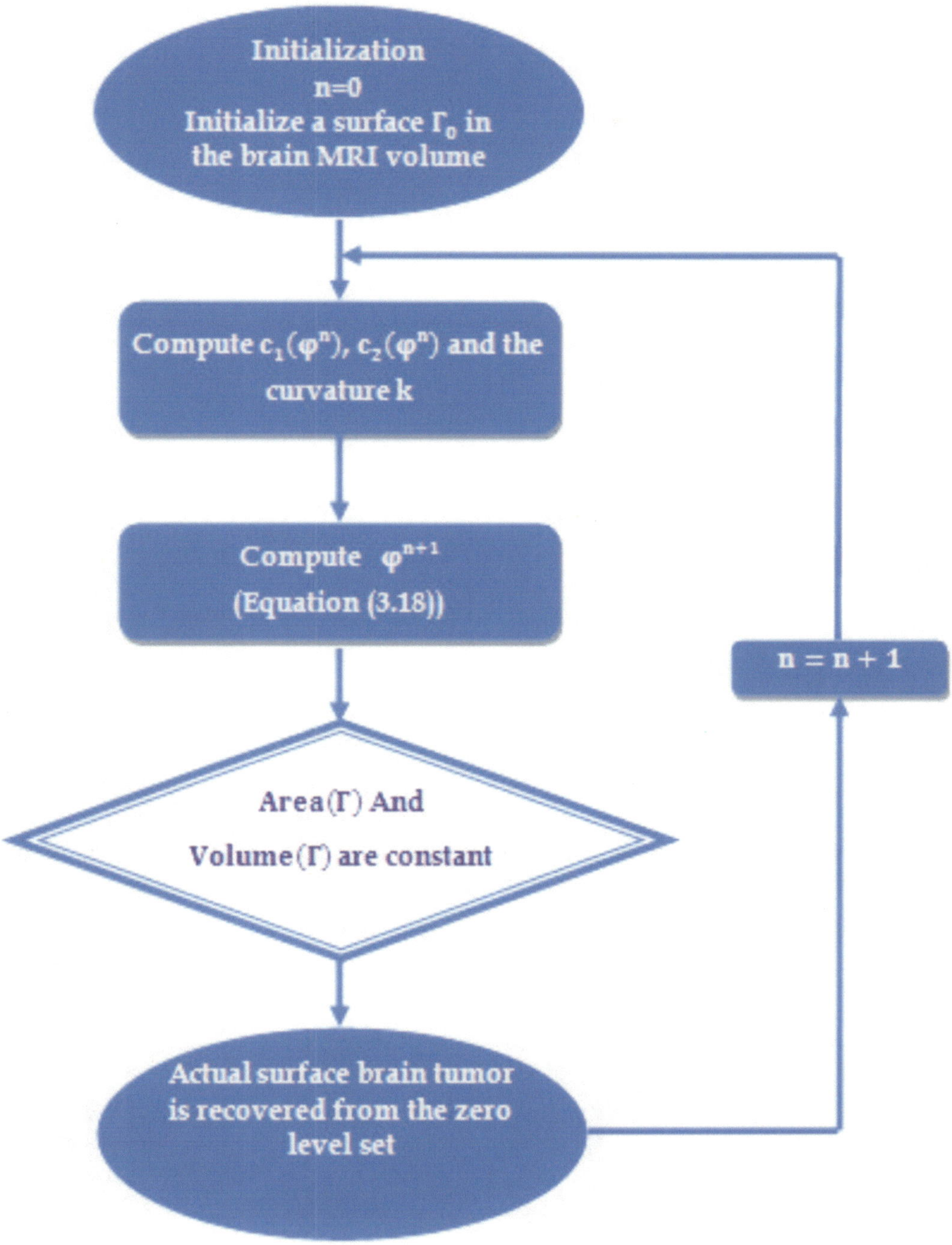

Fig. 14. Flowchart designed to isolate a brain tumor using the level-Sets method based on region informations.

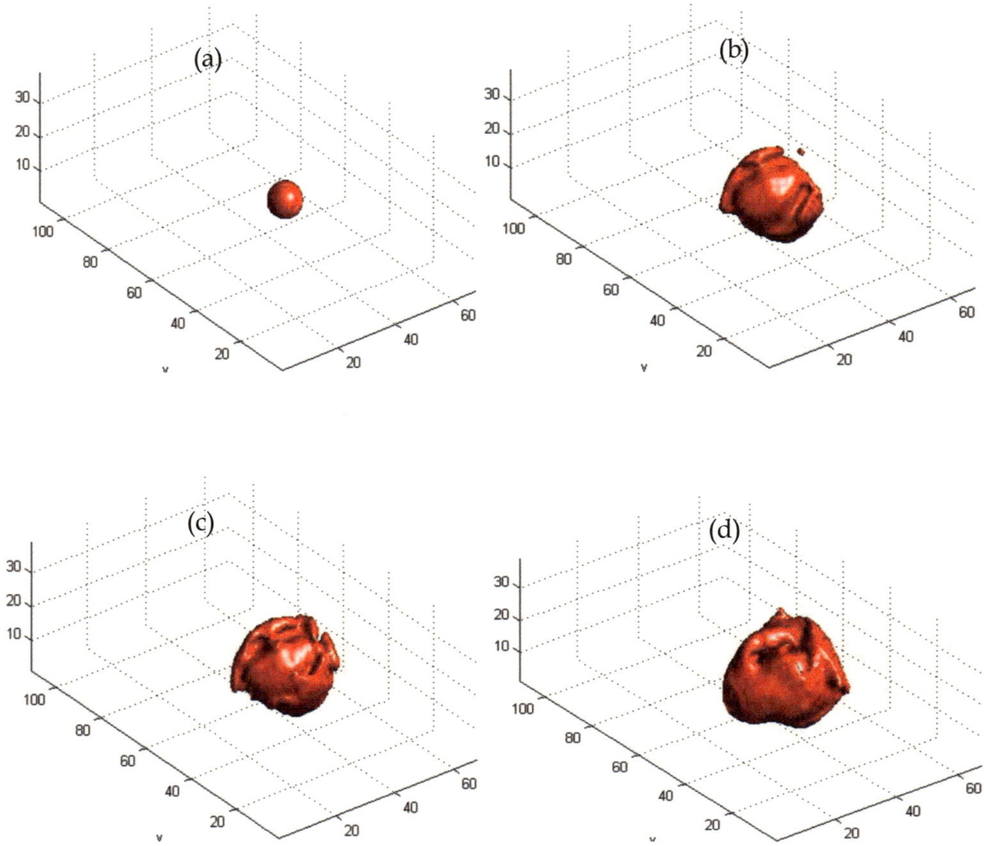

Fig. 15. 3D visualization of the surface of the brain tumor obtained by level-Sets method: (a) initialization, (b) iteration 80, (c) iteration 180, (d) iteration 300.

The following representation (Fig. 16) shows the segmentation result on some slicers.

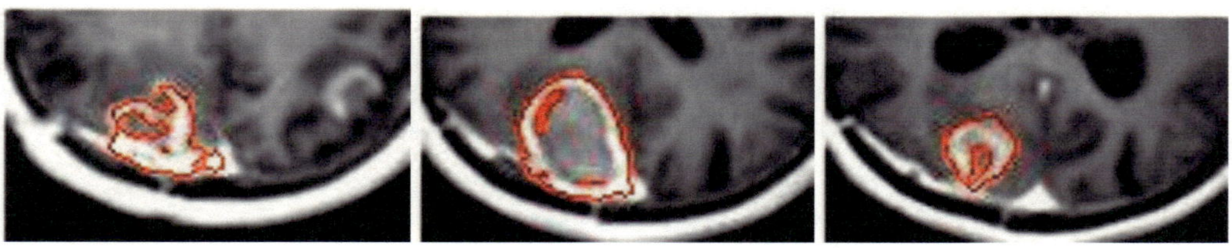

(a) (b) (c)

Fig. 16. Result of 2D segmentation: (a) slice 30, (b) slice 50, (c) slice 70.

5. Summary and discussion

Presented research was provided with a general goal to develop 3D segmentation algorithms of brain tumor from volumetric MRI images. We have presented a variational method, 3D level-Sets applied to automatic segmentation of brain tumor in MRIs, using boundary and region based information of tumor to control the deformable surface propagation. The first approach used, is the 3D reconstruction from its 2D contours using a sequence of 2D contours, detected by 2D level-Sets method in the parallel cross-sectional MRI images. This method goes very well but it has two major defects, there is no interaction between the slices and surface must be cylindrical. This approach is the most simple that one can make. It makes it possible to use active contours in the field 2D method which showed its robustness. However, an evolution was necessary to the glance of its defects related to the results obtained and the tumor shapes that were being able to be treated. The second approach comes to improve the segmentation quality, based on carrying out the computation in 3D space and detecting the brain tumor region directly using 3D level-Sets method. In the first volumetric approach 3D level-Sets model evolves according to information related to contours on IRM volume. In the second level -Sets model evolves according to related regions descriptors in the volumetric MR image. Evaluations were performed on a set of volumetric MRI images obtained from (MeDEISA) database.

6. References

Kass, M.; Witkin, A. & Terzopoulos, D. (1988). Snakes: Active contour models. International Journal of Computer Vision V. 1, no. , pp. 321-331, 1988.

Terzopoulos, D.; Witkin, A.; & Kass, M. (1988). Constraints on deformable models: Recovering 3D shape and nonrigid motion. Artificial Intelligence, vol. 36, pp. 91. -1 23.1988.

Amini, A.; Weymouth, T.; & Jain, R. (1990). Using dynamic programming for solving variational problems in vision. IEEE Trans. Patt. Anal. Mach. Intell., vol. 12, no. 9, pp. 855–867, 1990.

Cohen, L. (1991). On active contour models and balloons. CVGIP: Imag. Under., vol. 53, no. 2, pp. 211–218, 1991.

McInerney, T. & Terzopoulos, D. (1995). A dynamic finite element surface model for segmentation and tracking in multidimensional medical images with application to cardiac 4D image analysis. Comp. Med. Imag. Graph., vol. 19, no. 1, pp. 69–83, 1995.

Caselles, V.; Catte, F.; Coll, T. & Dibos, F. (1993). A geometric model for active contours. Numerische Mathematik, vol. 66, pp. 1–31, 1993.

Malladi, R.; Sethian, J. & Vemuri, B. (1995). Shape modeling with front propagation: A level set approach," IEEE Trans. Patt. Anal. Mach. Intell., vol. 17, no. 2, pp. 158–175, 1995.

Caselles, V.; Kimmel, R. & Sapiro, G. (1995). Geodesic active contours. 5th International Conf. Comp. Vis., pp. 694–699, 1995.

Whitaker, R. (1994). Volumetric deformable models: active blobs. Tech. Rep. ECRC-94-25, European Computer-Industry Research Centre GmbH, 1994.

Sapiro, G. & Tannenbaum, A. (1993). Affine invariant scale-space," International Journal Computer Vision, vol. 11, no. 1, pp. 25–44, 1993.

Kimia, B.; Tannenbaum, A. & Zucker, S. (1995). Shapes, shocks, and deformations: the components of two-dimensional shape and the reaction-diffusion space. International Journal Computer Vision. vol. 15, pp. 189–224, 1995.

Kimmel, R.; Amir, A. & Bruckstein, M. (1995). Finding shortest paths on surfaces using level sets propagation. IEEE Trans. Patt. Anal. Mach. Intell., vol. 17, no. 6, pp. 635–640, 1995.

Alvarez, L.; Guichard, F.; Lions, P. & Morel, J. (1993). Axioms and fundamental equations of image processing," Archive for Rational Mechanics and Analysis, vol. 123, no. 3, pp. 199–257, 1993.

Osher, S. & Sethian, J. (1988). Fronts propagating with curvature-dependent speed: algorithms based on Hamilton-Jacobi formulations. J. Computational Physics, vol. 79, pp. 12–49, 1988.

Sethian, J. (1999). Level Set Methods and Fast Marching Methods: Evolving Interfaces in Computational Geometry, Fluid Mechanics. Computer Vision, and Material Science. Cambridge, UK: Cambridge University Press, 2nd ed., 1999.

Kimia, B. (1990). Conservation Laws and a Theory of Shape. Ph.D. thesis, McGill Centre for Intelligent Machines, McGill University, Montreal, Canada, 1990.

Grayson, M. (1985). Shortening embedded curves. Annals of Mathematics, vol. 129, pp. 71–111, 1989.

Sethian, J. (1985). Curvature and evolution of fronts. Commun. Math. Phys., vol. 101, pp. 487–499, 1985.

Sethian, J. (1989). A review of recent numerical algorithms for hypersurfaces moving with curvature dependent speed. J. Differential Geometry, vol. 31, pp. 131–161, 1989.

Williams, D. & Shah, M. (1992). A fast algorithm for active contours and curvature estimation. CVGIP: Imag. Under., vol. 55, no. 1, pp. 14–26, 1992.

Malladi, R., Sethian, J. & Vemuri, C. (1995). Shape Modeling with Front Propagation: A Level Set Approach, IEEE Trans. on Pattern Analysis and Machine Intelligence, 17, 2, pp. 158–175, 1995.

Sethian, J. (1982). An Analysis of Flame Propagation. Ph.D. thesis, Dept. of Mathematics, University of California, Berkeley, CA, 1982.

Sethian, J. (1994). Curvature flow and entropy conditions applied to grid generation.

Journal of Computational Physics, 115 : 440−454, 1994.

Sussman, M.; Fatemi, E.; Smereka, P. & Osher, S. (1997). An improved level set method for incompressible two-phase flows. Computers and Fluids, vol. 27, 5-6, pp. 663-680, 1997.

Perona, P. & Malik, J. (1990). Scale-space and edge detection using anisotropic diffusion. IEEE Trans. Pattern Anal. Machine Intell., 12 :629.639, 1990.

Chan, T. & Vese, L. (1999). An Active Contour model without Edges. In LNCS, edited by M. Neilsen, P. Johanson, O.F. Olson and J. Weickert, Springer-Verlag, Berlin/New York. Vol. 1687, 141-151,1999.

Angelini, E. (2005). Segmentation of Real-Time Three-Dimensional Ultrasound for Quantification of Ventricular Function: A Clinical Study on Right and Left Ventricles, Ultrasound in Med. & Biol., Vol. 31, No. 9, pp. 1143–1158, 2005.

Sahoo, K.; Soltani, S.; Wong, C. & Chen, Y. (1988). A survey of thresholding techniques. Computer Vision Graphics Image Processing 1988; 41: pp233 - 260.

Moon, N.; Bulitt, E.; Leemput, K. and Gerig, G (2002). Model-based brain and tumor segmentation. Proceedings of ICPR 2002; 1: 528-531.

Wang, Z.; Hu, Q.; Loe, K.; Aziz, A. & Nowinski, L. (2004) Rapid and Automatic Detection of Brain Tumors in MR Images. Proceeding of SPIE 2004; 5369: 602 - 612.

Michael, K.; Simon, W.; Arya, N.; Peter, B.; Ferenc, J. & Ron, K. (2001) Automated Segmentation of MR Images of Brain Tumors. Radiology 2001; 218: 586 - 591.

Taheri, S.; Ong, S. & Chong, V. (2009). Level-set Segmentation of Brain Tumors using a Threshold-based Speed Function," Image and Vision Computing (IVC) Elsevier Journal, 2009.

Taheri, S.; Ong, S. & Chong, V. (2007). Threshold-based 3D Tumor Segmentation using Level Set (TSL). In Proc. IEEE Workshop on Application of Computer Vision (WACV), 2007.

Lefohn, A.; Cates, J. & Whitaker, R. (2003). Interactive, GPU- Based Level Sets for 3D Brain Tumor Segmentation, MICCAI 2003.

Lynn, F.; Lawrence, H.; Dmitry, G. & Murtagh, R. (2001). Automatic segmentation of non-enhancing brain tumors in magnetic resonance images. Artificial Intelligence in Medicine 2001; 21(1-3): pp 43 - 63.

MeDEISA, (2010). Medical Database for the Evaluation of Image and Signal processing (MeDEISA), http://www.medeisa.net.

Lima, P.; Bonarini, A. & Mataric, M. (2004). *Application of Machine Learning,* InTech, ISBN 978-953-7619-34-3, Vienna, Austria

Li, B.; Xu, Y. & Choi, J. (1996). Applying Machine Learning Techniques, *Proceedings of ASME 2010 4th International Conference on Energy Sustainability*, pp. 14-17, ISBN 842-6508-23-3, Phoenix, Arizona, USA, May 17-22, 2010

Siegwart, R. (2001). Indirect Manipulation of a Sphere on a Flat Disk Using Force Information. *International Journal of Advanced Robotic Systems,* Vol.6, No.4, (December 2009), pp. 12-16, ISSN 1729-8806

Arai, T. & Kragic, D. (1999). Variability of Wind and Wind Power, In: *Wind Power,* S.M. Muyeen, (Ed.), 289-321, Scyio, ISBN 978-953-7619-81-7, Vukovar, Croatia

Van der Linden, S. (June 2010). Integrating Wind Turbine Generators (WTG's) with Energy Storage, In: *Wind Power,* 17.06.2010, Available from http://sciyo.com/articles/show/title/wind-power-integrating-wind-turbine-generators-wtg-s-with-energy-storage

7

Deformable Model-Based Segmentation of Brain Tumor from MR Images

Sami Bourouis and Kamel Hamrouni
University Tunis El-Manar, National Engineering School of Tunis
Tunisia

1. Introduction

Segmentation of brain tumors is an important task for treatment planning and therapy evaluation. This task could also lead to new applications, including data compression, robust registration, and effective content based image retrieval in large medical databases. Accurate delineation of tumor can also be helpful for general modeling of pathological brains and the construction of pathological brain atlases Toga et al. (2001). Nevertheless, precise delineation of brain Tumor in MRI is a challenging problem that depends on many factors. Indeed, there is a large class of tumor types which vary greatly in size and position, have a variety of shape and appearance properties, have intensities overlapping with normal brain tissue, may deform and defect the surrounding structures giving an abnormal geometry also for healthy tissue. Moreover, MR images segmentation widely depends on the specific application and image modality. These images contain sometimes various amounts of noise and/or artifacts due to patient's motion and soft tissue boundaries are sometimes not well defined.

Traditionally manual brain tumors segmentation - usually performed by marking the tumor regions slice-by-slice by human expert - is time-consuming (hence impractical for processing large amounts of data), non- reproducible, difficult, and highly subjective. On the other hand, fully automatic and robust segmentation is highly required for clinical settings because it reduces significantly the computing time and generates satisfactory segmentation results.

The existence of several MR acquisition protocols provides different information on the brain. Each image usually highlights a particular region of the tumor. In visualizing brain tumors, a second T1-weighted image is often acquired after the injection of a 'contrast agent'. These 'contrast agent' usually contain an element whose composition causes a decrease in the T1 time of nearby tissue (gadolinium is one example) Brown & Semeka (2003). The presence of this type of 'enhancing' area can indicate the presence of a tumor. Figure 1 illustrates an example of T1-weighted image before and after the injection of a contrast agent.

Conventionally, it is difficult to segment a tumor by a simple technique like thresholding or classic edge- detection. These methods may not allow differentiation between non-enhancing tumor and normal tissue due to overlapping intensity distributions of healthy tissue with tumor and surrounding edema. Also, they are unable to exploit all information provided by MRI. Therefore, advanced image analysis techniques are needed to solve the problem.

Various promising works have studied the tumor segmentation, offering a diversity of methods and evaluation criteria. In particular, pattern classification techniques refer to a

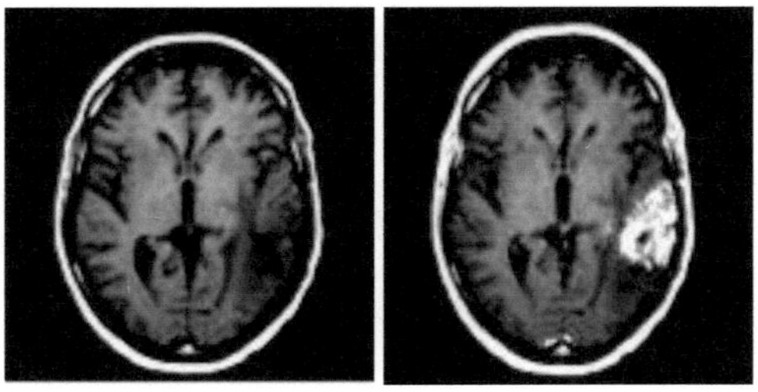

Fig. 1. Effects of contrast agent. (a): T1-weighted image, (b) T1-weighted image after contrast injection

large class of methods Corso et al. (2008); Liu et al. (2005); Prastawa et al. (2004); Zhang et al. (2001). For example, in a more recent publication, a Bayesian generative model Corso et al. (2008) is applied to brain tumor detection. This model is incorporated into the graph-based image segmentation. Fuzzy-connectedness Liu et al. (2005) and Markov random fields (MRFs) Zhang et al. (2001) are also ones of a useful method for medical image segmentation.

Other approaches were proposed in literature for brain tumor segmentation and the most of them focused on the use of a combinational strategy of several conventional techniques such as : mathematical morphological operations, registration methods, deformable models, anatomical information and voxel-based techniques Cobzas et al. (2007); Cuadra et al. (2004); Moon et al. (2002); Warfield et al. (2000). For instance, Warfield et al. Warfield et al. (2000) have proposed an ATM SVC algorithm that overcomes the limitations of intensity-based classification and Template based non-linear registration techniques by embedding both image and model information into a higher dimensionality space in which a k-Nearest Neighbors (k-NN) classification is performed. Cuadra et al. Cuadra et al. (2004) have presented an efficient tool for pathological brain segmentation. The idea is to deform the atlas in presence of large space-occupying tumors, based on an a priori model of lesion growth. Authors in Cobzas et al. (2007) have proposed a region-based variational method for brain tumor segmentation. They define a set of multidimensional features and use them to calculate statistics for 'tumor' and 'normal brain' area from labeled MRI data.

Many of these published works have been successfully applied to segment some tumor types. However, some of them fail when the ROI to be identified have overlapping spectral properties. It is also too difficult to differentiate between normal and abnormal tissues when dealing with only one modality (such as T1-weighted MR image) because the acquisition of tissue parameters is insufficient due to the lack of contrast. They are also very computationally expensive and the accuracy of the segmentation depends on the initial parameters. For instance, the use of atlas is problematic because tumor structures have no equivalent in the atlas. Moreover, algorithmic complexity is another disadvantages of some approaches cited above.

Deformable models are other popular methods that are widely used for a wide range of applications and have proved to be a successful segmentation technique Bourouis et al. (2008); Liew & Yan (2006). They have become used for medical image processing and especially for brain segmentation, implicitly in the form of a level set function Sethian (1999) or explicitly as a snake function Kass et al. (1987).

In the recent years, the level set method has become popular thanks to its ability to handle complex geometries and topological changes. Unlike the traditional deformable models, the level set method does not depend on the parameterizations of the surface. Moreover, they constitute an appropriate framework for merging heterogeneous information and they provide a consistent geometrical representation suitable for a surface-based analysis. These advantages make level-set technique very attractive and flexible in shape modeling and image segmentation.

A region-based speed function Ho et al. (2002) have been developed for automatic 3D segmentation of brain tumors by combining region based level sets and fuzzy clustering. An initial surface is used to guide an automatic initialization by calculating the difference image of T1-weighed images with and without gadolinium enhancement. The proposed speed function overcomes classical level-set functions by modulating the propagation term with a signed statistical force, leading to a stable solution. However, this method only segments the enhanced section of tumors in contrast enhanced T1-weighted image. A more recent approach was presented in Taheri et al. (2010), combining the threshold-based method and level sets. This method is similar to the method of Chen & Metaxas (2003) but it works in 3D and uses a threshold method to construct the speed function in level sets. The algorithm is started by selecting one or several ROI in the tumor region. An initial threshold value is calculated using these ROIs and a level set with the proposed threshold-based speed function is deformed using ROI(s) as zero level set. A semi-automatic algorithm in Bourouis & Hamrouni (2010) was applied to delineate tumor volume based on deformable model approach. Authors proposed a new function speed modulated by both boundary and regional information in order to have a more robust process for segmentation.

Unfortunately, there are difficulties in using level sets. One problem is that level set algorithm requires accurate initialization and robust attraction force to converge successfully. Another problem is that level set formulation needs the updating of several parameters. The main parameter in the level set equation is the speed function, whose design is the most important step in the level set approach. Consequently, this approach becomes less desirable in some circumstances.

In general, precise and reproducible segmentation of brain tumors are still a challenging and difficult task which is far from being solved, even if much effort has been spent in the medical imaging community.

As with most other works, we focus on the development of a generic algorithm that could help in the automation of medical image analysis tasks. Our work takes place in this growing area and we are mainly motivated by the deformable model approaches. This chapter extends some works and proposes an unsupervised method that incorporates additional information to better disambiguate the tumor from the surrounding deformed brain tissue. Unlike our previous method Bourouis & Hamrouni (2010), we propose here a fully automatic and more robust procedure for tumor segmentation.

2. Brief mathematical formulation of level sets

In the present section we provide a brief overview of some of the requisite mathematics that are needed to understand level-set technique. While detailed proofs are not included, the interested reader can refer to citations and detailed descriptions in Osher & Sethian (1988); Sethian (1999).

The level set method, developed by Osher and Sethian Osher & Sethian (1988), is an emerging method to represent shapes and track moving interfaces. The basic idea is to change the movement of a planar curve into the movement track of 3D surface.
Theoretically, the level set boundary is defined as a zero level set of an implicit representation ϕ of an evolving front $\Gamma(t)$. The implicit level set function ϕ can be evolved by solving the following PDE (partial differential equations) :

$$\frac{\partial \phi}{\partial t} = F.|\nabla \phi| \tag{1}$$

Where F is a scalar velocity (speed) function depending on the local geometric properties (e.g curvature) and on the external parameters related to the input data (e.g image gradient). ∇ denotes the gradient operator. The speed function F may be expressed as $F = F(k)$, where the local curvature k is given by:

$$k = div(\frac{\nabla \phi}{|\nabla \phi|}) = \nabla.\frac{\nabla \phi}{|\nabla \phi|} = \frac{\phi_{xx}\phi_y^2 - 2\phi_x\phi_y\phi_{xy} + \phi_{yy}\phi_x^2}{(\phi_x^2 + \phi_y^2)^{\frac{3}{2}}} \tag{2}$$

At time t the zero level set ($\phi = 0$) describes the evolved of front. Thereby, $\Gamma(t)$ (see Figure 2) deforms iteratively according to its normal direction with the speed function F, and its position is given at each iteration step by the equation:

$$\Gamma(x, y, t) = \{(x, y)/\phi(x, y, t) = 0\} \tag{3}$$

The initial function ϕ_0 is calculated based on the signed measure to the initial front Γ_0. It can be simply the Euclidean distance between one image point and the boundary the front. That is:

$$\phi_0(x, y) = \pm d((x, y), \Gamma_0) \tag{4}$$

The sign of the distance $d(x, y), \Gamma_0)$ is chosen such that the point inside the boundary has a negative sign and the one outside has a positive sign.

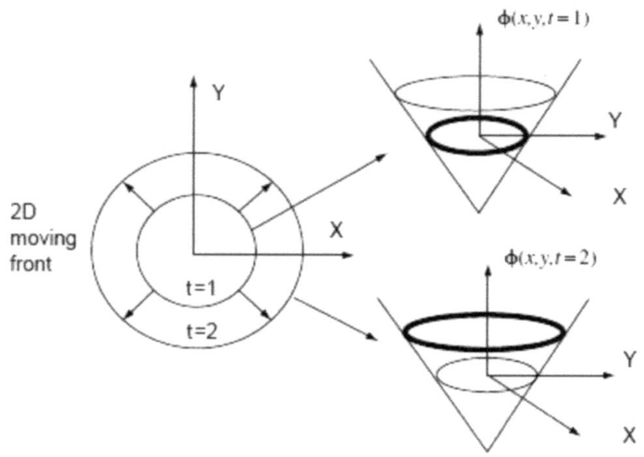

Fig. 2. The level set function.

For image segmentation purposes and in order to solve the shape recovery problem, Malladi et al. Malladi et al. (1995) and Caselles et al. Caselles et al. (1997) have introduced two kinds of speed functions, among others. To stop the evolution at the edge, F can be multiplied by a value that is a function of the image gradient Malladi et al. (1995). However, if the edge is missed, the surface cannot propagate backward. Hence, relying mainly on the edge is not sufficient for an accurate segmentation and other information from image should be used.
Because the initialization of the model through Eq. (2) is computationally expensive, there is an efficient way to solve the initial value of the level set problem: The Narrow Band method Sethian (1999). The key idea of this technique is to constrain the computation only to the pixels that are close to the zero level set. Therefore, by performing a narrow band update of the level set, we need only construct the speed function at a small set of points in the neighborhood close to the zero level set instead of constructing it at all the points on the image domain. We present below the basic pseudo-code of the Narrow-Band, and readers are referred to Sethian (1999) for details.

1. Initialize the signed distance function ϕ_0 of the initial front Γ_0,
2. Find the narrow band points: determine those points whose distance $|\phi(t)|$ is less than the specified narrow bandwidth, and mark them as the narrow band points,
3. Update: resolve level set equation, and track the zero level set curve; update the level set function value $|\phi(t + \Delta t)|$ in the narrow band,
4. Reinitialize: reinitialize the narrow band when the zero level set reaches the boundary of the narrow band. Repeat steps 3 and 4.
5. Convergence test: check whether the iteration converges or not. If so, stop; otherwise, enter the calculation of the next step, and go to step 3.

3. Methods and materials: Tumor segmentation

Our aim is to provide a stable and accurate solution for the segmentation of brain tumor. In this work, we propose two procedures for tumor segmentation: the first is a semi-automatic algorithm whereas the second is completely automatic.

3.1 Semi-automatic algorithm : single modality image

At this stage, we propose an algorithm (Algorithm: 1) that is able to detect tumor volume with a semi-automatic method based mainly on a partial derivative equation described below. Indeed, the user initializes the algorithm by manually selecting one voxel (we need only the position of the seed point) which belongs to the tumor area. This process could lead to generate the initial deformable model for the tumor area. Hence, this first model is defined as a set of neighbor's voxels having the same of intensity properties with the selected voxel. In the following stage, the initial deformable model will be deformed until extracting all tumor region.
The different steps of the current algorithm are summarized as follows:

3.2 Fully automatic algorithm : multimodality images

The fully automatic segmentation process is often a necessary task for medical applications. However, it has been proven to be problematic, both due to the high complexity of anatomical structures as well as their large variability. We think that it would be possible to automate our

Algorithm 1

1. Preprocessing step: Volume smoothing.

2. Manual selection of an initial voxel v_T.

3. Initial model estimation for tumor area: a set of neighbor's voxels $\vartheta(v_T)$ define this model ; calculation the mean value m_T in order to initialize the evolution of the deformable model.

4. Segmentation of the tumor under the action of the evolving level-set equation.
   - Taking into some evolution constraints (such as epsilon parameter ϵ_T and the maximum number of iterations).

method if we take account of more of MRI images such as weighted pre- and post-contrast 3D images. Indeed, the injection of gadolinium is used to differentiate tumor contrast from other close tissues. Under these conditions, we propose to use for example the same idea which was developed by other researchers such as Ho et al. Ho et al. (2002).
Operations performed by the current algorithm are summarized in figure 3.

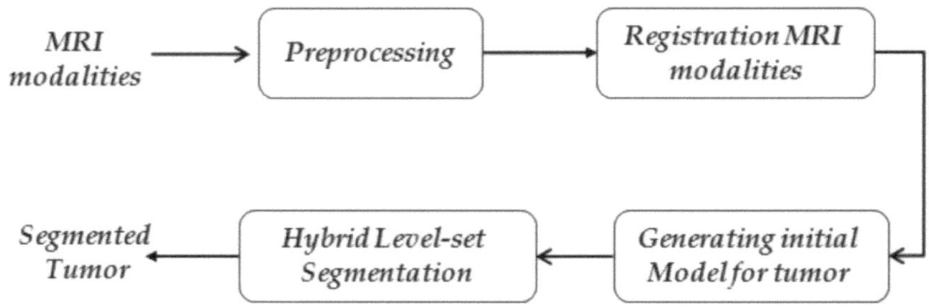

Fig. 3. The proposed algorithm.

Preprocessing step: (Smoothing and Edge Preserving)
We perform a pre-processing step that reduces the effect of noise and intensity variations within and between images. Here we use an anisotropic diffusion filter Perona & Malik (1990), which can remove only high-frequency noise, preserve edge, and should not affect relevant major geometrical features.

Affine registration step:
An alignment of different modalities is carried out using mutual information criterionMaes et al. (1997) to globally match different MRI modalities.

Initialisation step:
The aim of this step is to create an initial model that must be able to derive an automatic initialization of the surface and to locally guide the level set surface.

Level-Set evolution step:
The intention of this step is to extract accurately brain tumor volume by applying an efficient deformable model. As the evolution process can be guided by a combination of several information, we propose here an hybrid framework which controlled by a new evolution speed function. This function is able to take into account simultaneously the local spatial context and the global one. This mechanism may lead the algorithm to a stable and precise solution.

3.2.1 Initialization step

T1-weighted pre- and post-contrast 3D images are the inputs to perform an automatic initialization for our procedure. The use of T1-weighted pre- and post-contrast shows different aspects of the tumor region. T1-weighted MRI is commonly used for detailed imaging of anatomy, but do not distinguish tumor tissue well. At this stage, we calculate the difference image of T1-weighed images with and without contrast enhancement. This initial map is then used to derive an automatic initialization of the surface and to locally guide the level set surface. However, the obtained difference image from the last operation includes tumor voxels and some normal tissues. As we need only pathological voxels to initialize the level-set function, we apply a post-processing based on mathematical morphology operations. A binary morphological erosion process is applied to eliminate noise as well as normal tissue structures while retaining the brain tumor areas. This process requires the definition of the radius size of the neighbourhood associated with the structuring element. Finally, the mean and epsilon values of the obtained tumor area are calculated in order to start the evolution of the deformable model with the best parameters.

3.2.2 Adaptive, hybrid level-set evolution

In this section we detail the second step of the proposed approach: the previous detection of the tumor is used to initialize a deformable model.
Construction of a speed function is crucial in applying the level set method to medical image segmentation. The speed function is designed to control movement of the curve. In this section we focus on the construction of a novel speed function. Our intention is to exploit the advantage of the combination/cooperation of different information in the same framework. So, we propose basically to constrain our deformable model by both boundary and regional information.
To speed up the implemented algorithm, we propose the use of Narrow Band Sethian (1999). We remember that the contour of an object is defined as the zero level set of an implicit function ϕ. This function will change with time according to the evolution force F.
The partial differential equationSethian (1999) of ϕ is defined as follows:

$$\frac{\partial \phi}{\partial t} = F|\nabla \phi| \tag{5}$$

The classical evolution force is defined like in Malladi et al. (1995):

$$F = g(I)(\nu + k) \tag{6}$$

Where the curvature k and the constant force ν propagate the curve to image edges. $g(x)$ is a stopping function that limits the propagation force at edges.

The design of the velocity F plays a major role in the evolutionary process. Recently Bourouis & Hamrouni (2010), we have proposed the following formulation for the evolution equation (7):

$$\frac{\partial \phi}{\partial t} = [\alpha_r F_{region}(I) + \alpha_b F_{boundary}(I)]|\nabla \phi| \tag{7}$$

Where F_{region} and $F_{boundary}$ define the propagation term.
F_{region} is a region-based propagation term and $F_{boundary}$ is a boundary-based term. These two terms force the model to expand or contract toward desirable features in the input data. The constants α_r and α_b control the degree of evolution and smoothness in the solution.
$F_{boundary}$ causes the evolving of the front to be more strongly attracted to image edges. It is expressed as :

$$F_{boundary}(I) = sign(F_{boundary}).\frac{c+k}{1+|\nabla I|} \tag{8}$$

$$sign(F_{boundary}) = \begin{cases} +1 \; if & F_{region} < 0 \\ -1 \; otherwise & \end{cases} \tag{9}$$

The curvature k forces the surface to have smooth area.
F_{region} controls the evolution of the model and segments tumor tissue based on intensity values. We define F_{region} as:

$$F_{region}(I) = \begin{cases} I - (m_T - \epsilon_T) \text{ if } I < m_T \\ (m_T + \epsilon_T) - I \text{ otherwise} \end{cases} \tag{10}$$

Where ϵ_T is a constant parameter, and m_T is the mean value of the tumor region.
ϵ_T controls the brightness of the region to be segmented and define a range of greyscale values that could be considered inside the object.
In this way a model situated on voxels with greyscale values in the interval $[m_T - \epsilon_T, m_T + \epsilon_T]$ will expand to enclose that voxel, whereas a model situated on greyscale values outside that interval will contract to exclude that voxel. So, intensity values between $m_T - \epsilon_T$ and $m_T + \epsilon_T$ yield positive values in F_{region} (i.e the model expands), while outside intensities yield negative values in F_{region} (i.e the model contracts).
Finally, the algorithm will stop if the maximum number of iterations is terminated or if the convergence criterion is reached. The convergence criterion is defined in terms of the root mean squared error (RMSE). If the maximum RMSE value is reached, the solution is considered to have converged.

$$RMSE = \sqrt{\frac{1}{N \times M} \sum_{i=1}^{N} \sum_{j=1}^{M} (\phi_{i,j}^{n+1} - \phi_{i,j}^{n})^2}$$

Wher $N \times M$ is the matrix size of ϕ and **n** indicates the nth iteration.

In this work, we propose to improve our previous deformable model by introducing new parameters which help the evolution stability. More details will be introduced in the next section.

3.2.3 Threshold updating parameter

To improve the performance of the level set equation, we propose to change our previous region-based speed function (eq. 10) by an adaptive scheme which is better than the static one. This idea was already proposed by Taheri et al. Taheri et al. (2010).

Modified Region-based speed Function :

We introduce the bellow modifications to redefine the region speed term in order to segment also "non-homogeneous" tumor tissues. So, we propose to define a threshold updating parameter τ as:

$$\begin{cases} \epsilon_T = \sigma_T \\ \tau^{i+1} = m_T^i - sign(I).k.\sigma_T^i \end{cases} \tag{11}$$

Where

$$sign(x) = \begin{cases} +1 \text{ if } x < m_T^i \\ -1 \text{ otherwise} \end{cases} \tag{12}$$

τ^{i+1} : the threshold estimation for the (i+1)th iteration.
m_T^i : the mean value of the tumor region.
σ_T^i : the standard deviation of the tumor region.
k : is the factor which determines the confidence level and must be chosen properly.

The new formulation for the region-based speed term will define as:

$$\widetilde{F}^{i+1}_{region}(I) = \begin{cases} I - \tau^{i+1} \text{ if } I < m_T^i \\ \tau^{i+1} - I \text{ otherwise} \end{cases} = \begin{cases} I - (m_T^i - k.\sigma_T^i) \text{ if } I < m_T^i \\ (m_T^i + k.\sigma_T^i) - I \text{ otherwise} \end{cases} \tag{13}$$

At each iteration, the mean value m_T^i and the standard deviation σ_T^i are updating according to the equations below:

$$m_T^i = \frac{1}{n}\sum_{j=1}^{n} x_j \qquad \sigma_T^i = \frac{1}{n-1}\sum_{j=1}^{n}(x_j - m_T^i)^2 \tag{14}$$

Where n is the number of accepted tumor samples $\{x_j\}$.
The convergence of the algorithm is related to the choice of τ and k. Indeed, for a small value of k, the level set may never grow while for a relatively large value of k, convergence may not be possible.

4. Validation

The brain tumor MR images used in this work were generated by the simulator: *Simulated Brain Tumor MRI Database* Prastawa et al. (2009). The main advantage of these simulations is the existence of ground truth about the true tumor extent (in form of probability maps for the distribution of tumor and edema). We used five volumes: each volumetric image contained 256 x 256 x 181 voxels. Moreover, Three different imaging modalities (T1-weighted with and without gadolinium enhancement and T2-weighted) are provided.

Our experimental MRI data consists of T1 and T1w (T1 after injection with contrast agent - gadolinium). To evaluate the segmentation results, we compute the similarity index known as the kappa statistics (Dice similarity coefficient that is equivalent to Jaccard similarity measure) Zijdenbos et al. (1994a). It measures the normalized intersection in voxel space of two segmentations: in general the manual segmentation (GT) (Ground Truth) and another one (S). This metric is formulated as following:

$$KI = \frac{2|GT \cap S|}{|GT| + |S|} \tag{15}$$

Where $|.|$ is the cardinal of the segmentation result. The operator $\cap$ represents the intersection of two sets. This metric gives a score of 1 for perfect agreement and 0 for complete disagreement. Zijdenbos et al. Zijdenbos et al. (1994b) state that any value of KI above 0.7 indicates a strong agreement.

It should be noted that the overlap measure depends on the size and the shape complexity of the object. On the other hand, It is sensitive to the difference between two sets since both denominator and numerator change with increase or decrease in the overlap. Thus, we also computed error measures by using another metric called "Hausdorff distance". This second metric (HD) represents the maximum surface distance measure, which measures the largest difference between two tumor volumes. It defines the maximum surface distance as :

$$HD = \max(h(S, GT), h(GT, S)) \tag{16}$$

Where

$$h(S, GT) = \max_{x \in S} \min_{y \in GT} |x - y| \tag{17}$$

Some obtained results are given in figure 4 showing the initialization step. Indeed, the first and the second columns of this figure includes T1-weighted image before and after contrast injection. The third column presents the obtained contrast absolute difference images and the last column shows the effect of binary morphological erosion operator (i.e: initial model for the tumor region).

Concerning segmentation step, some segmented tumors are given in figure 6. Indeed, the first column includes T1-weighted image befor contrast injection, the second column shows the extraction of tumor boudaries and the third column shows the comparison between our segmentation (red color) and the ground truth (green color).

From a global point of view, we observed that the contours of the automated segmentations closely follow those of the ground truth labels as shown in figure 6. This observation can be explained by the merging of different source of information in the evolving model and the performing of a post-processing step that refine the segmentation result. Following these experiments, we can deduce that the obtained results are qualitatively strongly acceptable compared to the ground truth.

Quantitative segmentation results, which are performed on some data sets, are also given in Table 1. As we can see in this table, the results for the kappa measure (KI) indicate that the segmentation is reliable.

However, we have noticed some poor results in some cases. For example, it should be noted that the large values of HD in some cases is due to the presence of outliers. This observation can be explained also by the poor image quality, the complexity of the tumor shapes, and the effect of the τ (threshold estimation) and the smoothness parameter on the level set speed function.

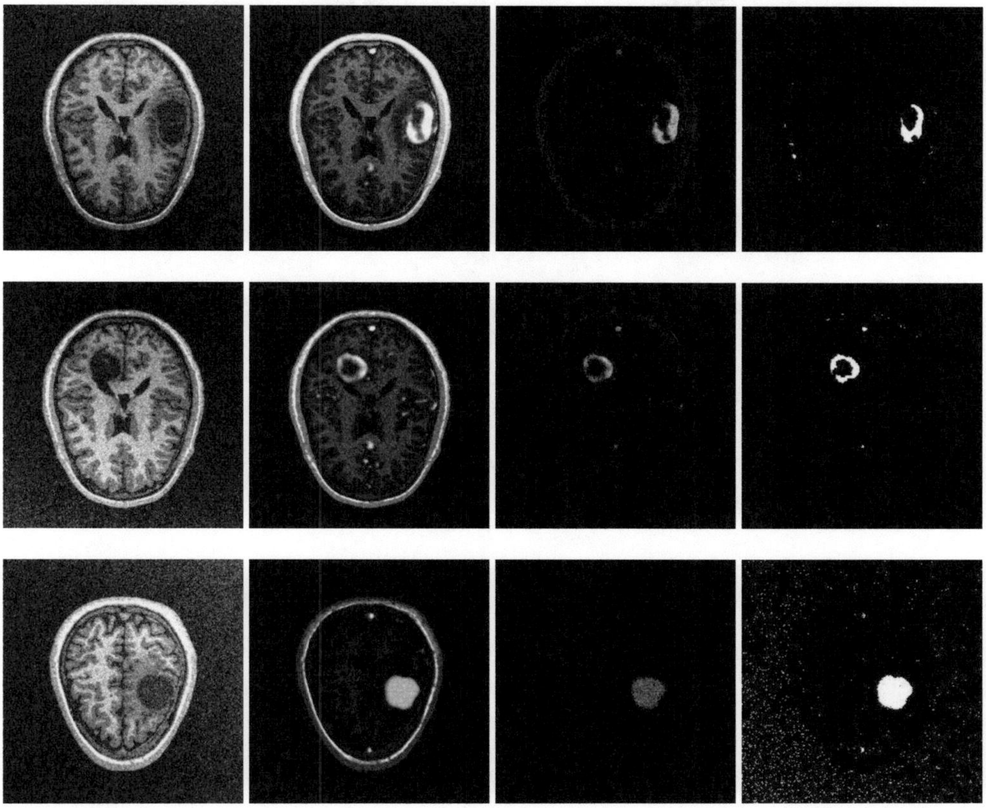

Fig. 4. Active model initialization : The first column includes T1-weighted image. The second column shows T1-weighted image after contrast injection. The third column are contrast absolute difference images. The last column shows the effect of binary morphological erosion operator (i.e: initial model for the tumor region)

Volume	KI (%)	HD (mm)
SimTumor001_Slice090	76,4	9.434
SimTumor001_Slice122	77,5	9.055
SimTumor001_Slice180	83,1	8.062
SimTumor002_Slice090	83,8	5.00
SimTumor002_Slice171	80,2	6.708

Table 1. Kappa measure and Hausdorff distance obtained on some brain tumor scans.

At this stage, the obtained image from the last operation includes a tumor, some tissues with intensities as high as the tumor voxels, and some noisy structures. However, only pathological voxels are needed. For this purpose, we apply a post-processing based on mathematical morphology operations. A binary morphological erosion and dilation process is applied to eliminate noise as well as normal tissue structures while retaining the brain tumor areas.

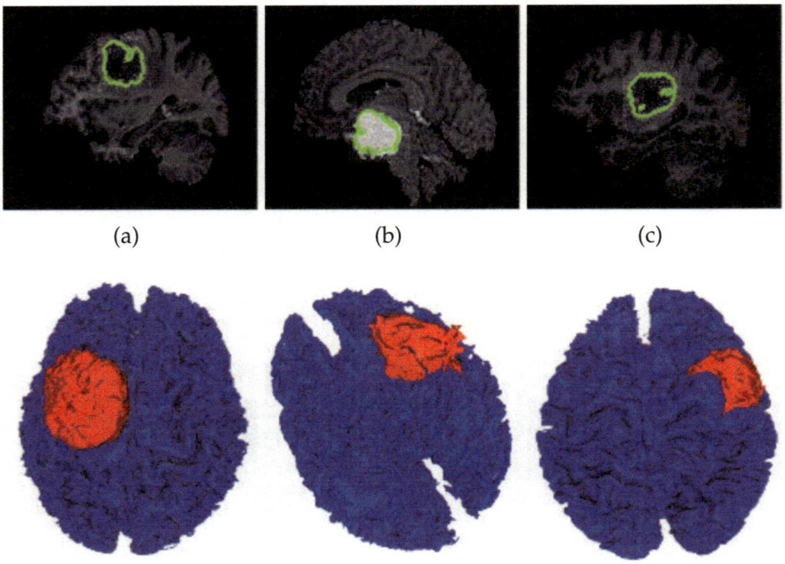

(a) (b) (c)

(d) (e) (f)

Fig. 5. 3D visualization of some tumors (red) within the cerebral cortex (blue). These results are obtained by the semi-automatic algorithm on real T1-weighted MR images

This process requires the definition of the radius size of the neighborhood associated with the structuring element. Once this process is done, we move to the next step to initialize the active model and to refine more and more the segmented tumor area.

We note that we have tested our method on some other real MRI images. Some 3D obtained results are given in figure 5. This figure shows the obtained 3D tumor surface which is superposed on 3D gray matter surface. Indeed, once isolated, the detected tumor can be further processed for volume measurement and three-dimensional rendering.

The mean computation time for the segmentation of a complete 3D image volume takes approximately 3 minutes on a Windows environment with a 2.8 GHz CPU and 512 MB RAM. The algorithm is implemented with C++ language.

5. Summary and discussion

The automatic brain tumor segmentation is an important problem in medical imaging. Although much effort has been spent on finding a good solution to this problem, it is far from being solved.

This chapter surveyed existing methods for brain tumor segmentation in MRI. It presents also a new deformable model based on level-set concept for 3D tumor segmentation. Our proposed deformable model uses both boundary and regional information to define the speed function. We have also proposed a fully automatic initialization process to start our algorithm by considering images with and without contrast enhancement. The segmentation quality in the borders of tumor is relatively good due to the combination of local and global information. Some issues are discussed in this section, including the influence of different parameters on the final segmentation results.

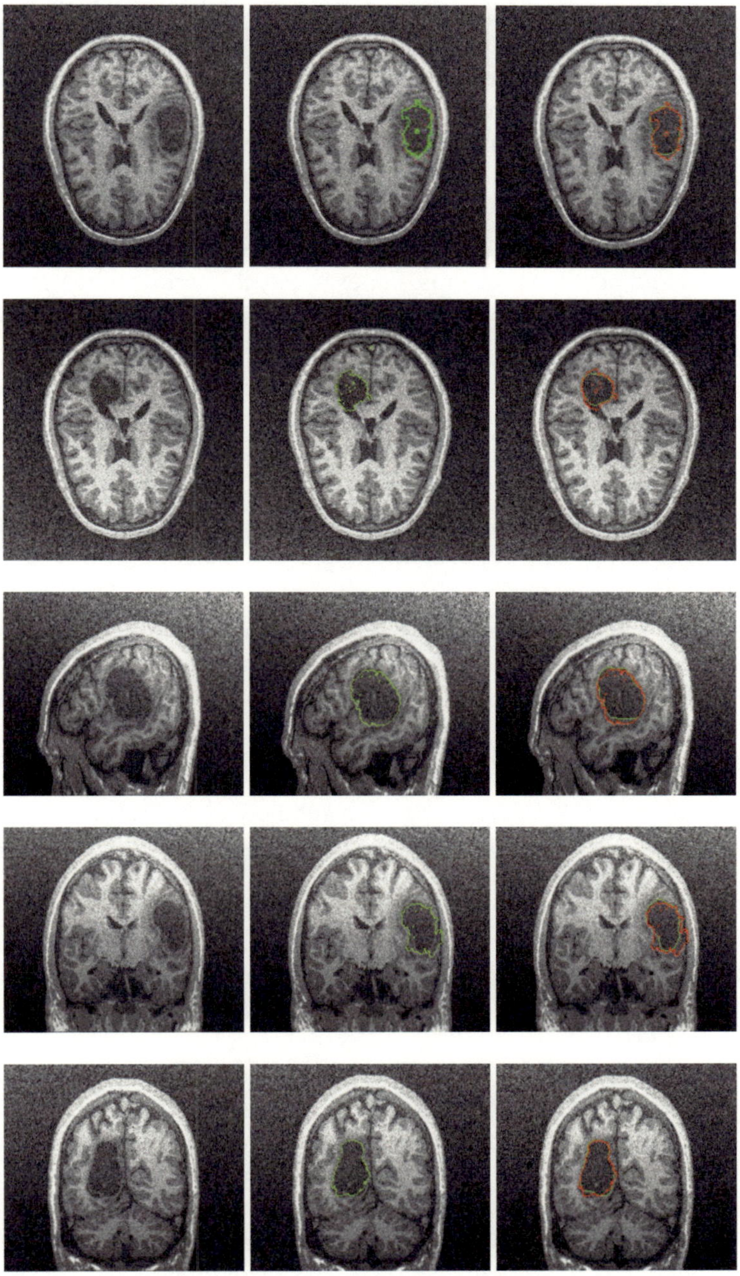

Fig. 6. Brain tumor segmentation: The cross-sections of extracted tumor surfaces with some of their image slices. The first column includes T1-weighted image befor contrast injection. The second column shows the extraction of tumor boudaries. The third column shows the comparison between our segmentation (red color) and the ground truth (green color).

- First of all, the purpose of the proposed method is to surmount limitations of some mentioned methods in the section 1 (Introduction). In particular, it tried to overcome the problem of quality, stability, precision, and to propose an automatic process for segmentation. This is done by the combination of regional and boundary information into the same deformable model formalism. However, the current work can not overcome all limitations and there are improvements to do in our future work.
- In the present study, we didn't consider the influence of non-brain tissue removal, the bias field correction and the partial volume averaging. However, these steps should be considered to avoid possible problems. For example, the brain volume could be extracted by removing the skull by using one of the best known method such as the "Brain Extraction Tool (BET)" Smith (2002).
- Unfortunately, only syntetic tumor types have been considered in this paper. Therefore, the method should be tested on more real data sets containing different kind and size of lesions in order to better validate. Also, further investigations are required to present the effect of tumor size, color, and location.
- Although the presence of this 'enhancement' can be a strong indicator of tumor location, there exist a large variety of types of brain tumors, and their appearance in MR images can vary considerably.

Although the presence of this 'enhancement' can be a strong indicator of tumor location, there exist a large variety of types of brain tumors, and their appearance in MR images can vary considerably.

6. References

Bourouis, S. & Hamrouni, K. (2010). 3d segmentation of mri brain using level set and unsupervised classification, *International Journal in Image and Graphics (IJIG)* Vol. 10(No. 1): 135–154.

Bourouis, S., Hamrouni, K. & Betrouni, N. (2008). Automatic mri brain segmentation with combined atlas-based classification and level-set approach, *5th International Conference on Image Analysis and Recognition, ICIAR,LNCS(5112)* pp. 770–778.

Brown, M. & Semeka, R. (2003). *MRI: Basic Principles and Applications*, John Wiley and Sons, Inc., 3rd edition.

Caselles, V., Kimmel, R. & Sapiro, G. (1997). Geodesic active contours, *International Journal on Computer Vision* Vol. 22(No. 1): 61–97.

Chen, T. & Metaxas, D. (2003). Gibbs prior models, marching cubes, and deformable models: A hybrid framework for 3d medical image segmentation, *Medical Image Computing and Computer-Assisted Intervention (MICCAI)* Springer LNCS 2879: 703–710.

Cobzas, D., Birkbeck, N., Schmidt, M., Jagersand, M. & Murtha, A. (2007). A 3d variational brain tumor segmentation using a high dimensional feature set, *IEEE 11th International Conference on Computer Vision (ICCV)* pp. 1–8.

Corso, J., Sharon, E., Dube, S., El-Saden, S., Sinha, U. & Yuille, A. (2008). Efficient multilevel brain tumor segmentation with integrated bayesian model classification, *IEEE Transactions on Medical Imaging* Vol. 27(No. 5): 629–640.

Cuadra, M., Pollo, C., Bardera, A., Cuisenaire, O., Villemure, J. & Thiran, J. (2004). Atlas-based segmentation of pathological mr brain using a model of lesion growth, *IEEE Transactions on Medical Imaging* 23: 1301–1314.

Ho, S., Bullitt, E. & Gerig, G. (2002). Level set evolution with region competition: Automatic 3-d segmentation of brain tumors, *International Conf on Pattern Recognition ICPR* Vol. 20(No. 8): 532–535.

Kass, M., Witkin, A. & Terzopoulos, D. (1987). Snakes: Active contour models, *Int. J. Comput. Vis.* Vol. 1: 321–331.

Liew, A. & Yan, H. (2006). Current methods in the automatic tissue segmentation of 3d magnetic resonance brain images, *Current Medical Imaging Reviews* Vol. 2: 91–103.

Liu, J., Udupa, J., Odhner, D., Hackney, D. & Moonis, G. (2005). A system for brain tumor volume estimation via mr imaging and fuzzy connectedness, *Computerized Medical Imaging and Graphics* Vol. 29(No. 1): 21–34.

Maes, F., Collignon, A., Meulen, D., Marchal, G. & Suetens, P. (1997). Multi-modality image registration by maximization of mutual information, *IEEE Trans. on Med. Imaging* Vol. 16: 187–198.

Malladi, R., RC., J. S. & Vemuri (1995). Shape modeling with front propagation: A level set approach, *IEEE Trans. Pattern Anal. Machine Intell* Vol. 17(No. 2): 158–174.

Moon, N., Bullitt, E., Leemput, V. & Gerig, G. (2002). Automatic brain and tumor segmentation, *MICCAI* pp. 372–379.

Osher, S. & Sethian, J. (1988). Fronts propagating with curvature-dependent speed: Algorithms based on Hamilton-Jacobi formulations, *Journal of Computational Physics* Vol. 79: 12–49.

Perona, P. & Malik, J. (1990). Scale-space and edge detection using anisotropic diffusion, *IEEE Trans. Med. Imaging* 12: 629–639.

Prastawa, M., Bullitt, E. & Gerig, G. (2009). Simulation of brain tumors in mr images for evaluation of segmentation efficacy, *Medical Image Analysis (MedIA)* Vol. 13(No. 2): 297–311.

Prastawa, M., Bullitt, E., Ho, S. & Gerig, G. (2004). A brain tumor segmentation framework based on outlier detection, *Medical Image Analysis (MedIA)* Vol. 8: 275–283.

Sethian, J. (1999). *Level Set Methods and Fast Marching Methods: Evolving Interfaces in Geometry, Fluid Mechanics, Computer Vision, and Materials Science*, second ed., Cambridge University Press, Place of publication.

Smith, S. (2002). Robust automated brain extraction, *Human Brain Mapping* Vol. 17: 143–155.

Taheri, S., Ong, S. & Chong, V. (2010). Level-set segmentation of brain tumors using a threshold-based speed function, *Image and Vision Computing* Vol. 28: 26Ű–37.

Toga, W., Thompson, A., Mega, P., Narr, M., KL. & Blanton, R. (2001). Probabilistic approaches for atlasing normal and disease-specific brain variability, *Anatomy and Embryology* Vol. 204(No. 4): 267–282.

Warfield, S., Kaus, M., Jolesz, F. & Kikinis, R. (2000). Adaptive, template moderated, spatially varying statistical classification, *Med Image Anal* Vol. 4: 43–55.

Zhang, Y., Brady, M. & Smith, S. (2001). Segmentation of brain mr images through a hidden markov random field model and the expectation-maximization algorithm, *IEEE Transactions on Medical Imaging* Vol. 20: 45–57.

Zijdenbos, A., Dawant, B., Margolin, R. & Palmer, A. (1994a). Morphometric analysis of white matter lesions in mr images: Method and validation, *IEEE Trans. on Medical Imaging* Vol. 13(No. 4): 716–724.

Zijdenbos, A., Dawant, B., Margolin, R. & Palmer, A. (1994b). Morphometric analysis of white matter lesions in mr images: Method and validation, *IEEE Trans. on Medical Imaging* 13(4): 716–724.

8

Current Optical Imaging Techniques for Brain Tumor Research: Application of *in vivo* Laser Scanning Microscopy Imaging with a Cranial Window System

Kyuha Chong[1], Taeyun Ku[1], Kyungsun Choi[1], Myunghwan Choi[2], Jonghee Yoon[1] and Chulhee Choi[1]
[1]*Korea Advanced Institute of Science and Technology (KAIST), Yuseong-gu, Daejeon,*
[2]*Wellman Center for Photomedicine, Massachusetts General HospitalCambridge, Massachusetts,*
[1]*Republic of Korea*
[2]*United States of America*

1. Introduction

"Seeing is believing." This may not be true in all areas of biomedical research, but identifying cellular characteristics of tumors and specifying their anatomical locations are the most important processes for diagnosing and treating tumors. Furthermore, various imaging techniques with various modalities have been introduced to investigate disease progression, track the pharmacokinetic behavior of drugs, and in clinical applications.

Reconstructing images at the molecular level has been realized with the dramatic advancement in energy sources, detectors, computational methods, and instruments. Computed tomography (CT), magnetic resonance imaging (MRI), positron emission tomography (PET), and ultrasound imaging are well-known imaging techniques that have tremendously improved not only preclinical research but also clinical treatment. Contrast-enhanced CT, MRI and PET have permitted non-invasive detection of abnormal tissues, particularly for tumor research and clinical applications.

Imaging techniques currently used for brain tumor research vary with purpose and imaging characteristics. The techniques can be grouped by three aspects: (1) energy, (2) spatial resolution, and (3) type of information obtained (Weissleder & Pittet, 2008). The energies generally used for these techniques are X-rays (e.g., classic X-ray imaging, CT, multi-detector CT), magnetic fields (e.g., MRI and diffusion MRI), positrons (e.g., PET), sound waves (e.g., ultrasound imaging, interventional ultrasound imaging), photons (e.g., bioluminescence imaging, fluorescence reflectance imaging, fluorescence-mediated tomography, and laser scanning microscopy imaging), and combinations of such modalities (e.g., PET-CT, PET-MRI, CT, or MRI with fluorescence-mediated tomography). The techniques can also be distinguished by spatial resolution and the information obtained: (1) macroscopic, (2) mesoscopic, and (3) microscopic or (1) anatomical, (2) physiological, and (3) cellular and molecular.

Optical imaging techniques (OITs) are a subset of imaging modalities that mainly use photons as their energy source. The beauty of these techniques is that the cellular or molecular level of the target can be visualized and target location or texture can be identified with different dyes (Kovar et al., 2007; Massoud & Gambhir, 2003). Although OITs have limited imaging depth and procedure accessibility, they have become indispensable in many fields of research and clinical applications, including brain tumor research.

2. OITs for brain tumor research

Tremendous technological improvements and an increase in the number of OIT applications have occurred with advances in optics and probes. Visualization of the structures and functions of the brain has become possible with microscopic and macroscopic imaging techniques. Because of these advances, OITs have been actively utilized in the field of brain research.

Ultraviolet, visible, and infrared light are the main spectrums of the light used in OITs. The energy (E) of photons is denoted by wavelength (λ). Photons with a shorter wavelength have higher energy than those with a longer wavelength, which is given by the following equation:

$$E = \frac{hc}{\lambda}$$

where h is Planck's constant and c is the speed of light.

Spectrum Spatial resolution	Visible light (380-780nm)	Near-infrared (650-1400nm)
Macroscopic	Bioluminescence imaging (BLI)	Near-infrared fluorescence (NIRF) imaging
Microscopic	Confocal laser scanning microscopy (CLSM) imaging	Multi-photon laser scanning microscopy (MPLSM) imaging

Table 1. Frequently used optical imaging techniques for *in vivo* studies

Although tissue penetration by photons varies with the type of tissue, longer wavelength light generally penetrates deeper; less than 1 mm at 400 nm (blue), 0.5 to 2 mm at 514 nm (green), 1 to 6 mm at 630 nm (red), and 1 to 2 cm at 800 nm (near-infrared) (Barolet, 2008; Kalka et al., 2000; Wilson & Patterson, 1986). Penetration depth for a human brain tumor was reported to be 1 mm at 514 nm, 2.5 mm at 635 nm, and 6 mm at 1060 nm (Svaasand & Ellingsen, 1985).

Spatial resolution and the biological level of information should also be considered for imaging. The primary macroscopic imaging information is physiological, cellular, and molecular, and screening of molecular events or cell tracking is possible with OITs. Higher resolution images to obtain anatomical and quantitative information can be attained with microscopic imaging. But both macroscopic and microscopic imaging have depth and coverage limitations, which are regulated by the chosen wavelength and fluorophore (Wiesner et al., 2009).

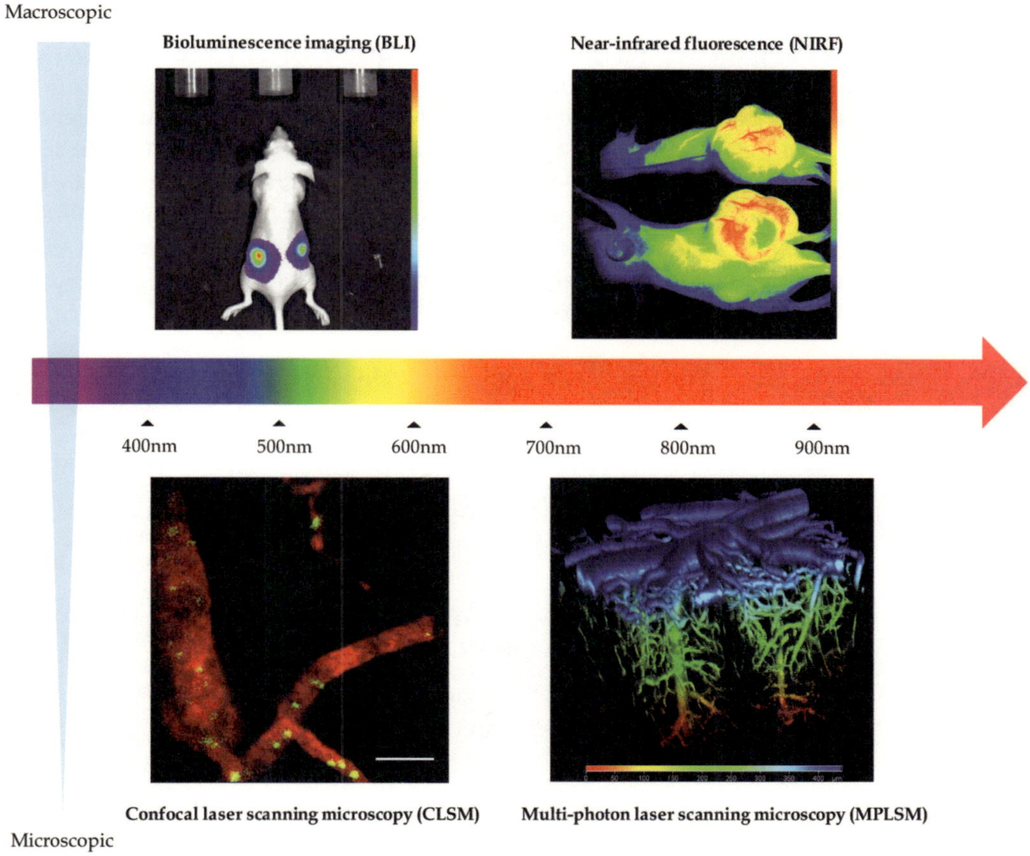

Fig. 1. Schematization of the most frequently used optical imaging techniques for *in vivo* studies. The bar in the middle indicates the light spectrum.

The most frequently used OITs for *in vivo* brain tumor studies are bioluminescence imaging (BLI), near-infrared fluorescence (NIRF) imaging, confocal laser scanning microscopy (CLSM) imaging, and multi-photon laser scanning microscopy (MPLSM) imaging (Table 1 and Fig. 1). These OITs are categorized by light spectrum and spatial resolution. Using a particular technique is determined by the needs and purposes of the research and by considering the technique characteristics (Table 2).

2.1 BLI

BLI is a non-invasive macroscopic imaging technique that uses luminescence for imaging. The chemical reaction between luciferase and luciferin (d-(-)-2-(60-hydroxy-20-benzothiazolyl)-thiazone-4-carboxylic acid) in the presence of oxygen and adenosine triphosphate transforms chemical energy into luminescence at a wavelength of 560 nm. Cells engineered to express luciferase emit light in the presence of luciferin (Ozawa & James, 2010; Sun et al., 2010).

A luciferin substrate is administered via an intraperitoneal injection, and images obtained 10 to 20 minutes after injection for tumor imaging in luciferase-expressing tumor xenograft models. The beauty of this technique is not only that it is non-invasive and rapid but that it is highly sensitive, because there is no inherent light background noise (Wiesner et al., 2009). Tumor development, growth, and location can be quantitatively and noninvasively analyzed with BLI (Rehemtulla et al., 2000).

Although BLI has many benefits, there are several drawbacks. The transmission efficiency of bioluminescence largely depends on the type of tissue and the depth of origin, due to the scattering properties of visible light. Disturbances in the light transmission due to light absorption by hemoglobin and signal attenuation by melanin and fur also limit application of BLI (O'Neill et al., 2010). Additionally, even though advances have been made to translate BLI data into three-dimensional (3D) tomographic imaging (Chaudhari et al., 2005; Slavine et al., 2006), commonly used BLI has limited use for 3D reconstruction.

Technique	Resolution	Depth	Time	Imaging agent	References
BLI	Several mm	cm	Minutes	Luciferin	(O'Neill et al., 2010; Rehemtulla et al., 2000; Sun et al., 2010)
NIRF	Several hundred µm	cm	Minutes	Near-infrared fluorophore	(Choi et al., 2011; Kircher et al., 2003; Veiseh et al., 2007)
CLSM	0.5-1.0 µm	< 100-200 µm	Second to hours	Fluorophore, photoprotein	(Centonze & White, 1998; Gratton, 2011)
MPLSM	0.5-1.0 µm	< 500-1,000 µm	Second to hours	Fluorophore, photoprotein	(Calabrese et al., 2007; Farrar et al., 2010; Levene et al., 2004; Theer et al., 2003; Winkler et al., 2009; Winkler et al., 2004)

Table 2. Overview of optical imaging techniques for *in vivo* studies

2.2 NIRF imaging

NIRF imaging is an efficient, non-invasive, and high-throughput modality useful for *in vivo* imaging (Hsu et al., 2006). NIRF imaging uses near-infrared fluorophores, whether the reflectance technique is applied or not. Because NIRF (650–900 nm) penetrates deeper into tissue than luminescence (Shah & Weissleder, 2005) and does not require cellular transfection, NIRF imaging is regarded as a more effective technique for brain tumor studies than that of BLI.

However, because data acquisition is based on a two-dimensional planar image, NIRF imaging is limited for 3D reconstruction. Additionally, NIRF imaging has problems of light scattering and low quantum efficiency, due to longer wavelengths, which leads to lower signal intensity (Amiot et al., 2008). Although NIRF penetrates deeper than BLI (up to several centimeters), the depth is not adequate to analyze deeper targets within a large animal. Thus, at present, this imaging modality, which uses traditional NIRF fluorophores, is suitable only for small animals such as rodents.

Currently used NIRF materials are fluorescent dyes, quantum dots, single-walled carbon nanotubes, and rare earth metal reagents (Amiot et al., 2008). Because such fluorophores do not have specific targets, molecular modifications are required to specify targets. Specificity is achieved by combining targeting molecules with fluorophores such as Cy5.5-chlorotoxin

(Veiseh et al., 2007). Vascular leakiness can be utilized for brain tumor imaging. Indocyanine green (ICG), an NIR fluorophore, has been used to analyze blood perfusion and permeability of tumors (Choi et al., 2011). Most ICG is bound to albumin in serum, so it does not normally leak into the extravascular space, but it does pass into highly leaky tumor vasculature. Rapid vascular normalization with neutralizing vascular endothelial growth factor was identified with this novel dynamic fluorescence imaging technique using ICG.

2.3 Laser scanning microscopy (LSM) imaging

Since CLSM was introduced in the late 1980s (Brakenhoff et al., 1985; Centonze & White, 1998), the acquisition of high resolution sectional imaging data has become practical, even with thick samples. CLSM collects information from selected foci using a pin-hole, which eliminates out-of-focus information. Phototoxicity in the area that is not the region of interest (ROI) and short penetration depth are major limitations of this technology.

MPLSM is a revolutionized fluorescence microscopy modality that uses non-linear optical properties such as multi-photon absorption. Near-infrared light, which is delivered with a high-power femtosecond pulse, excites fluorophores or molecules in a small specific spot with longer wavelength light (Gratton, 2011). MPLSM has been applied to intra-vital studies since the discovery of molecular excitation by simultaneous absorption of two photons (Denk et al., 1990).

Because MPLSM utilizes longer wavelength photons, image information can be acquired with minimal phototoxicity to the samples and with deeper penetration compared with conventional CLSM. Up to 800–1,000 µm depth resolution is achievable with an MPLSM system (Theer et al., 2003; Weissleder & Pittet, 2008), but typically < 500 µm depth of resolution is achievable for brain imaging (Levene et al., 2004).

However, it remains technically challenging, as significant decreases in resolution occur at greater depths. So, these techniques are inappropriate for deep tissue (> 1 cm depth) imaging. Furthermore, samples or specimens must be prepared with more invasive methods for *in vivo* brain tumor imaging, such as the dorsal skin-flap chamber or cranial window methods, as compared with BLI or NIRF imaging. Although lower energy photons are transmitted into the sample than with BLI or NIRF, fluorophore photo-bleaching frequently occurs, particularly with repetition.

3. Animal models for brain tumor research

In vivo animal model studies are very important for translating biological assessments. Many methods and techniques are available to create animal models that mimic the pathology and tumor environment of a human brain tumor. The tumor model type is chosen depending on the experimental conditions and study purposes.

The xenograft tumor model (XM) is one of the most common and powerful methods to mimic tumor status. XM has been widely used for interventional studies due to convenience. However, the genetically engineered mouse model (GEMM) is preferred for results because of the difference between cell origin and an inability to represent the mechanism of tumor development. However, difficulty producing the model, late onset, insufficient representation of the evolving microenvironment with additional stochastic genetic events, and the inherent difficulty of tumor diagnosis in a timely fashion makes GEMM less desirable (de Vries et al., 2010; Huse & Holland, 2009). Table 3 is an overview of the animal models currently used for brain tumor studies.

Type	Subtype	Realization	Lead time	Relevance	Imaging technique used	References
Genetically engineered mouse model (GEMM)	Germline modification	Highly difficult	Several months to years	High	BLI, NIRF	(Fomchenko & Holland, 2006; Huse & Holland, 2009)
	Somatic cell gene transfer	Difficult	Weeks to months	Intermedate to high	BLI, NIRF	(de Vries et al., 2010; Wiesner et al., 2009)
Xenograft tumor model (XM)	Subcutaneous transplant	Easy	Weeks to months	Low	BLI, NIRF	(Choi et al., 2011; O'Neill et al., 2010)
	Dorsal skin flap chamber	Intermediate	Several weeks	Low	LSM	(Hoffman, 2002; Tozer et al., 2005)
	Orthotopic, non-cranial window	Intermediate	Several weeks	Intermediate	BLI, NIRF	(Hashizume et al., 2010; Ozawa & James, 2010; Szentirmai et al., 2008)
	Orthotopic-cranial window	Difficult	Several weeks	Intermediate	LSM	(Calabrese et al., 2007; Farrar et al., 2010; Winkler et al., 2009; Winkler et al., 2004)

Table 3. Overview of animal models for brain tumor research ("imaging technique used" are those mainly used for *in vivo* imaging)

3.1 GEMM

GEMM is a tumor model generated by a particular genetic alteration. GEMM strongly recapitulates the tumorigenesis process and the nature of tumor progression. Thus, scientists appreciate the results that are obtained from this model. However, many GEMM express unexpected alterations in genes of other organs or tissues. In those cases, it is difficult to say whether GEMM fully presents tumorigenesis, so it is referred to as human cancer predisposition syndromes (Fomchenko & Holland, 2006). Because modifying a particular gene and achieving the target phenotype are very difficult to realize, this model is the first choice for an initial study.

GEMM includes transgene, knock-out, and knock-in mouse models. A transgenic mouse model contains additional genes for a certain purpose (Hanahan et al., 2007). A knock-out mouse model has one or more specific genes inactivated mainly by replacing or disrupting the coding exons, whereas a knock-in mouse model is one in which an endogenous sequence is exchanged with a mutated DNA sequence without disrupting any other genes (Manis, 2007).

There are many types of GEMMs that refer to brain tumors. These models mainly focus on gliomas and medulloblastomas, which are the most common brain tumors in humans. The main considerations for producing such models are as follows: genetics, tumorigenesis mechanism of the model (conventional and/or conditional, transgenic and/or knock-out), incidence of successful tumor development, histological or morphological grades (Huse & Holland, 2009), development type (*de novo* or progressive) (Kwon et al., 2008), the possibility of recapitulation, and organ or area specificity (Huse & Holland, 2010).

Advances have been made in production methods to overcome the inconveniences and uncertainties of traditional GEMM, which are derived from germline modification strategies. Somatic cell gene transfer is a method that generates a genetically altered tumor using viral or pegylated DNA plasmids. While traditional GEMM is used to spontaneously develop a tumor in any location, the somatic cell gene transfer model forces the alteration to a specific location, which is very important for imaging.

For example, de Vries et al. developed a high-grade glioma model using a stereotactic intracranial injection of lentiviral GFAP-Cre or CMV-Cre vectors into compound LoxP-conditional mice, p53;Ink4a/Arf;K-Ras^{v12} (de Vries et al., 2010). The mice developed a tumor within 25 days after injection. They obtained information about the existence of the tumor at an early stage using BLI. They also provided evidence for therapeutic interventional studies by comparing the alterations and differences in tumor growth between a control and a chemotherapy treatment group using longitudinal BLI analysis.

Although somatic cell gene transfer models can predict tumor location, the tumor usually originates in a deep brain structure. Therefore, the OITs are limited to BLI or NIRF imaging. It is affordable to use LSM imaging for GEMM; however, LSM imaging is mostly limited to sample slice imaging and is insufficient for *in vivo* studies.

3.2 XM

As mentioned previously, XM is the most frequently used model for *in vivo* tumor studies. The XM is created by implanting an established cell line or primary tumor cells into a particular location in the animal. The strengths and weaknesses of this technique are listed in Table 4 (Finkelstein et al., 1994; Fomchenko & Holland, 2006).

Strengths	Weaknesses
• Synchrony and reproducibility of tumor formation • Rapid tumor development • High penetrance • Easy tumor visualization	• Lack of stepwise genetic alteration • Alteration of the cells or cell line • Lack of histological accurate vascularization • Rare recapitulation of tumor-of-origin phenotype

Table 4. Strengths and weaknesses of the xenograft tumor model

The frequently used types of XM models for brain tumor studies can be summarized as follows: (1) subcutaneous transplant model, (2) dorsal skin-flap chamber model, (3) orthotopic, non-cranial window model, and (4) orthotopic-cranial window model. OITs can be used with these models, because of convenience and ability to specify the ROI.

3.2.1 Subcutaneous transplant model

The subcutaneous transplant model is simply made by injecting a tumor cell suspension in the flank or leg area of the animal. Tumor growth progression differs depending on cell characteristics but usually it takes several weeks to months to reach an adequate volume for study (Morton & Houghton, 2007). Usually 3×10^6–1×10^7 cells are needed for a successful implantation.

Interventional studies were classically performed by estimating tumor volume using direct length and width measurements (Jensen et al., 2008) or histopathological analysis such as immunohistochemistry. However, these estimates only provide relative values and are inherently biased, whereas histopathology can only be performed by excising the tumor. Because BLI and NIRF imaging provide non-invasive and semi-quantitative measurements, OITs have become a useful modality for longitudinal *in vivo* studies using this model.

In addition to quantifying tumor mass, an OIT modality can be used to measure functional vascular parameters (Choi et al., 2011). Vascular heterogeneity, density, and permeability of an implanted tumor can be estimated with a quantitative analysis of emitted signal intensity.

3.2.2 Dorsal skin-flap chamber model

Longitudinal *in vivo* optical studies are possible with minimal intervention if localized surgical implantation of the tumor is supported by fixing a transparent slide glass coverslip, such as in the dorsal skin-flap chamber (DSFC) model. More detailed and precise information can be obtained with the use of the LSM technique. Because MPLSM imaging has minimal phototoxicity and deeper penetration than some other modalities, minimally invasive and repetitive images are achievable with high resolution.

Using the LSM technique, the DSFC tumor model not only provides information about the tumor itself but also of the interaction between the tumor and tumor-associated vessels. Parameters such as inter-capillary distance, vessel length, and branching ratios can be analyzed (Tozer et al., 2005). Furthermore, 3D data facilitates a precise evaluation of tumor angiogenesis.

Implantation of the tumor is possible by either locating a tumor fragment or spheroid just above the upper tissue layer (Torres Filho et al., 1995) or by injecting a suspension of tumor cells above the fascia. The total cell count of the initial implantation is not fixed, and location and method of implantation can be varied depending on the study group. Regardless of which protocol is used, images can be acquired several weeks after injection.

3.2.3 Orthotopic, non-cranial window model

The orthotopic xenograft model offers more advanced synchrony of the brain tumor microenvironment than that of the subcutaneous transplant or DSFC models. Generally, a tumor is implanted with an inoculating cell line suspension containing 1×10^5–5×10^5 cells by stereotactic injection. Injection location varies among research groups. For example, implantation by Ozawa and James was 2 mm lateral to the bregma, 1 mm anterior to the coronal suture, and at a 3 mm depth from the underside of the skull (Ozawa & James, 2010); Hashizume et al. utilized an implantation protocol of 3 mm from the midline, just behind the bregma for supratentorial, and 3 mm from the midline, 1.5 mm behind the lambdoid suture for infratentorial, with a 3 mm depth from the bottom of the skull (Hashizume et al., 2010); and Szentirmai et al. performed surgery at 2.5 mm lateral and 0.5 mm posterior to the bregma and at a parenchymal depth of 3.5 mm (Szentirmai et al., 2008).

Implantation in deeper locations provides sufficient space and abundant vascular support for tumor growth but precludes intravital microscopic imaging. Early detection and time-series quantitative estimation of tumor growth are possible using BLI and NIRF imaging techniques.

3.2.4 Orthotopic-cranial window model

The orthotopic-cranial window model combines the benefits of window modeling, which enables microscopic evaluation, with the synchrony of an orthotopic xenograft. Complexity of realization is a drawback of this technique compared with other previously described xenograft models, but it is not as much as with GEMM. Researchers can efficiently achieve a model within several weeks with practice.

The tumor can be implanted by fragment or with a cell suspension. However, implantation methods vary between research groups, as compared to the non-cranial window model. We consider that the differences are mainly due to variations in the cranial window surgery method.

For example, Winker et al. attained the model by implanting 0.2–0.3 mm size tumor fragments at a depth of 0.4 mm (Winkler et al., 2004), whereas Farrar et al. injected 3×10^6–2×10^7 suspended cells at a depth of 1.75 mm with a 55° angle (Farrar et al., 2010). We believe that injecting a cell suspension volume of 3–5 µl containing 1×10^5–5×10^5 cells (Winkler et al., 2009) or up to 1×10^6 cells (Calabrese et al., 2007) at a depth of 0.5–2.0 mm from the bottom of the skull is adequate.

Theoretically, all OITs are applicable with this model, if cells and materials are properly prepared; however, MPLSM imaging is the first choice.

3.3 Metastatic brain tumor models

The brain tumor models discussed above are models for recapitulating primary or secondary brain tumors originating within the brain. Although most studies of primary and secondary brain tumors are ongoing, metastatic brain tumor studies are also conducted, because metastatic brain tumors have the highest incidence among all brain tumors. The XM is clearly more relevant to the metastatic process; therefore, model production methods are metaphysically the same as XMs.

A metastatic model can be produced by an entrancing method, as reported by Kienast et al. They realized a metastatic brain tumor model by injecting tumor cells via the carotid artery and demonstrated metastasis formation with MPLSM imaging and a cranial window (Kienast et al., 2010). Such a study was an excellent demonstration of how MPLSM imaging can be combined with the cranial window model.

4. Application of chronic cranial window model system with CLSM and TPLSM imaging for brain tumor research

An Orthotopic xenograft of a brain tumor with a cranial window system has emerged as a potent technique for brain tumor research because it is less costly and requires less lead time to manufacture an XM than a primary tumor model, and the researcher can select the ROI to perform the analysis in a time-dependent manner.

Thinned skull and open craniotomy (craniectomy) models are two types of cranial window systems. The main considerations relating to the two systems are invasiveness (Xu et al., 2007), feasible imaging depth, and maintenance duration of the window. Drew et al.

reported that chronic observations are possible with the thinned skull cranial window model (Drew et al., 2010). However, the thinned skull model can only be applied for metastatic brain tumor model which is created by intracardiac injection of metastatic tumor cells, or for some GEM brain tumor model which produces a tumor at the superficial cortical area. An open craniotomy is more suitable for LSM imaging of an orthotopic xenograft, regardless of whether dura matter must be removed (Orringer et al., 2010)

Now, we will introduce our xenograft model method, which we named the orthotopic xenograft-chronic cranial window (OxCCW) model. This model is based on previous studies and reports (Calabrese et al., 2007; Farrar et al., 2010; Winkler et al., 2009; Winkler et al., 2004). The OxCCW model preserves dura mater for avoidance of additional brain injury, convenience and a high success rate. The resulting images are obtained with CLSM and MPLSM imaging techniques.

4.1 OxCCW model

Red fluorescence protein (RFP) and green fluorescence protein (GFP) expressing U251 (U251-RFP and U251-GFP) tumor cells (human malignant glioma cell-line) were grown *in vitro* in Dulbecco's modified Eagle's medium (DMEM) with 10% fetal bovine serum, 1% non-essential amino acids, and 1% penicillin-streptomycin at 37°C under 20% O2 and 5% CO2. After harvesting, the cells were resuspended in serum-free DMEM medium for implantation into immunodeficient mice. The mouse head was fixed in a stereotactic frame. After the skin incision, a craniotomy was performed at the temporo-parietal area with a high-speed drill. A modified micropipette was introduced into a small incision in the dura at the trajectory point for the injection. In total, 2×10^5 cells in a 5 µl volume were injected at a depth of 0.5 mm from the bottom of the skull. After injection, the craniotomy area was covered with a slide glass coverslip and fixed with bone cement (Fig. 2).

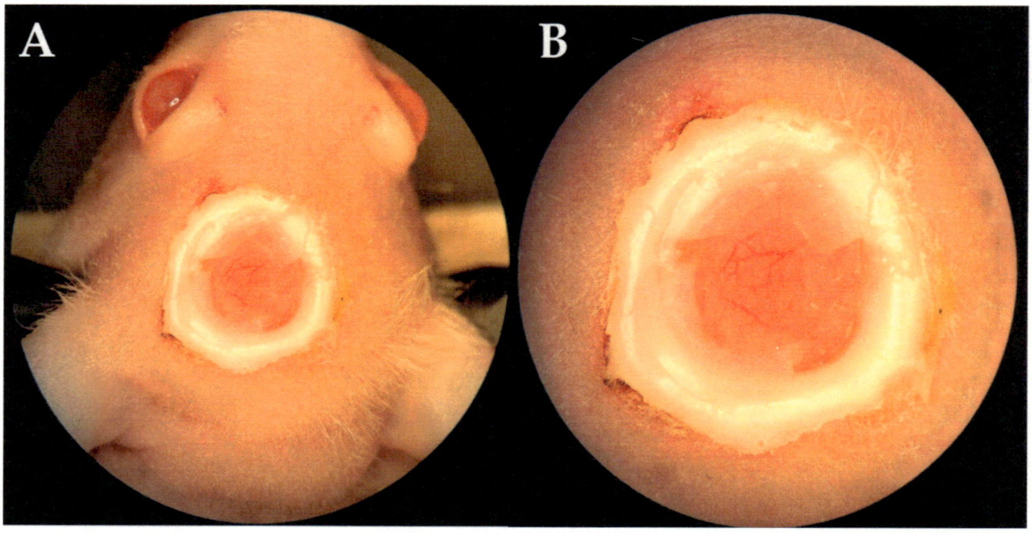

Fig. 2. Macroscopic inspection of orthotopic xenograft-chronic cranial window (OxCCW) model. A. 10X image. The cranial window was set at the left temporo-parietal area. B. 20X image. The slide glass coverslip was tightly fixed with bone cement. Pial vascular structures could be identified.

4.2 CLSM and MPLSM imaging of OxCCW

Time-series images using CLSM and MPLSM can be captured with the OxCCW model. CLSM images were obtained with 488 nm and 543 nm lasers, and MPLSM images were obtained with an 800 nm femtosecond pulsed laser. The growth and progression of the implanted tumor and vascular co-option processes were readily monitored. Vascular changes due to surgical injury (i.e., engorgement of superficial vessels), which were inevitable due to implantation, usually recovered within 1 week after the surgery (Fig. 3). Acquisition of acceptable CLSM images was limited to a depth of 100 μm in our OxCCW model. Imaging of an area deeper than 100 μm was not impossible, but deeper depths revealed poorer resolution, and photo-induced injury occurred more frequently due to a need for more laser power. This problem with CLSM imaging can be solved with MPLSM imaging (Fig. 4). Theoretically, imaging to a depth of 500–1,000 μm is possible with MPLSM. In our experience, acceptable imaging depth of the OxCCW model was extended up to 300 μm from the pial surface using MPLSM imaging.

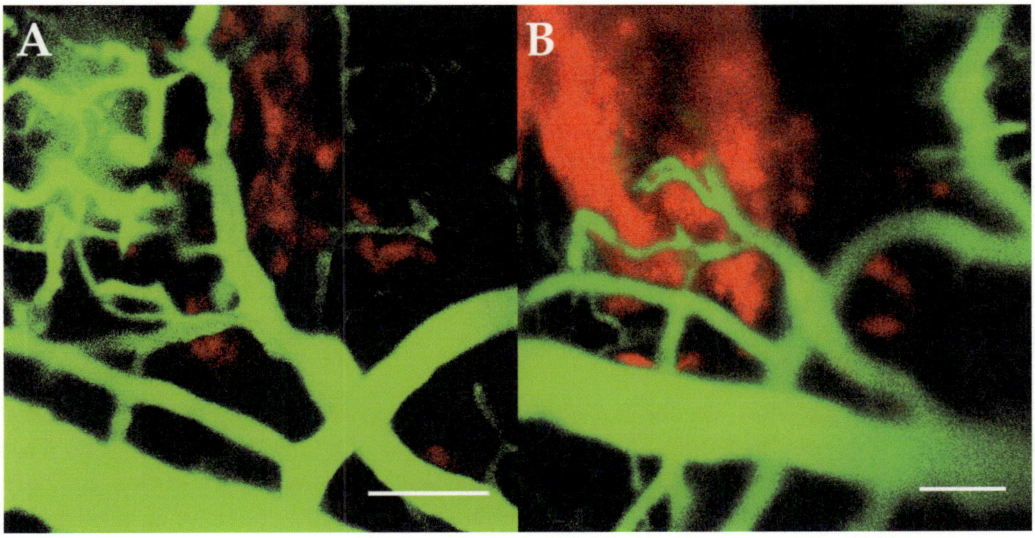

Fig. 3. Time-series confocal laser scanning microscopy images of the orthotopic xenograft-chronic cranial window (OxCCW) model. The images above are projections from the pial surface to a depth of 100 μm. In total, 2×10^5 U251-RFP cells were implanted 1 week before initial imaging. FITC-dextran (2 MDa) was intravenously injected for vascular imaging. (A, B) Tumor progression with the vascular co-option could be monitored with the imaging system. Red indicates emitted fluorescence from U251-RFP cells, and green indicates FITC-dextran. The interval between A and B was 1 week. Scale bar, 100 μm.

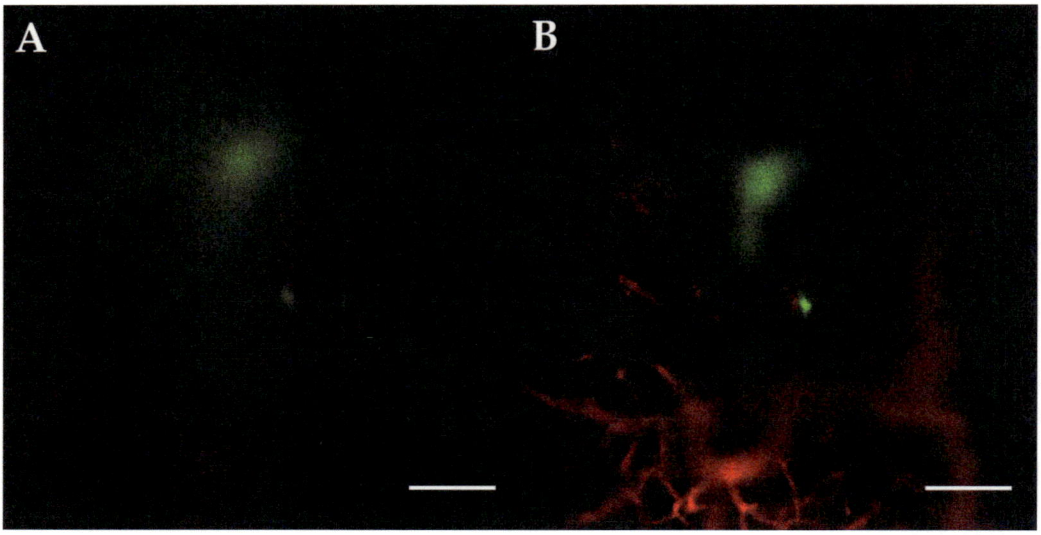

Fig. 4. Comparative confocal and multi-photon laser scanning microscopy images with the orthotopic xenograft-chronic cranial window model. In total, 2 x 10^5 U251-GFP cells were implanted 1 week before imaging. Rhodamin-dextran (70 kDa) was intravenously injected for vascular imaging. The imaging information was collected from a depth of 100–150 μm from the pial surface. Green indicates emitted fluorescence from U251-GFP cells and red indicates rhodamin-dextran. (A) Projection image from a confocal laser scanning microscope. (B) Projection image from a multi-photon laser scanning microscope. Scale bar, 100 μm.

5. Future perspectives

OIT applications are now beyond imaging itself and are not restricted by experimental boundaries. Intra-operative brain tumor imaging, to define the tumor area for resection, has already been applied in clinical settings. Fluorescence-guided surgical resection has been performed in an operating room using 5-aminolevulinic acid (5-ALA), a prodrug of fluorescent molecule protoporphyrin IX (PpIX), and useful statistical results were obtained (Stummer et al., 2006). In addition to the clinical application of OITs for diagnostic purposes, many attempts have been made to introduce therapeutic applications of OITs such as photodynamic therapy.

Combining optical technologies with OITs has been actively attempted for biomedical applications other than imaging. Our group recently reported utilizing a near-infrared femtosecond laser for minimally invasive molecular delivery into the brain (Choi et al. 2011). The delivery is acquired by optical modulation, which enhances the transient increase in vascular permeability (Fig. 5). Additionally, optical modulation of neurovascular coupling in combination with label-free optical activation of astrocytes was also demonstrated.

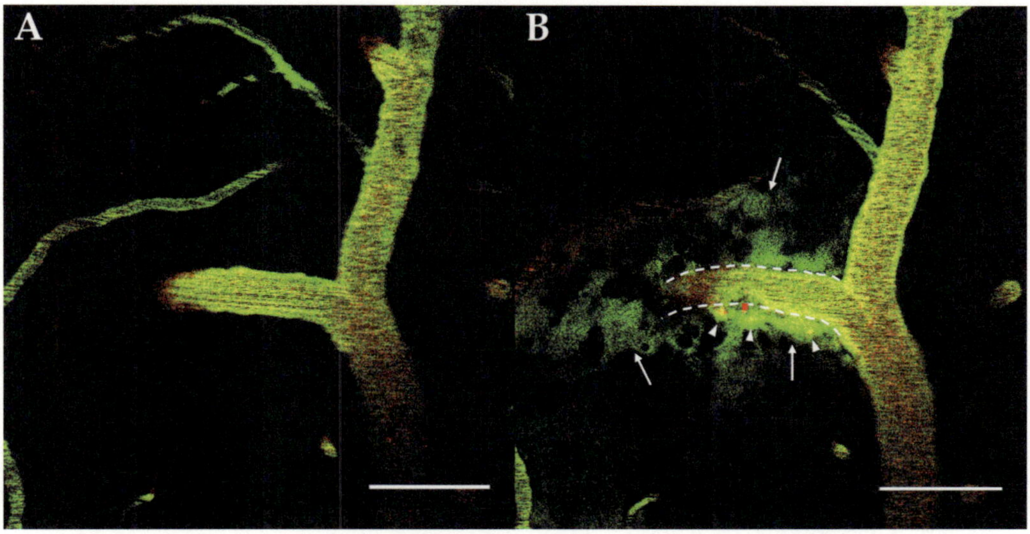

Fig. 5. Laser-induced vascular permeabilization. Imaging and optical modulation were performed with multi-photon laser scanning microscopy (800 nm, femtosecond pulsed laser). FITC-dextran (2 MDa) and fluorescent microspheres (FS03F/5147, Bangs Laboratories) were injected via the tail vein. Green and red indicate FITC-dextran and fluorescent microspheres, respectively. (A) Pre-permeabilization image. (B) Post-permeabilization image. Green dye (white arrows) and red fluorescent microspheres (white arrowheads) were extravasated after optical modulation. Red dot indicates the region that was optically modulated. White dotted line demarcates baseline lumen of the venule. Scale bar, 50 µm.

6. Conclusion

OITs have emerged as essential tools for intravital imaging. The most frequently used OITs are BLI, NIRF, and LSM imaging. Among them, MPLSM is the most potent imaging technique because it obtains precise intravital microscopic information. Translational and interventional studies are expected to be performed in a more efficient manner with the combination of MPLSM and the OxCCW system.

7. Acknowledgements

This research was supported by a grant (2009K001282) from the Brain Research Center of the 21st Century Frontier Research Program funded by the Ministry of Education, Science, and Technology, the Republic of Korea.
We are grateful to Prof. Gou Young Koh, Dr. Young Jun Koh and Junyeop Lee for their support of BLI imaging and their constructive discussions.

8. References

Amiot, C. L.; Xu, S. P.; Liang, S.; Pan, L. Y. & Zhao, J. X. J. (2008). Near-infrared fluorescent materials for sensing of biological targets. *Sensors,* Vol.8, No.5, pp. 3082-3105, ISSN 1424-8220

Barolet, D. (2008). Light-emitting diodes (LEDs) in dermatology. *Seminars in cutaneous medicine and surgery,* Vol.27, No.4, pp. 227-38, ISSN 1558-0768

Brakenhoff, G. J.; van der Voort, H. T.; van Spronsen, E. A.; Linnemans, W. A. & Nanninga, N. (1985). Three-dimensional chromatin distribution in neuroblastoma nuclei shown by confocal scanning laser microscopy. *Nature,* Vol.317, No.6039, pp. 748-9, ISSN 0028-0836

Calabrese, C.; Poppleton, H.; Kocak, M.; Hogg, T. L.; Fuller, C.; Hamner, B.; Oh, E. Y.; Gaber, M. W.; Finklestein, D.; Allen, M.; Frank, A.; Bayazitov, I. T.; Zakharenko, S. S.; Gajjar, A.; Davidoff, A. & Gilbertson, R. J. (2007). A perivascular niche for brain tumor stem cells. *Cancer cell,* Vol.11, No.1, pp. 69-82, ISSN 1535-6108

Centonze, V. E. & White, J. G. (1998). Multiphoton excitation provides optical sections from deeper within scattering specimens than confocal imaging. *Biophysical Journal,* Vol.75, No.4, pp. 2015-2024, ISSN 0006-3495

Chaudhari, A. J.; Darvas, F.; Bading, J. R.; Moats, R. A.; Conti, P. S.; Smith, D. J.; Cherry, S. R. & Leahy, R. M. (2005). Hyperspectral and multispectral bioluminescence optical tomography for small animal imaging. *Physics in medicine and biology,* Vol.50, No.23, pp. 5421-41, ISSN 0031-9155

Choi, M.; Choi, K.; Ryu, S. W.; Lee, J. & Choi, C. (2011). Dynamic fluorescence imaging for multiparametric measurement of tumor vasculature. *Journal of Biomedical Optics,* Vol.16, No.4, pp. 046008, ISSN 1560-2281

Choi, M.; Ku, T.; Chong, K.; Yoon, J. & Choi C. (2011). Minimally Invasive Molecular Delivery into the Brain Using Optical Modulation of Vascular Permeability. *Proceedings of the National Academy of Sciences,* Vol.108, No.22, pp. 9256-61, ISSN 1091-6490

de Vries, N. A.; Bruggeman S. W.; Hulsman D.; de Vries H. I.; Zevenhoven J.; Buckle T.; Hamans B. C.; Leenders W. P.; Beijnen J. H.; van Lohuizen M.; Berns A. J. M. & van Tellingen O. (2010). Rapid and Robust Transgenic High-Grade Glioma Mouse Models for Therapy Intervention Studies. *Clinical Cancer Research,* Vol.16, No.13, pp. 3431-3441, ISSN 1078-0432

Denk, W.; Strickler J. H. & Webb W. W. (1990). Two-photon laser scanning fluorescence microscopy. *Science,* Vol.248, No.4951, pp. 73-6, ISSN 0036-8075

Drew, P. J.; Shih A. Y.; Driscoll J. D.; Knutsen P. M.; Blinder P.; Davalos D.; Akassoglou K.; Tsai P. S.& Kleinfeld D. (2010). Chronic optical access through a polished and reinforced thinned skull. *Nature methods,* Vol.7, No.12, pp. 981-4, ISSN 1548-7105

Farrar, C. T.; Kamoun W. S.; Ley C. D.; Kim Y. R.; Kwon S. J.; Dai G. P.; Rosen B. R.; di Tomaso E.; Jain R. K. & Sorensen A. G. (2010). In vivo validation of MRI vessel caliber index measurement methods with intravital optical microscopy in a U87 mouse brain tumor model. *Neuro-oncology,* Vol.12, No.4, pp. 341-350, ISSN 1522-8517

Finkelstein, S. D.; Black P.; Nowak T. P.; Hand C. M.; Christensen S. & Finch P. W. (1994). Histological characteristics and expression of acidic and basic fibroblast growth factor genes in intracerebral xenogeneic transplants of human glioma cells. *Neurosurgery,* Vol.34, No.1, pp. 136-43, ISSN 0148-396X

Fomchenko, E. I. & Holland E. C. (2006). Mouse models of brain tumors and their applications in preclinical trials. *Clinical Cancer Research,* Vol.12, No.18, pp. 5288-5297, ISSN 1078-0432

Gratton, E. (2011) Applied physics. Deeper tissue imaging with total detection. *Science,* Vol.331, No.6020, pp. 1016-7, ISSN 1095-9203

Hanahan, D.; Wagner E. F. & Palmiter R. D. (2007). The origins of oncomice: a history of the first transgenic mice genetically engineered to develop cancerle. *Genes & development,* Vol.21, No.18, pp. 2258-2270, ISSN 0890-9369

Hashizume, R.; Gupta N.; Berger M. S.; Banerjee A.; Prados M. D.; Ayers-Ringler J.; James C. D. & VandenBerg S. R. (2010). Morphologic and molecular characterization of ATRT xenografts adapted for orthotopic therapeutic testing. *Neuro-oncology,* Vol.12, No.4, pp. 366-76, ISSN 1523-5866

Hoffman, R. (2002). Green fluorescent protein imaging of tumour growth, metastasis, and angiogenesis in mouse models. *The lancet oncology,* Vol.3, No.9, pp. 546-56, ISSN 1470-2045

Hsu, A. R.; Hou L. C.; Veeravagu A.; Greve J. M.; Vogel H.; Tse V. & Chen X. (2006). In vivo near-infrared fluorescence imaging of integrin alphavbeta3 in an orthotopic glioblastoma model. *Molecular imaging and biology : MIB : the official publication of the Academy of Molecular Imaging,* Vol.8, No.6, pp. 315-23, ISSN 1536-1632

Huse, J. T. & Holland E. C. (2009). Genetically Engineered Mouse Models of Brain Cancer and the Promise of Preclinical Testing. *Brain Pathology,* Vol.19, No.1, pp. 132-143, ISSN 1015-6305

--- (2010). Targeting brain cancer: advances in the molecular pathology of malignant glioma and medulloblastoma. *Nature reviews. Cancer,* Vo.10, No.5, pp. 319-31, ISSN 1474-1768

Jensen, M. M.; Jorgensen J. T.; Binderup T. & Kjaer A. (2008). Tumor volume in subcutaneous mouse xenografts measured by microCT is more accurate and reproducible than determined by 18F-FDG-microPET or external caliper. *BMC medical imaging,* Vol.8, pp. 16, ISSN 1471-2342

Kalka, K.; Merk H. & Mukhtar H. (2000). Photodynamic therapy in dermatology. *Journal of the American Academy of Dermatology,* Vol.42, No.3, pp. 389-413; quiz 414-6, ISSN 0190-9622

Kienast, Y.; von Baumgarten L.; Fuhrmann M.; Klinkert W. E.; Goldbrunner R.; Herms J. & Winkler F. (2010). Real-time imaging reveals the single steps of brain metastasis formation. *Nature Medicine,* Vol.16, No.1, pp. 116-22, ISSN 1546-170X

Kircher, M. F.; Mahmood U.; King R. S.; Weissleder R. & Josephson L. (2003). A multimodal nanoparticle for preoperative magnetic resonance imaging and intraoperative optical brain tumor delineation. *Cancer research,* Vol.63, No.23, pp.8122-5, ISSN 0008-5472

Kovar, J. L.; Simpson M. A.; Schutz-Geschwender A. & Olive D. M. (2007). A systematic approach to the development of fluorescent contrast agents for optical imaging of mouse cancer models. *Analytical biochemistry,* Vol.367, No.1, pp. 1-12, ISSN 0003-2697

Kwon, C. H.; Zhao D.; Chen J.; Alcantara S.; Li Y.; Burns D. K.; Mason R. P.; Lee E. Y.; Wu H. & Parada L. F. (2008). Pten haploinsufficiency accelerates formation of high-grade astrocytomas. *Cancer research,* Vol.68, No.9, pp. 3286-94, ISSN 1538-7445

Levene, M. J.; Dombeck D. A.; Kasischke K. A.; Molloy R. P. & Webb W. W. (2004). In vivo multiphoton microscopy of deep brain tissue. *Journal of neurophysiology,* Vol.91, No.4, pp. 1908-12, ISSN 0022-3077

Manis, J. P. (2007). Knock out, knock in, knock down - Genetically manipulated mice and the Nobel Prize. *New England Journal of Medicine,* Vol.357, No.24, pp. 2426-2429, ISSN 0028-4793

Massoud, T. F. & Gambhir S. S. (2003). Molecular imaging in living subjects: seeing fundamental biological processes in a new light. *Genes & development,* Vol.17, No.5, pp. 545-80, ISSN 0890-9369

Morton, C. L. & Houghton P. J. (2007). Establishment of human tumor xenografts in immunodeficient mice. *Nature protocols,* Vol.2, No.2, pp. 247-50, ISSN 1750-2799

O'Neill, K.; Lyons S. K.; Gallagher W. M.; Curran K. M. & Byrne A. T. (2010). Bioluminescent imaging: a critical tool in pre-clinical oncology research. *The Journal of pathology,* Vol.220, No.3, pp. 317-27, ISSN 1096-9896

Orringer, D. A.; Chen T.; Huang D. L.; Armstead W. M.; Hoff B. A.; Koo Y. E. L.; Keep R. F.; Philbert M. A.; Kopelman R. & Sagher O. (2010). The Brain Tumor Window Model: A Combined Cranial Window and Implanted Glioma Model for Evaluating Intraoperative Contrast Agents. *Neurosurgery,* Vol.66, No.4, pp. 736-743, ISSN 0148-396X

Ozawa, T. & James C. D. (2010). Establishing Intracranial Brain Tumor Xenografts With Subsequent Analysis of Tumor Growth and Response to Therapy using Bioluminescence Imaging. *Journal of Visualized Experiments*. No.41, ISSN 1940-087X

Rehemtulla, A.; Stegman L. D.; Cardozo S. J.; Gupta S.; Hall D. E.; Contag C. H. & Ross B. D. (2000). Rapid and quantitative assessment of cancer treatment response using in vivo bioluminescence imaging. *Neoplasia,* Vol.2, No.6, pp. 491-495, ISSN 1522-8002

Shah, K. & Weissleder R. (2005). Molecular optical imaging: applications leading to the development of present day therapeutics. *NeuroRx : the journal of the American Society for Experimental NeuroTherapeutics,* Vol.2, No.2, pp. 215-25, ISSN 1545-5343

Slavine, N. V.; Lewis M. A.; Richer E. & Antich P. P. (2006). Iterative reconstruction method for light emitting sources based on the diffusion equation. *Medical physics,* Vol.33, No.1, pp. 61-8, ISSN 0094-2405

Stummer, W.; Pichlmeier U.; Meinel T.; Wiestler O. D.; Zanella F. & Reulen H. J. (2006). Fluorescence-guided surgery with 5-aminolevulinic acid for resection of malignant glioma: a randomised controlled multicentre phase III trial. *The lancet oncology,* Vol.7, No.5, pp. 392-401, ISSN 1470-2045

Sun, A.; Hou L.; Prugpichailers T.; Dunkel J.; Kalani M. A.; Chen X. Y.; Kalani M. Y. S. & Tse V. (2010). Firefly Luciferase-Based Dynamic Bioluminescence Imaging: A

Noninvasive Technique to Assess Tumor Angiogenesis. *Neurosurgery,* Vol.66, No.4, pp. 751-757, ISSN 0148-396X

Svaasand, L. O. & Ellingsen R. (1985). Optical Penetration in Human Intracranial Tumors. *Photochemistry and Photobiology,* Vol.41, No.1, pp. 73-76, ISSN 0031-8655

Szentirmai, O.; Baker C. H.; Bullain S. S.; Lin N.; Takahashi M.; Folkman J.; Mulligan R. C. & Carter B. S. (2008). Successful inhibition of intracranial human glioblastoma multiforme xenograft growth via systemic adenoviral delivery of soluble endostatin and soluble vascular endothelial growth factor receptor-2: laboratory investigation. *Journal of neurosurgery,* Vol.108, No.5, pp. 979-88, ISSN 0022-3085

Theer, P.; Hasan M. T. & Denk W. (2003). Two-photon imaging to a depth of 1000 microm in living brains by use of a Ti:Al2O3 regenerative amplifier. *Optics letters,* Vol.28, No.12, pp. 1022-4, ISSN 0146-9592

Torres Filho, I. P.; Hartley-Asp B. & Borgstrom P. (1995). Quantitative angiogenesis in a syngeneic tumor spheroid model. *Microvascular research,* Vol.49, No.2, pp. 212-26, ISSN 0026-2862

Tozer, G. M.; Ameer-Beg S. M.; Baker J.; Barber P. R.; Hill S. A.; Hodgkiss R. J.; Locke R.; Prise V. E.; Wilson I. & Vojnovic B. (2005). Intravital imaging of tumour vascular networks using multi-photon fluorescence microscopy. *Advanced Drug Delivery Reviews,* Vo.57, No.1, pp. 135-152, ISSN 0169-409X

Veiseh, M.; Gabikian P.; Bahrami S. B.; Veiseh O.; Zhang M.; Hackman R. C.; Ravanpay A. C.; Stroud M. R.; Kusuma Y.; Hansen S. J.; Kwok D.; Munoz N. M.; Sze R. W.; Grady W. M.; Greenberg N. M.; Ellenbogen R. G. & Olson J. M. (2007). Tumor paint: a chlorotoxin:Cy5.5 bioconjugate for intraoperative visualization of cancer foci. *Cancer research,* Vol.67, No.14, pp. 6882-8, ISSN 0008-5472

Weissleder, R. & Pittet M. J. (2008). Imaging in the era of molecular oncology. *Nature,* Vol.452, No.7187, pp. 580-9, ISSN 1476-4687

Wiesner, S. M.; Decker S. A.; Larson J. D.; Ericson K.; Forster C.; Gallardo J. L.; Long C.; Demorest Z. L.; Zamora E. A.; Low W. C.; SantaCruz K.; Largaespada D. A. & Ohlfest J. R. (2009). De novo Induction of Genetically Engineered Brain Tumors in Mice Using Plasmid DNA. *Cancer research,* Vol.69, No.2, pp. 431-439, ISSN 0008-5472

Wilson, B. C. & Patterson M. S. (1986). The physics of photodynamic therapy. *Physics in medicine and biology,* Vol.31, No.4, pp. 327-60, ISSN 0031-9155

Winkler, F.; Kienast Y.; Fuhrmann M.; Von Baumgarten L.; Burgold S.; Mitteregger G.; Kretzschmar H. & Herms J. (2009). Imaging glioma cell invasion in vivo reveals mechanisms of dissemination and peritumoral angiogenesis. *Glia,* Vol.57, No.12, pp. 1306-15, ISSN 1098-1136

Winkler, F.; Kozin S. V.; Tong R. T.; Chae S. S.; Booth M. F.; Garkavtsev I.; Xu L.; Hicklin D. J.; Fukumura D.; di Tomaso E.; Munn L. L. & Jain R. K. (2004). Kinetics of vascular normalization by VEGFR2 blockade governs brain tumor response to radiation: role of oxygenation, angiopoietin-1, and matrix metalloproteinases. *Cancer cell,* Vol.6, No.6, pp. 553-63, ISSN 1535-6108

Xu, H. T.; Pan F.; Yang G. & Gan W. B. (2007). Choice of cranial window type for in vivo imaging affects dendritic spine turnover in the cortex. *Nature Neuroscience,* Vol.10, No.5, pp. 549-551, ISSN 1097-6256

9

The Dosimetry Calculation for Boron Neutron Capture Therapy

Li Deng, Chaobin Chen, Tao Ye and Gang Li
Beijing Capture Tech Co., Ltd.
Institute of Applied Physics and Computational Mathematics
China

1. Introduction

BNCT incorporates the targeting principles of chemotherapy and the anatomical localization principles of conventional radiotherapy but with three distinct advantages:

- Current boron compounds at the required concentrations are non-toxic.
- The time interval between drug administration and neutron irradiation can be chosen to maximize the concentration differential between tumour and normal tissue.
- Only the tissues located around the tumour volume are exposed to significant neutron activated boron damage.

Following the earliest suggestions that BNCT might be useful for the treatment of human cancers, interest developed regarding the application of BNCT to primary high-grade brain tumours – glioblastoma multiforme (GBM). It was postulated that the reduction of the blood brain barrier (BBB) in the vicinity of tumour could be exploited to selectively increase the concentration of boron in the brain tumour over normal brain. Initially sodium tetraborate (borax), was used as the vehicle for boron. Perhaps the early interest in applying BNCT to high-grade primary brain tumours stemmed from the fact that this was a cancer with a very poor prognosis. This would ensure that BNCT, even if minimally successful, would nevertheless appear superior to ineffective conventional therapies.

In addition to the considerations of beam quality, the beam should also be sufficiently intense to ensure that treatment times remain within reasonable limits. This facilitates the procedure for the patient and reduces the problem of patient motion during treatment. It should be realized that whereas conventional radiotherapy fractions are administered within a period of about 10 minutes, current clinical BNCT treatments often extend to a few hours per fraction (2001)[1].

In order for BNCT to be successful, a sufficient amount of ^{10}B must be selectively delivered to the tumor (~20μg/g weight or ~10^9 atoms/cell), and enough thermal neutrons must be absorbed by them to sustain a lethal $^{10}B(n,\alpha)^{7}Li$ capture reaction. Since the high linear energy transfer (LET) particles have limited boron pathlengths in tissue (5-9μm), the destructive effects of these high energy particles are limited to cells containing boron. Clinical interest in BNCT has focused primmarily on the treatment of high grade gliomas, and either cutaneous primaries or cerebral metastases of melanoma, and most recently head， neck and liver cancer. Since BNCT is a biologically rather than physically targeted type of radiation treatment, the potential exists to destroy tumor cells dispersed in the normal tissue parenchyma, if sufficient amounts of ^{10}B and thermal neutrons are delivered to the target volume. At its simplest, this could be the two low molecular weight drugs borated phenylalanine (BPA) and containing polyhedral borane (BSH). However, the dose calculations become much more complicated when combinations of agents are used (2006)[2].

Clinical dose distributions can be significantly influenced by tissue inhomogeneities. The accuracy of the transport geometry is a key factor to predict the dose distribution with Monte Carlo method. The distribution of mass densities and chemical compositions, which express the patient's anatomical structure, are needed for the precalculation of the physical cross sections before the dose calculation is done by making direct simulation of the interactions between the radiation and the patient's body. There are two types of computerized anthropomorphic phantoms that can be defined either by mathematical functions or by voxel-based volume arrays. The former is referred to the MIRD Phantoms (1978)[3], the latter is always made from CT or MRI images and well known about Zubal Phantom (1994)[4] and Male Adult Voxel Phantom(2003)[5]. They both can be used to model the patients in internal or external radiotherapy. But in radiation treatment planning, phantoms, which are directly made from the patient's CT images, are essential for the prediction of dose distribution in patient's body. DeMarco *et al* (1998)[6] defined medias of air, lung, fat, water, muscle and bone to figure a patient's anatomical structure. WANG e*t al* (2001)[7] treated voxels from the CT images above a user-specified electron density as bone and below as water. Ma *et al* (2002)[8] used air, tissue and bone to describe a human body. W Schneider(2000)[9]gave a recommendation of 24 materials for the CT images.

In 3D radiation treatment planning a patient model is commonly simulated by dividing it into voxels (cuboids), which have individual mass densities and chemical compositions. There are two kinds of work to do to establish a CT based voxel phantom from a patient's CT images. One is to set up the calibration of CT numbers to mass densities by fitting a set of CT numbers and mass densities of real tissues from ICRP (1975)[10] or ICRU-44 (1989)[11]. The other is to correlate the CT numbers with the elemental weights, which is usually done by defining several threshold values in order to classify the CT scale in Hounsfiled unit (-1000~1500) into different groups and the elemental weights are then constant within each group.

In recent years, the importance of BNCT obviously increases. The relative researches have been done in America, Japan, Finland, Netherland, Argentina, China and Italy etc. Especial for Japan and Argentina, a large amount of clinical tests have been done and good effects have been achieved (1994, 2008)[12,13]. Development of treatment planning system (TPS) software is one of an important part of BNCT, where the physical dose calculation is a key. High precision and rapid computational time are the basic requirements for clinical trials.

This chapter, BNCT principle, TPS status, neutron beam, medical pro, post processor and dose calculation will be discussed.

2. BNCT principles

BNCT technique is used in treating brain tumors by artificially loading the tumor tissue with isotope Boron enriched compound and subsequently irradiation of brain by low energy neutrons. In recent ten years, BNCT has been used to treat the other tumors located at neck, liver and lung etc. The technique is based on the $^{10}B(n,\alpha)^{7}Li$ nuclear reaction emitting alpha particle and ^{7}Li nuclei with total kinetic energy of 2.79 *MeV*, which is high enough to destroy the tumor cells and avoids to hurt the normal tissue. A ^{10}B nucleus absorbs a thermal neutron and promptly emits a back to back ^{7}Li ion and a ^{4}He (alpha) particle. The combined range of 12–13 μm is similar to mammalian cell dimensions.

2.1 Main nuclear reactions

The doses are primarily from four parts: (1) thermal neutrons; (2) boron-10; (3) fast neutrons; and (4) photons. The relative nuclear reactions are given as following:

(1) Nitrogen capture reaction

$$^{14}_{7}N + ^{1}_{0}n \rightarrow ^{14}_{6}C + ^{1}_{1}H + 0.66MeV \qquad (1)$$

Most of neutrons come from the thermal neutron in nuclear reaction. The release energy is deposited locally. The deposited dose is called as thermal neutron dose or proton dose. It is written by D_P.

(2) Boron neutron capture reaction

$$^{10}B + ^{1}_{0}n(0.025eV) \rightarrow {}^{11}B \left\langle \begin{array}{l} ^{4}He_2 + ^{7}Li + 2.79(MeV)\ (6\%) \\ ^{4}He_2 + ^{7}Li + 2.31(MeV)\ (94\%) \end{array} \right.$$

$$\downarrow$$

$$^{7}Li + \gamma + 0.48\ MeV \qquad (2)$$

The release energy is deposited locally except for 0.48 MeV photon energy. The boron dose is written by D_B.

(3) Hydrogen capture gamma reaction

$$^{1}_{1}H + ^{1}_{0}n \rightarrow ^{1}_{0}D + \gamma + 2.224MeV \qquad (3)$$

The photons are from hydrogen capture gamma reaction, boron neutron capture reaction and the neutron beam. The gamma energy is deposited step by step by Compton scattering and photoelectricity absorption. So the photon dose has a wide space distribution. The photon dose is written by D_γ.

(4) Elastic scattering of the fast neutron

The recoil protons are released when the elastic scattering is happened as soon as the epithermal and thermal neutron capture reaction with nitrogen. The proton energy is deposited locally. Of course, the energy of fast neutron is deposited by the elastic scattering, where 90% is from the nuclear reaction with nitrogen. The dose which is produced by the fast neutron elastic scattering is written by D_n. When the biological weighting factors are selected, the total biologically weighted dose, in Gy, becomes:

$$D_{bw} = w_c.D_B + w_\gamma.D_\gamma + w_n.D_n + w_pD_p \qquad (4)$$

Where D_{bw} is dose components, w_c is compound efficacy of the boron. w_γ, w_n. and w_p are the relative biology efficacy of the photon, fast neutron and proton, respectively.

2.2 TPS status

TPS usually includes: (1) the medical pre-processor, i.e a 3-d model of patient's head, which is based on CT and MRI DICOM data, is created and then automatically produces a input file of Monte Carlo code; (2) the dose calculation and (3) the post-processor, which plots the dose lines and surfaces of different tissues. Furthermore, the irradiation time and irradiation location are determined. Most of TPSs are developed from MCNP program [14]. Figure 1 shows a process of TPS. Figure 2 shows the flow of a TPS.

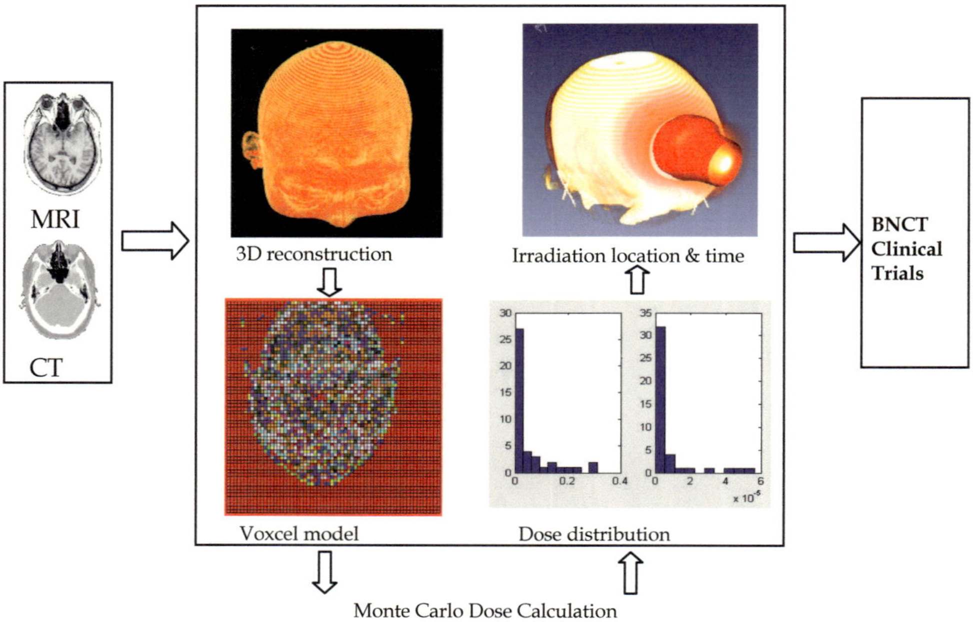

Fig. 1. Process of BNCT

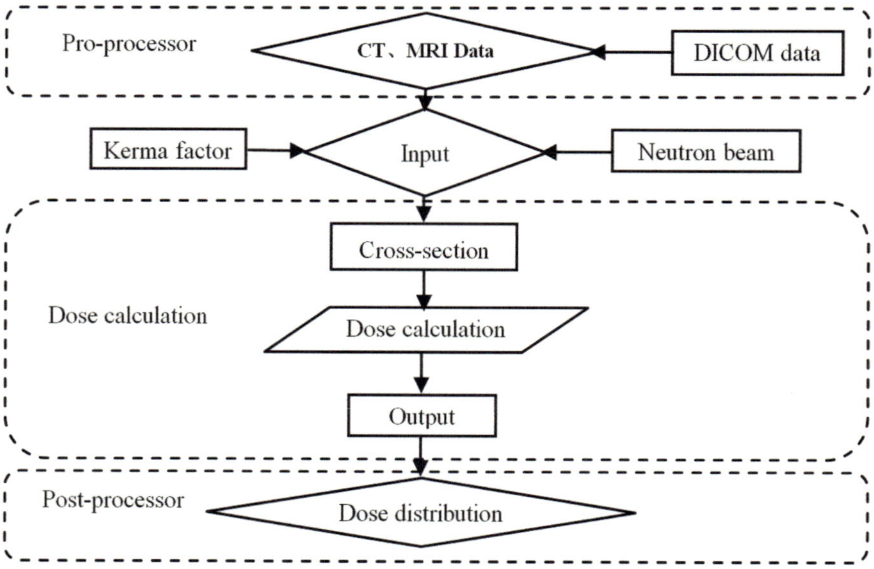

Fig. 2. Flow of BNCT TPS

Comparisons of BNCT TPSs have been limited in some scope. It is as far as know six TPSs, such as NCTPlan, MacNCTPlan (2002)[15], JCDS (2004)[16], BNCT-rtpe, SERA (2000)[17] and MCDB (2007)[18], have been used in the clinical trials, where the Idaho National Energy and Engineering Laboratory's SERA and Harvard-MIT's MacNCTPLAN are thought as the most valid.

3. Pro-processor and post-processor

3.1 Setting up of calibration curve

MDP is the pro-processor and post-processor of MCDB TPS. With a set of CT numbers and related mass densities of real tissues the calibration curve can be built by dividing the CT scale into a few groups and making linear fit in each group. While CT number in Housfiled Unit was first defined by Kouris et al (1982)[19] and can be calculated based on the energy spectrum of X-ray CT and the linear attenuation coefficient of the real tissues as a function of the photon energy. Uwe Schneider *et al* (1996)[20] developed the stoichiometric method to calculate the CT numbers of materials with their mass densities and chemical compositions known. In this paper the stoichiometric method is taken to acquire all the CT numbers of real tissues taken from ICRP (1975)[10].

Usually the CT scale is divided into two segments, which ranges from -1000 to 100 and from 100 to 1500, respectively, to make two linear calibration curves. In figure 3 the solid line is the calibration curve based on a GE 9000 CT scanner and the dash line is based upon a Siemens somatom plus 4 CT scanner. The X-ray tube kilovoltage is at 120kVp during the scans for the two scanners. Final calibration curves from the two type CT scanners fit close to each other for CT numbers below 100. The maximum deviation is about 5% at upper CT region.

3.2 Conversion of CT numbers to elemental weights

How to obtain the elemental weights for the CT based voxel phantoms is concerned here. Normally several thresholds values are chosen to divide the CT scale (-1000~1500) into a set of groups. Within each group, the CT numbers have the same elemental weights.

The distribution of CT numbers in Hounsfield unit from the CT image data of a man's head is shown in figure 4, on which some real tissues are marked. The following points of view are taken into consideration for the division of the CT scale. First, there will be more groups in regions with high proportion of CT numbers according to figure 4, by contraries, in the lower and upper CT regions there will be fewer groups. Secondly, the variation of the elemental weights, especially for calcium and phosphorus, whose weights have significant influence on the dose distribution of electron beams[8], is concerned during selection of the threshold values. Thirdly, the final weights of elements for each CT group is approximately represented by that of the real tissues, whose CT numbers calculated with the stoichiometric method are about in the middle of the CT group (see figure 3 and 4). The CT scale is divided into 24 groups in this paper, which is far exceeded the numbers of groups either from DeMarco (1998)[6] or from Ma (2002)[8], and each group correlates to a real tissue from ICRP publication (1975)[10]. Mass density distribution comes from the calibration curve based on GE 9000 (solid line in figure 4). A CT based voxel phantom can be generated easily by converting the CT numbers into mass densities and elemental weights voxel by voxel.

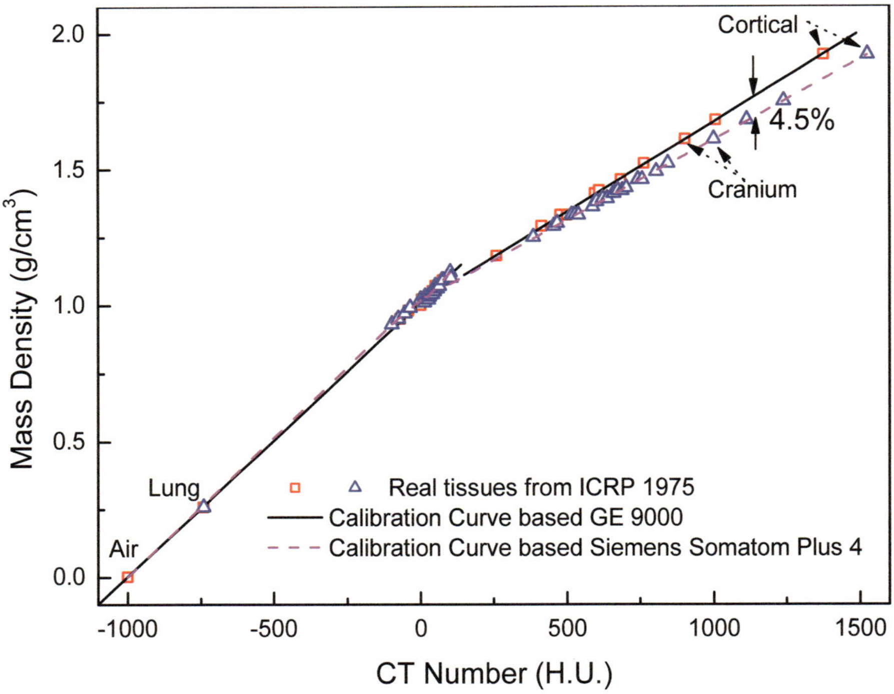

Fig. 3. Relationship between CT numbers and mass densities of real tissues

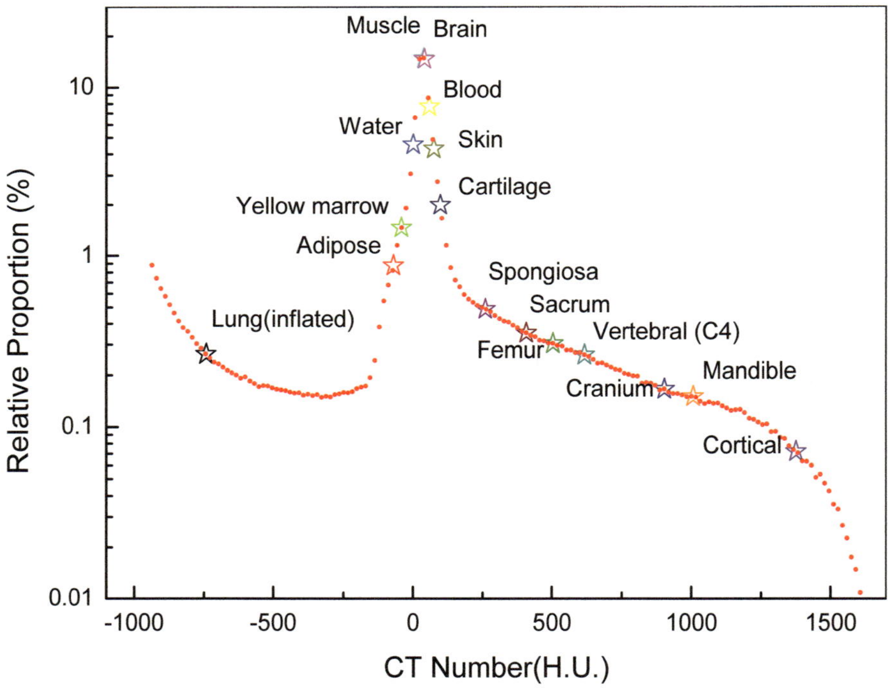

Fig. 4. Proportion of CT numbers for a human head

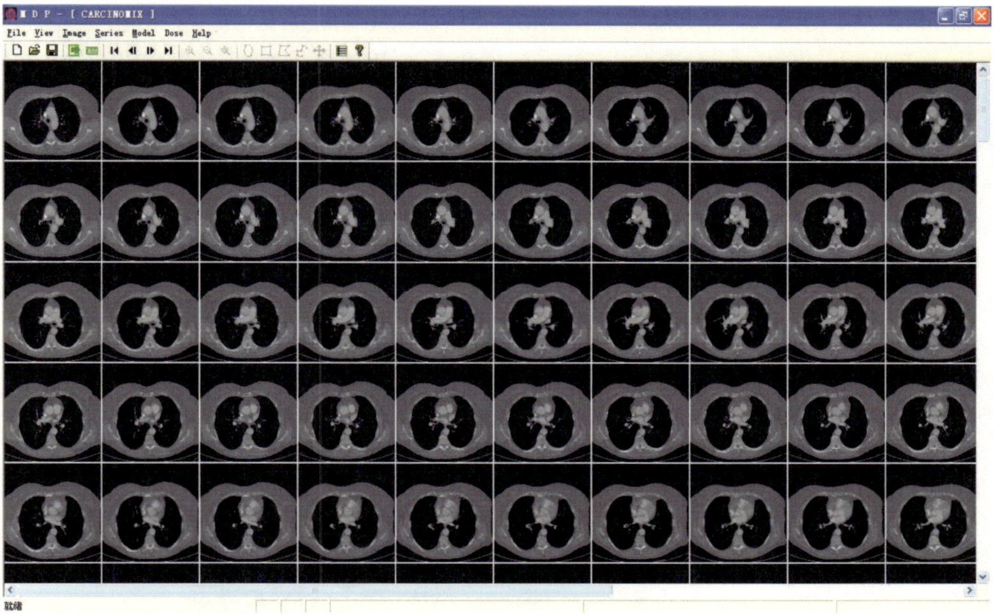

Fig. 5. Main interface of MDP

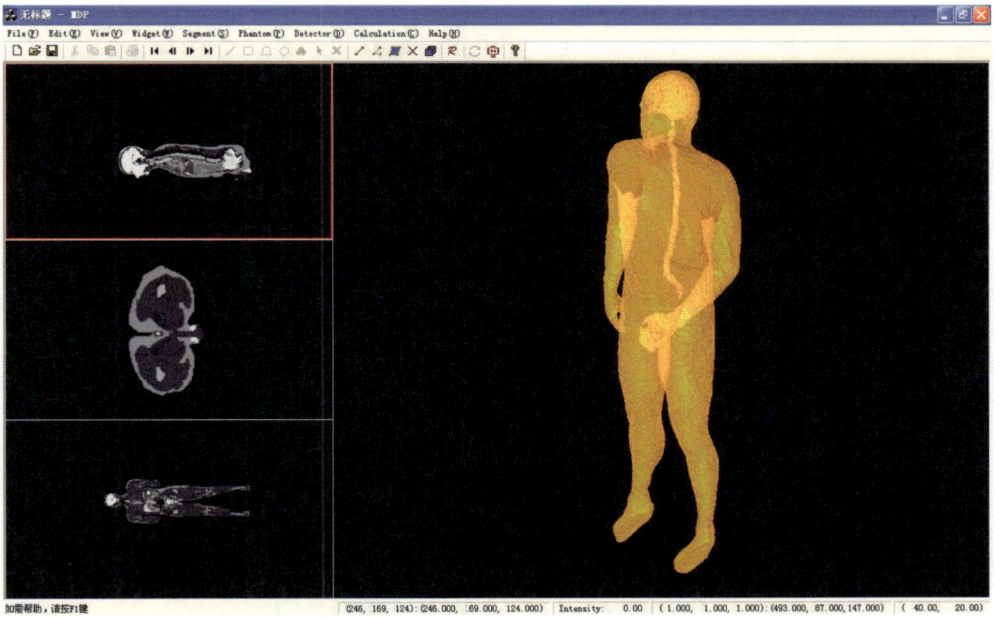

Fig. 6. Rendering of Zubal phantom

In MDP, the pro-processor processes volume data of a patient in DICOM or RAW format into an anthropomorphous phantom and translates it into an acceptable format for a Monte Carlo transport code. Of course, you can explore the patient's medical images in client window with a self-defined window level and window width. Surface rendering function based on MITK package supports extracting surface and rendering it for volume imaging data or volume dose data from dose calculator. Figure 6 shows the profile (Sagittal, Transverse, Coronary) of Zubal phantom and surface rendering results.

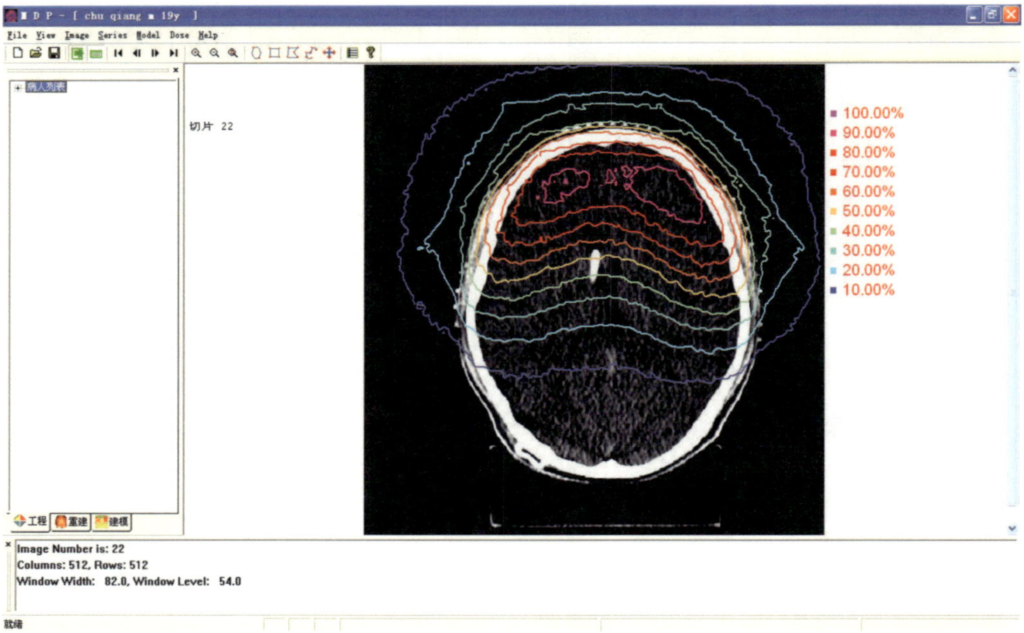

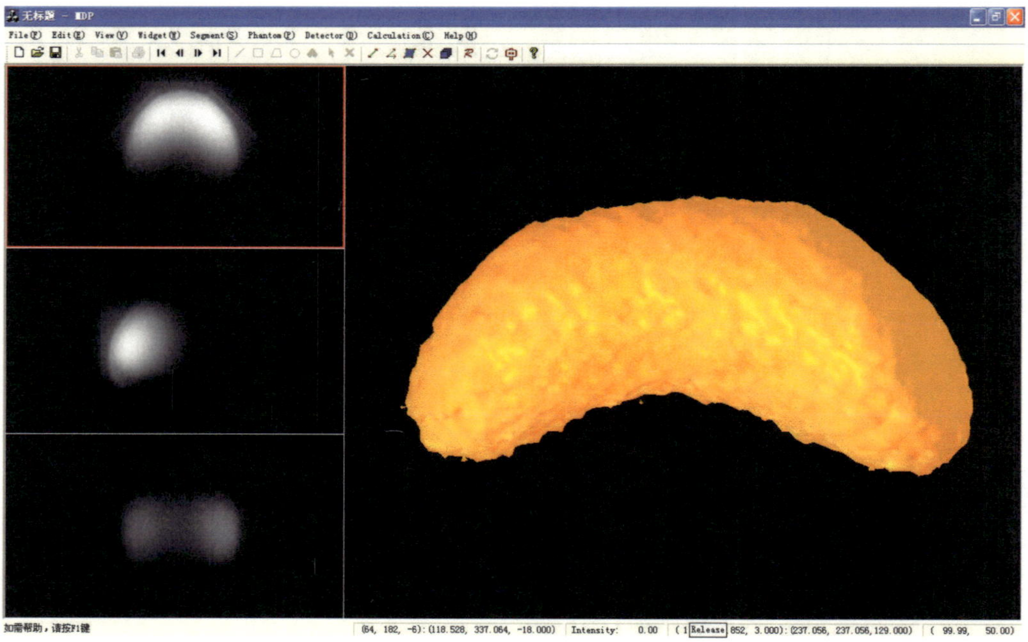

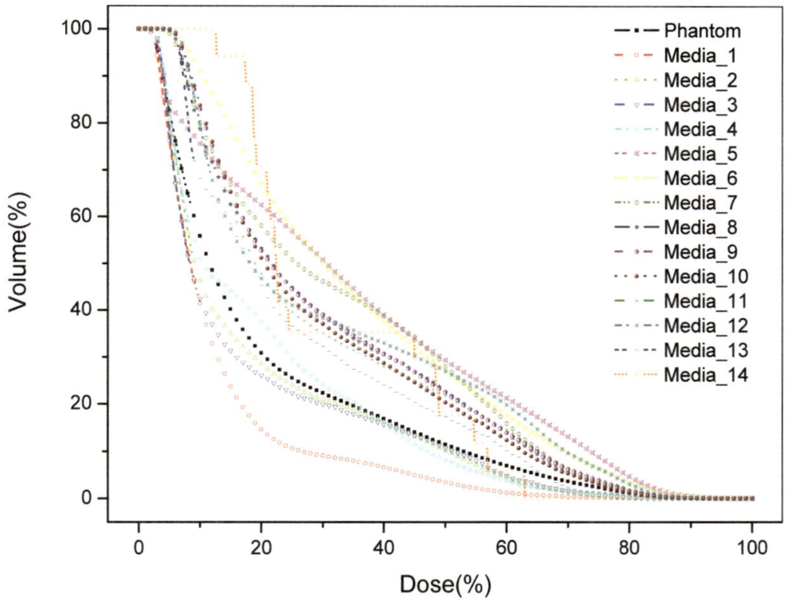

Fig. 7. Results processed by MDP, isoline, iso-surface and DVH

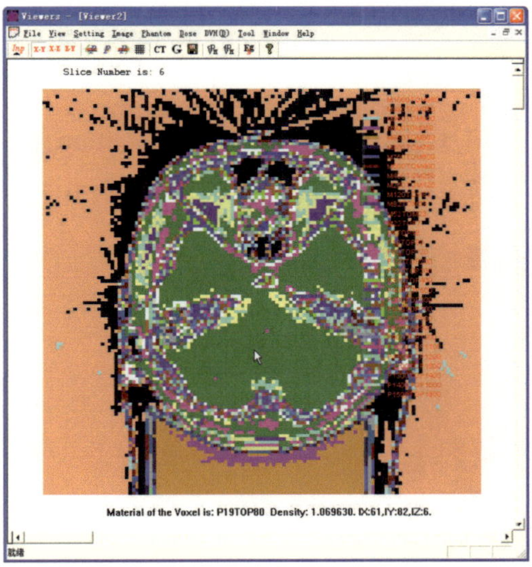

Fig. 8. Materials distribution for one slice

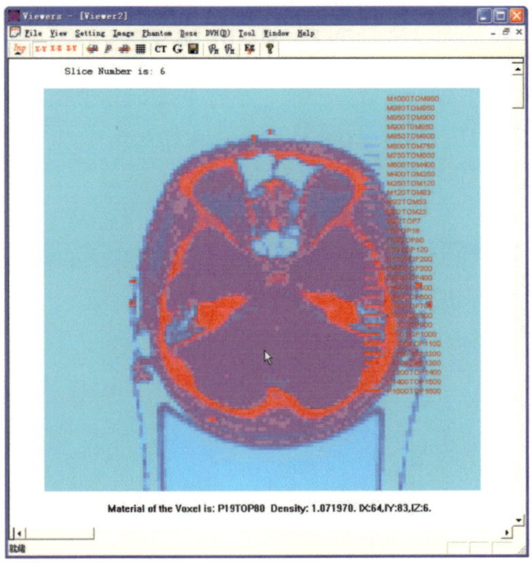

Fig. 9. Density distribution for one slice

At present, the dose calculation mainly represents general purpose Monte Carlo transport codes, such as MCNP[14], EGS[21] and GEANT4[22], etc. MCDB[18] can output an eligible input file for absorbed dose calculation. In case of BNCT, absorbed doses from thermal neutron, fast neutron and gamma will be scored separately. Also, volume dose related to 1ppm boron-10 and other interesting values will be scored.

The post-processor processes dose volume into all kinds of readable style, such as isoline, iso-surface and dose-volume-histogram, etc. An example is introduced to test the main techniques that have been carried out in MCDB. We use a typical spectrum from a research reactor and an approximate angular profile (current/flux=0.65) as incident neutron source. The beam lights on the phantom from three direction (left, top, right) with weight of 0.3, 0.4 and 0.3 respectively. Isoline of one slice, iso-surface rendering of volume dose for 1ppm boron-10 and dose-volume-histogram for different medias are shown in figure 7 from left to right. Some figures for geometry viewer and dose viewer are listed as below.

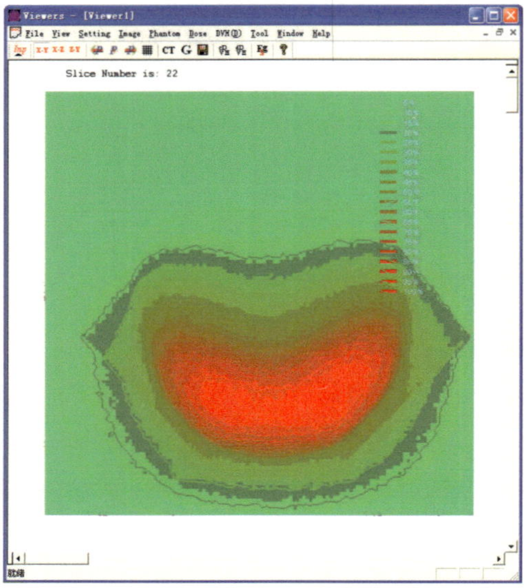

Fig. 10. Dose from thermal neutron distribution for one slice

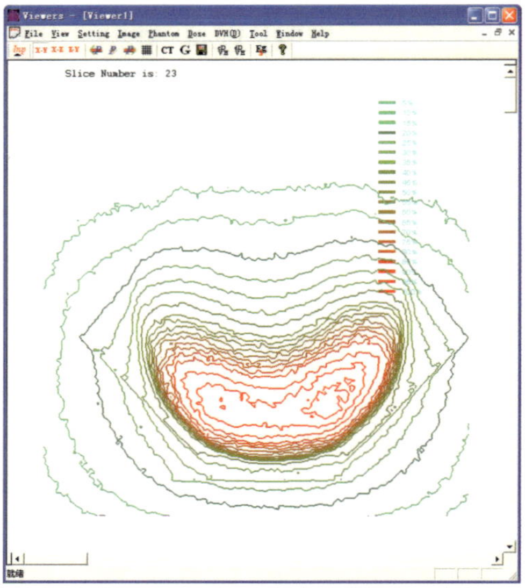

Fig. 11. Dose from 1ppm ^{10}B distribution for one slice

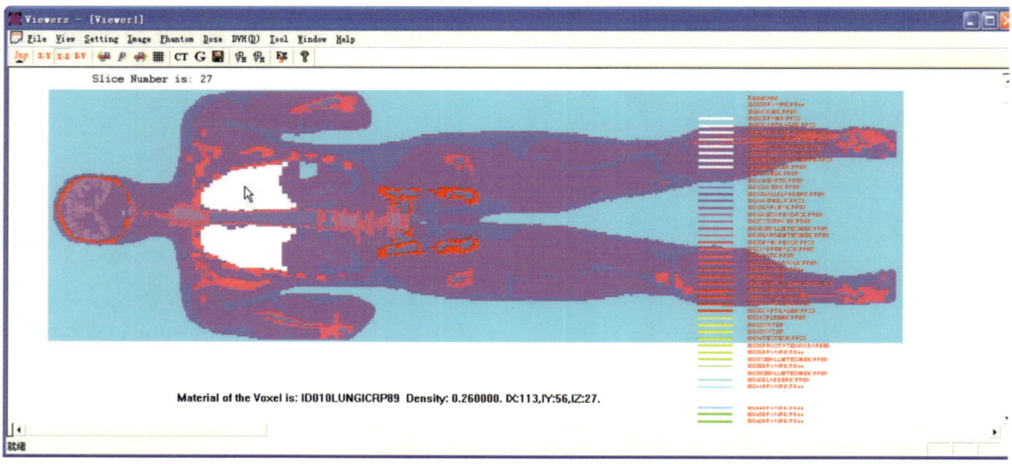

Fig. 12. Materials distribution (mouse clicked on lung) for one slice of Zubal Phantom (Geometry viewer of MDP)

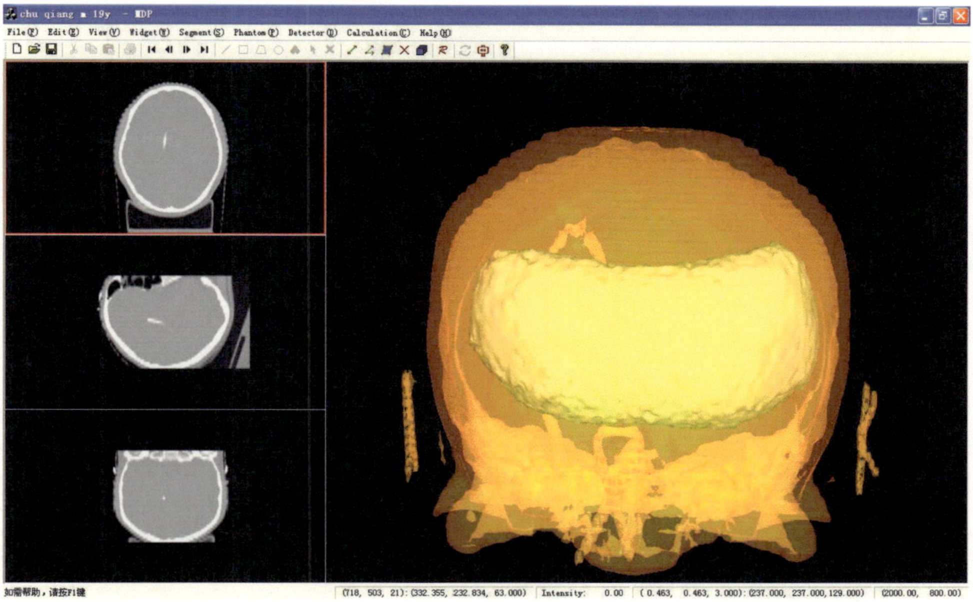

Fig. 13. Rendering results for dose from 1ppm ^{10}B distribution with 60% iso-surface

4. Reactor and neutron beam

Being the first step to start the BNCT studies, the neutron source has to be set up with the proper characteristics, which can create proper irradiation dose deposited at a desired position of the human body. The "proper" means the intensity of neutron flux or dose and the high ratio of useful flux or dose to harmful one requested by a reasonable treatment time. Thermal neutrons are the most wanted irradiation at tumor tissue in the BNCT treatment because of $^{10}B(n,\alpha)$ reaction. However, the thermal neutron beam cannot penetrate tissues. The epithermal neutron beam is preferred to produce thermal neutrons at a certain depth inside tissues, because its average energy is higher than the thermal neutron beam. So, both thermal and epithermal neutron beams are necessary in the BNCT treatment.

To date, a number of facilities have been used for BNCT studies or clinical trials around the world. And they can be roughly classified as 3 types, general purpose research reactors using spectrum shifting and filtering or fission converters, accelerator-based neutron sources, and the dedicated single-purpose reactors.

Eight of such facilities are listed as examples, the epithermal facility at the BMRR of the Brookhaven National Laboratory in USA, the HFR at JRC in Pettern in the Netherlands, KURRI in Japan, the fission converter beam at MIT in USA, RA-6 facility in Bariloche in Argentina, epithermal beam at WSU in USA, the mixed mode beam at JRR-4 at JAEA in Japan, and the epithermal beam at FiR at VTT in Finland [23].

In this session, a newly designed dedicated single-purpose reactor will be introduced [24, 25]. The first In-Hospital Neutron Irradiator (IHNI) in the world was set up in China Institute of Atomic Energy (CIAE) in Beijing, China, in 2009. The IHNI with thermal power 30 kW is developed by Beijing Capture Technology Company (BCTC) which consists of GuoRun Construction Company, China Zhongyuan Engineering Coporation and China Institute of Atomic Energy.

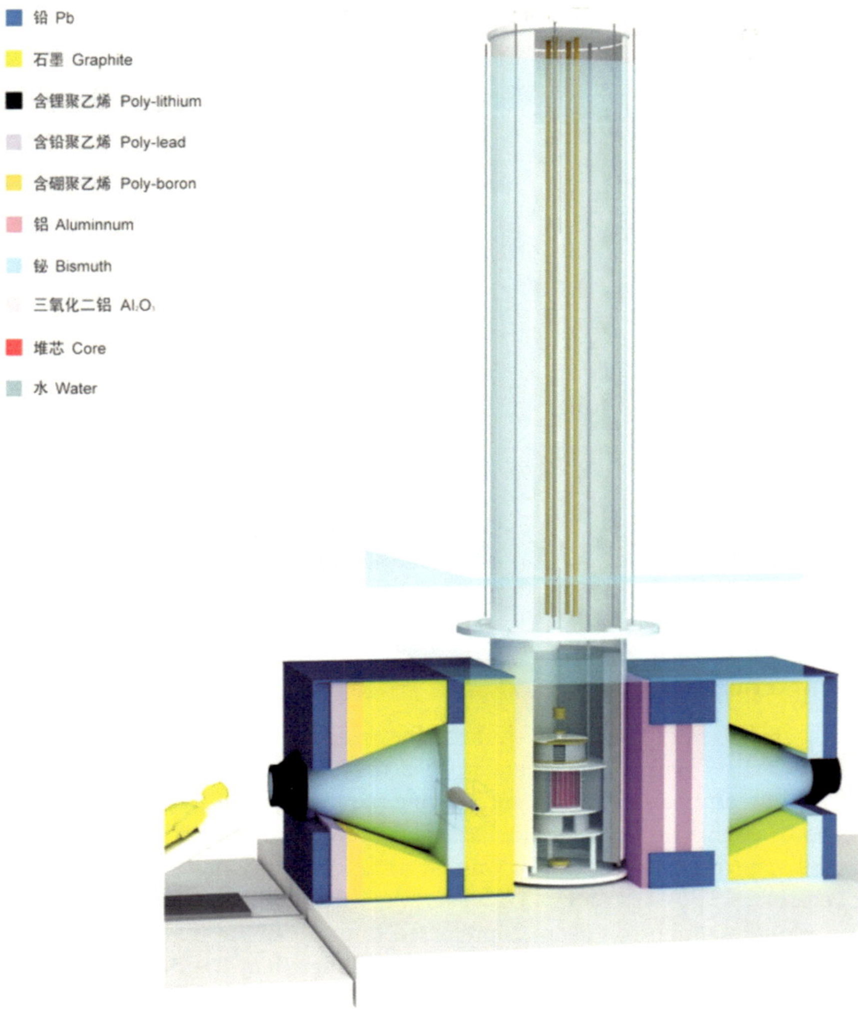

Fig. 14. In-hospital neutron irradiator (IHNI)

Based on modified Miniature Neutron Source Reactor (MNSR) techniques, the IHNI is an undermoderated reactor of pool-tank type with low enriched uranium (LEU) core, and can be installed on the basement floor of the main building or in an independent building. The IHNI uses UO_2 with enrichment of 12.5% ^{235}U as fuel, light water as coolant and moderator, and metallic beryllium as reflector. The IHNI has inherent safety with big negative temperature feedback, and its operation is done without any radioactive medium daily discharge to the environment. The fission heat produced by the reactor is removed by fully natural circulation cooling, and it includes no engineering operation facilities.

As a high efficiency neutron beam irradiation facility, the IHNI includes three beams, Epithermal neutron beam, Thermal neutron beam, and Blood-boron concentration measurement beam. The epithermal beam facility is equipped with the advanced energy spectrum regulator and high efficiency radiation shielding device. And the thermal beam Beam facility is equipped with thermalized neutron field and penumbra elimination device.

The last beam is designed for real time measurement of prompt gamma-ray neutron activation spectrometry analysis.

The IHNI also includes the complete medical treatment outfits for clinical trials and physics studies. The thermal neutron beam irradiation treatment room has full swivel bed for irradiation treatment of shallow focus while patients are in seating or laying positions and in-beam irradiation study of cells and small animals. The epithermal neutron beam irradiation treatment room has full swivel bed for irradiation treatment of deep focus while patients are in seating or laying positions. The treatment observation room is equipped with remote TV monitor, irradiation monitor and emergency treatment button. And the irradiation dosage detecting room is designed for gold foil activation detection, thermoluminescence brightness detection as well as blood-boron concentration gamma spectrometry analysis and assessment. The IHNI includes the boron compound batching and delivering room and computer software for treatment plan, too.

For treatment, the IHNI can provide ≥ 1×10^9 n_{epi}/cm^2 s for deep focus irradiation of 30 minutes, ≥ 2×10^9 $n_{th}/cm^2 \cdot s$ for shallow focus irradiation up to four hours, and a homogeneous thermal neutron field with neutron fluence of ≈ 10^{13} n/cm^2 for irradiation within beam facility. Meanwhile, the contamination irradiation dose rate is low at the beam port and in the air, in which the fast neutron contamination and the gamma ray contamination are smaller than 6×10^{-11}cGy $\cdot cm^2/n$ and 3×10^{-11} cGy $\cdot cm^2/n$, respectively.

The construction cost of the IHNI is equal to the price of importing a set of advanced CT or MRI scanning diagnosis system (approximate Five Million Euros). Shown in figure 15, the

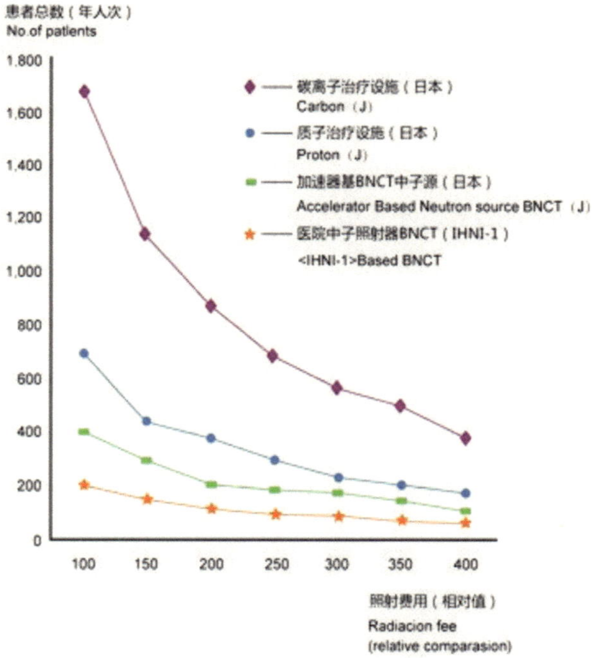

Fig. 15. Total cost of irradiation by IHNI

IHNI has the lowest operating cost comparing with the investment estimated by Japan to heavy ion beam irradiation treatment, proton beam treatment and the scheduled accelerator neutron beam treatment on the basis of the providing irradiation treatment capacity for 200 patients per year. For these reasons, the IHNI is suitable for the clinical trials and studies in the large and medium-sized professional hospitals or comprehensive hospitals, the large and medium-sized medical colleges or medical research centers, and High efficiency pharmaceuticals research center or pharmaceutical factories.

5. Dose calculation

5.1 Physical dose distribution

The doses are primarily from four parts: (1) thermal neutrons; (2) boron-10; (3) fast neutrons; and (4) photons.

(1) Boron dose

The reaction of boron with neutron gives in equation (1). The ^{10}B dose is primarily from $^{10}B(n,\alpha)^{7}Li$ capture reaction with thermal neutron. The reaction releases the secondary gamma according to the probability of 94%. Since ^{10}B has been isotope of choice due to the big thermal neutron capture cross-section of 3840 *barns*, a high Q-value of 2.79 *MeV*, the contribution of the boron dose is a big part of the total dose in spite of the boron consistence small (2002)[26].

(2) Thermal neutron dose

The thermal neutron dose primarily arises from the $^{14}N(n,p)^{12}C$ thermal neutron capture reaction, comprise 96% of the neutron kerma for ICRU-46 (1992)[27] brain tissue below 0.5 *eV* energy cutoff for thermal neutron.

(3) Fast neutron dose

The fast neutron dose tallies the full deposited energy from elastic neutron collision with hydrogen $^{1}H(n,n)^{1}H$ and represents 90% of adult brain kerma between energies of ~600 *eV* to ~3 *MeV*. The remain dose about 4-8% is from the other neutron reactions, primarily with ^{12}C、^{31}P and ^{16}O (2002)[26].

(4) Photon dose

The photon dose component originates from two parts: (1) the contaminating photons from neutron beam incident on the target; and (2) the prompt gammas produced by the neutron capture in the target, primarily by $^{1}H(n,\gamma)^{1}H$ reaction in tissue of brain.

(5) Kerma factor

The kerma (kinetic energy released in material) is a conversion factor from the flux to dose. The data is from ICRU-63 (2000)[28], where the neutron is based on ENDF/B-VI library (1991) [29].The key problem is how to treat the neutron of the energy lower 0.0253 *eV*.

(6) Flux

The flux in voxel *j* is obtained by Monte Carlo track length estimator.

$$\begin{cases} \phi(j,E) \approx \dfrac{S_0}{N}\displaystyle\sum_{n=1}^{N}\sum_{m} w_m^{(n)}(j,E)d_m^{(n)}(j), \\ w_m^{(n)}(j,E) = w_{m-1}^{(n)}(j,E)\left[1-\Sigma_a^{(m-1)}(j,E)/\Sigma_t^{(m-1)}(j,E)\right] \end{cases} \tag{5}$$

Where S_0 is the source intensity, N is the sample number (i.e. histories), w_m is a particle weight in m-th collision (w_0=1), d_m is the track length in voxel j, Σ_a, Σ_t are the macroscopic absorption and total cross-section (1997)[14].

(7) Dose

When a particle passes through the voxel *j*, the dose tally of the voxel is:

$$dose(j) = \int \phi(j,E) \cdot kerma(j,E)dE \,/\, V(j) \tag{6}$$

where *V(j)* is the volume of the voxel *j*.

5.2 Some difficulties in dose calculation

Due to the complicated geometry and the neutron thermalization treatment, the Monte Carlo particle transport code with point-wise cross-sections is usually selected the first simulation tool. In the early, the general purpose MCNP Monte Carlo code (1997)[14] has been used for BNCT dose calculation, however the longer time consuming is the main drawback. In addition, MCNP is not for patient treatment planning. It is a general purpose, continuous energy, generalized geometry, time dependent, coupled neutron-photon-electron Monte Carlo transport code system. The flux and its response are obtained by an estimation of the track length. To obtain the track length, the intersection of a particle ray with the surface being traversed must be found. The collision point is sampled in each cell. The statistical data shows that the time percentage is over 60~70% in all transport computations. In addition, the initialization and tally times increase with decreasing voxel size. In article of Kiger et al.(2004)[30] showed the memory increase for variable size voxel, where the MCNP transport time increases in linear with decreasing of the voxel size. However, the tally and initialization times increase in exponent with deceasing of the voxel size. Tallies and their initialization time have a profound impact on the speed of voxel model calculations.

5.3 Voxel models

(1) Analytical models

In Goorley et al.'s paper(2002)[26], the Snyder head phantom model consists of three ellipses and four materials, where the inner region is the brain, the middle region is the skull and the outer region is skin. The area outside the head is air (see figure 16) . An ellipsoidal head phantom based on the Snyder model is used by the Harvard-MIT group for physical dosimetry of the two neutron beams at the MIT Research Reactor. The original Snyder head phantom consists of two ellipsoids, which divide the head into regions of cranium and adult brain. A third 5 mm thick shell representing skin has also been added. Equations (7)-(9), which locate the center of the head at the origin, specify these regions: the boundary between brain and skull:

$$\left(\frac{x}{6}\right)^2 + \left(\frac{y}{9}\right)^2 + \left(\frac{z-1}{6.5}\right)^2 = 1 \tag{7}$$

the boundary between skull and scalp:

$$\left(\frac{x}{6.8}\right)^2 + \left(\frac{y}{9.8}\right)^2 + \left(\frac{z}{8.3}\right)^2 = 1 \tag{8}$$

the boundary between scalp and air:

$$\left(\frac{x}{7.3}\right)^2+\left(\frac{y}{10.3}\right)^2+\left(\frac{z}{8.8}\right)^2=1 \tag{9}$$

The three different regions of the analytical modified Snyder head phantom are composed of adult whole brain, adult whole cranium, and adult skin materials, as defined by ICRU-46 (1992)[27] and listed in Table 1. Air, of composition described by Chadwick *et al.* surrounds the models. This geometry model is called in analytical model. It is used to test of treatment planning software.

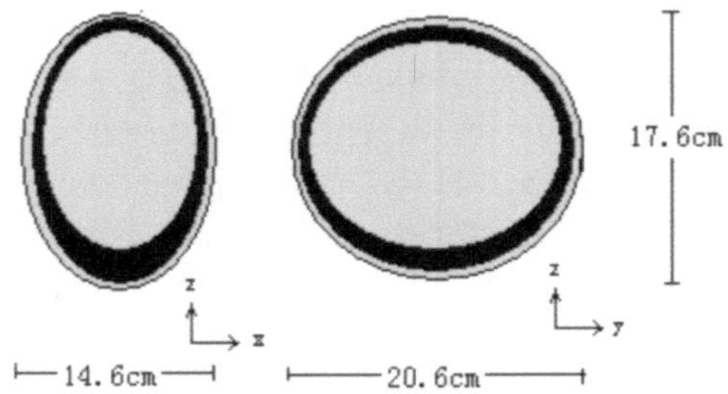

Fig. 16. Sections of the modified Snyder head phantom

Z	element	Air	Skeleton-Cranium	Adult whole brain	Adult skin
ρ (g/cm³)		0.001293	1.61	1.04	1.09
1	H	0	5.6	10.7	10
6	C	0.01	21.2	14.5	20.4
7	N	75.53	4	2.2	4.2
8	O	23.18	43.5	71.2	64.5
11	Na	0	0.1	0.2	0.2
12	Mg	0	0.2	0	0
15	P	0	8.1	0.4	0.1
16	S	0	0.3	0.2	0.2
17	Cl	0	0	0.3	0.3
19	K	0	0	0.3	0.1
20	Ca	1.28	17.6	0	0

Table 1. Material densities and compositions in mass percent.

(2) Benchmark voxel models

For analytical model, three voxel models of 16, 8, 4mm are constructed (see figure 17). The majority of voxels contain only one of the four materials: air, skin, skull or brain. However, some cells in the boundary contain more than two of these basic materials. They are mixed in 10% increments and that result in an additional 282 kinds of new materials. Therefore, there are a total of 286 different materials. The analytical model uses ellipse geometries. The materials are composed of brain, skull and skin of an adult, as defined by ICRU-46 (1992)[27].

The composition of air is described by Chadwick et al.(1999)[31]. Kerma data is from ICRU-63 (2000)[28]. At present, the Snyder head phantom analytical model and voxel models have been chosen as the benchmarks of BNCT. In general, the geometries of various organs are so complicated that they are difficult to describe by analytical geometry. Therefore, the analytical model represents a simplification of the actual physical geometry. In a clinical trial, CT and MRI image data, which are a group of discrete data, are used. It is then converted into a voxel model.

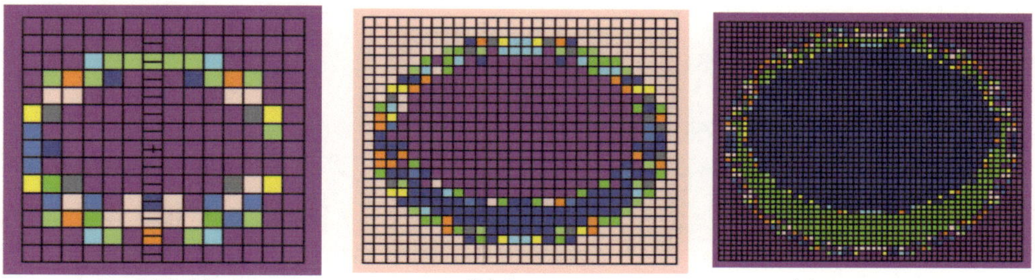

(a) 16mm (b) 8mm (c) 4mm

Fig. 17. Benchmark voxel models (mixture material)

(3) Modified voxel models

The mixture material is very complicated in a boundary voxel of interface because the volume ratio of different materials is usually very difficult to be determined. A simple treatment takes the material and density of the voxel center point as the material and density of this voxel. It does not increase the new materials and keeps the basic four materials. The memory is obviously reduced. Of course, the center point method is valid if and only if the mass conservation satisfies. The mass maximal error of each tissue is usually less than 1%. Figure 18 gives the modified voxel models being produced by the center point method. Three modified voxel models are tested. The contents include mass, memory and computational time. The simulation tool is MCNP code. Table 2 shows the test results of 50 million histories. The results indicate that the mass conservation is good for the 4mm model, with a maximum error of 0.93%. However, the maximum mass errors are 4.48% and 19.79% for the 8mm and 16mm models, respectively. Both of these errors appear in the skin. Figure 19 shows the calculation result comparison of benchmark 4mm voxel model and modified 4mm voxel model. Almost same results are achieved. Too long computational time is main drawback no matter how 8mm or 4mm model.

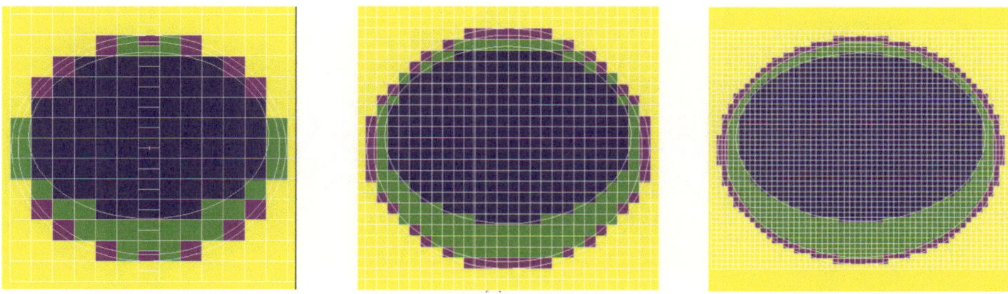

(a) 16mm (b) 8mm (c) 4mm

Fig. 18. Modified voxel and analytical models

mass (g) /model	brain error(%)	skull error(%)	skin error(%)	total mass error(%)	number of cubes	memory (MB)	cpu time (m)
Analytical	1529.1	1363.0	495.7	3387.8		6	326.01
Ben. 16mm	–	–	–	3394.7 (0.20)	2352	43	371.32
Ben. 8mm	–	–	–	3387.2 (-0.02)	16016	175	494.96
Ben. 4mm	–	–	–	3383.6 (-0.12)	94392	323	1208.60
Mod.16mm	1559.1 (1.96)	1266.2 (-7.10)	593.8 (19.79)	3419.1 (0.92)	2352	10	359.23
Mod. 8mm	1522.9 (-0.41)	1355.2 (-0.57)	517.9 (4.48)	3396.0 (0.24)	16016	37	489.36
Mod. 4mm	1528.0 (-0.07)	1370.4 (0.54)	491.1 (-0.93)	3389.5 (0.05)	94392	196	1206.81

Computer: Pentium IV 2.4 GHz PC machine and 50 million particles are simulated.

Table 2. Comparisons of mass, memory and computational time for different models

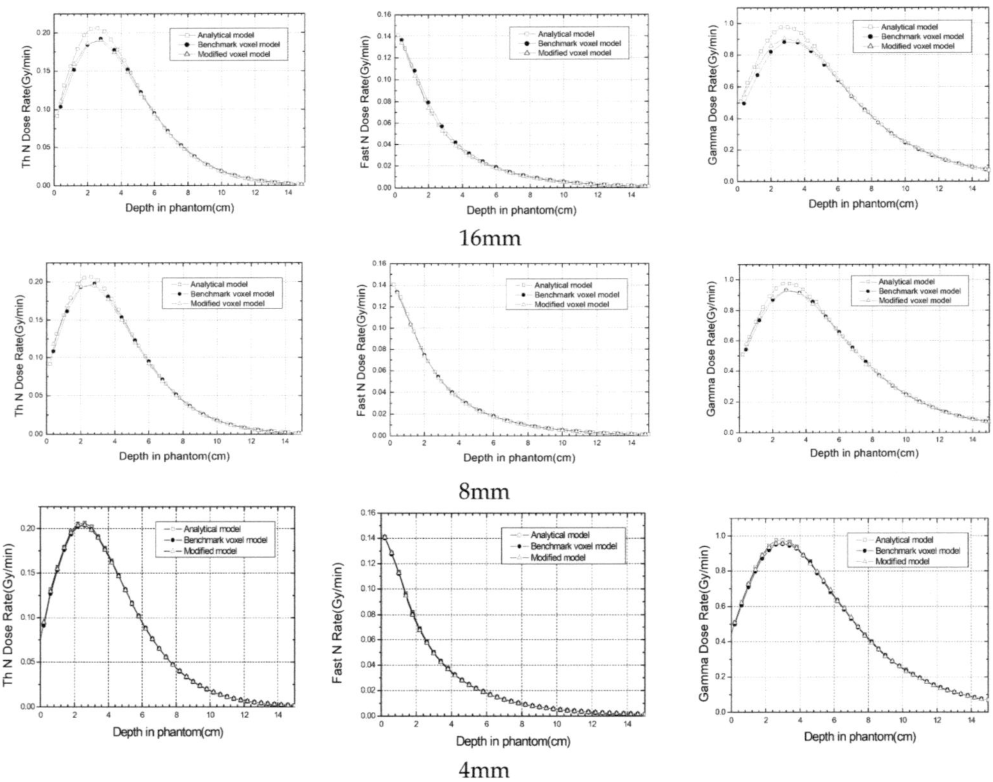

Fig. 19. Result comparisons of modified voxel, benchmark voxel and analytical models

(4) Optimized voxel models

Take the dose distribution of the thermal neutron as a example, we can see that it firstly goes up before 2.5cm and then goes down till zero with the depth, and the peak value appears at about 2.5cm depth. After the 6cm depth, the dose becomes lower than that it gets in the skin. For a generic epithermal beam, the therapy effect is good before 6 cm depth, and 77.65% of the thermal neutron kerma rate is before 5.6 cm (it is defined as region *I*). 21.50% between 5.6cm and 12cm (it is defined as region *II*), only 0.85% left beyond 12cm (it is defined as region *III*) (see table 3). So the dose precision of the region *I* is a key. Table 2 shows that the dose errors of 8mm and 4mm voxel model are small, but a long computational times are taken. However, the computational time of 8mm voxel model is only a half of the time of 4mm voxel model. On the other hand, although some error exists for 16mm model, due to the dose contribution very small in region III, the 16mm voxel can be used in region III. So some optimized voxel models are designed. Figure 20 shows three combinated voxel models. Figure 21 gives the comparison of thermal neutron calculation results and errors (fast neutron and photon similar case with thermal neutron). The big error appears in region III. Table 4 shows the comparison of the computational times. Table 5 shows the test of the mass. The results show that the 4+8mm combinated voxel model almost keep approach error of 4mm voxel model and the computational time is obvious shorter. But the computational time still exceeds 10 hours.

particles	depth (cm)		
	(I) 0-5.6	(II) 5.6-12.0	(III) 12.0--
thermal neutron	77.65%	21.50%	0.85%
fast neutron	85.53%	13.06%	1.29%
photon	63.26%	32.36%	4.00%

Table 3. Kerma rate of the analytical model

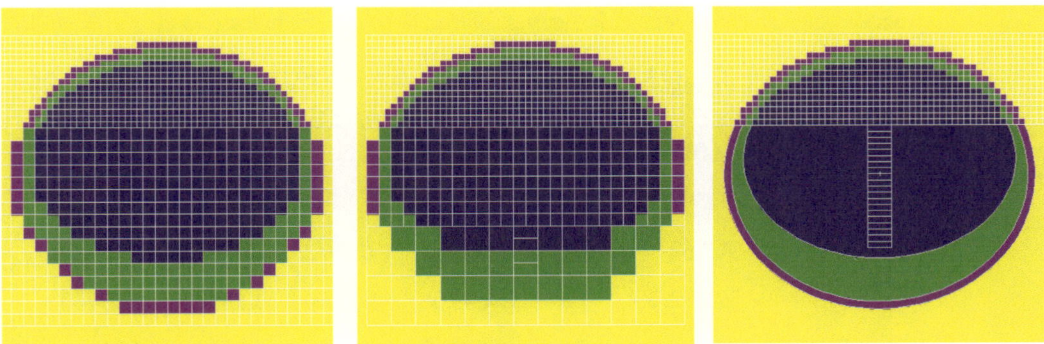

(a) 4+8mm (b) 4+8+16mm (c) 4mm+analysis

Fig. 20. The combinated voxel models

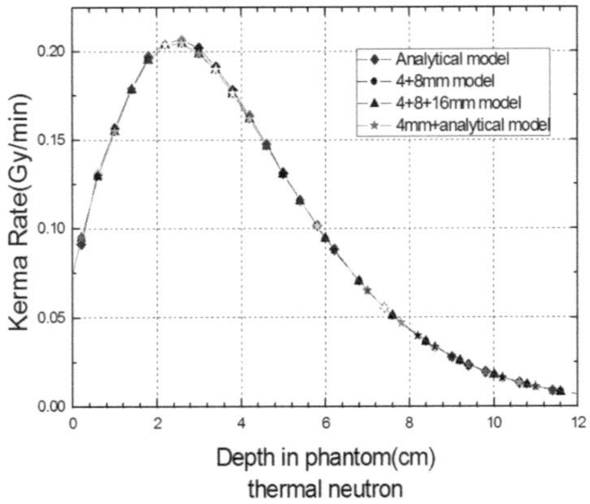

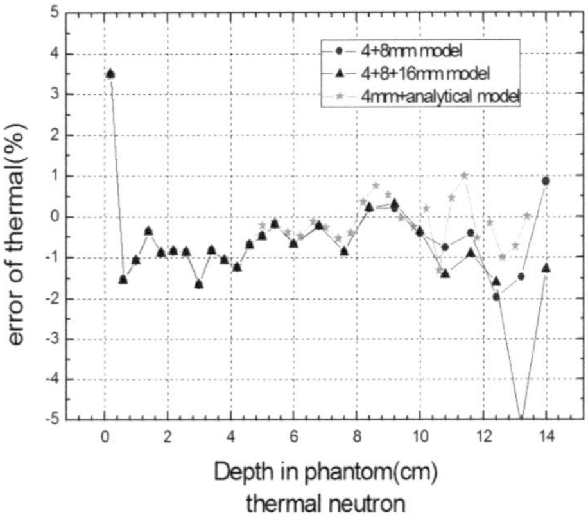

Fig. 21. Comparisons of doses and error of thermal neutron for combinated voxel models

Model	Number of voxels	Memory (MB)	Time (min)	error (%)		
				thermal n	fast n	photon
8mm	16016	37	489.36	3.2025	1.6388	2.7715
4mm	94392	196	1208.60	0.8754	0.9612	1.1683
4+8mm	42560	89	693.88	0.9972	1.1508	1.7015
4+8+16mm	32292	70	639.58	1.0150	1.1690	1.7404
4mm+analytical	28104	71	622.67	0.8684	0.9813	1.1209

Table 4. Comparison of computational times and errors for combinated models

Model	brain(g)	skull(g)	skin(g)	total(g)
analytical	1529.1	1363.0	495.7	3387.8
4+8mm	1524.2(-0.32)	1355.6(-0.54)	514.8(3.85)	3394.6(0.20)
4+8+16mm	1513.6(-1.01)	1398.5(2.60)	474.6(-4.26)	3386.7(-0.03)
4mm+analytical	1529.0(-0.01)	1363.3(0.02)	494.6(-0.22)	3386.8(-0.03)

Table 5. Tests of masses for combinated models

5.4 Algorithms for dose calculation

5.4.1 Mesh tally matrix and material matrix

Two matrixes are used to tally the dose and store the material of each voxel. They are similar to the CT threshold matrix. The orders of the matrix are $L \times M \times N$, where L, M and N are the mesh numbers in x, y and z directions, respectively. Every element in the matrix expresses the dose or material of a voxel. When the particle ray passes through voxel, the voxel tally is performed. The total computational time does not increase in relation to the local cell tally because searching the tally cell is unnecessary. The mesh tally is a new tally in MCNP and it uses the simple planes to tally. The track length is easily calculated relative to the cell tally. The mesh tally matrix is a tally of MCDB. It is very simple and also uses the planes as well as arithmetical relationships.

5.4.2 Fast track length techniques

Firstly, each voxel is mapped on a unit cube. Then, the relationship among neighboring voxels is established. Each grid of every voxel is expressed as (i, j, k) in integer. It is also the voxel's ID. The interval range of the present voxel is defined by $[i-1,i)\times[j-1,j)\times[k-1,k)$ (half open and half closed). Since each surface of every voxel belongs only to one side of another voxel, losing a particle can be avoided. The total number of neighbor voxels for the present voxel is twenty-seven, but only six voxels: $[i\pm1,j,k)$, $[i,j\pm1,k)$ and $[i,j,k\pm1)$ maintain the surface link relation. The other voxels only maintain the vertex link relation. When a ray passes through the vertex (i.e. $f = 0$), the neighbor relation is valid. This case requires special treatment. When the material changes according to the Ids, the collision point is resampled.

For the voxel model, a cube is used and most of the voxels are of the same material. Once the direction of the ray is known, the ID of the next voxel and the track length are rapidly determined and calculation of the intersection is unnecessary. The details are described in reference [17,32].

6. Example

This example is from a patient, which consists of 43 CT pictures (figure 22(a)). Firstly the 3-D reconstruction is done (figure 22(b)), then the two voxel models are designed, where one of model is CT8 which is consisted by 8×8 pixels (the total cubes = 64×64×43=176128, the size = $0.3703\times 0.3703\times0.3mm^3$) and another model is CT4 which is consisted by 4×4 pixels (the total cubes=128×128×43=704512, the size=$0.1852\times 0.1852\times0.3mm^3$, Fig.22(c)). The neutron beam is same as benchmark models. 10 million histories are simulated and all meshes are tallied. The figure 23 gives the comparison of the dose between MCDB and MCNP, where figure 23 gives the dose distributions of the thermal neutron, fast neutron and secondary photon of each voxel. The almost same results of MCDB and MCNP are obtained. Table 6 shows the comparison of MCDB and MCNP in computing time. The figure 24 and 25 show the neutron dose surface and the photon dose surface. It is used to direct the irradiation.

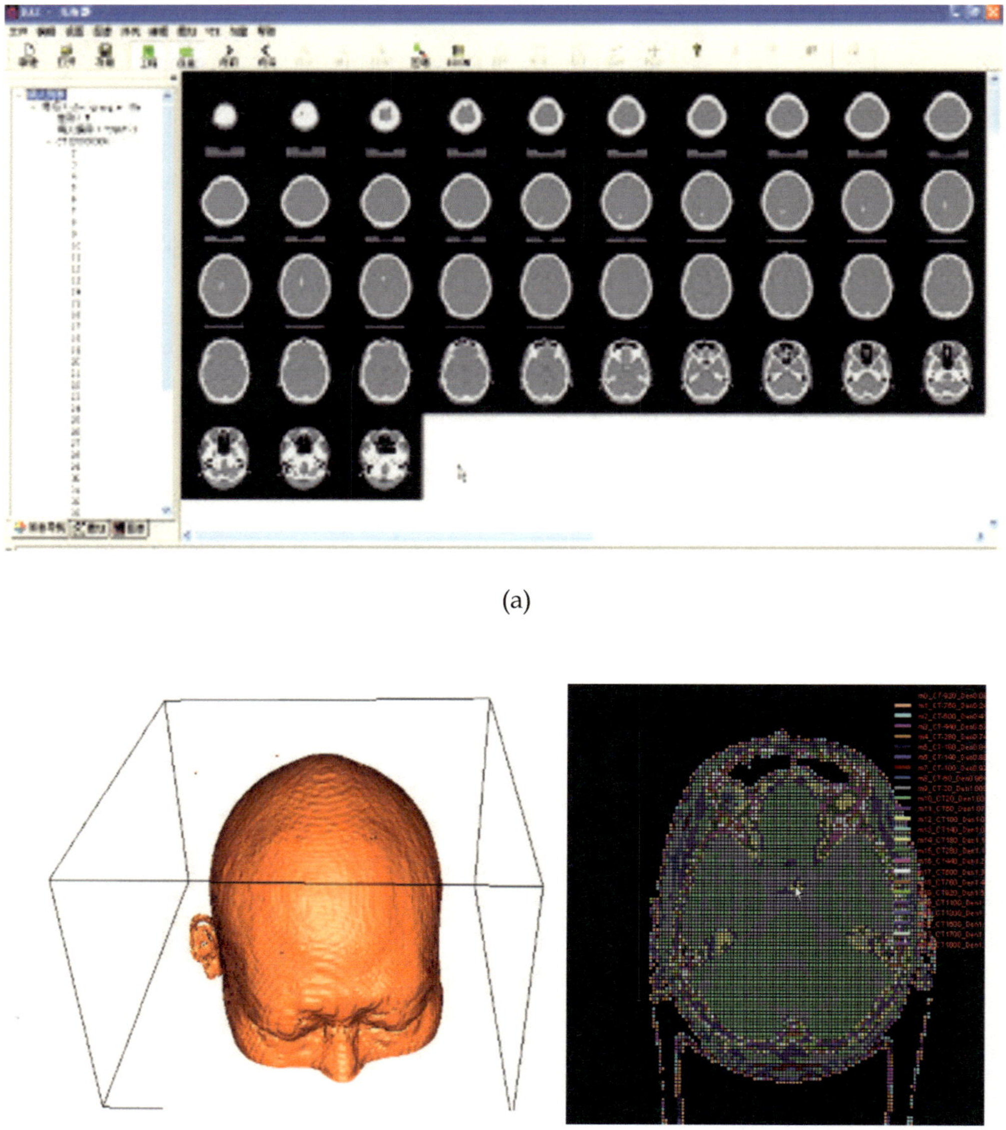

(a)

(b)

(c)

Fig. 22. Cross section view of CT image and CT4 voxel model

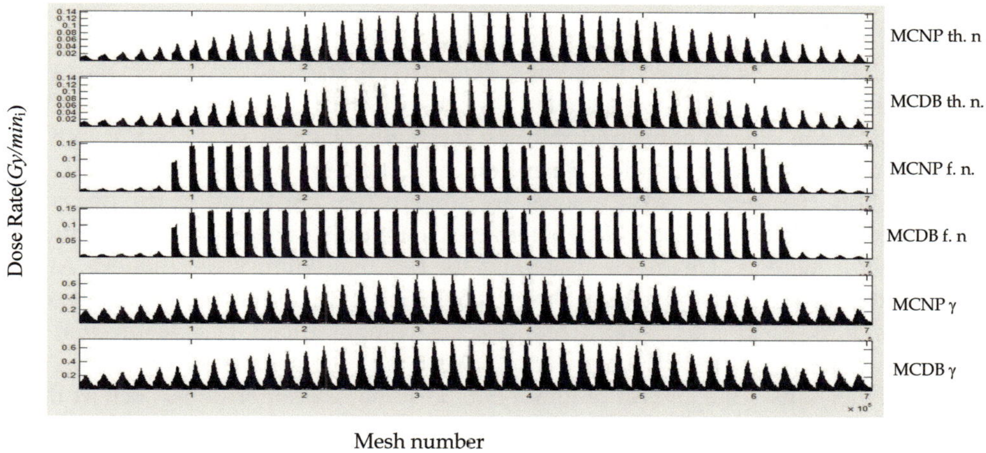

Fig. 23. Comparison of MCDB and MCNP result

model	voxel number	geometry	tally	code	time(m)	speedup
CT8	176128	lattice	mesh tally	MCNP	185.26	
		material Matrix	mesh tally matrix	MCDB	60.34	3.07
CT4	704512	lattice	mesh tally	MCNP	276.34	
		material Matrix	mesh tally matrix	MCDB	81.26	3.40

Computer: Pentium IV 3.0 GHz PC machine.

Table 6. Comparison of computing times based on the CT image model

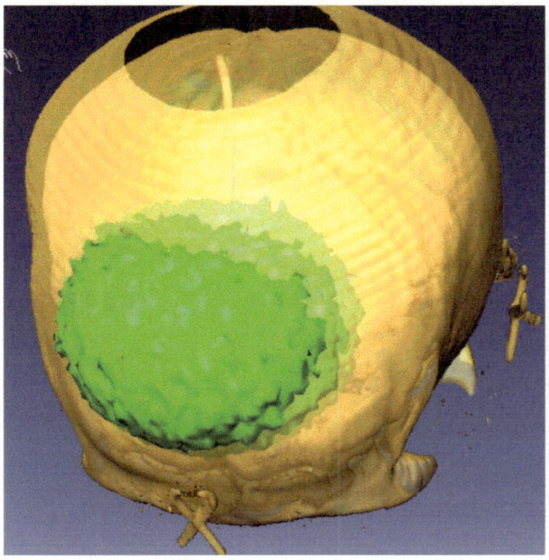

Fig. 24. Neutron dose surface

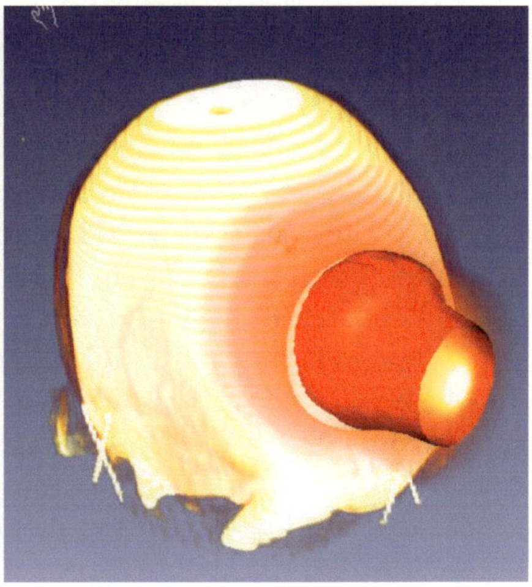

Fig. 25. Photon dose surface

7. Conclusions

The status of TPS recalls in this article. For a general TPS, the medical pro-processor, dose calculation and post-processor are included. In pro-processor, the basic data from CT and MRI DICOM image data is converted into the input file of voxel model for Monte Carlo dose calculation. The reactor device and neutron beam are a important part of BNCT. In the dose calculation, the several voxel models are constructed. For avoid to the difficulty of mixture material treatment in boundary interface, the modified voxel model is produced by the center point method. This method is valid for less than 4mm voxel models. At same time, the combinated voxel models are design according to the dose varies with the depth. The test result is good and greatly reduces the computational time. However, these measures only partly decrease the simulation time if uses the general Monte Carlo MCNP code. It does not satisfy the clinical requirement. So some new algorithms, such as the fast track technique, material and tally matrix etc., are developed. These algorithms are written into the MCDB TPS. It makes the MCDB speed is fast about 3 times with respect to the MCNP. It basicly satisfies the clinical requirement.

8. Acknowledgment

This research is supported by Capture Technology Ltd.. The authors also wish to thank Prof. Y. M. Zhou. This project is supported by CAEP fund (No. 2011A0103006).

9. References

[1] Rorer, A., Wambersie, G., Whitmore, et al. (2001). Current status of neutron capture therapy, *IAEA-TECDOC-1223*

[2] Rolf F. Barth, Jeffrey A. Coderre, Vicente, M. G. H.(2006). Boron neutron Capture therapy, *Encycloped of Medical Devices and Instrumentation,* Second Edition, edited by John G. Webster

[3] Snyder W S, et al.(1978). Estimates of absorbed fractions for monoenergetic photon sources uniformly distributed in various organs of a heterogeneous phantom MIRD Pamphlet no 5 (revised). *Society of Nuclear Medicine,* New York, USA

[4] Zubal I G, et al.(1994). Computerized three-dimensional segmented human anatomy. *Med. Phys.* 21: 299

[5] Kramerl R, et al.(2003). All about MAX: a male adult voxel phantom for Monte Carlo calculations in radiation protection dosimetry. *Phys. Med. Biol.,* 48: 1239

[6] DeMarco J J, et al.(1998). A CT based Monte Carlo simulation tool for dosimetry planning and analysis Med. Phys. 25: 1-11

[7] WANG, L. et al.(2001). Monte Carlo Evaluation Of Tissue Inhomogeneity Effects In the Treatment ff the Head And Neck. *Int. J. Radiation Oncology Biol. Phys.* 50: 1339

[8] C-M Ma, et al.(2002). A Monte Carlo dose calculation tool for radiotherapy treatment planning. *Phys. Med. Biol.* 47: 1671

[9] Schneider W, et al.(2000). Correlation between CT numbers and tissue parameters needed for Monte Carlo simulations of clinical dose distributions. *Phys. Med. Biol.* 45: 459

[10] ICRP Publication 23 (1975). Report of the Task Group on Reference Man. *ICRP Publication 23*
[11] ICRU-44(1989). Tissue Substitutes in Radiation Dosimetry and Measurement. *ICRU Reports 44*
[12] Hatanaka, Y. and Nakagawa, Y.(1994). Chinical results of long-surviving brain tumor patients who underwent boron neutron capture therapy, *Int. J. Radiation Oncology Biol. phys.* ,1061
[13] Zonta, A., Altier, S., Roveda, L., *et al.*(2008). Neutron Capture Therapy. *Proceedings of 13th International Congress on Neutron Capture Therapy*. Florence, Italy
[14] Briesmeister, J. F., (Ed.) (1997). MCNP-A general Monte Carlo code for N-particle transport code, *LA-12625-M*
[15] Gonzàlez , S., J., Santa Cruz, Kiger III, W., et al.(2002). NCTPlan, the New PC version of MacNCTPlan: Improvements and Verification of a BNCT Treatment Planning System, *Proceedings of the 10th International Congress on Neutron Capture Therapy for Cancer*, Essen, Germany
[16] Kumada, H., Yamamoto, K., Matsumura, A., et al.(2004). Verification of the computational dosimetry system in JAERI(JCDS) for boron neutron capture therapy, *Phys. Med. Biol.* 49, 3353-3365
[17] Seppälä , Kankaanranta, L., Serėn , T., et al.(2000). BNCT_RTPE and SERA Dose Planning Programs: Phantom and Patient Studies, *In Program and abstracts of 9th International Symposium on Neutron Capture Therapy for Cancer*, 175-176. ISNCT: Osaka
[18] Li DENG, Gang LI, Tao YE, et al.(2007). MCDB Monte Carlo Code with Fast Track Technique and Mesh Tally Matrix for BNCT. *J. Nucl. Sci. Tech.* 44, 1518–1525
[19] Kouris K, Spyrou N M and Jackson D F.(1982). *Imaging with Ionizing Radiations*. Surrey University Press, Glasgow
[20] Schneider U, et al.(1996). The calibration of CT Hounsfield units for radiotherapy treatment planning. *Phys. Med. Biol.*, 41: 111
[21] Kawrakow, I. and Rogers, D. W. O.(2000). The EGSnrc Code System: Monte Carlo simulation of electron and photon transport, Technical Report PIRS–701, National Research Council of Canada, Ottawa, Canada
[22] www.cern.ch/geant4; www.ge.infn.it/geant4
[23] Auterinen, I., Seren, T., Anttila, K.,*et al.*(2004). Measurement of free beam neutron spectra at eight BNCT facilities worldwide. *Appl. Radiati. Isot.* 61, 1021-1026 (2004).
[24] Ke, G., Sun, Z., Lv, Z., *et al.*(2008). The study of Physics and Thermal Characteristics for In-hospital neutron irradiator (IHNI), *Proceedings of 13th International Congress on Neutron Capture Therapy*, 474 , Florence, Italy
[25] Li, Y., Xia, P. Zou, S. *et al.*(2008). The physics experimental study for In-hospital neutron irradiator, *Proceedings of 13th International Congress on Neutron Capture Therapy*, 474, Florence, Italy

[26] Goorley, J.T., Kiger III, W.S., Zamenhof, R.G.(2002). Reference dosimetry calculations for neutron capture therapy with comparison of analytical and voxel models, *Med. Phys.*, 29(2), 145-156

[27] ICRU-46(1992). Photon, Electron, Proton and Neutron Interaction Data for Body Tissues. International Commission on radiation Units and Measurements, *Bethesda*, MD

[28] ICRU-63(2000). Nuclear data for neutron and proton radiotherapy and for radiation protection, *ICRU Report No. 63, International Commission on Radiation Units and Measurements*, Bethesda, MD

[29] Cross Section Evaluation Working Group(1991). ENDF/B-VI Summary Documentation, *BNL-NCS-17541(ENDF-201)*, 4-th edition, National Nuclear Data Center, Brookhaven National Laboratory, Upton, NY

[30] Kiger III, W.S., Albritton, J.R., Hochberg A.G., et al.(2004). Performance Enhancements of MCNP4B, MCNP5, and MCNPX for Monte Carlo Radiotherapy Planning Calculations in Lattice Geometries, *LA-UR-04-6972*

[31] Chadwick, M., Barschall, H., Caswell, R., *et al.*(1999). A consistent set of neutron kerma coefficients from thermal to 150 *MeV* for biologically important materials, *Med. Phys.* 26, 974-991

[32] Frandsen, M.W.(2001). Rapid Geometry Interrogation for Uniform Volume Element-Based BNCT Monte Carlo Particle Transport Simulation, *Proceedings of the Eighth International Symposium on Neutron Capture Therapy,* Plenum Press, New York

10

Magnetic Resonance Tractography in Neuroradiological Diagnostic Aspects

Jaroslaw Paluch, Jaroslaw Markowski, Tatiana Gierek, Przemyslaw Pencak, Malgorzata Witkowska, Maciej Kajor, Agnieszka Gorzkowska and Agnieszka Piotrowska
Medical University of Silesia in Katowice
Poland

1. Introduction

Diffusion tensor imaging (DTI) is an Magnetic Resonance (MR) method used for analysis of diffusion anisotropy in central nervous system (CNS). It provides the anatomic details of brain white matter. At present, it is also a very useful method in neuro-radiology, providing morphological markers of disease progression or reaction to treatment [1]. In the last 10-15 years, the studies concerning magnetic resonance imaging technique focused more on the phenomenon of diffusion in living tissues [2]. The graphic representation of diffusion in MR is a pretty valuable observation method when dealing with nervous tissue structures, and due to its non-invasive character [2, 3] it is perfectly suited for assessment of brain throughout its development, from birth until reaching complete biological maturity, and further on to elderly age and senility. Human brain, from the embryonic stage on, is subject to transformations due to development, differentiation, and proliferation of neurons, improvement of synaptic junctions, while maintaining those junctions is related to a long process of myelinization, lasting until 25 years of age [4]. Diffusion imaging in magnetic resonance investigation (DT-MRI) allowed for calculations of nerve fibre pathways, within the properly arranged structure of the white matter of brain.

2. Discussion of the method: mathematical and physical aspect

Diffusion is a process based on the movement of particles of a substance dissolved in the solution, all well as movement of particles of the very solution (medium) [6], leading to levelling of concentrations of substrates contained in the solution (of liquid or gas). That phenomenon is related to the chaotic movement of particles of the solution, depending on the thermal energy of the system, also labelled as 'random movement of particles' also – historically "Brownian movements" [4]. In human body structures anisotropic centres are usually present, the nature of which results mainly from the fact of occurrence of many membranes, both cellular ones, and intracellular ones, which interfere with free diffusion. Human body may be divided into many centres, one different from another, which may be classified as one of the three basic areas, namely: extracellular space, intracelullar space, third space. Extracellular space is characterized by isotropy and relatively high values of diffusion coefficient [4]. Due to the homogeneous properties of the basilar medium (extracellular fluid), and proportionally large (in comparison with translocations of particles due to chaotic thermal motion) distances between cell membranes. Intracellular space, due to the medium (cytosol, formerly referred to as cytoplasm), as well as the occurrence of numerous cellular and intracellular membranes, as well as their arrangement (spatial arrangement in the form of "dense packing"), is anisotropic and has a relatively lower level of effective diffusion coefficient (absolute level of diffusion of the medium, corrected due to the barriers present) [2]. Some of the existing processes may cause reduction of the extracellular space, in favour of intracellular space, which is followed by changes in averaged values of the diffusion coefficient within the voxel. The third space is anisotropic, while the diffusion coefficient value depends on the composition of the medium (e.g. mucous serous content, purulent content, etc.) [4].

The bio-structure of brain belongs to anisotropic structures, thus the diffusion tensor is used to describe the coefficient of diffusion (highly differentiated, depending on the location and direction), instead of single scalar value [7]. The tensor, being a mathematical concept, independent on the selection of the coordinate system is, to simplify, similar to the notion of "vector". It enables presentation of physical quantity, the value of which depends on direction. The application of diffusion tensor allows to provide an approximate description of the distribution of diffusion coefficient values, taking into account its direction in anisotropic spaces.

Complementing the theoretical model, which solely takes diffusion into consideration, by phenomena occurring in the bio-structures, perfusion and micro-circulation among others, influencing the size of signal change in the sequence utilizing diffusion coding gradients, led to the formulation of the notion of "apparent diffusion coefficient" (ADC), calculated and presented in the form of ADC maps [4]. The principle has been assumed that in diffusion-weighted imaging (DWI), areas of low diffusion are shown as bright ones. However, in interpreting them, one should always take into account the b value. In case of low values of b, the image contrast is strongly dependent on the time of transverse relaxation, T. That phenomenon is called T shining (T-dependent shining) [2].

Data calculated from measurements taken with the application of at least two sequences, with different values of b, is used for developing of ADC images. The contrast in ADC images is in proportion to diffusion – tissues with low diffusion are shown as dark areas, whereas tissues or spaces with high diffusion are encoded as bright ones [4]. In humans, anisotropic areas prevail, where the multi-directional differentiation of diffusion calls for more complex description, in the form of diffusion tensor. For the purpose of computing the tensor, it is indispensable to take measurements of diffusion in at least six, at best nine or more (in newest MRI system up to 265) directions.

Besides the notion of "diffusion coefficient", also the notion of "diffusivity" is used [3], being correspondent to diffusion per time unit. One of the values used for describing the diffusion tensor is a scalar value of total diffusion, labelled as "trace" (D), as well as mean diffusivity (MD), being dependent on the former. Both those values represent the total value of diffusion in a given point in space, yet do not contain any information about its differentiation depending on direction.

To express the level of anisotropy of the examined structure, the notion of fractional anisotropy (FA) is applied, which is a scalar quantity, and has values in the 0-1 range. The value of 0 corresponds to isotropic structure, whereas the value of 1 to a structure, in which diffusion is possible in one direction only [2, 4]. Due to the degree of organization, the white matter of brain has high values of FA (the highest in the *corpus callosum* and pyramidal tracts), as well as relatively low value of MD. The grey matter is characterized by relatively low values of FA and MD [4, 8]. For cerebrospinal fluid, very low values of FA are typical (close to 0), at the same time the MD values occur to be high. There are different ways of imaging the diffusion tensor (DTI) distribution. Among the most popular ones are the MD images in various shades of grey, FA images in grey shading scale, and colour-coded FA images and tractography. There is a rule, according to which in FA mapping using scale of grey, the areas of high anisotropy are presented as bright, whereas isotropic centres - as dark. In case of parametric colour-coded FA maps, the colour is determined by the direction of the maximum component of diffusion tensor (red: right-left, green: forward-backward, blue: up-down), while the intensity depends on the FA value [4, 5]. In tractography, the algorithm of plotting the tract of fibres from a selected point is used, based on the principle of continuity of voxels, as well as selection of every next point, depending on the direction determined by the dominating component of diffusion tensor in the current voxel [6]. In other words, starting with the initial point, the line goes towards the maximum diffusion, until it encounters the first voxel [1]. Then it changes the direction to the maximum diffusion of the next new voxel. That process is continued until the critical end moment is reached [4]. The end point may be a relatively low level of anisotropy, indicating the necessity of terminating the tract in the white matter. Depending on the starting point, one can code the colours for specific tracts, thus the multi-coloured imaging [3, 8]. It should be remembered that the hypothetical tract of fibres, plotted in tractography, results from a mathematical model developed on the basis of diffusion tensor, averaged for a given voxel, not from the actual fibre route [2, 4].

3. Application of DTI – MR

Tractography, treated as a way of imaging nerve tracts, has been used in clinical studies and diagnostics of brain diseases [5]. Tractography techniques enable showing the structures in white matter, and nerve tract [7, 9]. That allowed, among other things, to study the tracts running in the major point of connection between cerebral hemispheres, which is the *corpus callosum*, and to discover new tracts between distant regions [1, 3, 6, 10], as well as development of a 3D model of nerve fibre bundles [5, 11]. Changes in fractional anisotropy or mean diffusivity in brain diseases enable accurate location of topical lesion. Finding out, which nerve tracts are visible, one may determine the degree of development and progression of the disease, as well as to select the intervention method [12]. That has been used in studies on epilepsy [13], where the impairment of nerve tract connections in both hemispheres have been shown. Also in neuro-oncology, radiological imaging by means of tractography provides information about the functions of specific nerve tracts, as well as their relations with the tumour being subject of surgical intervention [10]. That has found applications for pre-surgical mapping of tracts, as well as planning the scope and type of surgical intervention [12]. In Poland, neuro-surgical procedures are already carried out with simultaneous following the functions of nerve tracts. Thanks to modern software for tractography, available since December 2008, it was possible to visualize in real time - during the surgical procedure of tumour excision - the activity and functions of nerve fibres. The data obtained were subsequently utilized by the system for neuro-surgical navigation, to enable more precise excision of tumour, which significantly enhanced the safety of surgical procedure, and reduced the risk of complications [12].

Tractography also allowed imaging of lesions in the brain in patients with multiple sclerosis (SM), as well as with amyotrophic lateral sclerosis (Charcot's disease), where changes in diffusion and anisotropy, degeneration of cortico-spinal tract became visible [13]. Moreover, that type of investigation allows to diagnose not only changes related to defect, but also increased compensatory myelinization in case of brain with unilateral injury. Tractography served the purpose of proving the possibility of fibre regeneration or change in the of nerve tract around the place of lesion in experimental studies carried out on Apes with injury of a part of brain [11]. DT-MRI adreno-leucodystrophy allows to identify degenerated white matter, which is not possible in conventional magnetic resonance (MR) [2]. The paper describing the results of studies on Alzheimer's disease, describes using the DT-MRI method for independent imaging of the degree of defect of white matter, by measuring diffusivity and anisotropy, in comparison with control [14].

To sum up, tractography enables reconstruction of the alignment of nerve fibres, in colourful 3D projection, in accordance with the highest level of diffusivity, fibres that connect one region with another in the brain [2, 11, 15]. It is based on imaging the diffusion tensor, and is a quickly developing method of examining the central nervous system [1]. In order to validate that technique, objective methods are required, which compare white matter tracts, as well as diameters of alignment of tracts in biological assays [2]. It is essential to be aware of the limitations resulting from application of that method. Due to the fact that the size of voxel is a few millimetres [13] it may contain dozens of thousands of axons with different arrangement/ arrangement [3, 6, 13]. What is more, one should take into account the fact that the image of fibre alignment (track) does not provide the answer about the direction of the fibres [8, 13]. In case of fibres having similar size, yet oriented in opposite directions, no path will be marked. In turn, when a pathway having bigger size passes next to smaller tracts, it may happen that the latter will be imaged as part of the former pathway, and true data about the alignment will be lost [1]. Difficulties may also arise from differentiating between crossing pathways, which form a bigger route [3]. The direction that we get image of is then analogical, despite differences in anisotropy. The inter-penetration of pathways also distorts the regular/ regular image provided by DT-MRI [10]. It would seem that voxel size reduction would allow avoiding the limitations [10]. Unfortunately, that will increase costs and extend the examination time [3], which is connected with the occurrence of artefacts resulting from breathing, flow of fluids in brain, as well as eye movement, or movement of the entire head during examination [2].

In future, the method of diffusion imaging in MRI may be applied in other tissues containing fibres, such as heart, where it would provide information concerning correct development of the organ or diagnosing of the disease [1, 2]. The application of fibre tract visualization methods with the application of contrast media, such as manganite, together with DT-MRI shall provide additional possibilities in both diagnosing diseases, as well as observation of regular brain structures, as well as structures of other fibrous tissues. That, in turn, will explain the dependency of connections with central and peripheral nervous systems [1].

DT-MRI is a method of imaging the structures of brain white matter [1, 5]. Disclosure of the connection system allows to get the understanding of how the brain organization works, it also provides information on irregularities in those structures [16]. Dissemination of that method shall enable imaging nerve tract connections in the entire body.

In otolaryngological diagnosing, particularly in otoneurological diagnosing, the following application possibilities are perceived:

- assessment of hearing, olfactory, and gustatory tracts, in the aspect of physiological development;
- disturbances in functions of tracts belonging to senses in the course of neuro-degenerative diseases (Alzheimer's disease, Parkinson's disease, atherosclerotic syndromes, diabetes, metabolic diseases, neuropathies of renal origin);
- diagnostics in patients with peripheral or central lesion of the organ of hearing, before surgical treatment, as well as post-surgery monitoring;
- determination of morphological parameters on the basis of analysis of hearing tract image, in the treatment of patients with cochlear implants and bone anchored hearing aid (BAHA).

4. References

[1] Basser PJ, Pajevic S, Pierpaoli C, Duda J, Aldroubi A. In vivo fiber tractography using DT-MRI data. Magn Reson Med. 2000 Oct;44(4):625-32.

[2] Melhem ER, Mori S, Mukundan G, Kraut MA, Pomper MG, van Zijl PC. Diffusion tensor MR imaging of the brain and white matter tractography. AJR Am J Roentgenol. 2002 Jan;178(1):3-16.

[3] Watts R, Liston C, Niogi S, Uluğ AM. Fiber tracking using magnetic resonance diffusion tensor imaging and its applications to human brain development. Ment Retard Dev Disabil Res Rev. 2003;9(3):168-77.

[4] Walecki J., Pawłowska- Detko A., Adamczyk M., Rola współczesnych metod obrazowania w rozpoznaniu i monitorowaniu otępienia. Polaski Przegląd Neurologiczny 2007; 3,2.

[5] Yamada K, Kizu O, Mori S, Ito H, Nakamura H, Yuen S, Kubota T, Tanaka O, Akada W, Sasajima H, Mineura K, Nishimura T. Brain fiber tracking with clinically feasible diffusion-tensor MR imaging: initial experience. Radiology. 2003 Apr;227(1):295-301.

[6] Maddah M, Mewes AU, Haker S, Grimson WE, Warfield SK. Automated atlas-based clustering of white matter fiber tracts from DTMRI. Med Image Comput Comput Assist Interv. 2005;8(Pt 1):188-95.

[7] Behrens T.E.J., Johansen Berg H., Jbabdi S., Rushworth M.F.S., Woolrich M.W. Probabilistic diffusion tractography with multiple fibre orientations: What can we gain? Neuroimage 2007 (34): 144-155.

[8] Behrens T.E.J., Johansen Berg H., Woolrich M.W., Smith S.M., Wheeler- Kingshott C.A., Boulby P.A. Non- invasive mapping of connections between human thalamus and cortex using diffusion imaging. Nat- Neurosc 2003, Jul; 6(70, 750-7.

[9] Corouge I., Gouttard S., Gerig G. Towards a shape model of white fiber bundles using diffusion tensor MRI. Interantion symposium on Biomedical Imaging 2004 Vol 1, 334-347.

[10] Lazar M, Weinstein DM, Tsuruda JS, Hasan KM, Arfanakis K, Meyerand ME, Badie B, Rowley HA, Haughton V, Field A, Alexander AL. White matter tractography using diffusion tensor deflection. Hum Brain Mapp. 2003 Apr;18(4):306-21.

[11] Maddah M., Wells W.M., Warfield S.K., Westin C., F., Eric W., Grimson L.A.: A spation model of White Matter Fiber Tracts
[12] http://web.mit.edu/mmaddah/www/mahnaz_ISMRM2007_clusteringfibertracts.pdf.
[13] Witwer BP, Moftakhar R, Hasan KM, Deshmukh P, Haughton V, Field A, Arfanakis K, Noyes J, Moritz CH, Meyerand ME, Rowley HA, Alexander AL, Badie B. Diffusion-tensor imaging of white matter tracts in patients with cerebral neoplasm. J Neurosurg. 2002 Sep;97(3):568-75.
[14] Johansen-Berg H, Behrens TE. Just pretty pictures? What diffusion tractography can add in clinical neuroscience. Curr Opin Neurol. 2006 Aug;19(4):379-85. Review.
[15] Taoka T, Iwasaki S, Sakamoto M, Nakagawa H, Fukusumi A, Myochin K, Hirohashi S, Hoshida T, Kichikawa K. Diffusion anisotropy and diffusivity of white matter tracts within the temporal stem in Alzheimer disease: evaluation of the "tract of interest" by diffusion tensor tractography. AJNR Am J Neuroradiol. 2006 May;27(5):1040-5.
[16] Catani M, Jones DK, Donato R, Ffytche DH. Occipito-temporal connections in the human brain. Brain. 2003 Sep;126(Pt 9):2093-107. Epub 2003 Jun 23.
[17] Lazar M., Weinstein D., Hasan K., Alexander A.L. Axon tractography with tensorlines. Proc. Intl. Soc. Mag. Reson. Med. 8, 2000.

11

Pediatric Brain Tumors: Magnetic Resonance Spectroscopic Imaging

A. Aria Tzika, Loukas Astrakas and Maria Zarifi
Department of Surgery, Massachusetts General Hospital
Harvard Medical School, Boston
USA

1. Introduction

The incidence of cancer in the United States in children under 15 years of age has risen in recent years (Ries et al., 1991). This is largely due to the increased incidence of lymphoblastic leukemia and tumors of the brain and nervous system, as opposed to Wilms tumors, soft tissue and bone sarcomas, lymphomas and Hodgkin's disease or other malignancies of childhood. Between 1973 and 1988, the incidence of childhood nervous system tumors jumped by 30% (Bleyer, 1993). Every year, more than 1,500 children are diagnosed with brain tumors (Pollack, 1994). Because a child is more likely to develop cancer during the first 5 years of life, the etiology of these early cancers is likely different from those later in life and of different factors. While childhood tumors are more aggressive, their long-term control is often possible (Albright, 1993). Cancer Statistics Review reports an overall decrease in childhood cancer mortality, although brain and nervous system cancer deaths have decreased less than those due to other malignancies (Ries et al., 1991). These results indicate the need for useful *in vivo* biomarkers to allow the evaluation of treatment protocols for pediatric brain tumors. Given the inherent difficulties of sequential biopsies to monitor therapeutic response in children with brain tumors, non-invasive and non-irradiating imaging methods are needed to provide additional diagnostic indices or biomarkers beyond simple tumor volume measurements. Brain tumor treatment in most modern centers is managed through a tumor board, which typically rely in part on available proton Magnetic Resonance Spectroscopic Imaging (MRSI) results, especially for inoperable tumors that can be difficult to biopsy. Additionally, where progression or treatment response is questioned, serial *in vivo* MRSI is preferred over serial biopsy or PET/SPECT, which is irradiating, expensive and often unavailable. Non-invasive and non-irradiating *in vivo* MRSI can be performed as an adjunct to Magnetic Resonance Imaging (MRI), and is thus cost effective and the method of choice in children under 5 years, when radiation is a serious concern. Although MRSI does not obviate the utility of biopsy, it is suggested that it has the potential to replace serial biopsy and is an excellent alternative to biopsy in inoperable or unbiopsied tumors. The MRSI data when combined with anatomical or other type MR images provide unique information regarding brain tumor biochemistry in inoperable tumors and, might complement neuropathology, guide biopsies, and monitor therapy for operable brain tumors. The combination of such non-invasively acquired prognostic information and the high-resolution anatomical imaging provided by conventional MR imaging will surpass molecular analysis or DNA microarray gene profiling, which although promising depend on invasive biopsy.

2. Application of brain tumor proton MRSI in children

Localized MR spectroscopy studies in children are increasing (Tzika et al., 1993a; Lazareff et al., 1996; Tzika et al., 1997; Lazareff et al., 1998; Lazareff et al., 1999; Warren et al., 2000; Tzika et al., 2001; Tzika et al., 2002; Tzika et al., 2003; Astrakas et al., 2004; Tzika et al., 2004). Brain tumors are usually heterogeneous and complicated by edema and necrosis of the adjacent brain parenchyma, yet their spectra are critically impacted by precision in voxel size and position. Single-voxel MR spectroscopy has the inherent disadvantage that spectral data is not simultaneously collected from the tumor and its surrounding tissue, which greatly hinders the incorporation of valuable information in assessing therapeutic response (Kurhanewicz et al., 1996; Nelson et al., 1997a; Wald et al., 1997; Dillon and Nelson, 1999; Nelson, 2001). Due to technical difficulties, a limited number of adult brain tumor studies using advanced localized MR spectroscopy have been reported (Wald et al., 1995; Nelson et al., 1997a; Nelson et al., 1997b; Wald et al., 1997; Graves et al., 2001a; Vigneron et al., 2001a; Li et al., 2002), and even fewer studies have been carried out in children, employing advanced localized MRSI (Lazareff et al., 1996; Tzika et al., 1997; Lazareff et al., 1998; Taylor et al., 1998; Gonen et al., 1999; Lazareff et al., 1999; Tzika et al., 2001; Tzika et al., 2002; Tzika et al., 2003; Astrakas et al., 2004; Tzika et al., 2004).

3. Biological aspects of selected metabolites detected by proton MRSI

Proton MR spectroscopy has identified several metabolites that are biomarkers of tumor growth and apoptosis (Tzika et al., 1997). To this end, brain tumor proton MR spectroscopy studies **(Fig. 1)** consistently demonstrate: (1) reduced or absent n-acetylaspartate (NAA) and total creatine (tCr) attributed to edema and necrosis; (2) increased Cho-containing compounds possibly due to cell membrane disruption (Griffin et al., 2001) and altered phospholipid metabolism (Aboagye and Bhujwalla, 1999; Podo, 1999; Ackerstaff et al., 2001); and (3) increased lactate due to metabolic acidosis (Bruhn et al., 1989; Alger et al., 1990; Arnold et al., 1990; Segebarth et al., 1990; Luyten et al., 1991; Nelson et al., 1997a; Nelson et al., 1997b; Wald et al., 1997; Aboagye et al., 1998). Reduced NAA is expected in glial tumors, since NAA is primarily localized to neurons. Therefore NAA detection within glial tumors corresponds to either partial volume averaging with adjacent normal tissue, or tumor infiltration of normal tissue. Since NAA occurs in cell cultures of oligodendroglia progenitors (Urenjak et al., 1992), NAA in childhood tumors may also reflect immature oligodendroglia. A reduction in tCr resonance may indicate cell loss due to necrosis, and correspond to exhausted energy reserves resulting from rapid cell proliferation and ischemia. It is also possible that tCr may be a valuable independent predictor of tumor response to therapy (Tzika et al., 2001).

The Cho peak consists of water-soluble Cho-containing compounds, such as phosphocholine (PCho) and glycerophosphocholine (GPC), and free choline (Barker et al., 1994), versus membrane-bound phospatidylcholine (Miller et al., 1996a). *In vivo* MRS reveals that phosphomonoesters (PME), such as phosphocholine (PCho) and phosphoethanolamine (PEth), are elevated in tumors and rapidly proliferating tissues (Daly et al., 1987; Daly and Cohen, 1989; Gillies et al., 1994a). Furthermore, elevations in PCho and PEth correlate with increased cell growth or increased cell degradation, and have been shown to occur in human tumors, as well as in animal tumor models and cell lines. For instance, actively proliferating cultures show dramatically lower PCho/PEth as compared to stationary cultures (Aiken and Gillies, 1996). Gillies et al., found that PCho levels are lowest, and PEth levels are highest in non-proliferating cells and concluded there is a decrease in the biosynthesis of PCho concomitant with a reduction in culture growth (Gillies et al., 1994b). Mahmood et al., found a strong radiation dose-dependent response in the relative PCho/PEth ratio, suggesting that changes in the PCho levels may be related to cell proliferation and/or radiation-induced membrane damage (Mahmood et al., 1994). Aiken et al., suggested that growth stimulation in rat-2 fibroblasts increases phosphomonoesters suggesting that growth stimulation increases PCho levels (Aiken et al., 1996). Together, these data suggest the hypothesis that PCho, which can be measured with either phosphorous or proton MRS, is elevated in actively proliferating cells. Indeed, *in vivo* proton MRS studies suggest the Cho peak reflects proliferative activity in gliomas (Shimizu et al., 2000; Tamiya et al., 2000). Furthermore, PCho concentration correlates with the number of S-phase cells, with depletion corresponding to growth arrest (Smith et al., 1991), and the PCho/GPC ratio corresponding to oncogenic transformation (Bhakoo et al., 1996). Also, the PCho-produced Cho signal has been proposed to also depend on local cellularity (Chang et al., 1995; Miller et al., 1996b). Recently, using a high-resolution magic angle spinning proton MRS technique, it has been shown that PCho levels in glioblastoma multiforme correlate to the percentage of highly cellular malignant glioma (Cheng et al., 2000b). Also, altered phospholipid metabolism, such as PCho and GPC accumulation, has been reported to reflect early stages of growth arrest or apoptosis (Smith et al., 1991). In addition, GPC levels were found to increase in cultured mammalian cells exhibiting perturbed energetic metabolism during acidosis (Galons et al., 1995). In general, the consensus is that tissues with high proliferative potential or tissues that are oncogenically transformed are also highly cellular in the absence of compensating apoptotic mechanisms or limitations of vascular supply. Consistent with this, many studies strongly have suggested that the Cho peak detected by *in vivo* MRS may be elevated because the volume of interest is highly cellular (Chang et al., 1995; Miller et al., 1996b; Cheng et al., 2000b) or includes cells with high PCho which may be due to increased proliferative potential (Daly et al., 1987; Daly and Cohen, 1989; Gillies et al., 1994a; Mahmood et al., 1994; Aiken and Gillies, 1996; Aiken et al., 1996) or includes cells which are oncogenically transformed (Bhakoo et al., 1996; Aboagye and Bhujwalla, 1999; Ackerstaff et al., 2001). It was recently reported that in *ex vivo* high resolution MR spectra (which show much higher than the spectra obtained *in vivo*) of a biopsy from a cerebellar primitive neuroectodermal tumor, myo-inositol, taurine and phosphorylethanolamine contribute to the *in vivo* signal at 3.2 ppm, usually attributed to Cho-containing compounds (Tugnoli et al., 2001).

Cancer cells are apoptotic, and thus typically die upon conventional chemotherapy, radiation (Thompson, 1995) and experimental approaches such as antiangiogenic (Holmgren et al., 1995) and ganciclovir treatments (Freeman et al., 1993; Wei et al., 1998). Recently, it was shown that *in vivo* proton MR spectroscopy detects a substantial accumulation of polyunsaturated fatty acids associated with gene therapy-induced apoptosis (Hakumaki et al., 1999). Furthermore, PCho depletion, a major constituent of the Cho peak detected *in vivo* in tumors, coincides with growth arrest (Smith et al., 1991). Therefore, facilitation of apoptosis by selective chemotherapeutic agents or gene therapy could be a future strategy for human cancer treatment (Thompson, 1995). It has also been

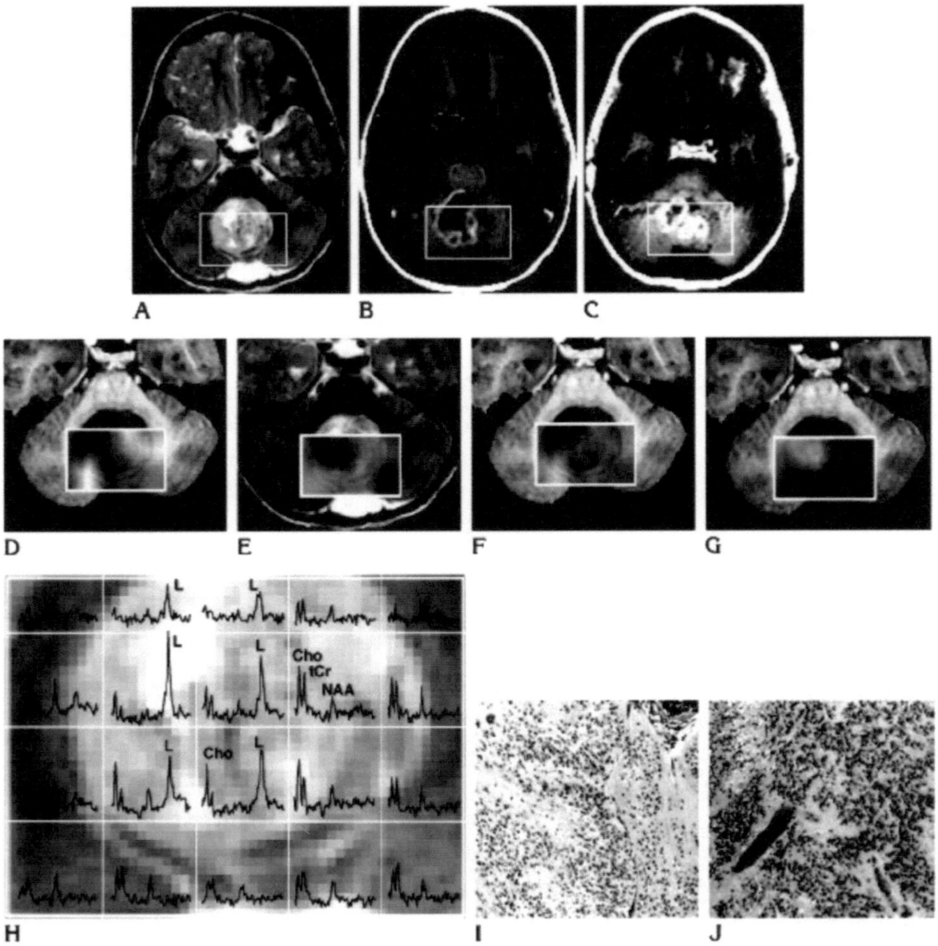

Fig. 1. MR imaging and MR spectroscopy in a 4-year-old boy with a large posterior fossa anaplastic ependymoma. *A*, Axial T2-weighted MR image shows a large cystic posterior fossa tumor. *B* and *C*, Two contiguous axial T1-weighted MR sections after injection of contrast material show a large cyst and nonhomogeneous enhancement. *Rectangles* indicate the volume selected for MR spectroscopy. *D–G*, Composite images represent Cho (*D*), NAA (*E*), tCr (*F*), and lactate/lipids (*G*) metabolite distributions (*rectangles*) superimposed on the T2-weighted MR images. Increased brightness corresponds to higher metabolite levels and decreased brightness to lower levels. In *D*, *F*, and *G*, the T2-weighted image contrast has been reversed so that the tumor is dark and does not interfere with the intensity of the metabolite image. Note that the cyst (clearly seen as a dark region in *B*) corresponds to low or no NAA and high lactate/lipids, which suggests that lactic acid has been concentrated in the cyst. *D* shows two regions of high Cho corresponding to the solid portion of the tumor. *H*, The spectral grid has been superimposed on a zoomed T2-weighted image. The metabolic heterogeneity of the tumor as depicted by multivoxel MR spectroscopy is illustrated. *I* and *J*, Histologic sections show certain regions of the tumor are "typical" ependymoma (*I*), whereas other regions had more anaplastic features, including increased cellularity (*J*).

inferred that prior to volume loss, the treatment response is associated with an increase in tissue water diffusion and T2 relaxation time (Poptani et al., 1998), which suggests increased water content and bulk diffusibility. Also, reduced diffusion of Cho-containing compounds in gliomas undergoing apoptosis has been reported (Hakumaki et al., 1998). These observations imply an increased viscosity and restriction within cells, to reflect cell shrinkage. Also, flow-cytometric studies demonstrate that gene therapy-induced apoptosis (Freeman et al., 1993) is preceded by an irreversible arrest in the late S- or G2-plase of the cell cycle (Wei et al., 1998). The MRS-visible lipids not only correlate with apoptosis or necrosis (Cheng et al., 2000a; Tugnoli et al., 2001), but also with the proportion of cells in these S- or G2 stages (Veale et al., 1997). Finally, the ceramide resonance region has been associated with the differential diagnosis of high and low malignancy of brain gliomas (Lombardi et al., 1997). This observation deserves further investigation, since apoptotic stimuli such as ceramide, a second messenger related to apoptosis, disrupt electron transport in mitochondria (Kyriakis and Avruch, 1996; Susin et al., 1997; Kolesnick and Kronke, 1998; Schwandner et al., 1998; Williams et al., 1998; Yasuhara et al., 1999), which acts as an important site for apoptosis initiation (Ashkenazi and Dixit, 1998; De Laurenzi and Melino, 2000; Tournier et al., 2000).

4. Methodology for acquiring proton MRSI data in the clinical setting

It is important to note that the methodological aspects of MRSI are not standardized and may vary among investigators or clinical sites. Typically, for MRSI, a large volume of interest can be selected and then phase encoding is applied to obtain multiple voxels in a single plane (Tzika et al., 1997) or in three-dimensions (Nelson et al., 1997c; Vigneron et al., 2001b). The advantage of obtaining multivoxel data is that it is possible to observe not only heterogeneity within the lesion but to examine surrounding tissue that may appear normal on MR images. This provides a reference for comparing metabolite levels in the tumor and makes it possible to identify regions of abnormal metabolism outside the morphological lesion (Nelson et al., 1999; Graves et al., 2000; Graves et al., 2001a; Tzika et al., 2002). According to our experience with MRSI in children, multilevel two-dimensional MR spectroscopy data acquisitions with no gap may be rather used than three-dimensional methods. This approach improves the signal-to-noise ratio, because adjustments for magnetic field homogeneity and water suppression may be performed in each section; with a large volume, these adjustments often fail in the clinical MR setting (Tzika et al., 2002). The two most common methods used for volume pre-selection is point-resolved spectroscopy (PRESS) (Bottomley, 1984; Bottomley, 1987) or stimulated echo acquisition mode (STEAM) (Bruhn et al., 1989), with PRESS being preferred when the echo time allows because of its intrinsically higher signal to noise ratio (Tzika et al., 1996b). Briefly, after a 50–100-mL volume is selected and after shimming and water suppression adjustments are made, a large data set is obtained by using phase-encoding gradients in two or three directions. The following parameters may be used for 2 dimensional acquisitions: 1000/65 (TR/TE), 16 X 16 phase-encoding matrix, 160-mm FOV, section thickness of 10 mm, 1250-Hz spectral width, two averages, and 512 points. Using these parameters, data sets of 1–1.2-cm^3 resolution are acquired. The decision to use a TE of 65 milliseconds may be made for the following reasons. If one is not as interested in the lactic acid detection as in the presence of lipids, which might be important, because lipids are related to tumor necrosis or apoptosis; this, in turn, is a determining factor of tumor activity. Our current notion is that a TE of 65 milliseconds provides us with the opportunity to 1) null lactic acid; 2) increase sensitivity in

lipid detection, and 3) prevent diffusion artifacts and water-suppression failures with PRESS performed at TEs shorter than 65 milliseconds. Thus, the four prominent peaks of biologic importance in our studies were those of NAA, Cho, tCr, and lipids (and/or lactate). An advantage of the above stated approach is that the volume of interest can be selected to eliminate as much of the subcutaneous lipids as possible and to avoid regions likely to cause large variations in susceptibility such as the sinuses. This permits improved shimming and provides spectra with narrower peaks and higher signal to noise. **Fig. 1** shows examples of multivoxel spectra from normal brain tissue, necrosis, and different regions from brain tumors (Tzika et al., 1997). The normal brain has N-acetylaspartate that is approximately twice the intensity of choline and creatine. Tumor generally has decreased N-acetylaspartate and increased choline and variable levels of creatine. Peaks corresponding to lipid and/or lactate may be present in regions of necrosis (Tzika et al., 1997; Tzika et al., 2002).
MRSI is more demanding in magnetic field homogeneity than MRI. In many circumnstances (e.g. close to the sinus or to cavities of resected tumors, or close to permanent radioactive seeds) shimming fails and water and lipid suppression become inadequate compromising the quality of the data obtained. Also due to the low spatial resolution of MRSI (about 1-cm^3 per voxel at 1.5 T) the spectra may reveal a mixed metabolic profile of tumor, necrosis, and normal brain tissue. Finally MRSI sequences are time consuming because usually they lack the most rapid form of gradient spatial enconding, namely the frequency enconding performed by the readout gradient. Many new approaches have been developed to improve the performance of conventional MRSI (Nelson et al., 1997b). Special alternative radiofrequency pulses are able to provide improved spatial and frequency selection (Star-Lack et al., 1997a; Star-Lack et al., 1997b) and better volume selection can be achieved with spatially selective saturation bands (Tran et al., 2000). Multislice and multiple echo time techniques (Spielman et al., 1992; Duyn et al., 1993) can be used to acquire multivoxel MRSI data in a time efficient manner. Also a fast three dimension multivoxel MRSI can be achieved with echo planar methodology with good quality data (Posse et al., 1994; Adalsteinsson et al., 1995; Posse et al., 1995). In the future the development of a hybrid PRESS-echo planar spectroscopic imaging technique with spatially selective saturation bands may speed up MRSI and overcome its present limitations in water suppression, volume selection and susceptibility artifacts (Nelson, 2003).

5. Processing and analysis of proton MRS data in the clinical setting

The processing and analysis of the resulting proton MR spectra combines fourier transforms and apodization with automated methods of spectral processing to provide data that can be interpreted by visual inspection or quantified to generate maps of the spatial distribution of different metabolites (Nelson, 2001). Different MR system manufacturers offer different packages for proton MRS analysis. Typically, the data are transferred off-line to the remote Sun workstation, converted into a standard data format, fourier-transformed and phased using appropriate spectroscopic packages. To reliably and reproducibly quantify *in vivo* spectra, requires removal of baseline components, identification of peaks, and estimation of peak parameters, which can be accomplished using several different approaches (Barkhuijsen et al., 1985; Hore, 1985; Laue et al., 1985; Nelson and Brown, 1987; Spielman et al., 1988; Van der Veen et al., 1988; Derby et al., 1989; Nelson and Brown, 1989). Characteristics of the proton MR spectroscopy data that guide the choice of methodology are the larger number of spectra that need to be considered, and the need for whatever method is chosen to be robust to differences in signal to noise and peak configurations corresponding to different tissue types. Additionally, more sophisticated fitting algorithms can be applied to spectra that have sufficient signal to noise for the optimization routines to be reliable (e.g., (Provencher, 1993)). The output of the analysis is a number of spatial maps of metabolite parameters that can be applied to identify regions of normal and abnormal metabolism.

We have used a software application we have written in IDL that employs the PIQUABLE algorithm, which has the advantages (Nelson and Brown, 1987; Nelson and Brown, 1989) of being automated, uses non-parametric methods for objective identification of peaks, and can remove broad baseline components. This algorithm has been tested using simulated data (Nelson and Brown, 1987; Nelson and Brown, 1989) and data from human volunteers and patients (Nelson et al., 1997a). We have calibrated our software with simulated spectra, and spectra from phantom and patients, to result in reliable and reproducible results, within the accuracy of random noise. Additional corrections for spatial variations in intensity caused by the data acquisition procedures may also be required if comparing relative intensities of metabolites such as choline, creatine, N-acetylaspartate, lactate, and lipid (Nelson, 2001). When the PIQUABLE algorithm fails, we use alternative quantitation algorithms (AMARES, HLSVD, etc) in the MRUI package.

Several approaches may be used to display the information from multivoxel MRSI data sets and to correlate the anatomy with spatial variations in metabolites, including: (1) A grid superimposed on the MR image and plotting of the corresponding array of spectra. This approach does not require quantification and can be quickly performed after data collection; and (2) Metabolite images formed from arrays of estimated peak parameters. The primary resonances of interest are NAA, Cho, tCr, as well as lipid resonances at: 0.9 ppm (methyl groups), 1.3 ppm (methylene groups and lactate); 2.8 ppm (bisallylic methylene fatty acids); and a resonance at 5.4 ppm which arises from vinyl protons and includes ceramide. In addition, other metabolites, such as glutamate, glutamine, γ-aminobutyric acid, scyllo-inositol, aspartate, taurine, N-acetylaspartylglutamate, glucose and branched amino acids, may be detected (Tkac et al., 2001; Di Costanzo et al., 2003). To visualize the spatial distributions that correspond to the metabolites of interest, gray-level images mapping the peak area of these metabolites may be obtained; (3) Color metabolite images overlaid on gray-level MR images. This aids the estimation of the anatomic correlation of the varying levels of color metabolite images; (4) Selected spectra may be extracted from the MRSI data sets to be correlated with data from other modalities or with the *ex vivo* high resolution magic angle spinning proton MR spectra of tumor biopsies that correspond to the same anatomic location.

6. Contribution of proton MRSI in clinical tumor grading

Whether proton MRSI is able to contribute to defining tumor type and grade remains an open question. Although elevated Cho and low NAA before therapy may be a reliable indicator of pediatric brain tumor malignancy (Sutton et al., 1992; Tzika et al., 1993b; Tzika, 1995; Byrd et al., 1996b; Tzika et al., 1996a; Tzika et al., 1997; Taylor et al., 1998; Tzika et al., 2004), the consensus is that proton MR spectroscopy results may not be used alone to classify tumors, as some studies have shown considerable overlap in proton MRSI results among different tumor types (Warren et al., 2000; Warren, 2004). In our experience, the different MR spectral patterns may suggest that proton MRSI can be used to distinguish at least three different tissue compartments —normal, tumor, and necrosis— (Naidich, 1995; Tzika et al., 1997), whereas mixed MR spectral patterns were due to the known heterogeneity of tumors, as confirmed by the histopathologic features (Tzika et al., 2002). This notion is in agreement with other reports (Ott et al., 1993; Wald et al., 1997; Star-Lack et al., 1998; Li et al., 2002). MR spectral patterns with elevated Cho and lipid levels in the absence of NAA that are histologically verified to represent regions of active tumor with extensive areas of necrosis suggest that such MR spectral patterns contribute additional information that is not available with conventional MR imaging. Because glial tumors are graded according to their cellularity, proliferative activity, and degree of necrosis, Cho mapping (increased cellularity and proliferative activity), may contribute added value to MR neuroimaging in patients with brain tumors, especially when it is combined with lipid mapping (necrosis and/or apoptosis). Indeed, contrast-enhancing regions with high lipid levels and low or no Cho levels, as shown in 11 patients with malignant or inoperable tumors, have been suggested to represent areas of high neoplastic potential intermingled with microscopic necrosis; this finding was verified at biopsy (Tzika et al., 2002). Low-grade tumors not enhancing on the T1-weighted Gd-enhanced images exhibit prominent peaks corresponding to Cho; although tCr and NAA peaks are occasionally detected the absence of lipids and or lactate is demonstrated **(Fig 2).**

A successful classification of pediatric patients with posterior fossa tumors was published by Arle *et al.,* (Arle et al., 1997) using single voxel proton MR spectroscopy and a computer-based neural network. The network combined MR spectroscopy data (ratios of N-acetyl-aspartate, choline, and creatine) with 10 characteristics of tumor tissue obtained from MR images, as well as tumor size and the patient's age and sex, and improved diagnostic accuracy by identifing 95% of the tumors correctly. However, given the differences in spatial extent of tumors, the question arises as to whether the single voxel MR spectroscopy is able to contribute to defining tumor type and grade. To this end, an excellent classification of adult patients with brain tumors was reported by Preul *et al.,* (Preul et al., 1996) who used two-dimensional proton MRSI and a multivariate pattern recognition analysis of peaks corresponding to choline, creatine, N-acetylasparate, lactate, lipid, and alanine. Grade 2 gliomas tended to have low lactate and lipid, some N-acetylaspartate, and some creatine. Grade 3 gliomas tended to have low lactate and lipid, less N-acetylaspartate and creatine, with higher choline. Grade 4 gliomas tended toward high lactate and lipid, with very low N-acetylaspartate. Upon visual inspection of spectral patterns and metabolite levels in each class, it was clear that meningiomas were distinguished as they were the only lesions that had alanine. Although these results were very promising, there has not yet been a prospective study using the statistical classification that these authors derived. One of the complications in analyzing data obtained with a multivoxel data acquisition technique is in determining which spectrum to consider for each lesion. Suggestions that have been made include using the most abnormal voxel and the average of all voxels within the lesion. Both of these approaches involve a subjective decision that takes the anatomical appearance of the lesion into account. For example, does the lesion include the entire T2 abnormality or is it restricted to the enhancing volume. As seen in the study by Li *et al.,* the spectral characteristics of these regions may be quite different (Li et al., 2002). The same issue is present with single voxel analysis, but in that case, the decision is made implicitly at the time of data acquisition by the choice of the selected volume. The studies from Dr. Nelson's group at UCSF have suggested that although it may be possible to detect mean differences between populations of gliomas with different grades based upon metabolite levels, there is considerable overlap, both for mean metabolite levels or for the most abnormal voxels within the T2 lesion (Li et al., 2002).

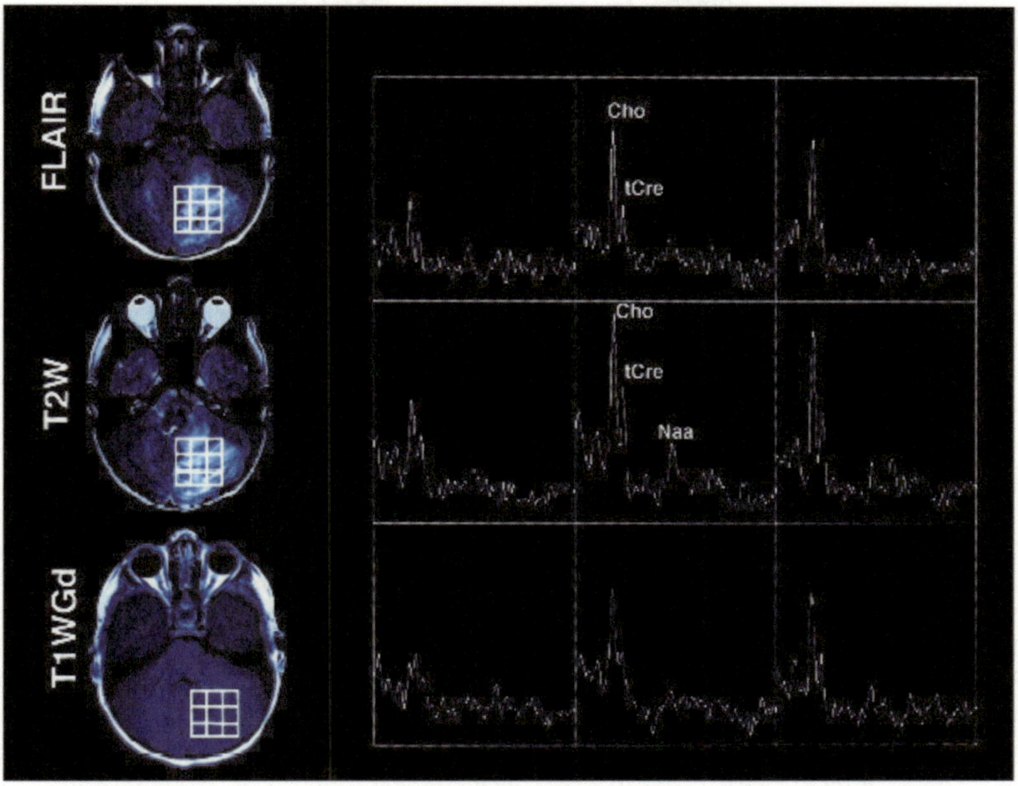

Fig. 2. Axial FLAIR, T2-weighted (T2W), and T1-weighted Gd-enhanced (T1WGd) MR images and selected proton MR spectra from a multivoxel MR spectroscopic data set in a 10-year-old girl with a cerebellar tumor. The lesion appears inhomogeneously hyperintense on the FLAIR and T2-weighted images and is not enhancing on the T1-weighted Gd-enhanced image. Prominent peaks corresponding to Cho are detected. Also, tCr and NAA peaks are occasionally detected. The Figure illustrates that no relationship existed between Cho detection and contrast enhancement on T1-weighted Gd-enhanced images and that spectral patterns devoid of lipid and/or lactate peaks are characteristic of low grade tumors. .

In our experience, information such as relative cerebral blood volume or apparent diffusion coefficient may also help in grading tumors and in distinguishing between tumors and other types of mass lesions (Tzika et al., 2003). Because brain tumors can be characterized according to their physiological parameters, including proton MR spectral metabolites (NAA, Cho, tCr, L), hemodynamic indices (i.e., rCBV) and physicochemical measures (ADC) the notion is that relationships among these parameters may reflect the biochemical state of tumors and this notion was supported by our findings so far (Tzika et al., 2003). Finally, age and tumor location in addition to anatomic factors seem likely to be relevant for classification and that which ever procedure is considered should ensure that the influence of all factors explicitly considered in the analysis.

7. Clinical role of proton MRSI in predicting response to therapy

A number of studies suggest that proton MRS spectroscopy promises an early prediction of whether a lesion has responded to therapy (Byrd et al., 1996a; Lazareff et al., 1998; Warren et al., 2000; Tzika et al., 2001; Tarnawski et al., 2002; Tzika et al., 2004). In a study involving 75 children with brain tumors, Byrd et al., found elevated Cho and elevated lactate and or lipids (Byrd et al., 1996a), which agrees with our data and data in adults. Another study involving 11 pediatric patients with low-grade gliomas, the tumors that progressed during a 2-year period displayed higher normalized Cho than those that remained stable (Lazareff et al., 1998). Warren et al., found in 27 children with recurrent or progressive tumors that the maximum tumor Cho:NAA ratio was predictive of outcome; Cho:NAA greater than 4.5 correpsonded to survival time of 22 weeks and all 13 patients died by 63 weeks; Cho:NAA less or equal to 4.5 corresponded to more than 50% survival at 63 weeks (Warren et al., 2000). Since proton MR spectroscopy detects total creatine (creatine, phosphocreatine; tCr) in addition to Cho and NAA in tumors, we hypothesized that we might be able to use proton MRSI to measure tCr to predict treatment response of pediatric brain tumors. To this end, 24 patients aged 10 months to 24 years were studied using MRI and point-resolved spectroscopy (PRESS) with volume preselection and phase encoding in 2-dimensions on a 1.5-T MR imaging system (TR-2000ms; TE-65ms). Multiple logistic regression was performed to establish the independent predictors of active tumor growth. Biologically vital cellular metabolites such as tCr, N-acetyl-aspartate (NAA), choline-containing compounds (Cho), and lipid or lactate (L), were seen to differ between tumor and control tissues ($P< 0.05$). Brain tumors (n=8), while responding to treatment (radiation or chemotherapy), exhibited decreased Cho ($P=0.05$), increased tCr ($P=0.02$), decreased NAA ($P=0.50$), and decreased L ($P=0.04$) when compared to untreated tumors (except surgery) or to tumors not responding to treatment (n=16), although the only significant independent predictor of active tumor growth was tCr ($P<0.01$). We concluded that Cho was the strongest metabolite signal detected in tumors, and tumor tCr was the only independent predictor of active tumor growth, and suggested that tCr is biological important metabolite useful in brain tumor assessment (Tzika et al., 2001). Other investigators have used other metabolite ratios such as lactate/NAA ratios to evaluate the prognostic value of MRS in brain tumors; for lactate/NAA ratios greater than 2.0 have been associated with 1-year survival rate of 20%, whereas for lactate/NAA values less than 2.0, the 1-year survival rate was 85% (Tarnawski et al., 2002).

In our experience, percent change in Cho/NAA is the most promising prognostic index in children with brain tumors (Tzika et al., 2004). From the serial proton MRSI exams of 27 children with neuroepithelial tumors we calculated and plotted the maximum percent change in Cho/NAA ratios versus clinical outcome. Each exam was rated either as stable or as progressive disease, according to the evaluation of the clinical oncologist who was blinded to the MRSI results. We used the Mann-Whitney U-test (since the Kolmogorov-Smirnov test detected significant skewness) and our results showed that percent change in Cho/NAA is significantly higher in the progressive (n = 18) as compared to the stable (n = 32) disease group ($P < 0.001$). Logistic regression confirmed that percent change in Cho/NAA is an important predictor of tumor progression (likelihood ratio test = 33.4, $P <0.001$). Using a 20% increase as a cutoff, Cho/NAA correctly classifies 16 out of 18 progressing cases (sensitivity = 0.89, 95% confidence limits = 0.65 - 0.99) and 27 out of 32 stable cases (specificity = 0.88, 95% confidence limits = 0.71 - 0.97). The odds of tumor progression are estimated to be approximately 55 times higher for cases showing at least a 20% change in Cho/NAA (odds ratio = 55.1, 95% confidence interval = 9.2 to 140.3). We also found significant differences between progressing and stable outcomes with respect to Cho/ntCr (progressing: median = 2.03, range 0.83 to 3.17; stable 1.53, range 0.74 to 6.81, P = 0.03). Furthermore, significant differences are seen between progressing and stable outcomes in percent change of Cho/ntCr (progressing: median +63%, range -14% to +140%; stable: median +9%, range -57% to +166%, P = 0.04).

For proton MRSI to be included in the clinical management of the patient it is important that MRSI improves the assessment of pediatric brain tumors by adding independent information regarding tumor involvement. For instance, if it were possible for proton MRS to assist in defining tumor borders since in gadolinium-enhanced MR images the relation between tumor cell extent and contrast-enhanced regions is unclear, it would allow modifying an ineffective treatment strategy before the tumor progresses further. To this end, we analyzed MRI and MRSI data in 31 children with brain tumors and we found that tumor spectral patterns were detected in tumor regions and outside enhancing tumor beds in patients with clinical progression; these were confirmed at neuropathologic analysis. This study demonstrates the importance of mapping out both the temporal and spatial distribution of metabolite changes in response to the therapy of interest. Such mapping requires the use of two or three-dimensional proton MRSI and is most easily achieved for the case of focal therapies such as surgery or radiation. The incorporation of multiple imaging modalities into therapy planning offers the potential to improve identification of regions of pathology. To this end, multiparametric and/or multimodality imaging has been proposed (Graves et al., 2001b; Tzika et al., 2003). Registration of the MR images and proton MRS data are critical for correlating data from such examinations. To this end excellent results from the studies in adults undergoing brain tumor therapy at the University of California San Francisco have been already reported (Wald et al., 1997; Dowling et al., 2001; Graves et al., 2001a; Graves et al., 2001b). In our opinion, multivoxel proton MRSI is more powerful than conventional or some of the recently promising types of MRI such as perfusion MRI for prediction of tumour behaviour (Tzika et al., 2004). Although proton MRSI generally agrees with perfusion MRI **(Fig. 3),** it may be superior to perfusion MRI in the case where perfusion MRI is limited **(Fig. 3).**

8. Clinical relevance of proton MRSI

The therapeutic approach to pediatric patients with malignant brain tumors is multifaceted and takes into account the location and resectability of the tumor, as well as the patient's age (Allen and Siffert, 1997). Surgery continues to be the treatment of choice for most patients, although overall effectiveness is often limited by disease dissemination or primary location (Mickle, 1997; Tomita, 1998). Radiation therapy has a documented role in the treatment of children with brain tumors (Buatti et al., 1997; Kalapurakal and Thomas, 1997), although most high-grade glial tumors show only temporary responses. Furthermore, the deleterious effects of radiation therapy on the developing nervous system often prevent the use of this modality. Finally, effective chemotherapy has been predominantly observed in neural

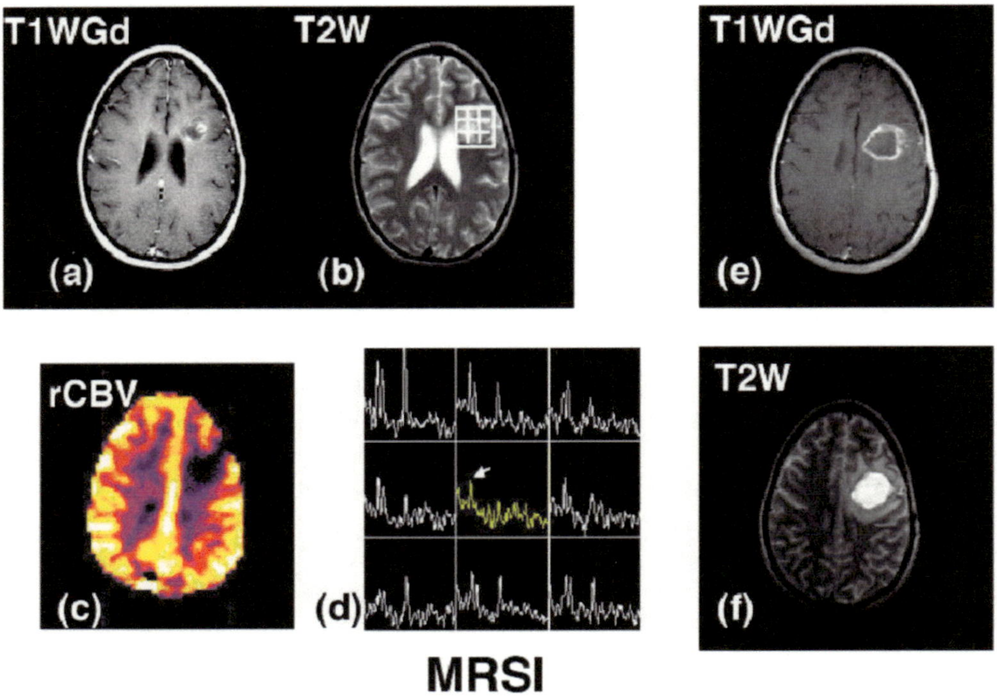

Fig. 3. Baseline magnetic resonance (MR) images and MR spectroscopic imaging (MRSI) (a–d) and 1-month follow-up MR images (e,f) from a female patient age 13 years with an anaplastic ependymoma during therapy. Gadolinium (Gd)-enhanced, T1-weighted (T1WGd) MR image (a) after Gd injection shows a region of enhancement within the left frontal lobe that is hyperintense on T2-weighted (T2W) image (b) and hypointense on a relative cerebral blood volume (rCBV) image (c). These findings may suggest tumor recurrence or radiation necrosis. The MRSI image (d) distinguishes radiation necrosis from tumor recurrence (middle voxel with a prominent choline [Cho] peak at arrow) and predicted tumor progression, which was evident on the T1WGd and T2W MR images (e,f) 1 month later. The rCBV image in c does not illustrate true relative tumor blood volume values, because the rCBV quantitation failed in the tumor region (most likely because of the leaky vasculature of the tumor), which is a limitation of the perfusion technique.

tumors and low-grade gliomas, but not in patients with high-grade glial or recurrent/progressive disease (Kedar, 1997). Given the difficulties inherent with sequential biopsy to monitor response to therapy in children with brain tumors, non-invasive and non-irradiating imaging methods are needed to provide additional diagnostic and/or prognostic indices or biomarkers beyond simple tumor volume measurements. Moreover, an important unresolved issue in brain tumor therapy is that dying or necrotic tissue within the CNS is difficult to differentiate from viable recurring tumor (Nelson et al., 1997a). By both clinical and standard CT or MRI scan criteria, necrosis or recurring tumor can appear to be identical. In time, tumor cell death will resolve, and thus the capability to differentiate between growing tumor and necrotic tissue at an early point in time is of great importance for both patient management and access to the biologic activity of tumorigenesis inhibitors or chemotherapeutic drugs. Advanced neuroimaging MR techniques, such as proton MRSI, promise to help differentiate between these two entities at an early stage. Also, the spatial extent of the metabolic lesion by MRS is different from the gadolinium-enhancing region and hyperintensity on T2-weighted images (Tzika et al., 2002). Since there is such a distinction there may be added value for the proton MRSI data over and above conventional MRI. More importantly, the general consensus is that proton MRSI might be able to make an early prediction of whether a lesion has responded to therapy (Byrd et al., 1996a; Lazareff et al., 1998; Warren et al., 2000; Tzika et al., 2001; Tarnawski et al., 2002; Tzika et al., 2004). If this were possible, it would allow tailoring therapy to each individual patient and modifying an ineffective treatment strategy before the tumor progresses. It would also be possible to avoid giving unnecessary treatment in the case that an increase in tumor volume is attributable to treatment-induced necrosis as opposed to recurrent or residual tumor.

9. Conclusion

Although the clinical relevance of proton MRSI has not been decided yet, in our opinion, it is clear that proton MRSI improves the assessment of pediatric brain tumors by adding independent biochemical information regarding tumor type or grade, tumor involvement and by depicting residual or recurrent tumor outside the gadolinium-enhancing tumor bed. More importantly it is an invaluable adjunct to MRI and other modalities. To this end, it may provide biomarkers predicting tumor response earlier than conventional MRI. We believe that in the near future, and since higher field MR systems have been approved by the FDA and are being introduced in the clinical setting high-field, higher resolution proton MRSI, will provide unique biomarkers regarding brain tumor biochemistry in inoperable tumors and, might complement neuropathology, guide biopsies and monitor the success and failure of therapy, for operable brain tumors. Correlative studies with genomic biomarkers will strengthen the biological and clinical relevance of proton MRS.

10. Acknowledgments

We thank our colleagues from the Departments of Radiology, Neurosurgery and Radiation Oncology Children's Hospital Boston, especially Tina Young Poussaint (neuroradiologist), Liliana Goumnerova (neurosurgeon), Michael R. Scott (Chief of Pediatric Neurosurgery), Nancy J. Tarbell (Chief of Pediatric Radiation Oncology), Peter McL Black (Chairman of Neurosurgery) and David Zurakowski (Biostatistics) for their contributions to the work presented here. We also thank our colleagues Dr. Sarah J. Nelson and Daniel B. Vigneron from the Magnetic Resonance Science Center at the University of California, San Francisco for their collaboration and consulation over the years.

11. References

Aboagye, E.O. and Bhujwalla, Z.M.: Malignant transformation alters membrane choline phospholipid metabolism of human mammary epithelial cells. Cancer Res 59 (1999) 80-4.

Aboagye, E.O., Bhujwalla, Z.M., He, Q. and Glickson, J.D.: Evaluation of lactate as a 1H nuclear magnetic resonance spectroscopy index for noninvasive prediction and early detection of tumor response to radiation therapy in EMT6 tumors. Radiation Research 150 (1998) 38-42.

Ackerstaff, E., Pflug, B.R., Nelson, J.B. and Bhujwalla, Z.M.: Detection of increased choline compounds with proton nuclear magnetic resonance spectroscopy subsequent to malignant transformation of human prostatic epithelial cells. Cancer Res 61 (2001) 3599-603.

Adalsteinsson, E., Irarrazabal, P., Spielman, D.M. and Macovski, A.: Three-dimensional spectroscopic imaging with time-varying gradients. Magn Reson Med 33 (1995) 461-6.

Aiken, N.R. and Gillies, R.J.: Phosphomonoester metabolism as a function of cell proliferative status and exogenous precursors. Anticancer Res 16 (1996) 1393-7.

Aiken, N.R., Szwergold, E.S., Kappler, F., Stoyanova, R., Kuesel, A.C., Shaller, C. and Brown, T.R.: Metabolism of phosphonium choline by rat-2 fibroblasts: effects of mitogenic stimulation studied using 31P NMR spectroscopy. Anticancer Res 16 (1996) 1357-63.

Albright, A.L.: Pediatric Brain Tumors. CA Cancer J Clin 43 (1993) 272-288.

Alger, J., Frank, J., Bizzi, A., Fulham, M., DeSouza, B., Duhaney, M., Inscoe, S., Black, J., van Zijl, P., Moonen, C. and Di Chiro, G.: Metabolism of human gliomas: assessment with H-1 MR spectroscopy and F-18 flourodeoxyglucose PET. Radiology 177 (1990) 633-641.

Allen, J.C. and Siffert, J.: Contemporary issues in the management of childhood brain tumors. Current Opinion in Neurology 10 (1997) 137-41.

Arle, J.E., Morriss, C., Wang, Z.J., Zimmerman, R.A., Phillips, P.G. and Sutton, L.N.: Prediction of posterior fossa tumor type in children by means of magnetic resonance image properties, spectroscopy, and neural networks. Journal of Neurosurgery 86 (1997) 755-61.

Arnold, D., Shoubridge, E., Villemure, J. and Feindel, W.: Proton and phosphorus magnetic resonance spectroscopy of human astrocytomas in vivo. Preliminary observations on tumor grading. NMR Biomed 3 (1990) 184-9.

Ashkenazi, A. and Dixit, V.M.: Death receptors: signaling and modulation. Science 281 (1998) 1305-8.

Astrakas, L.G., Zurakowski, D., Tzika, A.A., Zarifi, M.K., Anthony, D.C., De Girolami, U., Tarbell, N.J. and Black, P.M.: Noninvasive magnetic resonance spectroscopic imaging biomarkers to predict the clinical grade of pediatric brain tumors. Clin Cancer Res 10 (2004) 8220-8.

Barker, P., Breiter, S., Soher, B., Chatham, J., Forber, J., Samphilipo, M., Magee, C. and Anderson, J.: Quantitative proton spectroscopy of canine brain: *in vivo* and *in vitro* correlations. Magn Reson Med 32 (1994) 157-163.

Barkhuijsen, H., de Beer, R., Bovee, W. and van Ormondt, D.: Retrieval of frequencies. Amplitudes, damping factors, and phases from time-domain signals using a linear least-squares procedure. J Magn Reson 61 (1985) 465-481.

Bhakoo, K.K., Williams, S.R., Florian, C.L., Land, H. and Noble, M.D.: Immortalization and transformation are associated with specific alterations in choline metabolism. Cancer Res 56 (1996) 4630-5.

Bleyer, W.: What can be learned about childhood cancer from "Cancer Statistics Review 1973-1988". Cancer 71 (1993) 3229-3236.

Bottomley, P.A.: Selective volume method for performing localized NMR spectroscopy. U S patent 4 480 228 (1984).

Bottomley, P.A.: Spatial localization in NMR spectroscopy *in vivo*. Ann N Y Acad Sci 508 (1987) 333-348.

Bruhn, H., Frahm, J., Gungell, M., Merboldt, K., Hanicke, W., Sauter, R. and Hamburger, C.: Noninvasive differentiation of tumors with use of localized H-1 MR spectroscopy *in vivo*: initial experience in patients with cerebral tumors. Radiology 172 (1989) 541-548.

Buatti, J.M., Meeks, S.L., Marcus, R.B., Jr. and Mendenhall, N.P.: Radiotherapy for pediatric brain tumors. Semin Pediatrc Neurol 4 (1997) 304-319.

Byrd, S.E., Tomita, T., Palka, P.S., Darling, C.F., Norfray, J.P. and Fan, J.: Magnetic resonance spectroscopy (MRS) in the evaluation of pediatric brain tumors, Part II: Clinical analysis. Journal of the National Medical Association 88 (1996a) 717-23.

Byrd, S.E., Tomita, T., Palka, P.S., Darling, C.F., Norfray, J.P. and Fan, J.: Magnetic resonance spectroscopy (MRS) in the evaluation of pediatric brain tumors, Part II: Clinical analysis. J Natl Med Assoc 88 (1996b) 717-23.

Chang, L., McBride, D., Miller, B.L., Cornford, M., Booth, R.A., Buchthal, S.D., Ernst, T.M. and Jenden, D.: Localized in vivo 1Hmagnetic resonance spectroscopy and in vitro analyses of heterogeneous brain tumors. J Neuroimaging 5 (1995) 157-163.

Cheng, L., Anthony, D., Comite, A., Black, P., Tzika, A. and Gonzalez, R.: Quantification of microheterogeneity in glioblastoma multiforme with ex vivo high-resolution magic-angle spinning (HRMAS) proton magetic resonance spectroscopy. Neuro-Oncology 2 (2000a) 87-95.

Cheng, L.L., Anthony, D.C., Comite, A.R., Black, P.M., Tzika, A.A. and Gonzalez, R.G.: Quantification of microheterogeneity in glioblastoma multiforme with ex vivo high-resolution magic-angle spinning (HRMAS) proton magnetic resonance spectroscopy. Neuro-oncol 2 (2000b) 87-95.

Daly, P.F. and Cohen, J.S.: Magnetic resonance spectroscopy of tumors and potential in vivo clinical applications: a review. Cancer Res 49 (1989) 770-9.

Daly, P.F., Lyon, R.C., Faustino, P.J. and Cohen, J.S.: Phospholipid metabolism in cancer cells monitored by 31P NMR spectroscopy. J Biol Chem 262 (1987) 14875-8.

De Laurenzi, V. and Melino, G.: Apoptosis. The little devil of death. Nature 406 (2000) 135-6.

Derby, K., Hawryszko, H. and Troop, J.: Baseline deconvolution, phase correction and signal quantification in fourier localized spectroscopic imaging. Magn Reson Med 12 (1989) 235-240.

Di Costanzo, A., Trojsi, F., Tosetti, M., Giannatempo, G.M., Nemore, F., Piccirillo, M., Bonavita, S., Tedeschi, G. and Scarabino, T.: High-field proton MRS of human brain. Eur J Radiol 48 (2003) 146-53.

Dillon, W.P. and Nelson, S.: What is the role of MR spectroscopy in the evaluation and treatment of brain neoplasms? AJNR Am J Neuroradiol 20 (1999) 2-3.

Dowling, C., Bollen, A.W., Noworolski, S.M., McDermott, M.W., Barbaro, N.M., Day, M.R., Henry, R.G., Chang, S.M., Dillon, W.P., Nelson, S.J. and Vigneron, D.B.:

Preoperative proton MR spectroscopic imaging of brain tumors: correlation with histopathologic analysis of resection specimens. AJNR Am J Neuroradiol 22 (2001) 604-12.

Duyn, J.H., Gillen, J., Sobering, G., van Zijl, P.C. and Moonen, C.T.: Multisection proton MR spectroscopic imaging of the brain. Radiology 188 (1993) 277-82.

Freeman, S.M., Abboud, C.N., Whartenby, K.A., Packman, C.H., Koeplin, D.S., Moolten, F.L. and Abraham, G.N.: The "bystander effect": tumor regression when a fraction of the tumor mass is genetically modified. Cancer Research 53 (1993) 5274-83.

Galons, J.P., Job, C. and Gillies, R.J.: Increase of GPC levels in cultured mammalian cells during acidosis. A 31P MR spectroscopy study using a continuous bioreactor system. Magnetic Resonance in Medicine 33 (1995) 422-6.

Gillies, R.J., Barry, J.A. and Ross, B.D.: In vitro and in vivo 13C and 31P NMR analyses of phosphocholine metabolism in rat glioma cells. Magnetic Resonance in Medicine 32 (1994a) 310-8.

Gillies, R.J., Barry, J.A. and Ross, B.D.: In vitro and in vivo 13C and 31P NMR analyses of phosphocholine metabolism in rat glioma cells. Magn Reson Med 32 (1994b) 310-8.

Gonen, O., Wang, Z., Viswanathan, A., Molloy, P. and Zimmerman, R.: Three-dimensional multivoxel proton MR spectroscopy of the brain in children with neurofibromatosis type 1. AJNR 20 (1999) 1333-1341.

Graves, E.E., Nelson, S.J., Vigneron, D.B., Chin, C., Verhey, L., McDermott, M., Larson, D., Sneed, P.K., Chang, S., Prados, M.D., Lamborn, K. and Dillon, W.P.: A preliminary study of the prognostic value of proton magnetic resonance spectroscopic imaging in gamma knife radiosurgery of recurrent malignant gliomas. Neurosurgery 46 (2000) 319-26; discussion 326-8.

Graves, E.E., Nelson, S.J., Vigneron, D.B., Verhey, L., McDermott, M., Larson, D., Chang, S., Prados, M.D. and Dillon, W.P.: Serial proton MR spectroscopic imaging of recurrent malignant gliomas after gamma knife radiosurgery. AJNR Am J Neuroradiol 22 (2001a) 613-24.

Graves, E.E., Pirzkall, A., Nelson, S.J., Larson, D. and Verhey, L.: Registration of magnetic resonance spectroscopic imaging to computed tomography for radiotherapy treatment planning. Med Phys 28 (2001b) 2489-96.

Griffin, J.L., Mann, C.J., Scott, J., Shoulders, C.C. and Nicholson, J.K.: Choline containing metabolites during cell transfection: an insight into magnetic resonance spectroscopy detectable changes. FEBS Lett 509 (2001) 263-6.

Hakumaki, J.M., Poptani, H., Puumalainen, A.M., Loimas, S., Paljarvi, L.A., Yla-Herttuala, S. and Kauppinen, R.A.: Quantitative 1H nuclear magnetic resonance diffusion spectroscopy of BT4C rat glioma during thymidine kinase-mediated gene therapy in vivo: identification of apoptotic response. Cancer Research 58 (1998) 3791-9.

Hakumaki, J.M., Poptani, H., Sandmair, A.M., Yla-Herttuala, S. and Kauppinen, R.A.: 1H MRS detects polyunsaturated fatty acid accumulation during gene therapy of glioma: implications for the in vivo detection of apoptosis. Nature Medicine 5 (1999) 1323-7.

Holmgren, L., O'Reilly, M.S. and Folkman, J.: Dormancy of micrometastases: balanced proliferation and apoptosis in the presence of angiogenesis suppression [see comments]. Nature Medicine 1 (1995) 149-53.

Hore, P.: Data processing using the maximum entropy method. J Magn Reson 62 (1985) 561-567.

Kalapurakal, J.A. and Thomas, P.R.: Pediatric radiotherapy. An overview. Radiologic Clinics of North America 35 (1997) 1265-1280.

Kedar, A.: Chemotherapy for pediatric brain tumors. Semin Pediatr Neurol 4 (1997) 320-332.

Kolesnick, R.N. and Kronke, M.: Regulation of ceramide production and apoptosis. Annu Rev Physiol 60 (1998) 643-65.

Kurhanewicz, J., Vigneron, D.B., Hricak, H., Parivar, F., Nelson, S.J., Shinohara, K. and Carroll, P.R.: Prostate cancer: metabolic response to cryosurgery as detected with 3D H-1 MR spectroscopic imaging. Radiology 200 (1996) 489-96.

Kyriakis, J.M. and Avruch, J.: Protein kinase cascades activated by stress and inflammatory cytokines. Bioessays 18 (1996) 567-77.

Laue, E., Skilling, J., Staunton, J., Sibisi, S. and Bretereton, R.: Maximum entropy method in Nuclear Magnetic Resonance Spectroscopy. J Magn Reson 62 (1985) 437-452.

Lazareff, J.A., Bockhorst, K.H., Curran, J., Olmstead, C. and Alger, J.R.: Pediatric low-grade gliomas: prognosis with proton magnetic resonance spectroscopic imaging. Neurosurgery 43 (1998) 809-17; discussion 817-8.

Lazareff, J.A., Gupta, R.K. and Alger, J.: Variation of post-treatment H-MRSI choline intensity in pediatric gliomas. J Neurooncol 41 (1999) 291-8.

Lazareff, J.A., Olmstead, C., Bockhorst, K.H. and Alger, J.R.: Proton magnetic resonance spectroscopic imaging of pediatric low-grade astrocytomas. Childs Nerv Syst 12 (1996) 130-5.

Li, X., Lu, Y., Pirzkall, A., McKnight, T. and Nelson, S.J.: Analysis of the spatial characteristics of metabolic abnormalities in newly diagnosed glioma patients. J Magn Reson Imaging 16 (2002) 229-37.

Lombardi, V., Valko, L., Valko, M., Scozzafava, A., Morris, H., Melnik, M., Svitel, J., Budesinsky, M., Pelnar, J., Steno, J., Liptaj, T., Zalibera, L., Budinska, J., Zlatos, J., Giuliani, A., Mascolo, L., Leibfritz, D., Troncone, A., Marzullo, F., Mazur, M., Klener, J. and Zverina, E.: 1H NMR ganglioside ceramide resonance region on the differential diagnosis of low and high malignancy of brain gliomas. Cell Mol Neurobiol 17 (1997) 521-35.

Luyten, P., Marien, A. and den Hollander, J.: Acquisition and quantitation in proton spectroscopy. NMR in Biomed 4 (1991) 64-69.

Mahmood, U., Alfieri, A.A., Thaler, H., Cowburn, D. and Koutcher, J.A.: Radiation dose-dependent changes in tumor metabolism measured by 31P nuclear magnetic resonance spectroscopy. Cancer Res 54 (1994) 4885-91.

Mickle, J.P.: Neurosurgery for pediatric brain tumors. 4 (1997) 273-281.

Miller, B.L., Chang, L., Booth, R., Ernst, T., Cornford, M., Nikas, D., McBride, D. and Jenden, D.J.: In vivo 1H MRS choline: correlation with in vitro chemistry/histology. Life Sci 58 (1996a) 1929-35.

Miller, B.L., Chang, L., Booth, R., Ernst, T., Cornford, M., Nikes, D., McBride, D. and Jenden, D.: In vivo 1H MRS choline: correlation with in vitro chemistry/histology. Life Sci 58 (1996b) 1929-1935.

Naidich, T.: The American Society of Neuroragiology First Derek Harwood-Nash Award Winner: A. Aria Tzika. Int J Neuroradiology 1 (1995) 115-116.

Nelson, S. and Brown, T.: A study of the accuracy of quantification which can be obtained from 1-D NMR spectra using the PIQABLE algorithm. J Magn Reson 84 (1989) 95-109.

Nelson, S.J.: Analysis of volume MRI and MR spectroscopic imaging data for the evaluation of patients with brain tumors. Magn Reson Med 46 (2001) 228-39.

Nelson, S.J.: Multivoxel magnetic resonance spectroscopy of brain tumors. Mol Cancer Ther 2 (2003) 497-507.

Nelson, S.J. and Brown, T.R.: A new method for automatic quantification of 1-D spectra with low signal to noise ratio. J Magn Reson 75 (1987) 229-243.

Nelson, S.J., Huhn, S., Vigneron, D.B., Day, M.R., Wald, L.L., Prados, M., Chang, S., Gutin, P.H., Sneed, P.K., Verhey, L., Hawkins, R.A. and Dillon, W.P.: Volume MRI and MRSI techniques for the quantitation of treatment response in brain tumors: presentation of a detailed case study. Journal of Magnetic Resonance Imaging 7 (1997a) 1146-52.

Nelson, S.J., Vigneron, D.B. and Dillon, W.P.: Serial evaluation of patients with brain tumors using volume MRI and 3D 1H MRSI. NMR Biomed 12 (1999) 123-38.

Nelson, S.J., Vigneron, D.B., Star-Lack, J. and Kurhanewicz, J.: High spatial resolution and speed in MRSI. NMR in Biomedicine 10 (1997b) 411-22.

Nelson, S.J., Vigneron, D.B., Star-Lack, J. and Kurhanewicz, J.: High spatial resolution and speed in MRSI. NMR Biomed 10 (1997c) 411-22.

Ott, D., Hennig, J. and Ernst, T.: Human Brain Tumors: Assessment with in Vivo Proton MR Spectroscopy. Radiology 186 (1993) 745-752.

Podo, F.: Tumour phospholipid metabolism. NMR Biomed 12 (1999) 413-39.

Pollack, I.: Brain tumors in children. N Engl J Med 331 (1994) 1500-1507.

Poptani, H., Puumalainen, A.M., Grohn, O.H., Loimas, S., Kainulainen, R., Yla-Herttuala, S. and Kauppinen, R.A.: Monitoring thymidine kinase and ganciclovir-induced changes in rat malignant glioma in vivo by nuclear magnetic resonance imaging. Cancer Gene Therapy 5 (1998) 101-9.

Posse, S., DeCarli, C. and Le Bihan, D.: Three-dimensional echo-planar MR spectroscopic imaging at short echo times in the human brain. Radiology 192 (1994) 733-8.

Posse, S., Tedeschi, G., Risinger, R., Ogg, R. and Le Bihan, D.: High speed 1H spectroscopic imaging in human brain by echo planar spatial-spectral encoding. Magn Reson Med 33 (1995) 34-40.

Preul, M.C., Caramanos, Z., Collins, D.L., Villemure, J.G., Leblanc, R., Olivier, A., Pokrupa, R. and Arnold, D.L.: Accurate, noninvasive diagnosis of human brain tumors by using proton magnetic resonance spectroscopy. Nat Med 2 (1996) 323-325.

Provencher, S.W.: Estimation of metabolite concentrations from localized in vivo proton NMR spectra. Magn Reson Med 30 (1993) 672-9.

Ries, L., Hankey, B., Miller, B., Hartman, A. and Edwards, B.: Cancer statistics review 1973-88, NIH publication no. 91-2789, 1991.

Schwandner, R., Wiegmann, K., Bernardo, K., Kreder, D. and Kronke, M.: TNF receptor death domain-associated proteins TRADD and FADD signal activation of acid sphingomyelinase. J Biol Chem 273 (1998) 5916-22.

Segebarth, C., Baleriaux, D., Luyten, P. and den Hollander, J.: Detection of metabolic heterogeneity of human intracranial tumors in vivo by H-1 NMR spectroscopic imaging. Magn Reson Med 13 (1990) 62-76.

Shimizu, H., Kumabe, T., Shirane, R. and Yoshimoto, T.: Correlation between choline level measured by proton MR spectroscopy and Ki-67 labeling index in gliomas. AJNR Am J Neuroradiol 21 (2000) 659-65.

Smith, T.A., Eccles, S., Ormerod, M.G., Tombs, A.J., Titley, J.C. and Leach, M.O.: The phosphocholine and glycerophosphocholine content of an oestrogen-sensitive rat mammary tumour correlates strongly with growth rate. British Journal of Cancer 64 (1991) 821-6.

Spielman, D., Webb, P. and Macovski, A.: A statistical framework for in vivo spectroscopic imaging. J Magn Reson 79 (1988) 66-77.

Spielman, D.M., Pauly, J.M., Macovski, A., Glover, G.H. and Enzmann, D.R.: Lipid-suppressed single- and multisection proton spectroscopic imaging of the human brain. J Magn Reson Imaging 2 (1992) 253-62.

Star-Lack, J., Nelson, S.J., Kurhanewicz, J., Huang, L.R. and Vigneron, D.B.: Improved water and lipid suppression for 3D PRESS CSI using RF band selective inversion with gradient dephasing (BASING). Magnetic Resonance in Medicine 38 (1997a) 311-21.

Star-Lack, J., Spielman, D., Adalsteinsson, E., Kurhanewicz, J., Terris, D.J. and Vigneron, D.B.: In vivo lactate editing with simultaneous detection of choline, creatine, NAA, and lipid singlets at 1.5 T using PRESS excitation with applications to the study of brain and head and neck tumors. J Magn Reson 133 (1998) 243-54.

Star-Lack, J., Vigneron, D.B., Pauly, J., Kurhanewicz, J. and Nelson, S.J.: Improved solvent suppression and increased spatial excitation bandwidths for three-dimensional PRESS CSI using phase-compensating spectral/spatial spin-echo pulses. Journal of Magnetic Resonance Imaging 7 (1997b) 745-57.

Susin, S.A., Zamzami, N., Castedo, M., Daugas, E., Wang, H.G., Geley, S., Fassy, F., Reed, J.C. and Kroemer, G.: The central executioner of apoptosis: multiple connections between protease activation and mitochondria in Fas/APO-1/CD95- and ceramide-induced apoptosis. J Exp Med 186 (1997) 25-37.

Sutton, L., Wang, Z., Gusnard, D., Lange, B., Perilongo, G., Bogdan, A., Detre, J., Rorke, L. and Zimmerman, R.: Proton magnetic resonance spectroscopy of pediatric brain tumors. Neurosurgery 31 (1992) 195-202.

Tamiya, T., Kinoshita, K., Ono, Y., Matsumoto, K., Furuta, T. and Ohmoto, T.: Proton magnetic resonance spectroscopy reflects cellular proliferative activity in astrocytomas. Neuroradiology 42 (2000) 333-8.

Tarnawski, R., Sokol, M., Pieniazek, P., Maciejewski, B., Walecki, J., Miszczyk, L. and Krupska, T.: 1H-MRS in vivo predicts the early treatment outcome of postoperative radiotherapy for malignant gliomas. Int J Radiat Oncol Biol Phys 52 (2002) 1271-6.

Taylor, J.S., Ogg, R.J. and Langston, J.W.: Proton MR spectroscopy of pediatric brain tumors. Neuroimaging Clin N Am 8 (1998) 753-79.

Thompson, C.B.: Apoptosis in the pathogenesis and treatment of disease. Science 267 (1995) 1456-62.

Tkac, I., Andersen, P., Adriany, G., Merkle, H., Ugurbil, K. and Gruetter, R.: In vivo 1H NMR spectroscopy of the human brain at 7 T. Magn Reson Med 46 (2001) 451-6.

Tomita, T.: Neurosurgical perspectives in pediatric neurooncology. Childs Nervous System 14 (1998) 94-96.

Tournier, C., Hess, P., Yang, D.D., Xu, J., Turner, T.K., Nimnual, A., Bar-Sagi, D., Jones, S.N., Flavell, R.A. and Davis, R.J.: Requirement of JNK for stress-induced activation of the cytochrome c- mediated death pathway. Science 288 (2000) 870-4.

Tran, T.-K., Vigneron, D., Sailasuta, N., Tropp, J., Le Roux, P., Kurhanewicz, J., Nelson, S. and Hurd, R.: Very selective suppression pulses for clinical MRSI studies of brain and prostate cancer. Magn Reson Med 43 (2000) 22-33.

Tugnoli, V., Tosi, M.R., Tinti, A., Trinchero, A., Bottura, G. and Fini, G.: Characterization of lipids from human brain tissues by multinuclear magnetic resonance spectroscopy. Biopolymers 62 (2001) 297-306.

Tzika, A.: Localized MR spectroscopy of neurodegenerative disease and tumors. In: Faerber, E. (Ed.), MRI of the central nervous system in infants and children. Mac Keith Press, London, 1995, pp. 307-328.

Tzika, A., Vigneron, D., Dunn, R., Nelson, S. and Ball, W.: Intracranial tumors in children: small single-voxel proton MR spectroscopy using short and long-echo sequences. Neuroradiology 38 (1996a) 254-263.

Tzika, A., Zurakowski, D., Poussaint, T., Goumnerova, L., Astrakas, L., Barnes, P., Anthony, D., Billet, A., Tarbell, N., Scott, R. and Black, P.: Proton magnetic resonance spectroscopic imaging of the child's brain: the response of tumors to treatment. Neuroradiology 43 (2001) 169-177.

Tzika, A.A., Astrakas, L.G., Zarifi, M.K., Petridou, N., Young-Poussaint, T., Goumnerova, L., Zurakowski, D., Anthony, D.C. and Black, P.M.: Multiparametric MR assessment of pediatric brain tumors. Neuroradiology 45 (2003) 1-10.

Tzika, A.A., Astrakas, L.G., Zarifi, M.K., Zurakowski, D., Poussaint, T.Y., Goumnerova, L., Tarbell, N.J. and Black, P.M.: Spectroscopic and perfusion magnetic resonance imaging predictors of progression in pediatric brain tumors. Cancer 100 (2004) 1246-56.

Tzika, A.A., Vajapeyam, S. and Barnes, P.D.: Multivoxel proton MR spectroscopy and hemodynamic MR imaging of childhood brain tumors: preliminary observations. Ajnr: American Journal of Neuroradiology 18 (1997) 203-18.

Tzika, A.A., Vigneron, D.B., Ball, W.S., Jr., Dunn, R.S. and Kirks, D.R.: Localized proton MR spectroscopy of the brain in children. Journal of Magnetic Resonance Imaging 3 (1993a) 719-29.

Tzika, A.A., Vigneron, D.B., Ball, W.S., Jr., Dunn, R.S. and Kirks, D.R.: Localized proton MR spectroscopy of the brain in children. J Magn Reson Imaging 3 (1993b) 719-29.

Tzika, A.A., Vigneron, D.B., Dunn, R.S., Nelson, S.J. and Ball, W.S., Jr.: Intracranial tumors in children: small single-voxel proton MR spectroscopy using short- and long-echo sequences. Neuroradiology 38 (1996b) 254-63.

Tzika, A.A., Zarifi, M.K., Goumnerova, L., Astrakas, L.G., Zurakowski, D., Young-Poussaint, T., Anthony, D.C., Scott, R.M. and Black, P.M.: Neuroimaging in pediatric brain tumors: Gd-DTPA-enhanced, hemodynamic, and diffusion MR imaging compared with MR spectroscopic imaging. AJNR Am J Neuroradiol 23 (2002) 322-33.

Urenjak, J., Williams, S.R., Gadian, D.G. and Noble, M.: Specific expression of N-acetylaspartate in neurons, oligodendrocyte-type-2 astrocyte progenitors, and immature oligodendrocytes in vitro. J Neurochem 59 (1992) 55-61.

Van der Veen, J., de Beer, R., Luyten, P. and van Ormondt, D.: Accurate quantification of in vivo ^{31}P nmr signals using the variable projectio method and prior knowledge. Magn Reson Med 6 (1988) 92-98.

Veale, M.F., Roberts, N.J., King, G.F. and King, N.J.: The generation of 1H-NMR-detectable mobile lipid in stimulated lymphocytes: relationship to cellular activation, the cell cycle, and phosphatidylcholine-specific phospholipase C. Biochemical & Biophysical Research Communications 239 (1997) 868-74.

Vigneron, D., Bollen, A., McDermott, M., Wald, L., Day, M., Moyher-Noworolski, S., Henry, R., Chang, S., Berger, M., Dillon, W. and Nelson, S.: Three-dimensional magnetic resonance spectroscopic imaging of histologically confirmed brain tumors. Magn Reson Imaging 19 (2001a) 89-101.

Vigneron, D., Bollen, A., McDermott, M., Wald, L., Day, M., Moyher-Noworolski, S., Henry, R., Chang, S., Berger, M., Dillon, W. and Nelson, S.: Three-dimensional magnetic resonance spectroscopic imaging of histologically confirmed brain tumors. Magn Reson Imaging 19 (2001b) 89-101.

Wald, L.L., Moyher, S.E., Day, M.R., Nelson, S.J. and Vigneron, D.B.: Proton spectroscopic imaging of the human brain using phased array detectors. Magnetic Resonance in Medicine 34 (1995) 440-5.

Wald, L.L., Nelson, S.J., Day, M.R., Noworolski, S.E., Henry, R.G., Huhn, S.L., Chang, S., Prados, M.D., Sneed, P.K., Larson, D.A., Wara, W.M., McDermott, M., Dillon, W.P., Gutin, P.H. and Vigneron, D.B.: Serial proton magnetic resonance spectroscopy imaging of glioblastoma multiforme after brachytherapy. Journal of Neurosurgery 87 (1997) 525-34.

Warren, K.E.: NMR spectroscopy and pediatric brain tumors. Oncologist 9 (2004) 312-8.

Warren, K.E., Frank, J.A., Black, J.L., Hill, R.S., Duyn, J.H., Aikin, A.A., Lewis, B.K., Adamson, P.C. and Balis, F.M.: Proton magnetic resonance spectroscopic imaging in children with recurrent primary brain tumors. J Clin Oncol 18 (2000) 1020-6.

Wei, S.J., Chao, Y., Hung, Y.M., Lin, W.C., Yang, D.M., Shih, Y.L., Ch'ang, L.Y., Whang-Peng, J. and Yang, W.K.: S- and G2-phase cell cycle arrests and apoptosis induced by ganciclovir in murine melanoma cells transduced with herpes simplex virus thymidine kinase. Experimental Cell Research 241 (1998) 66-75.

Williams, S.N., Anthony, M.L. and Brindle, K.M.: Induction of apoptosis in two mammalian cell lines results in increased levels of fructose-1,6-bisphosphate and CDP-choline as determined by 31P MRS. Magnetic Resonance in Medicine 40 (1998) 411-20.

Yasuhara, S., Kanakubo, E., Perez, M.E., Kaneki, M., Fujita, T., Okamoto, T. and Martyn, J.A.: The 1999 Moyer award. Burn injury induces skeletal muscle apoptosis and the activation of caspase pathways in rats. J Burn Care Rehabil 20 (1999) 462-70.

12

Intraoperative Photodynamic Diagnosis of Brain Tumors Using 5-Aminolevulinic Acid

Satoshi Utsuki, Hidehiro Oka and Kiyotaka Fujii
Department of Neurosurgery, Kitasato University School of Medicine
Japan

1. Introduction

Glioma is a type of invasive brain tumor, and the properties of the center region of the tumor differ from those of normal brain tissue. Accordingly, the macroscopic differences from normal brain tissue or differences in terms of properties such as hardness allow one to recognize that the glioma is, in fact, tumor tissue. The difference from normal brain tissue in the periphery of the tumor, i.e., the tumor's region of infiltration, does not show glioma to be as evident, making it difficult to make any objective determination as to whether there is any tumor infiltration. The margin between the normal brain tissue and tumor tissue is not clearly discernible in the band of infiltration around the malignant brain tissue, often preventing the gross-total resection (GTR) of a malignant brain tumor. Researches have shown that GTR of a malignant brain tumor has a significant impact on patient survival (Filippini et al., 2006; Gorlia et al., 2006). Accordingly, any surgery on malignant glioma is performed for the purpose of GTR, and objectively determining the region of infiltration to perform GTR on malignant glioma is necessary to significantly affect patient survival. Photodynamic diagnosis (PDD) using 5-aminolevulinic acid (5-ALA) has enabled the objective assessment of tumor infiltration whenever surgery on glioma is to be performed (Stummer et al., 1998a, 1998b). When 5-ALA is administered, protoporphyrin IX (PpIX), which is a metabolite of 5-ALA, accumulates to a greater extent in the tumor cells than in normal brain cells. The PpIX used in the procedure reacts to light within the UV range, and emits a red fluorescent hue. Irradiation of tumor-infiltrated regions with UV-range light results in the regions appearing fluorescent red if tumor cells containing an accumulation of PpIX have infiltrated. This effectively allows for an objective assessment of tumor infiltration. Resection utilizing the fluorescence of the glioma after administration of 5-ALA has been shown to assist in the visualization of the tumor tissue during surgery. As a result, the use of 5-ALA is currently being praised as a new approach that allows for a significant increase in the potential to successfully perform GTR of malignant brain tumors (Stummer et al., 1998a, 1998b, 2006, 2011).

This chapter will cover the principles of PDD using 5-ALA and provide commentary on the usefulness of this procedure for brain tumors. This will be followed by further commentary on the potential for PDD in regard to brain tumors, and finally a synopsis on the current limitations of and perspectives on this promising technique.

2. 5-ALA metabolic pathway

2.1 5-ALA metabolism in normal cells

5-ALA is a substance that naturally exists in the body. In the first stage, 5-Ala is produced via the condensation of glycine and succinyl-CoA by ALA synthetase (ALAS) in the mitochondria. This process receives negative feedback from heme, which is the end-product. 5-ALA is actively transported via cytoplasm. In the next step, porphobilinogen (PBG) is created from ALA via ALA dehydratase. The actions of PBG deaminase (PBGD) and uroporphyrinogen III synthase compress 4 PBG molecules, effectively cyclizing a tetrapyrrole chain and producing uroporphyrinogen III. Uroporphyrinogen III is converted by uroporphyrinogen decarboxylase into coproporphyrinogen III, which is exposed to coproporphyrinogen oxidase in the mitochondrial intermembrane space. Decarboxylation and oxidation of the propionic side chains of the vinyl groups' rings A and B ultimately form protoporphyrinogen IX in the cell nucleus. PpIX is synthesized from protoporphyrinogen IX via protoporphyrinogen oxidase activity, and heme is synthesized via the uptake of iron into the tetrapyrrole structure by ferrochelatase in the mitochondrial membrane (Fig. 1). Regarding mitochondrial ferrochelatase, all of the enzymes in the heme pathway that are dependent on mitochondrial energy generation display irreversibleactions and are partially adjusted via ALAS feedback control (Rimington & Riley, 1993). ALAS has the next lowest level of activity after PBGD, as the other enzymes display much high degrees of activity. When administered, 5-ALA is incorporated into cells. PBGD

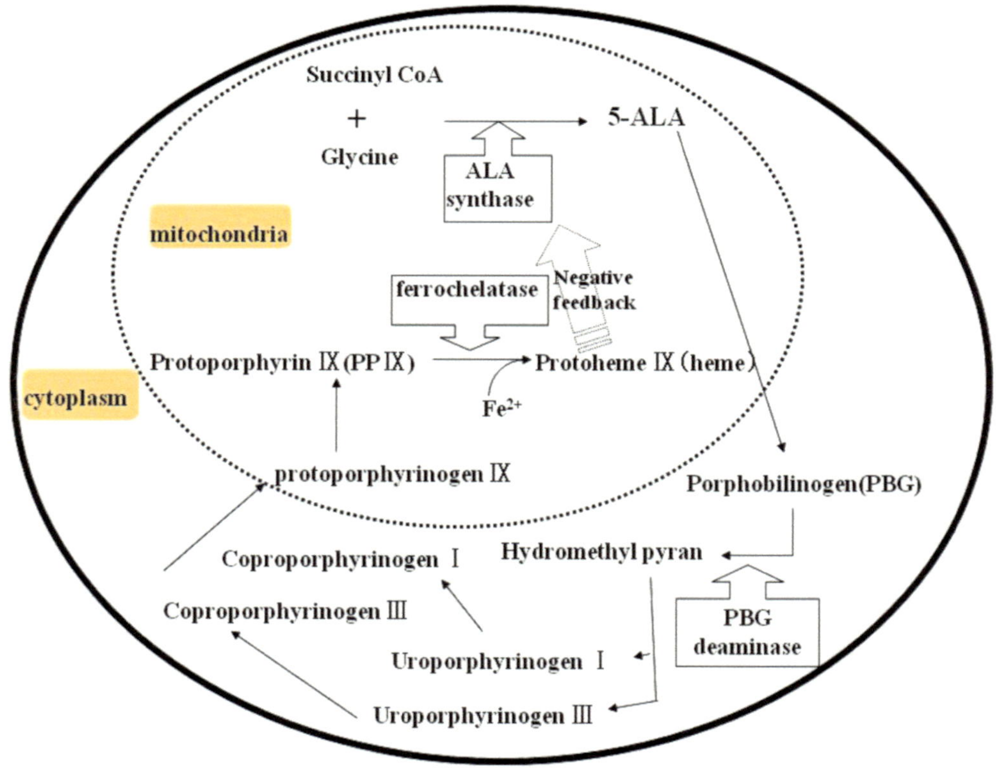

Fig. 1. Simplified metabolic pathway of 5-ALA-induced heme in cells

however, is rate-limiting, and the reactions do not proceed any further. Excessive 5-ALA is not metabolized and ALAS feedback control occurs, effectively controlling even the synthesis of 5-ALA in the cell. The resulting physiological state does not allow for synthesis of significant volumes of porphyrin or heme. External administration of a large volume of 5-ALA, however, prevents feedback control from having any additional effect and results in generation of more porphyrin than normal. The level of activity is lowest after that of PBGD, however, so extremely excessive generation of porphyrin does not occur (Mustajoki P et al., 1992).

2.2 5-ALA metabolism in tumor cells

5-ALA synthesis is the same in tumor cells as in normal cells, however, differences in enzyme activity, have been cited. In tumor cells, PBGD is not rate-controlling and metabolism is increased, so more heme is synthesized than in normal cells. Moreover, tumor cells show a relatively decreased level of ferrochelatase activity (Kaneko, 2008). Accordingly, administration of a large volume of extrinsic 5-ALA results in the 5-ALA being incorporated into tumor cells, progression of metabolism beyond PBG, and more porphyrin being produced than in normal cells (Utsuki et al., 2009).

It has been reported that in patients whose normal brain cells do not display PpIX fluorescence, glioblastoma tissue, which displays intense PpIX fluorescence, shows an increase in all porphyrins from 5-ALA to PpIX (Kaneko, 2008). However, ferrochelatase is rate-limiting, so the PpIX is not converted to heme and excessively accumulates in the tumor cells. Actually, the only enzyme activity from 5-ALA to PpIX that has a negative correlation with PpIX is the ferrochelatase activity (Kaneko, 2008). These processes show that abnormal growth of malignant glioma cells causes increased cellular uptake of 5-ALA, resulting in an increase in heme intermediate metabolites containing PpIX and a decrease in heme-synthesizing enzymes; particularly enzymes such as ferrochelatase. Accordingly, administration of 5-ALA results in increased concentration and accumulation of PpIX in tumor cells, making it an effective substance for photosensitivity (El-Sharabasy et al., 1992).

The details concerning why ferrochelatase activity is relatively low in tumor cells are unknown. Downregulation of ferrochelatase mRNA expression has been identified in tumor tissue (Teng et al., 2011). Moreover, it is also known that generation of nitric oxide in tumor cells reduces ferrochelatase in the mitochondria and increases PpIX accumulation (Yamamoto et al., 2007). These processes likely represent the cause for the relatively low ferrochelatase activity in tumor cells.

3. PDD using 5-ALA

PDD using 5-ALA was used by the authors at Kitasato University Hospital on 204 patients with brain tumor or suspected of brain tumor. 5-ALA was administered after approval by the IRB. Approval was obtained to administer 5-ALA to all patients prior to surgery. It was administered in 78 cases with glioblastoma (including 22 relapse cases), 25 cases with glioma grade III (including 6 relapse cases), 18 cases with glioma grade II (10 astrocytomas, 8 oligodendrogliomas), 2 cases with pilocytic astrocytoma, 2 cases with ependymoma, 2 cases with subependymal giant cell astrocytoma (SEGA), 1 case with choroid plexus papilloma, 1 case with atypical teratoid/rhabdoid tumor (AT/RT), 1 case with central neurocytoma, 9 cases with hemangioblastoma, 6 cases with germinoma, 20 cases with malignant lymphoma, 6 cases with pituitary adenoma, 10 cases with meningioma, 4 cases with neurilemmoma, 15 cases with metastatic brain tumor, and 4 cases with pseudotumor.

3.1 Administration of the 5-ALA

When 5-ALA is orally administered, PpIX begins to accumulate at the lesion 1 hour later. The accumulation peaks 4 to 6 hours after administration, declining afterwards. To enable accumulation of PpIX within the tumor to a peak level 1 hour after anesthesia and coincide with initiation of tumor excision, each patient was orally administered 1 g of 5-ALA (5-ALA hydrochloride, Cosmo Bio Co., Let., Tokyo, Japan) that was dissolved in 20 ml of 5% glucose solution 2 hours prior to initiation of the anesthesia. Regarding steroid administration, betamethasone (8-16 mg) was administered 1 hour prior to initiation of the anesthesia only in cases of severe cerebral edema.

3.2 Excitation light and fluorescent observation

PpIX reacts to UV light by displaying a red fluorescent hue. To explain, irradiation of the PpIX with excitation light results in absorption of light energy and a change from a ground state to a singlet excited state. Then, fluorescence is emitted when there is the shift from the singlet excited state to the ground state. The more PpIX in a tissue and the more intense the excitation light, the stronger the display of fluorescence by PpIX. Among the wavelengths that excite PpIX are 410 nm, 510 nm, 545 nm, 580 nm, and 630 nm. PpIX is most intensely excited by light around of ~405 nm. We used a semiconductor laser device (VLD-V1 version 2 M & M Co., Ltd., Tokyo, Japan) to provide the excitation light. This device was used to irradiate the tumor tissue via optical fiber as close to the tumor as possible with excitation light at a wavelength of 405 nm and an output of 120 mW (Fig. 2). This was observed using a cut-off filter that blocks the transmission of light at a wavelength < 430 nm and is attached to a microscope. The wavelengths included in the microscope's irradiation light near 400 nm are blocked, which lowers the PpIX photobleaching effect of the irradiation light. It blocks the excitation light, allowing for easier observation of PpIX fluorescence.

A neurosurgical microscope for fluorescence incorporated into a microscope system was developed to irradiate with excitation light, and was the principal instrument used. The device could switch from conventional white light to violet-blue excitation light and was very convenient to use (Stummer et al., 1998a). This system also provided a favorable contrast because, after image processing, it displayed fluorescence which was detected via a CCD camera.

One advantage of these methods compared to the laser method is that they allow for detection of fluorescence over the entire area observed by the microscope. When irradiating excitation light with a laser, the scope of irradiation is narrow and allows for detection of fluorescence only within the narrow area observed by the microscope (Haj-Hosseini et al., 2010; Utsuki et al, 2006). Laser methods, however, do have benefits over systems incorporated into microscopes. The biggest advantage is that use of this technology allowsfor excitation of fluorescence even with a low PpIX level. When excitation light is irradiated from a microscope, the distance to the target tumor tissue increases, effectively weakening the power of the excitation light that reaches the tumor tissue and resulting in weaker fluorescence. When optical fibers are used to irradiate with laser, the optical fiber is brought to a spot very near the tumor tissue, and this allows for irradiation of excitation light on the target tissue with a strong output. Also, even if this results in a low level of PpIX accumulation, the irradiation by strong excitation light allows for detection of fluorescence with a low level of PpIX.

3.3 Fluorescent analysis

PpIX reacts to light in the UV field, emitting fluorescence at two bimodal peaks, i.e., 636 nm and 704 nm. We perceive blood to be red, and may not be able to differentiate blood from the red coloring of PpIX. We usually perceive wavelengths between 610 and 750 nm to be red. Oxyhemoglobin has an absorption spectum of 400 - 630 nm. This differs from that of PpIX, so they can be differentiated via wavelength analysis. Moreover, if the PpIX level is low, the fluorescence can be confirmed macroscopically. Also, wavelength analysis allows for detection of minute levels of PpIX fluorescence that cannot be observed macroscopically. We used a spectrometer and accessory software (BW-Spec V3.09; B & W TEK, Inc., Newark, Del., U.S.A.) to analyze the spectrum waveform via PC (Fig. 2). Wavelength analysis when performing PDD is necessary to make objective determinations regarding PpIX fluorescence and to detect minute levels of PpIX fluorescence (Utsuki et al, 2006).

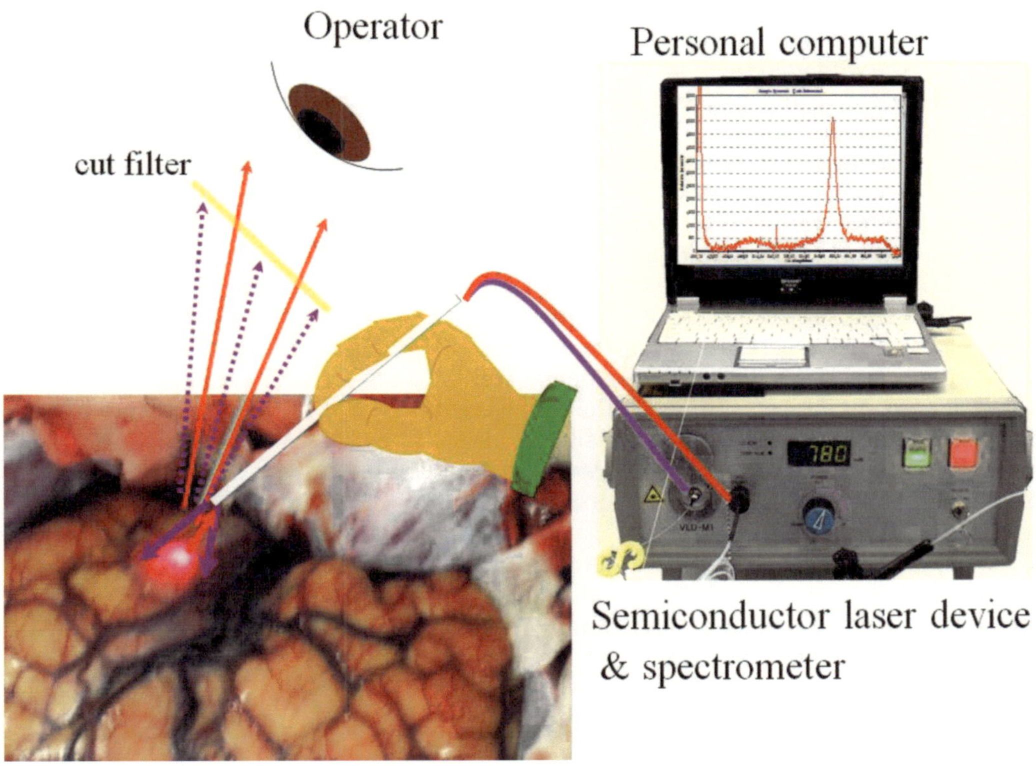

Fig. 2. Photo of intraoperative brain tumor fluorescence using a semiconductor laser device. The tumor emits red fluorescence upon exposure to a laser light with peak wavelength of 405 nm and a light output of 120 mW through optical fiber. Tumor emissions were analyzed by personal computer via spectrometer through a second optical fiber in parallel. PpIX-specific fluorescence and relative intensity were measured. The surgeons made observations via cut-off filter, so were unable to see the irradiated 405 nm blue light (blue arrows), yet the red hue of the PpIX was enhanced (red arrows).

3.4 Results of PDD for brain tumors

The strength of the perceived PpIX fluorescence is correlated with the relative strength measured with a spectrometer. When strong PpIX fluorescence is perceived, a bimodal spectrum for PpIX can be observed and the height of the 636 nm peak is at least 3,000. Weak PpIX fluorescence was observed at a height of 636 nm (the peak) between strengths of 3,000 and 1,000. Strong PpIX fluorescence was observed in 76 cases with glioblastoma (including all recurrent cases), 15 cases with glioma grade III (including all recurrent cases), 5 cases with glioma grade II (1 astrocytoma, 4 oligodendrogliomas), 2 cases with pilocytic astrocytoma, 2 cases with ependymoma, 1 case with SEGA, 1 case with choroid plexus papilloma, 1 case with AT/RT, 1 case with central neurocytoma, 9 cases with hemangioblastoma, 5 cases with germinoma, 12 cases with malignant lymphoma, 8 cases with meningioma, and 1 case with pseudotumor. Moreover, weak PpIX fluorescence was observed in 4 cases with glioma grade III, 6 cases with glioma grade II (3 astrocytomas, 3 oligodendrogliomas), 1 case with SEGA, 1 case with germinoma, 4 cases with malignant lymphoma, 1 case with meningioma, 11 cases with metastatic brain tumor, and 3 cases with pseudotumor. A clear enhancing effect of the entire/part of the tumor was observed in the magnetic resonance images (MRIs) in all of these cases except 4 cases with glioma grade II (3 astrocytomas, 1 oligodendroglioma).

PpIX fluorescence could not be macroscopically observed in 2 cases with glioblastoma, 6 cases with glioma grade III, 7 cases with glioma grade II (6 astrocytomas, 1 oligodendroglioma), 4 cases with malignant lymphoma, 6 cases with pituitary adenoma, 1 case with meningioma, 4 cases with neurilemmoma, or 4 cases with metastatic brain tumor. PpIX fluorescence was not observed even if there was a clear enhancing effect on the MRI in 2/74 cases with glioblastoma (not including 2 cases in which there was not an enhancing effect), 3/22 cases with glioma grade III (not including 3 cases in which there was not an enhancing effect), 4/18 cases with malignant lymphoma (not including 2 cases in which there was not an enhancing effect), 6/6 cases with pituitary adenoma, 1/6 cases with meningioma, 4/4 cases with neurilemmoma, and 4/15 cases with metastatic brain tumor. This said, among the cases in which the above mentioned PpIX fluorescence could not be macroscopically confirmed, it was possible to detect fluorescence of PpIX with a 636 nm peak using a spectrometer in 4 cases with glioma grade II (3 astrocytomas, 1 oligodendroglioma), 3 cases with malignant lymphoma, 1 case with meningioma, and 1 case with metastatic brain tumor.

These findings show that there may be some tumors (even benign tumors) that allow for PPD using 5-ALA in cases in which there is an enhancing effect on the MRI, but it may be difficult to use PDD with 5-ALA for pituitary adenoma or neurilemmoma, even if the MRI shows an enhancing effect.

4. The role of PDD in brain tumors

4.1 Tumor confirmation: Assisting tumor resection of invasive tumors

Glioma surgery probably receives the most benefits from PDD using 5-ALA. Even if the central region of a tumor in a malignant glioma case clearly displays different properties from normal brain cells, the peripheral region cannot be differentiated (normal brain from tumor). Also, even if there is an enhancing effect on MRI in that region, it can be difficult to determine whether there is tumor infiltration during surgery. A randomized controlled multicenter phase III trial on malignant gliomas showed a significantly higher percentage of GTR (gross-total resection) of the regions for which there was an enhancing effect on MRI among those who underwent surgery after PDD using 5-ALA, vs. those for whom 5-ALA was not used (Stummer et al., 2006). Accordingly, the 6-month progression-free survival (PFS) in the group in which 5-ALA was used was 46% as opposed to 28% in the control group, i.e., PFS in the group in which 5-ALA was used was significantly longer (Stummer et al., 2011). Moreover, the group in which 5-ALA was used showed lower cumulative reoperation rates. PDD using 5-ALA is very helpful in glioma surgery in order to determine tumor infiltration and for an objective determination on where (what region) to resect.

In the same patients, PpIX fluorescence and tumor cell density are roughly proportionate to each other. We will show you one example of our experience. In a case of anaplastic oligodendroglioma, tumor cells with heteromorphic nuclei proliferated in a sheet-like manner in the tumor's central region (Fig. 3 B). The distinct red fluorescence of PpIX was observed in this region (Fig. 3 A,in circle) and a PpIX spectrum with a relatively high peak of 636 nm was displayed (Fig. 3 A). The Ki-67 staining index (SI) for this region was 14% (Fig. 3 C). In the tumor's region of infiltration (Fig. 4 B), weak red fluorescence of the PpIX (Fig. 4 A, in circle) and a PpIX spectrum with a low peak at 636 nm were observed (Fig. 4 A). The Ki-67 SI of this region was 3% (Fig. 4 C). Moreover, in the peripheral region, infiltration of a very small number of tumor cells with heteromorphic nuclei on an edema-like background was observed (Figure 5 C) yet PpIX red fluorescence was not observed (Figure 5 B). However, a PpIX spectrum with a very low peak was observed at 636 nm (Figure 5 A). In this region, the PpIX fluorescence could not be confirmed macroscopically, but it was a region in which PpIX could be confirmed in the spectrum only.

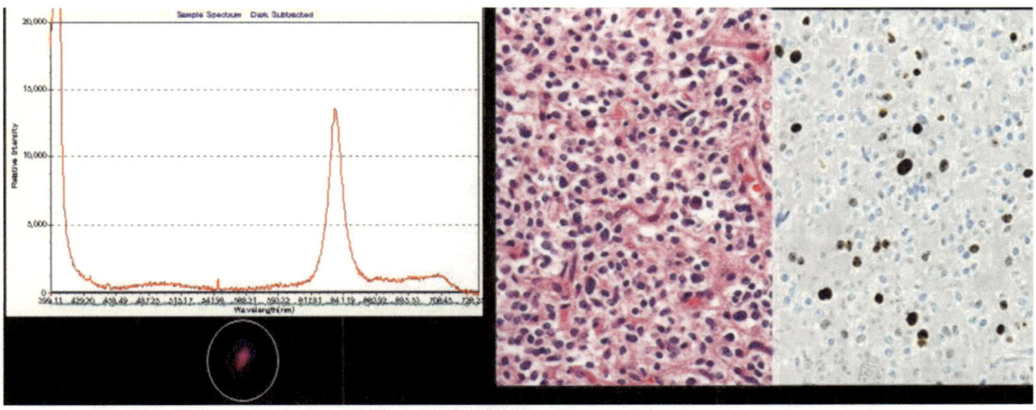

A B C

Fig. 3. Image of tissue from the central region of a tumor, the PpIX fluorescence for the region, and the fluorescence analysis results via spectrometer. It shows a proliferation of heteromorphic tumor cells with a halo around the nucleus (B, HE staining, original magnification X200). Irradiation of this region with laser showed a strong PpIX fluorescence (A, in circle). This spectrum of fluorescence featured a peak at 636 nm, indicating PpIX fluorescence (A). The relative intensity of this peak was 14000. At 14%, the Ki-67 staining index (SI) of this region was relatively high (C, Ki-67 staining, original magnification X200).

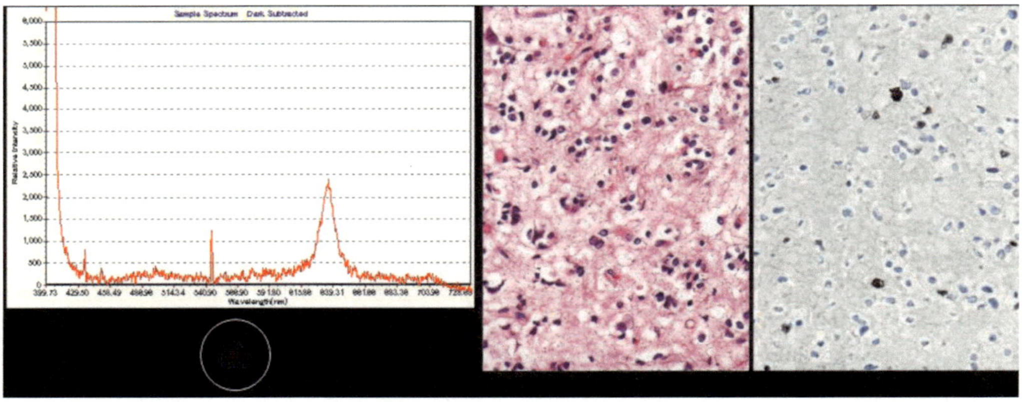

A B C

Fig. 4. Image of tissue from the region of infiltration into the brain around the tumor, the PpIX fluorescence for the region, and the fluorescence analysis results via spectrometer. Normal brain cells can be seen between the infiltrating tumor cells, so the tumor density is lower than in Fig. 3 (B, HE staining, original magnification X200). Weak PpIX fluorescence was observed (A, in circle) after irradiation of the region with a laser. The fluorescence spectrum peaks at 636 nm, with the relative intensity of the peak at 2500 (A). The Ki-67 staining index (SI) of this region was 3% (C, Ki-67 staining, original magnification X200).

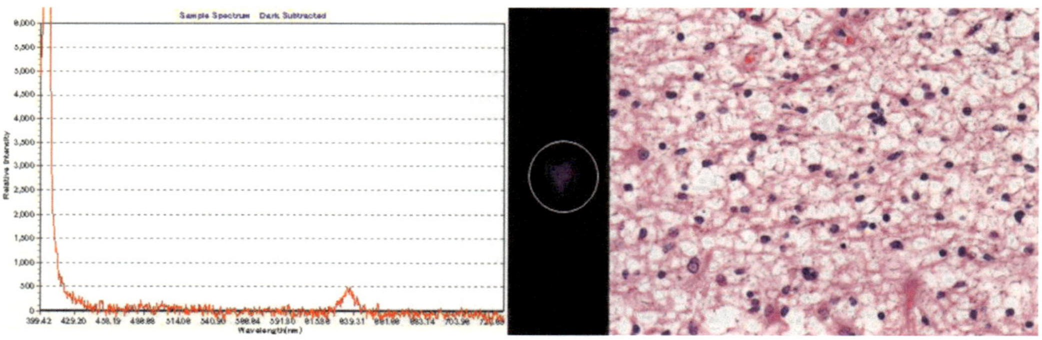

A B C

Fig. 5. Image of tissue featuring more of the peripheral region than in Fig. 3, the PpIX fluorescence for the region, and the fluorescence analysis results via spectrometer. A small number of tumor cells with heteromorphic nuclei have infiltrated edema-like brain cells, and disperse reactive astrocyte can also be seen (C, HE staining, original magnification X200). Irradiation of this region with laser did not allow for observation of the red fluorescence of PpIX (B). This fluorescence spectrum peaks at 636 nm, with fluorescence of a slight level of PpIX likely detected. The relative intensity of the peak was 500 (A).

Glioma surgery in eloquent areas is conducted using sensory-evoked potential (SEP), motor-evoked potential (MEP), awake surgery, and other methods. Cortical and subcortical stimulation must be conducted to identify the cortical pathway of the functional field/lesion periphery and determine the scope of resection. For example, if the permanent decrease in MEP amplitude obtained via transcranial electronic stimulation is at least 50% compared to baseline, tumor resection should be removed as an optio. (Feigl et al., 2010). This is because once this occurs; continuing with excision of the tumor significantly increases the percentage of post-surgical neuropathy and lowers patients' quality of life (QOL). However, there are limitations to the scope of identification for these monitoring. In particular, if tumor resection is the primary measure in a case where the eloquent areas and tumor body are proximal, it facilitates worsening of patient QOL, and excessive concern about post-surgical dysfunction can result in much of the tumor remaining after surgery. In such a case, if the strength of the PpIX fluorescence, even in the regions considered to have function differs, more detailed examination of the scope of the function of the region can enable additional resection of the region(s) with strong PpIX fluorescence (region with significant tumor infiltration) and increase the glioma excision rate.

4.2 Identification of tumor's malignant regions: Determination of glioma grading

Tissue heterogeneity is normal in diffuse infiltrating glioma (Coons et al., 1993; Paulus & Peiffer, 1989). One of the reasons is that genetic mutation occurs in a portion of the tumor, and this is also one reason for it becoming malignant. To accurately ascertain how malignant a tumor is, the region that has become malignant must be left as a specimen. Moreover, whether a tumor has become malignant in that region or not has an impact on the decision regarding the scope of surgical excision if the tumor is in the vicinity of eloquent areas. Contrast-enhanced MRI and image diagnostics such as positron emission tomography (PET) using an amino acid (e.g., methionine or 18F-F-fluoroethyl-L: -tyrosine) tracer represent examples of pre-surgical image diagnostics that can be used to determine the malignant regions of the tumor. Contrast-enhanced MRI often does not show an image of WHO grade II glioma, but it does display a "patchy and faint" enhancing effect and the tumor's most active cells may exist in this region (Pallud et al, 2009). In PET diagnosis, the region with the highest accumulation of tracer represents the region in which the tumor cell metabolism activity is highest (Goldman et al., 1997; Sadeghi et al., 2007). It is difficult to identify these regions during surgery. This is because even if a navigation system is used, craniotomy, brain shift due to CSF loss/gravity, as well as cerebral edema can result in targeted deviation. PDD using 5-ALA is useful for determining this factor (Widhalm et al., 2010). Fluorescence is observed in WHO grade III glioma regions with high cell mitotic activity, but less so in regions tantamount to WHO grade II glioma with low cell mitotic activity (Ishihara et al, 2007). It has been reported that the higher the grade of glioma, the higher the PpIX concentration tends to be in tissue (Kaneko , 2008; Johansson et al., 2010). The post-surgical treatment regimen changes according to whether or not the WHO grade III glioma region remains as a specimen. Those patients are initiated on radiation therapy and chemotherapy immediately after surgery if diagnosed with WHO grade III glioma. However, if those patients are diagnosed with WHO grade II glioma, watchful waiting without any treatment may be a temporary option (Mittal et al., 2008; van den Bent et al., 2005). This is because even if irradiation is used immediately after surgery, it has been shown that there is no significant difference in total survival if it is used when the patient's post-surgical status has worsened (van den Bent et al., 2005). Considering that use of irradiation immediately after surgery results in a significantly longer PFS, , when a cell group with high mitotic activity in a very small portion of the tumor is likely turning malignant, it is possible that worsening of progressive neurological deficit may immediately be observed. Accordingly, such a case legitimizes use of irradiation immediately after surgery. In this way, PDD using 5-ALA is useful for determining detailed treatment regimens for WHO grade II to III glioma.

4.3 Confirmation of tumor resection region: Confirmation of validity of biopsy region

If the targeted lesion is small when conducting a biopsy, a minute error can prevent accurate diagnosis. This makes it necessary to confirm whether the target region is being excised. CT or MRI during or after surgery can be used to confirm whether the targeted region has been removed, but this requires time and effort. In such a case, PDD with 5-ALA can be used on a real-time basis to confirm whether the targeted region has been excised. If PpIX fluorescence can be detected from the excised tissue sample, it allows for confirmation that the targeted lesion area has been excised.

Here, we will present an actual example of this. We used the Leksell Stereotactic System (Elekta, Stockholm, Sweden) under MRI-guidance to conduct biopsy, and used a side cut biopsy needle kit (Elekta, Stockholm, Sweden) as biopsy forceps. This forceps can excise specimens up to 1.4 mm in diameter and 10 mm of length. Prior to surgery, this was a suspected case of malignant lymphoma. We planned to obtain a biopsy of a 7mm lesion in the right-frontal lobe (Fig. 6 A). Irradiation of the tissue excised with forceps using a 405 nm laser allowed for observation of the red PpIX fluorescence in a portion of the tissue (Fig. 6 B). Tumor cell infiltration can be seen in the region of the tissue sample in which PpIX fluorescence was observed (Fig. 6 C). Moreover, the regions in which no PpIX fluorescence was observed did not show any tumor cell infiltration. Naturally, not all lesions allow for observation of PpIX fluorescence, so this method is not effective in lesions in which there is no PpIX accumulation. In such a case, image diagnostics after biopsy becomes necessary.

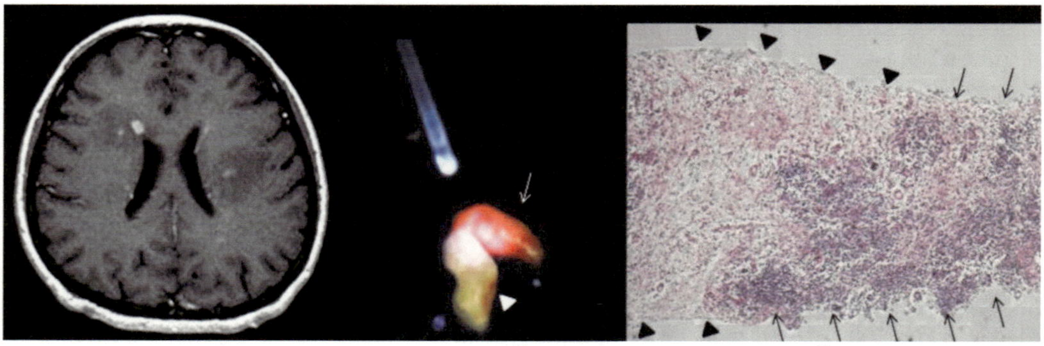

Fig. 6. Image shows a gadolinium-enhanced axial MRI image (A). A 7 mm lesion with a uniform enhancing effect can be seen proximal to the anterior horn of the lateral ventricle in the right frontal lobe. Irradiation with a 405 nm laser on the excised tissue showed the red fluorescence of PpIX over half of the tissue (arrow), but no fluorescence on the remaining of half (arrowhead) (B). The tissue image shows a clear distinction between the region infiltrated with tumor cells (arrow) and those not infiltrated (arrowhead) (C, HE staining, original magnification X40). In these regions, the portion showing PpIX fluorescence and that showing the tumor's region of infiltration concurred.

4.4 Significance of PDD using 5-ALA for benign tumor: Confirmation of remaining tumor

Recurrence is possible in benign brain tumors whereby the boundary with the periphery brain tissue is clear-cut. As is the case of meningioma, there are times in which GTR cannot be conducted in order to maintain the blood vessels/nerves in the region and within the tumor. However, there are cases of recurrence even after a surgeon has conducted GTR. The biggest reason for recurrence/relapse in such tumors is tumor remaining after excision. PDD using 5-ALA can be utilized to check for any remaining tumor after GTR procedures (Shimizu et al., 2006; Utsuki et al., 2008). PDD using 5-ALA can be used in most cases of meningioma, hemangioblastoma, and pilocytic astrocytoma, etc., because it serves as a useful detection method in such types of tumors (Coluccia et al., 2010).

Tumors in meningioma cases are mostly benign with a clear-cut boundary between the tumor and the brain, but there can be subpial infiltration even if WHO grade I, and this is quite common in recurrent cases. There are also some cases in which these tumors infiltrate bone and dura mater, creating difficulties in the resected region. if tumor infiltration into the skull base is detected, there are times in which the tumor will be left, because it cannot be adequately detached. In such cases, PDD using 5-ALA can be useful in meningioma in order to diagnose the tumor infiltration region (Kajimoto et al., 2007). In meningioma cases, dural tail sign can be observed in regions in which tumor is attached. These regions can show tumor infiltration, but also dilated blood vessels and inflammation (Rokni-Yazdi et al., 2009). Here, we have used PDD with 5-ALA to determine whether the meningioma has infiltrated the dura mater. If it has, PpIX fluorescence can be observed (Fig. 7 A). Tumor infiltration into this region can also be confirmed histologically (Fig. 7 B).

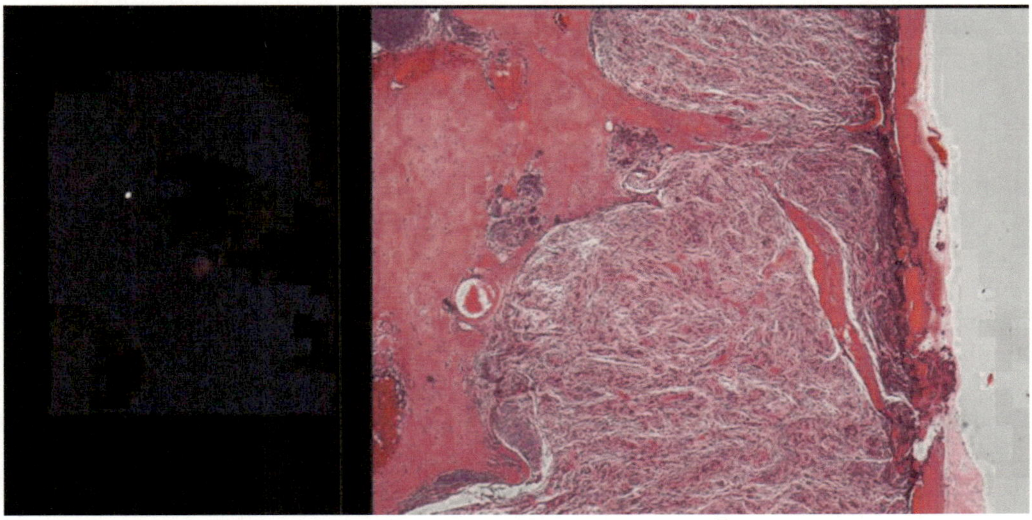

A B

Fig. 7. Image shows PDD during surgery on region of infiltration in a dura mater in a case of meningioma. In the tumor's region of infiltration into the dura mater, the PpIX in the tumor reacted to the laser, allowing for observation of fluorescence (A). The tissue sample from this region shows a tumor mass inside a thin layer of dura mater, indicating that the tumor has infiltrated the dura mater (B, HE staining, original magnification X40).

Hemangioblastoma is a type of cancer featuring benign tumors with frequent recurrence even after GTR. A part of recurrent hemangioblastoma cases include to occur by a genetic problem. Some recurrent cases in regard to the tumor can be due to the inability to resect tumor cells that have infiltrated brain parenchyma or a cyst wall accompanying the tumor (Bishop et al., 2008). Also, PDD using 5-ALA can be useful in diagnosing residual tumor, even when it is difficult to ascertain (Utsuki et al., 2010).

5. Precautions in regard to PDD using 5-ALA

5.1 Photobleaching effect

There is great variance in tumor excision rates among surgeons even when using PDD with 5-ALA, the same device, or the same reagents. This is largely because this technique depends on the skill level of the surgeon. While tumors can be visualized on an objective basis, there likely are many aspects that depend on a surgeon's knowledge and experience when it comes to the detailed regions. Also, one factor involves the characteristics of the device being used. Another is the PpIX photobleaching effect due to the relative light exposure (Stummer et al., 1998b). Light-sensitive substances such as PpIX absorb light energy when exposed to light for a certain period of time, causing a change from a ground state to a singlet excited state. PDD has been used so that light-sensitive substances in a singlet excited state emit a fluorescent hue and shift to a ground state. This process does not always occur however, e.g., a substance in a singlet excited state can be transformed into a triplet excited state, generating free radicals, radical ions, and singlet oxygen, and effectively damaging the periphery cells. Photodynamic therapy (PDT) has used this. In this situation, PpIX (the light-sensitive substance) is not visible. The lower the level of PpIX, the earlier photobleaching occurs, although, this tends not to occur very often in the central region of the tumor where the PpIX level is high. In a tumor's region of infiltration, the fluorescence of the PpIX fades before anybody notices due to the low PpIX level (Utsuki et al., 2007a). Light in the UV field does not reach deep areas, so there may be PpIX remaining in the tissue directly below the region in which photobleaching has occurred. To avoid overlooking fluorescence because of photobleaching, and particularly in the region of infiltration of an invasive tumor, when checking for residual tumor, it is necessary to remove a small amount of surface tissue to check for any PpIX fluorescence in the newly appearing tissue.

5.2 Pseudonegative fluorescence

Stummer et al have reported some cases of malignant glioma not showing PpIX fluorescence even after showing a gadolinium-enhancing effect in an MRI (Stummer et al., 1998b). The blood brain barrier (BBB) is one of the problems. Deterioration of the BBB is an important factor required to allow 5-ALA to reach tumor cells. If there is a tumor around which the BBB has not deteriorated, 5-ALA tends not to reach the tumor cells, preventing successful use of PDD (Miyatake et al., 2007). Moreover, steroids are often used on edema accompanying brain tumor. A tightening effect caused by the steroids makes it difficult for 5-ALA to leak from deteriorated BBB around the tumor, possibly resulting in a lower supply of 5-ALA to the tumor cells (Grabb & Gilbert , 1995). The extent of steroid use that impacts the BBB permeability to 5-ALA has yet to be identified. Dexamethasone (12 mg /daily) does not appear to impact 5-ALA permeability (Stummer et al., 2006). This said, there are some cases in which the tumor does not show PpIX fluorescence after 5-ALA, even in non-brain tumors (Hoda & Popken, 2009). This indicates that the BBB is not the only reason for failure of PDD using 5-ALA. Another cause may be in the tumor, but it must be noted that there are some cases in which PpIX fluorescence is not observed in tumors that normally should allow for PDD.

Moreover, the excitation light used when conducting PDD is light in the UV field, so PDD can usually only be used for the surface tissue. If necrotic tissue is on the surface, or a tumor is in a brain ventricle covered by brain ventricle ependyma, etc., there are cases in which tumor PpIX cannot be detected. If so, this tissue should be removed to conduct PPD.

5.3 Psudopositive fluorescence

PpIX fluorescence is observed in some cases even if a brain tumor is not present. Based on our experience, PpIX fluorescence is observed even when there are no tumor cells, for example, in cases with brain abscess, multiple sclerosis, or remarkable infiltration of reactive astrocytes and macrophages in relapsed tumors (Miyatake et al., 2007; Utsuki et al., 2007b). PpIX fluorescence is observed even in cases of radiation necrosis without tumor recurrence (Miyatake et al., 2007) or a metastatic brain tumor's edema field (Utsuki et al., 2007a). For whatever reason, PpIX fluorescence is observed even outside the brain in cases of strong inflammatory cell infiltration (Filbeck et al.; 1999). A gadolinium-enhancing effect on MRI often occurs in regions of inflammatory cell infiltration. There are also positive findings in regards to PET using L-[methyl-11C] methionine, which tends not accumulate in non-neoplastic brain lesions or be impacted by local inflammatory reaction, and the metabolism increases due to the inflammatory cells (Kawai et al., 2010). In such regions, heme synthesis is very common, as is the production of PpIX, which likely results in fluorescence being observed with PDD. Moreover, the PpIX produced by the tumor leaks to the periphery, resulting in PpIX being observed in the tumor's peripheral region, even if there is not tumor infiltration (Utsuki et al., 2007a). When employing PDD using 5-ALA, it is necessary to conduct surgery with the knowledge that tumor cells may not be present even if PpIX fluorescence is observed.

5.4 Toxicity and side effects of 5-ALA

5-ALA is an endogenous substance synthesized in the body, and is very safe. The only type of patients absolutely contraindicated for 5-ALA is porphyria patients. The most common side effect of oral administration of 5-ALA is temporary hepatic dysfunction (25%), with the incidence of nausea/vomiting being slightly lower. It causes virtually no other side effects, and there are no serious side effects as long as the oral dose of 5-ALA does not exceed 60 mg/kg and IV dose, 30 mg/kg (Mustajoki et al., 1992; Webber et al., 1997a). Erythema, edema, hyperpigmentation, etc occur in rare occasions, and require respective attention (Steinbauer et al., 2009). Excessively administered 5-ALA is completely excreted from the kidneys in 24 hours, but slower if the patient suffers from renal dysfunction (Webber et al., 1997b). Some 5-ALA is metabolized in the liver. If a patient suffers from renal dysfunction or hepatic dysfunction, the potential for phototoxocity may rise unless the dose of 5-ALA is either reduced or administration is discontinued.

Past research has shown that administration of ALA once or several times results in a high concentration of serum porphyrin among cancer patients or healthy volunteers, but no symptoms of porphyria (Mustajoki et al., 1992; Utsuki et al., 2009). Moreover, the porphyrin level was observed to be higher than the level that causes attacks among porphyria patients. Accordingly, even if administration of 5-ALA causes a high concentration of porphyrin, it will not result in symptoms often observed in cases of porphyria.

6. Conclusions and future directions

Utilization of PDD with 5-ALA in cases of invasive brain tumor increases the rate of GTR and promises improved prognosis. It allows for confirmation of residual tumor even in cases with a benign tumor, so PDD may be helpful in the reduction of recurrence. The extent of fluorescence in PDD differs according to the level of PpIX and the strength of excitation light. Moreover, measurement of the spectrum of fluorescence allows for detection of PpIX fluorescence that cannot be observed macroscopically. When performing PDD using 5-ALA, the surgeon must know to perform surgery, about the possibility of the photobleaching effect, pseudopositive, and pseudonegative, etc.

Further studies should focus on identifying tumors in which PpIX does not accumulate and the mechanism as well as the development of methods to enhance PpIX accumulation in benign glioma in which PpIX does not tend to accumulate. Moreover, a certain degree of success has been achieved from in vitro experiments on PDT using PpIX, so there is anticipation that it can be used as a part of therapy on tumors that are difficult to excise.

7. References

Coluccia, D., Fandino, J.; Fujioka, M.; Cordovi, S.; Muroi, C. & Landolt, H. (2010). Intraoperative 5-aminolevulinic-acid-induced fluorescence in meningiomas. *Acta Neurochir (Wien),* Vol.152, No.10, pp. 1711-1719, ISSN 0001-6268

Coons, S.W. & Johnson, P.C. (1993). Regional heterogeneity in the proliferative activity of human gliomas as measured by the Ki-67 labeling index. J Neuropathol Exp Neurol, Vol.52, No.6, pp. 609-618, ISSN 0022-3069

El-Sharabasy, M.M.H.; El-Waseef, A.M.; Hafez, M.M. & Salim, S.A. (1992). Porphyrin metabolism in some malignant diseases. *Br J Cancer,* Vol.65, No.3, pp. 409 - 412, ISSN 0007-0920

Feigl, G.C.; Ritz, R.; Moraes, M.; Klein, J.; Ramina, K.; Gharabaghi, A.; Krischek, B.; Danz, S.; Bornemann, A.; Liebsch, M. & Tatagiba, M.S. (2010). Resection of malignant brain tumors in eloquent cortical areas: a new multimodal approach combining 5-aminolevulinic acid and intraoperative monitoring. *J Neurosurg,* Vol.113, No.2, pp. 352-357, ISSN: 0022-3085

Filbeck, T.; Roessler, W.; Knuechel, R.; Straub, M.; Kiel, H.J. & Wieland, W.F. (1999). 5-aminolevulinic acid-induced fluorescence endoscopy applied at secondary transurethral resection after conventional resection of primary superficial bladder tumors. *Urology,* Vol.53, No.1, pp. 77-81, ISSN 0090-4295

Filippini, G.; Falcone, C.; Boiardi, A.; Broggi, G.; Bruzzone, M.G.; Caldiroli, D.; Farina, R.; Farinotti, M.; Fariselli, L.; Finocchiaro, G.; Giombini, S.; Pollo, B.; Savoiardo, M.; Solero, C.L. & Valsecchi, M.G.; Brain Cancer Register of the Fondazione IRCCS (Istituto Ricovero e Cura a Carattere Scientifico) Istituto Neurologico Carlo Besta. (2008). Prognostic factors for survival in 676 consecutive patients with newly diagnosed primary glioblastoma. *Neuro-oncol,* Vol.10, No.1, pp. 79-87, ISSN 1522-8517

Goldman, S.; Levivier, M.; Pirotte, B.; Brucher, J.M.; Wikler, D.; Damhaut, P.; Dethy, S.; Brotchi, J. & Hildebrand, J. (1997). Regional methionine and glucose uptake in high-grade gliomas: a comparative study on PET-guided stereotactic biopsy. *J Nucl Med,* Vol.38, No.9, pp. 1459-1462, ISSN 0161-5505

Gorlia, T,; van den Bent, M.J.; Hegi, M.E.; Mirimanoff, R.O.; Weller, M.; Cairncross, J.G.; Eisenhauer, E.; Belanger, K.; Brandes, A.A.;, Allgeier, A.; Lacombe, D. & Stupp, R. (2008). Nomograms for predicting survival of patients with newly diagnosed glioblastoma: prognostic factor analysis of EORTC and NCIC trial 26981-22981/CE.3. Lancet Oncol, Vol.9, No.1, pp. 29-38, ISSN 1470-2045

Grabb, P.A. & Gilbert, M.R. (1995). Neoplastic and pharmacological influence on the permeability of an in vitro blood-brain barrier. *J Neurosurg,* Vol.82, No.6, pp. 1053-1058, ISSN: 0022-3085

Haj-Hosseini, N.; Richter, J.; Andersson-Engels, S. & Wårdell K. (2010). Optical touch pointer for fluorescence guided glioblastoma resection using 5-aminolevulinic acid. *Lasers Surg Med,* Vol.42, No.1, pp. 9-14, ISSN 0196-8092

Hoda, M.R. & Popken, G. (2009). Surgical outcomes of fluorescence-guided laparoscopic partial nephrectomy using 5-aminolevulinic acid-induced protoporphyrin IX. *J Surg Res,* Vol.154, No.2, pp. 220-225, ISSN 0022-4804

Ishihara, R.; Katayama, Y.; Watanabe, T.; Yoshino, A.; Fukushima, T. & Sakatani, K. (2007). Quantitative spectroscopic analysis of 5-aminolevulinic acid-induced protoporphyrin IX fluorescence intensity in diffusely infiltrating astrocytomas. *Neurol Med Chir (Tokyo),* Vol.47, No.2, pp. 53-57, ISSN 0470-8105

Johansson, A.; Palte, G.; Schnell, O.; Tonn, J.C.; Herms, J. & Stepp, H. (2010). 5-Aminolevulinic acid-induced protoporphyrin IX levels in tissue of human malignant brain tumors. *Photochem Photobiol,* Vol.86, No.6, pp. 1373-1378, ISSN 0031-8655

Kajimoto, Y.; Kuroiwa, T.; Miyatake, S.; Ichioka, T.; Miyashita, M.; Tanaka, H. & Tsuji, M. (2007). Use of 5-aminolevulinic acid in fluorescence-guided resection of meningioma with high risk of recurrence. Case report. *J Neurosurg,* Vol.106, No.6, pp. 1070-1074, ISSN 0022-3085

Kaneko, S. (2008). A current overview: photodynamic diagnosis and photodynamic therapy using 5-arainolevulinic acid in neurosurgery. *J Jpn Soc Laser Surg Med,* Vol.29. No.2, pp. 135-146, ISSN 0288-6200

Kawai, N.; Okauchi, M.; Miyake, K.; Sasakawa, Y.; Yamamoto, Y.; Nishiyama, Y. & Tamiya, T. (2010). 11C-methionine positron emission tomography in nontumorous brain lesions. *No Shinkei Geka,* Vol.38, No.11, pp. 985-995, ISSN 0301-2603

Mittal, S.; Szlaczky, M.C., & Barger, G.R. (2008). Low-grade gliomas in adults. *Curr Treat Options Neurol,* Vol.10, No.4, pp. 271-284, ISSN 1092-8480

Miyatake, S.; Kuroiwa, T.; Kajimoto, Y.; Miyashita, M.; Tanaka, H. & Tsuji, M. (2007). Fluorescence of non-neoplastic, magnetic resonance imaging-enhancing tissue by 5-aminolevulinic acid: case report. *Neurosurgery,* Vol.61, No.5, pp. E1101–E1104, ISSN 0148-396X

Mustajoki, P.; Timonen, K.; Gorchein, A.; Seppäläinen, A.M.; Matikainen, E. & Tenhunen, R. (1992). Sustained high plasma 5-aminolaevulinic acid concentration in a volunteer, no porphyric symptoms. *Eur J Clin Invest,* Vol.22, No.6, pp. 407-411, ISSN 0014-2972

Pallud, J.; Capelle, L.; Taillandier, L.; Fontaine, D.; Mandonnet, E.; Guillevin, R.; Bauchet, L.; Peruzzi, P.; Laigle-Donadey, F.; Kujas, M.; Guyotat, J.; Baron, M.H.; Mokhtari, K. & Duffau, H. (2009). Prognostic significance of imaging contrast enhancement for WHO grade II gliomas. *Neuro Oncol,* Vol.11, No.2, pp. 176-182, ISSN 1522-8517

Paulus, W. & Peiffer, J. (1989). Intratumoral histologic heterogeneity of gliomas. A quantitative study. *Cancer.* Vol.64No.2, pp. 442-447, ISSN 0008-543X

Rimington, C. & Riley, P.A. (1993). The biochemical approach to cancer therapy: a short essay. *Int J Biochem,* Vol.25, No.10, pp. 1385 - 1393, ISSN 0020-7114

Roberts, D.W.; Valdes, P.A.; Harris, B.T.; Fontaine, K.M.; Hartov, A.; Fan, X.; Ji, S.; Lollis, S.S.; Pogue, B.W.; Leblond, F.; Tosteson, T.D.; Wilson, B.C. & Paulsen, K.D. (2011). Coregistered fluorescence-enhanced tumor resection of malignant glioma: relationships between δ-aminolevulinic acid-induced protoporphyrin IX fluorescence, magnetic resonance imaging enhancement, and neuropathological parameters. *J Neurosurg,* Vol.114, No.3, pp. 595-603, ISSN: 0022-3085

Rokni-Yazdi, H.; Azmoudeh Ardalan, F.; Asadzandi, Z.; Sotoudeh, H.; Shakiba, M.; Adibi, A.; Ayatollahi, H. & Rahmani, M. (2009). Pathologic significance of the "dural tail sign". *Eur J Radiol.* Vol.70, No.1, pp. 10-16, ISSN 0720-048X

Sadeghi, N.; Salmon, I.; Decaestecker, C.; Levivier, M.; Metens, T.; Wikler, D.; Denolin, V.; Rorive, S.; Massager, N.; Baleriaux, D. & Goldman, S. (2007). Stereotactic comparison among cerebral blood volume, methionine uptake, and histopathology in brain glioma. *AJNR Am J Neuroradiol,* Vol.28, No.10, pp. 455-461, ISSN 0195-6108

Shimizu, S.; Utsuki, S.; Sato, K.; Oka, H.; Fujii, K. & Mii, K. (2006). Photodynamic diagnosis in surgery for spinal ependymoma. Case illustration. *J Neurosurg Spine,* Vol.5, No.4, pp. 380-380, ISSN 1547-5654

Steinbauer, J., Schreml, S.; Karrer, S.; Ackermann, G.; Babilas, P.; Landthaler, M. & Szeimies, R.M. (2009). Phototoxic reactions in healthy volunteers following photodynamic therapy with methylaminolevulinate cream or with cream containing 5-aminolevulinic acid: a phase II, randomized study. *Photodermatol Photoimmunol Photomed,* Vol.25, No.5, pp. 270-275, ISSN 0905-4383

Stummer, W.; Stepp, H.; Moller, G.; Ehrhardt, A.; Leonhard, M. & Reulen, H.J. (1998a). Technical principles for protoporphyrin-IXfluorescence guided microsurgical resection of malignant Glioma tissue. *Acta Neurochir (Wien),* Vol.140, No.10, pp. 995-1000, ISSN 0001-6268

Stummer, W.; Stocker, S.; Wagner, S.; Stepp, H.; Fritsch, C.; Goetz, C.; Goetz, A.E.; Kiefmann, R. & Reulen, H.J. (1998b). Intraoperative detection of malignant gliomas by 5-aminolevulinic acidinduced porphyrin fluorescence. *Neurosurgery,* Vol.42, No.3 pp. 518-526, ISSN 0148-396X

Stummer, W.; Pichlmeier, U.; Meinel, T.; Wiestler, O.D.; Zanella, F. & Reulen, H.J. (2006). Fluorescence-guided surgery with 5-aminolevulinic acid for resection of malignant glioma: a randomised controlled multicentre phase III trial. *Lancet Oncol,* Vol.7, No.5, pp. 392-401, ISSN 1470-2045

Stummer, W.; Tonn, J.C.; Mehdorn, H.M.; Nestler, U.; Franz, K.; Goetz, C.; Bink, A. & Pichlmeier, U.; on behalf of the ALA-Glioma Study Group. (2011). Counterbalancing risks and gains from extended resections in malignant glioma surgery: a supplemental analysis from the randomized 5-aminolevulinic acid glioma resection study. *J Neurosurg,* Vol.114, No.3, pp. 613–623, ISSN: 0022-3085

Teng, L.; Nakada, M.; Zhao, S.G.; Endo, Y.; Furuyama, N.; Nambu, E.; Pyko, I.V.; Hayashi, Y. & Hamada, J.I. (2011). Silencing of ferrochelatase enhances 5-aminolevulinic acid-based fluorescence and photodynamic therapy efficacy. Br J Cancer, Vol.104, No.5, pp. 798-807, ISSN 0007-0920

Utsuki, S.; Oka, H.; Sato, S.; Suzuki, S.; Shimizu, S.; Tanaka, S. & Fujii, K. (2006). Possibility of using laser spectroscopy for the intraoperative detection of nonfluorescing brain tumors and the boundaries of brain tumor infiltrates. Technical note. *J Neurosurg,* Vol.104, No.4, pp. 618-620, ISSN 0022-3085

Utsuki, S.; Miyoshi, N.; Oka, H.; Miyajima, Y.; Shimizu, S.; Suzuki, S. & Fujii, K. (2007a). Fluorescence-guided resection of metastatic brain tumors using 5-aminolevulinic acid–induced porphyrins - pathological study. *Brain Tumor Pathol,* Vol.24, No.2, pp. 53-55, ISSN 1433-7398

Utsuki, S.; Oka, H.; Sato, S.; Shimizu, S.; Suzuki, S.; Tanizaki, Y.; Kondo, K.; Miyajima, Y. & Fujii, K. (2007b). Histological examination of false positive tissue resection using 5-aminolevulinic acid-induced fluorescence guidance. *Neurol Med Chir (Tokyo),* Vol.47, No.5, pp. 210-214, ISSN 0470-8105

Utsuki, S.; Oka, H.; Miyajima, Y.; Shimizu, S.; Suzuki, S. & Fujii, K. (2008). Auditory alert system for fluorescence-guided resection of gliomas. Technical Note. Neurol Med Chir (Tokyo), Vol.48, No.2, pp. 95-98, ISSN 0470-8105

Utsuki, S.; Oka, H.; Suzuki, S.; Sato, S.; Mabuti, I.; Kijima, C. & Fujii, K. (2009). Significance of porphyrins in blood and urine of brain tumor patients that underwent 5-ALA administration. *Neuro Oncol,*Vol.11, No.6, pp. 920-920, ISSN 1522-8517

Utsuki, S.; Oka, H.; Sato, K.; Shimizu, S.; Suzuki, S. & Fujii, K. (2010). Fluorescence diagnosis of tumor cells in hemangioblastoma cysts with 5-aminolevulinic acid. *J Neurosurg,* Vol.112, No.1, pp.130-132, ISSN 0022-3085

van den Bent, M.J.; Afra, D.; de Witte, O.; Ben Hassel, M.; Schraub, S.; Hoang-Xuan, K.; Malmstrom, P.O.; Collette, L.; Pierart, M.; Mirimanoff, R. & Karim, A.B.; EORTC Radiotherapy and Brain Tumor Groups and the UK Medical Research Council. (2005). Long-term efficacy of early versus delayed radiotherapy for low-grade astrocytoma and oligodendroglioma in adults: the EORTC 22845 randomised trial. *Lancet.* Vol.366, No.9490, pp. 985-990, ISSN 0140-6736

Webber, J.; Kessel, D. & Fromm, D. (1997a). Side effects and photosensitization of human tissues after aminolevulinic acid. *J Surg Res,* Vol.68, No.1, pp. 31-37, ISSN 0022-4804

Webber, J.; Kessel, D. & Fromm D. (1997b). Plasma levels of protoporphyrin IX in humans after oral administration of 5-aminolevulinic acid. *J Photochem Photobiol B,* Vol.37, No.1-2, pp. 151-153, ISSN 1011-1344

Widhalm, G.; Wolfsberger, S.; Minchev, G.; Woehrer, A.; Krssak, M.; Czech, T.; Prayer, D.; Asenbaum, S.; Hainfellner, J.A. & Knosp, E. (2010). 5-Aminolevulinic acid is a promising marker for detection of anaplastic foci in diffusely infiltrating gliomas with nonsignificant contrast enhancement. *Cancer,* Vol.116, No.6, pp. 1545-1552, ISSN 0008-543X

Yamamoto, F.; Ohgari, Y.; Yamaki, N.; Kitajima, S., Shimokawa, O.; Matsui, H. & Taketani, S. (2007) The role of nitric oxide in delta-aminolevulinic acid (ALA)-induced photosensitivity of cancerous cells. *Biochem Biophys Res Commun,* Vol.353, No.3, pp. 541-546, ISSN 0006-291X

13

Laser-Induced Autofluorescence as a Possible Diagnostic Tool for Use in Neurosurgery

Mihail - Lucian Pascu[1], Mihaela - Oana Romanitan[2], Alexandru Pascu[1], Josè - Maria Delgado[3] and Leon Danaila[4]
[1]*National Institute for Laser, Plasma and Radiation Physics, Laser Department, Bucharest*
[2]*Neurology Clinics, Emergency University Hospital, Bucharest*
[3]*Division de Neurociencias, Universidad Pablo de Olavide, Sevilla*
[4]*Neurosurgery Clinics, National Institute of Neurology and Neurovascular Diseases, Bucharest*
[1,2,4]*Romania*
[3]*Spain*

1. Introduction

One of the main neurosurgical problem consists in accurately identify the margins of brain tumors to allow a tumor's precise excision without destruction of the surrounding healthy tissue. Excision is optimal if the tumor mass is removed from the brain without affecting the surrounding healthy tissue or with minimum injury to it. The result of resection and the histopathological diagnosis of the extracted tumor tissue impose a therapeutic strategy to further treat the disease. Given these clinical requirements, it is highly recommended to accurately identify tumor tissue borders during the surgical operation proper, by means of specific methods and techniques. Identification is done in two steps: (a) a preoperative imaging of the tumor tissue and borders using CT, MRI, and/or ultrasound-based equipment; and (b) an intraoperative stage, in which the tumor borders are identified by direct visual inspection; the operating microscope, endoscopic techniques, and autofluorescence measurements of the tumor and healthy tissues are also available methods that may be associated with the visual observation/search.

Laser-induced autofluorescence is one of the main candidates for use in the operative field to identify tumor borders in both benign and malignant cases. It may allow, in principle, accurate identification of the interface between normal brain tissue and tumor tissue by measuring the optical fluorescence spectra emitted by these tissues after excitation with laser optical beams having suitable characteristics. Literature reports show that the autofluorescence method is promising for delineating brain tumor resection margins (Bottirolli et al., 1998; Lin et al., 2000; Lin et al., 2001; Croce et al., 2003; Cubillos et al., 2006). At the same time, more research needs to be devoted in order to develop the instruments, procedures, and clinical recommendations for intraoperative use of autofluorescence, at the level of both in vivo and in vitro measurements (Kremer et al., 2009).

Literature reports also show that progress was made stepwise to identify brain tumor tissues and to differentiate them from the normal brain tissues on the base of the laser induced fluorescence emitted by exogenous fluorophores (K. Svanberg and S. Svanberg 1983, J. Ankerst et al.1984, S. Montan, K. Svanberg and S. Svanberg 1985, K. Svanberg 1986, Andersson - Engels et al. 1989, 1994). An alternative is the measurement of the autofluorescence emitted by the brain tissues, i.e. by the endogenous fluorophores contained naturally in them. The autofluorescence experiments were approached and are still developed along two main lines: the measurements of the spectral properties of the autofluorescence beams and the contemporary or consecutive measurements of the lifetime of the autofluorescence radiation (Andersson-Engels, et al. 1990a,b, Marcu et al. 2004, Butte et al. 2011). Combinations of these techniques reflected in imaging spectroscopy are also experimented (Gebhart et al. 2006, Kantelhardt 2007, Butte et al. 2010, Sun et al. 2010).
This book chapter is conceived as a synthesis of the characteristics of the laser-induced autofluorescence method applied in neurosurgery for diagnostics and/or intraoperative procedures; at the same time relevant research contributions of the authors in this field are described in more detail and discussions are made on the place occupied by the autofluorescence method among the other methods/techniques used for real time differentiation between normal and tumor brain tissues.

2. Materials and methods

2.1 Autofluorescence definition: basic data

The autofluorescence emitted by a tissue (in particular the brain tissue) is that fluorescence emitted by it when exogenous fluorescent substances are not added to it; in other words the autofluorescence radiation is emitted only by the natural constituents of the tissue when an optical radiation of suitable wavelength falls on the tissue. Consequently, autofluorescence spectra give accurate information about the content and molecular structure of the emitting tissue. The autofluorescence is emitted by molecules that exist normally in the tissues, following their resonant interaction with optical radiation. The scheme that describes the fluorescence emission and the lifetime of the fluorescence radiation emitted by a molecule (usually named fluorophore) is shown in Fig.1 (Danaila and Pascu, 2001; Valeur, 2001).
The molecular de-excitation may also involve the energy transfer from an excited electronic singlet state to an excited triplet state by the process called "intersystem crossing", one system being formed by the singlet and other by the triplet states (v=0 of S_2 to v=4 of T_2, or v=2 of S_1 to v=0 of T_2, or v=0 of S_1 to v=4 of T_1). The de-excitation of the molecule may be also produced without changing the electronic state by passing without emission of radiation from excited vibrational levels to less excited vibrational levels; this process being called vibrational relaxation and is accompanied by the slight heating of the samples.
If the fluorophore interacts with an optical radiation emitted by an external light source in visible and/or ultraviolet, then the first process which takes place is the absorption of one (transition S_0 to S_1) or more (transition S_0 to S_1 followed by S_1 to S_2 etc) photons of this pumping radiation and the consequent excitation of the molecule due to the transition selection rules from the fundamental singlet state S_0 to the S_1, S_2,...S_n states; the time interval needed for that is one fsec i.e. the process is so fast that the excitation of the molecule takes place so quickly that the nuclei are found in the same position before and after the transition. Once excited on a vibrational (or rotational-vibrational) state of an excited singlet state, the molecule may pass to the fundamental singlet state on different

vibrational levels in different ways (Brewer et al., 2001). One is the internal conversion on the S_1 state which takes place in 10^{-6}s - 10^{-12}s followed by vibrational relaxation in 10^{-12}s - 10^{-13}s on the v=0 vibrational level of the S_1 excited singlet state. Both processes are nonradiative and the energy lost by the molecule is transformed in kinetic energy of it that may slightly increase the tissue temperature. From v=0 of S_1 the molecule falls radiatively on several vibrational levels of the S_0 state emitting fluorescence radiation in 10^{-6}s - 10^{-9}s. This is the main way in which the autofluorescence radiation is emitted, so that its characteristics such as wavelength, spectral range, time duration, polarization state are specific to the emitting molecules; i.e. the fluorescence radiation properties are related to the structural properties of the emitting molecules and with their environment which may influence the fluorescence emission. From the S_1 state the fluorophore molecule may decay with a much lower probability back to the S_0 fundamental singlet state by other mechanisms.

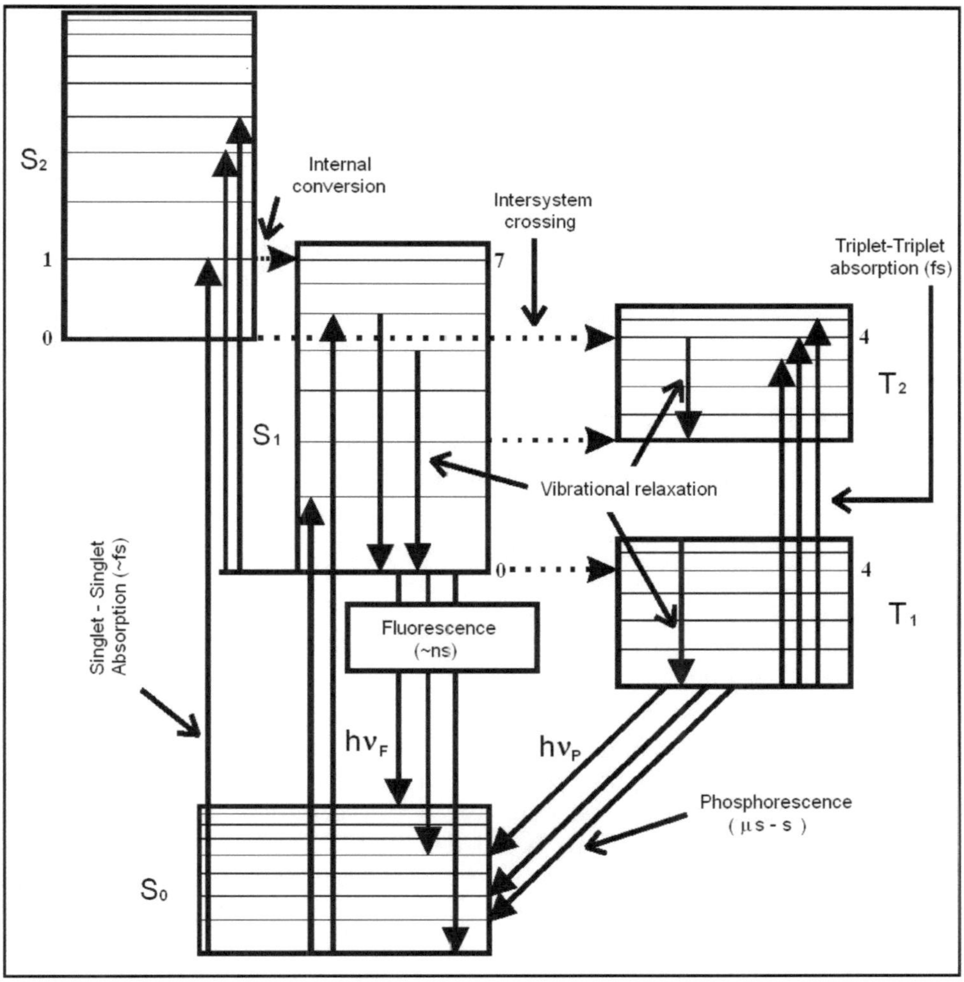

Fig. 1. Molecular diagram used to describe the emission of fluorescence radiation

The molecule may pass from the S_1 state to the first excited triplet state T_1 by intersystem crossing in 10^{-4}s - 10^{-13}s; so, the molecule may occupy a vibrational level of a triplet state after which a vibrational relaxation may occur in 10^{-12}s - 10^{-13}s at the end of which v=0 on T_1 state is populated. The first triplet state T_1 of the fluorophore molecule is metastable and consequently the lifetime of the molecule on it is much longer than on S_1. From it there are two possibilities for the molecule to further de-excite. One is the radiative transition on different vibrational levels of the fundamental singlet state S_0 which leads to the emission of phosphorescence radiation at longer time intervals than the fluorescence radiation with respect to the time moment at which the S_0 - S_n absorption occurs; usually, the phosphorescence takes place in 10^{-4}s - 10^{-2}s which is the lifetime of the molecule on the T_1 state. The phosphorescence radiation also differs from the autofluorescence by the wavelengths which are always longer in phosphorescence than in the fluorescence case.
The second possibility to de-excite T_1 to the S_0 state is the intersystem crossing process ($T_1 \rightarrow S_0$) followed by fluorescence quenching which takes place in 10^{-11}s-10^{-12}s. The fluorescence quenching is, in fact, the process of vibrational relaxation which leads to the nonradiative decay of the molecule on v=0 belonging to the S_0 singlet state.
As a rule, the autofluorescence emission is produced after absorbing one photon of radiation at a wavelength which is usually in the near UV or in the short wavelengths range of the visible. Due to the fact that the fluorophore molecules are surrounded by the other tissues components, which normally (but not only) act as a liquid environment of the molecules, the rotational-vibrational levels are broadened on the singlet and triplet states so that the absorption and the fluorescence emission spectra are broad and their structures are also broadened. Consequently, in the autofluorescence spectra a partial superposition between the emitted bands takes place but, nevertheless, the spectra characteristics are specific to the emitting molecules. At the same time, the fluorescence spectra ($S_1 \rightarrow S_0$ transitions) are more or less the mirror images of the corresponding absorption spectra. The pH of the tissue in which the emitting molecules are embedded may also influence the autofluorescence spectra characteristics, such as the spectral width, the shape etc. Some of the molecules found in the tissue alongside with the emitting fluorophores may absorb the emitted fluorescence; this leads to autofluorescence decrease and from here to errors in measuring/estimating the emitters' positions and concentrations in the tissue.

2.2 Autofluorescence experimental monitoring

The experimental system for measuring autofluorescence signals should be conceived taking into account that fluorescence excitation is always produced at shorter wavelengths than is the emitted fluorescence radiation. At even longer wavelengths, autophosphorescence is emitted, with a lifetime longer than that of autofluorescence. The spectral distribution of the autofluorescence emission is much broader and more structured than that of the pumping/excitation radiation; at the same time its duration is usually longer than, and its polarization state is different from, that of the pumping beam. The coherence state of the excitation beam is different from that of the autofluorescence radiation. Experimentally, it is possible to excite autofluorescence using a laser beam that is monochromatic, coherent, and highly polarized. The obtained fluorescence radiation is incoherent, broad-band, and nonpolarized.
Autofluorescence measures exclusively the properties of the tissues, because it is produced only by their endogenous molecules. It may provide, mainly, two types of information

(Sokolov et al., 2002): (a) image - allows obtaining a more or less extended image of a part of the studied tissue (Gebhart et al., 2006; Kantelhardt et al.,); and (b) fluorescence radiation - it is excited by focusing the pumping beam on the tissue (Lin et al., 2000, 2001, 2002; Kremer et al., 2009; Pascu et al., 2009). The fluorescence radiation has a spectral distribution and a specific intensity; it also has a polarization state, and is characterized by specific ratios between the spectrum peaks.

Autofluorescence is highly sensitive to endogenous emitters of the tissue, if properly excited. It allows identification of the molecular components of a tissue and their combinations, and investigation of the interaction between them and the surrounding media (usually described by the pH of the tissue); it also allows the monitoring of the modifications produced in the molecular composition of a tissue by the effect of natural and/or artificial factors.

The autofluorescence emission of a fluorophore may be characterized by the following properties (Pascu et al., 2009): overall intensity of the emitted spectrum; emission spectral range; spectral structure of the radiation described by the intensity peaks and their relative ratios and by the wavelength of the main intensity peak (if such peak exists); fluorescence lifetime, measured either by its full time width (FTW) or by the full time width at the half maximum of the fluorescence peak (FTWHM), if only one peak is involved (Yong et al., 2006).

The measurement of the lifetime requires excitation of the autofluorescence with a laser pulse that is short enough, i.e. it should have an FTWHM of 5 ns, at most. This parameter may be measured for each fluorescence peak if the autofluorescence spectrum exhibits more peaks.

Human brain tissues (both normal and tumor) contain endogenous fluorophores that belong to the following classes of biomolecules: aminoacids (tryptophan, tyrosine, phenylalanine); structural proteins (collagen, elastin); enzymes and co-enzymes (flavin adenine dinucleotide - FAD, the reduced form of the nicotinamide adenine dinucleotiode-NADH, flavins); lipids (phospholipids, lipofuscin, ceroids); porphyrins; and vitamins (A, K, and D). The autofluorescence emitted by the tissue contains signals originating from the active fluorophores and depends on their concentration and spatial distribution, as well as the properties of the surrounding environment, such as pH, optical properties, structure and organization, homogeneity, (an)isotropy, and turbidity.

The autofluorescence is, therefore, sensitive to the above mentioned properties, and may signal small modifications of any of them. Moreover, tissue histology and biochemistry leave their signatures on the autofluorescence spectra (Bottiroli et al., 1998; Toms et al., 2005). Consequently, variations in the health state of the tissue that modifies its histology and/or histochemical properties can be evidenced by autofluorescence measurements. Such is the case of tumor/malignant tumor tissues that have properties that differ from those of a normal tissue; autofluorescence may become a method to detect and investigate malignant tumor tissues (Svanberg, 1987).

In neurosurgery, it may assist the neurosurgeon to find, in real time, the borders of the malignant tumors. To do this, specialized equipment should be developed to detect the malignant tumors and/or their limits in the brain for early stages or more-developed tumor tissues.

This article brings together the autofluorescence measurements made by the authors in brain tissues in view of future specific equipment development.

2.3 Sample preparation

2.3.1 First type of sample preparation

This approach was exploratory and it was chosen initially to find the best procedures for sample processing and for their mounting in the optical system. The conclusions that resulted from the measurements were used to identify the conditions for reproducibility in: sample preparation and arrangement in the optical set-up utilized for autofluorescence spectra excitation and collection.

Accordingly, a protocol to conserve, transport, and treat tumor/normal tissues was established, to ensure unaltered samples. Once extracted using operative procedures, the brain tissue samples were kept immersed in natural saline at 20°C in a Dewar container. The time interval between tumor extraction and measurements was, at most, 60 min. The samples were irrigated from time to time with natural saline to prevent uncontrolled drying and to remove blood traces; the control and in any case the removal of the blood traces from the samples are important since blood fluorescence may superpose on the autofluorescence of the sample tissues (Andersson-Engels et al., 1990a,b). The working temperature was 20°C. To ensure the best possible conditions for reproducibility of the measurements and to prevent errors in the fluorescence excitation and collection, the samples were placed in direct contact with an optical quartz plate of 0.5 mm in thickness; each sample surface that was exposed to the excitation / fluorescence pumping radiation and from which the fluorescence was emitted was very well defined. The exposed surface was 1–2 mm in diameter (diameter of the excitation beam), and for each sample 5 such spots/discs were used in the measurements; the geometrical arrangement was reproducible, and the results obtained for each excitation wavelength were averaged.

2.3.2 Homogenate preparation

The results from the studies performed on samples processed as mentioned in the previous paragraph, have shown that there are variations in the reproducibility of the autofluorescence curves. To avoid this, samples were processed using a different method, namely, as homogenates: each sample was washed abundantly in natural saline, then ground and further exposed to ultra-sounds to obtain a homogeneous mixture. The preparing of the homogenates did not affect the molecular structures or concentrations of the constituent fluorophores in the samples. It was done to prevent errors due to the unhomogeneities occurring naturally in the collected samples and to the geometry at the interface between the tissue and the optical excitation/collection system.

The optical arrangement for autofluorescence excitation/ collection was the same as described in the paragraph above. For each measured sample (either tumor or normal tissue), three measuring points/spots were used, and the three signals were averaged. The autofluorescence excitation and detection system worked for all samples within the same spectral range (excitation between 337 and 500 nm, and emission measurement between 400 and 650 nm), so that no corrections related to variation in the sensitivity of the photodetectors with wavelength were needed from one sample to another.

2.4 Experimental set-up and sequence

The main goal of the measurements was to identify the spectral properties of the autofluorescence of brain tissues for two cases/types of samples: normal tissues and malignant tumor; by studying these spectra, one aimed to establish criteria to differentiate between the fluorescence radiations emitted by the two types of samples and to quantify the differences between them. The experiments were made in two steps: (a) measurement of the spectral characteristics of the autofluorescence emitted by the fluorophores existing in the brain tissues; and (b) comparative in vitro measurements of the spectral properties of the autofluorescence emitted by pairs of normal/malignant tumor tissue.

The experimental set-up (shown in Fig.2) consisted of a system adapted to measure laser-induced fluorescence (LIF).

In choosing the radiation source used to excite the autofluorescence, several variants previously reported in the literature were evaluated (Ramanujam et al., 1994; Ramanujam, 2000; Lin et al., 2002; Wu et al., 2003).

For the purpose of this work, a pulsed laser with emission in the near-ultraviolet and visible spectral ranges was developed. This has two advantages: (a) it generates short time-width laser pulses of relatively low energy, which produce a weak perturbation of the studied tissues and a higher overall efficiency of the fluorescence emission; and (b) it enables measurement not only of the spectral distribution of the autofluorescence radiation but also of the fluorescence emission lifetime.

The laser source is a frequency-doubled tunable dye laser pumped by a nitrogen pulsed laser (NPL), described elsewhere (Danaila and Pascu, 1999; Pascu, 2000; Danaila and Pascu, 2001). The main characteristics of the laser system unit used to pump the fluorescence are (a) NPL: emission at 337.1 nm, laser beam bandwidth < 0.1 nm, pulse FTW 1 ns, energy / pulse 50 μJ, peak power per pulse 500 kW, pulse repetition rate continuously adjustable between 1 and 10 pulses per second (pps), beam divergence 5 mrad x 10 mrad; and (b) tunable dye laser: NPL pumped, emits tunable radiation between 350 and 700 nm by using a succession of dyes, beam spectral bandwidth maximum 0.2 nm, pulse FTW 1 ns, energy per pulse typically 5 μJ, pulse repetition rate as driven by the NPL, and laser beam divergence 5 mrad. The dye laser beam focusing produces an irradiance of 10^8 W/m^2 on the sample. The dyes that were mostly used in the experiments are given in Table 1.

Laser dye	Synonymous	Chemical formula	Molec. weight	Solvent	Molar concentration
POPOP	2,2'-(1,4-phenylene)bis[5-phenyl-oxazole]	$C_{24}H_{16}N_2O_2$	364	toluene	$3.5 \cdot 10^{-3}$
Coumarin 540A (Coumarin 153)	2,3,6,7-tetrahydro-9-(trifluoromethyl)-1H,5H,11H-[1]benzopyrano[6,7,8-ij] quinolizin-11-one	$C_{16}H_{14}F_3NO_2$	309.29	ethanol	$5 \cdot 10^{-3}$
Rhodamine 590-Rh 590 (Rhodamine 6G-Rh 6G)	2-[6-(ethylamino)-3-(ethylimino)-2,7-dimethyl-3H-xanthen-9-yl]-benzoic acid, ethyl ester perchlorate	$C_{27}H_{29}ClN_2O_7$	543.01	ethanol	$5 \cdot 10^{-3}$

Table 1. Laser dyes used in the autofluorescence experiments

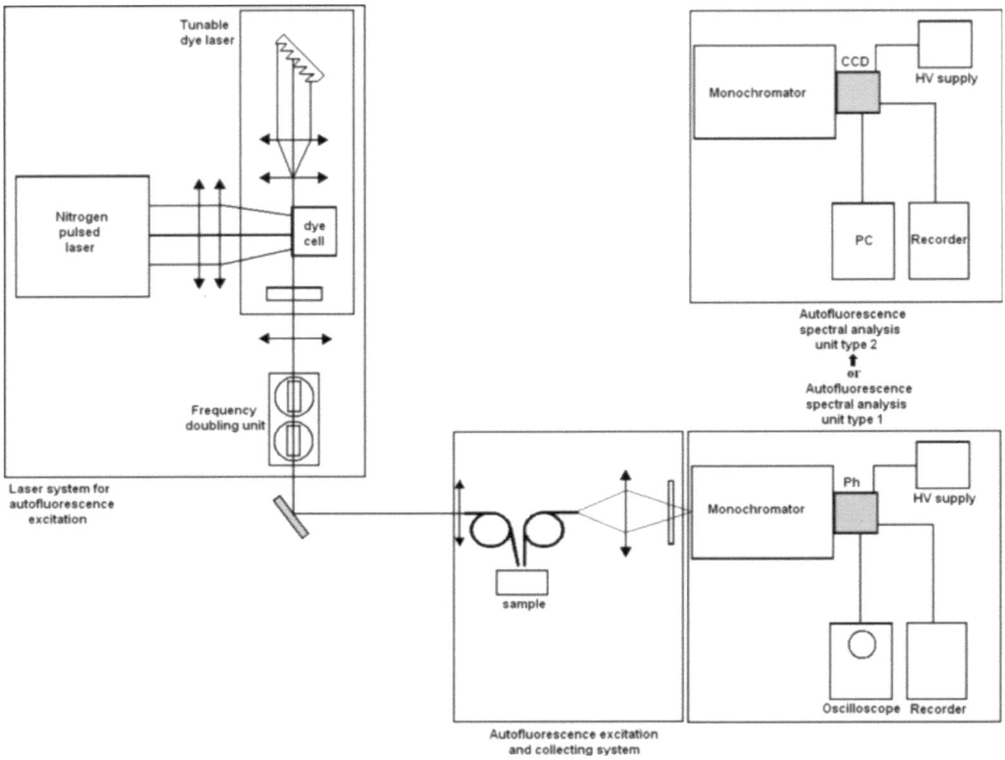

Fig. 2. The fluorescence/autofluorescence excitation set-up.

The frequency doubling crystal used to cover by second harmonic generation (SHG) the wavelength gap in the near-ultraviolet up to 337.1 nm is an ADP crystal; the obtained laser beam has with the following characteristics: tunability range 260 - 300 nm, spectral bandwidth 0.05 nm when the pumping dye laser beam has 0.1 nm full spectral bandwidth, pulse FTW ≤ 1 ns, pulse repetition rate as driven by the NPL, peak energy per pulse typically 0.5 μJ, which enables obtaining a peak irradiance of 5×10^6 W/m^2 at the focus. The system to excite and collect the autofluorescence signal (Fig. 2) consisted of a pair of optical fibers, one of which is used to excite the autofluorescence; it transmits the excitation beam with losses lower than 1%. The excitation optical fiber is a quartz fiber with a core of 1.5 mm in diameter; it has a transmission spectral range between 180 and 700 nm, and a numerical aperture NA = 0.22. The fiber used for the collection of the autofluorescence signal is a fiber bundle of 6 mm in diameter, transmitting between 400 and 700 nm. The sample is either a solution or a piece of brain tissue prepared for in vitro measurements. The autofluorescence radiation transmitted by the collection optical fiber is focused on the input slit of a monochromator; this is part of the spectral analyzing unit, and works between 220 and 800 nm at a linear dispersion of 0.4 nm/mm; signal detection is made by using a fast photomultiplier, sensitive between 180 and 800 nm and able to measure optical signals with rise times of up to 1 ns. With this system (Autofluorescence spectral analysis unit type 1 in Fig.2), the spectral distribution and the lifetime of the autofluorescence were measured.

The second variant (Autofluorescence spectral analysis unit type 2 in Fig.2) for signal detection was a computer- controlled, 2048 pixel CCD camera working between 300 and 800 nm, used only for spectral distribution measurements.

3. Results

3.1 Fluorophore measurements

The measured samples were primary endogenous fluorophores, such as aminoacids, structural proteins, enzymes and coenzymes, porphyrins, and riboflavins. Literature reports (for example Zuluaga et al., 1999; Drezek et al., 2001a, b) on the fluorescence properties of such fluorophores show sets of data measured in experimental conditions that differ slightly from one case to another; this prevents the construction of a reference system based on which the interpretation of the autofluorescence data measured in brain tissues could be made. In this chapter, are presented data measured on primary fluorophores that are potentially present in the brain tissues, aiming to have controllable comparison conditions for the autofluorescence measurements made on tissue samples. So, Figs. 3 - 5 show the fluorescence spectra of the, respectively, phenylalanine, tryptophan and tyrosine solutions are shown when excited at 266 nm.The samples for each substance were phosphate buffer aqueous solutions at pH = 7 and the concentrations were in each case 10^{-5}M.

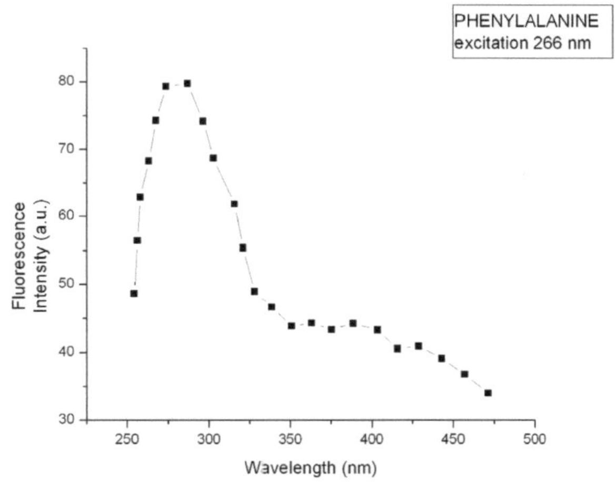

Fig. 3. The phenyalanine fluorescence emission spectrum

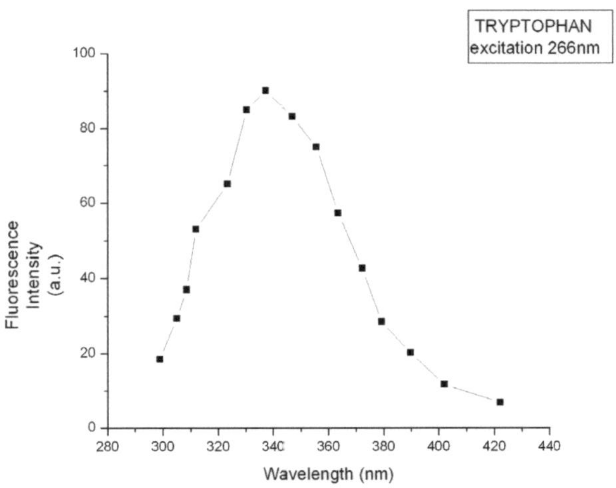

Fig. 4. The tryptophan fluorescence emission spectrum.

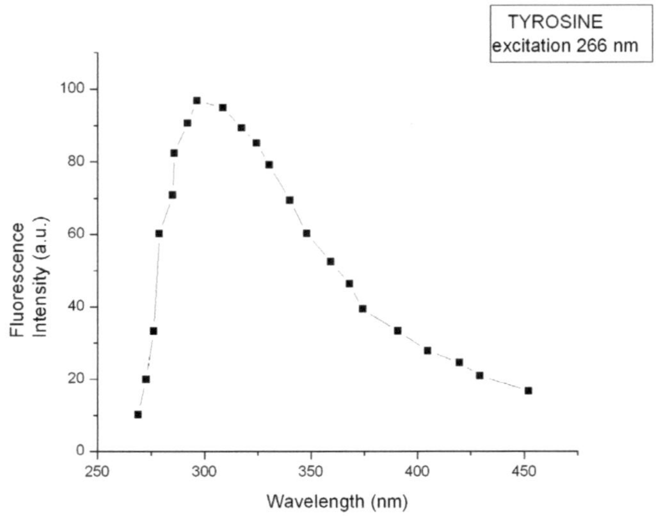

Fig. 5. The tyrosine fluorescence emission spectrum

The fluorescence peaks for each of these aminoacids are broad, have different intensities, are unstructured and constitute a superposition of narrower peaks originating in transitions between several specific pairs of electronic states. To obtain an objective base for the autofluorescence spectra, the LIF was measured for various fluorophores. Figs. 6–12 show fluorescence spectra emitted by fluorophores which are found in brain tissues as follows: in Fig.6 NADH excited at 337.1 nm with NPL laser beam; in Fig.7 and Fig.8 collagen excited at 266 nm with beam obtained by SHG from Rh6G emission at 532 nm, respectively at 337.1 nm; in Fig.9 elastin excited at 337.1 nm; in Fig.10 FMN (flavin mononucleotide) excited at 337.1 nm; in Fig.11 riboflavin excited at 440 nm; in Fig.12 protoporphyrin excited at 440 nm by laser beam emitted either by coumarine or by POPOP.

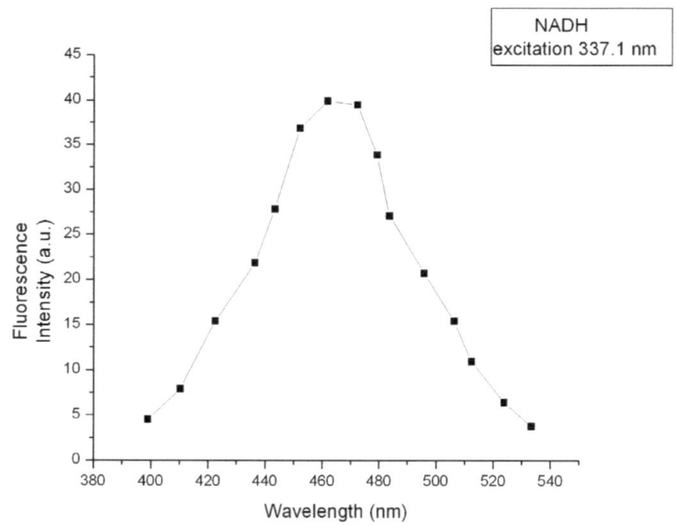

Fig. 6. Fluorescence emission of NADH

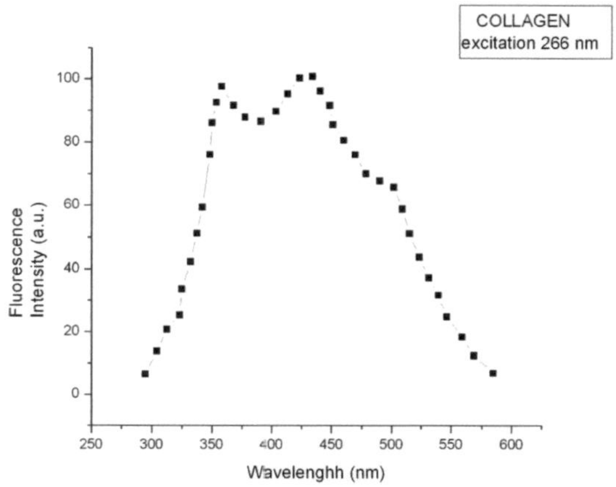

Fig. 7. Fluorescence emitted by collagen excited at 266 nm

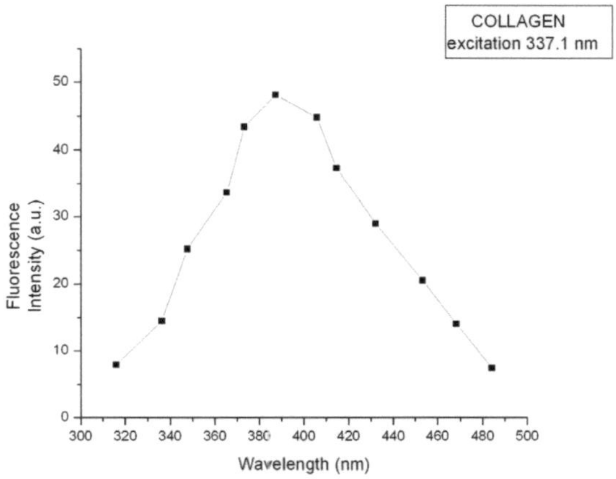

Fig. 8. Fluorescence emission by collagen excited at 337.1nm

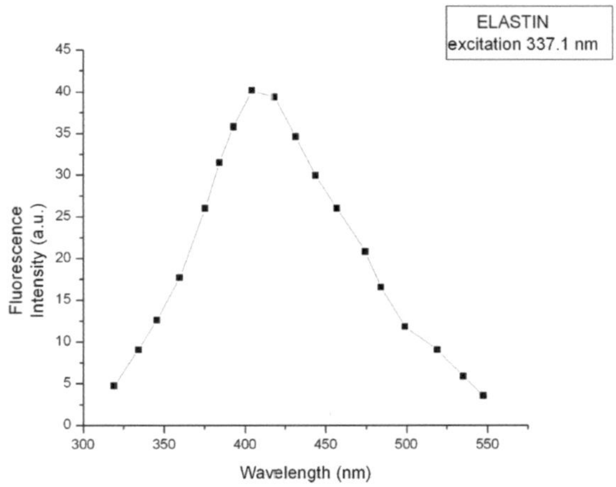

Fig. 9. Fluorescence emitted by elastin excited at 337.1 nm

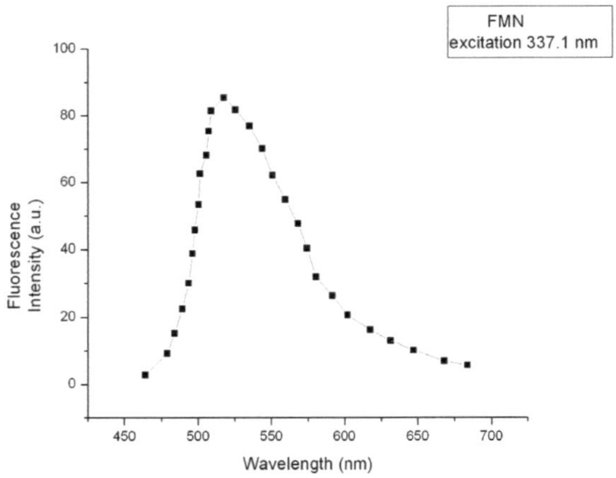

Fig. 10. Fluorescence emitted by FMN

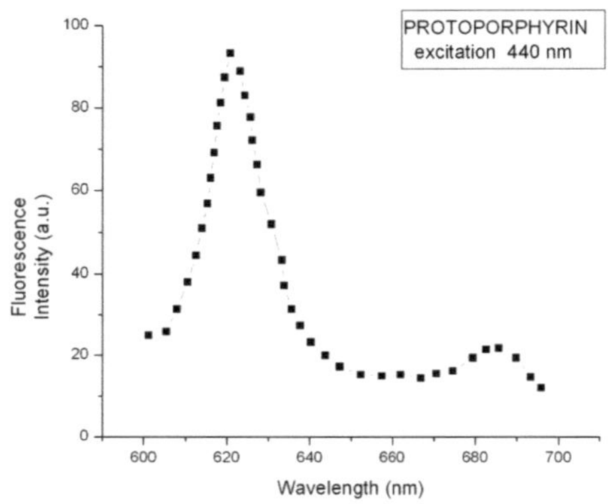

Fig. 11. Fluorescence emission of riboflavin

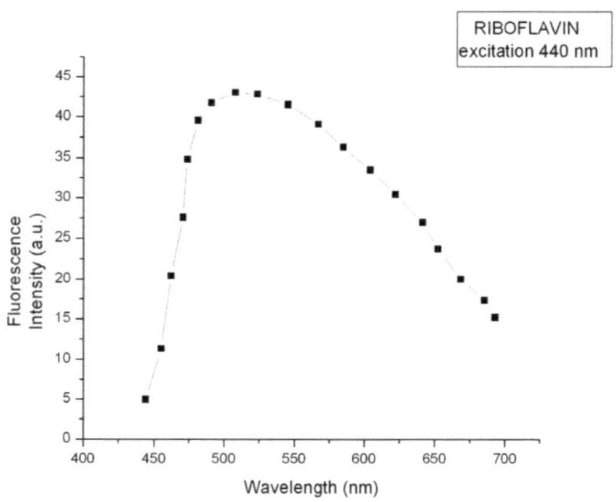

Fig. 12. Fluorescence emission of protoporphyrin

The results are given in Table 2, which shows the fluorescence peak positions, together with the corresponding excitation wavelengths.

Compound	Solvent / concentration	Excitation wavelength (nm) / utilized laser	Fluorescence wavelength peak
Collagen	10^{-5}M phosphate buffer aqueous solutions at pH = 7	270/SHG of dye laser at 540 nm	395
Collagen	10^{-5}M phosphate buffer aqueous solutions at pH = 7	285/SHG of dye laser at 570 nm	310
Collagen	10^{-5}M phosphate buffer aqueous solutions at pH = 7	337.1/NPL	395
NADH	10^{-5}M phosphate buffer aqueous solutions at pH = 7	290/SHG of dye laser at 580 nm	510
NADH	10^{-5}M phosphate buffer aqueous solutions at pH = 7	337.1/NPL	455
NADH	10^{-5}M phosphate buffer aqueous solutions at pH = 7	400/tunable dye laser (POPOP)	510

Table 2. Fluorescence peaks of several fluorophores

The lifetimes of the fluorescence radiation emitted by some fluorophores that are found in the brain tissues, measured as in Fig.2, are displayed in Table 3; most of the values are between 1ns and 10ns. As for NADH this value is very short and a p-i-n (PIN) fast photodiode was used, which was able to indicate only that the fluorescence lifetime is shorter than 0.5 ns. On the contrary for the FMN the lifetime is longer, around 45ns.
These values may be used as discriminating factors between different types of tissues.

Compound	Fluorescence lifetime (FTWHM) ns	Compound	Fluorescence lifetime (FTWHM) ns
Tryptophan	2.9	Collagen	5.5
Tyrosine	4.1	Flavin monocleotide (FMN)	45
Phenylalanine	6.0	Porphyrin	12
NADH	< 0.5		

Table 3. Fluorescence lifetimes for several brain tissue compounds

The autofluorescence measurements performed on some of the main molecular components of the brain tissues allow to conclude as follows: (a) the autofluorescence spectra of the fluorophores strongly depend on the absorption characteristics of the fluorophores molecules, which–in turn–depend on the solvent, solution pH, and concentrations in the samples; this is a rather general conclusion in LIF but, in this case, it becomes particularly critical; (b) the fluorescence excitation and emission spectra are mainly obtained by excitation with laser radiation in the near-ultraviolet and visible (200–500 nm) and are emitted in the visible; (c) each of the fluorophore molecules has a specific fluorescence pattern/trace which depends on the excitation wavelength. The spectral distribution of the fluorescence radiation and the number, relative intensities and shapes of the peaks are strongly dependent on the excitation wavelength. For qualitative analysis, the use is recommended of more successive wavelengths in order to accurately identify the specific peaks for each fluorescence source; (d) if fluorescence peaks, that are very close to each other in the spectrum, are emitted by different fluorophores, one possibility to reveal the emitting molecules and to differentiate between them is to measure the fluorescence lifetime, which may differ from one fluorophore to another.

3.2 Brain tissue measurements

The data reported above can be used to reveal alterations of normal brain tissues towards tumor tissues (either benign or malignant). For such cases, the first factors to be considered are related to the interaction between the laser beam and the tissue on which it is falling (Pascu, 2000; Danaila and Pascu, 2001; Pascu et al., 2009). Figure 13 describes the processes of laser beam interaction with brain tissues which derive from the general case of the laser beam-target tissues interaction. At the point of contact with the tissue border (i.e. the interface of the tissue with the environment form which the laser beam comes), the laser beam (of intensity I_0) is reflected in part (I_R) and backscattered ($I_{b.s}$) by elastic scattering (Gong et al., 2008); a non-negligible part of it is sent back to the environment without interacting with the tissue. The beam penetrating the tissue is refracted (I_r), depending on the tissue's optical properties and changes its propagation direction with respect to the incident beam. A part of it is scattered forward ($I_{f.s}$) the light spreading around the incidence point inside the tissue in all directions, function of the unhomogeneities of the tissue. Another part (I_a) is absorbed by resonant interaction. The rest (I_{rem}) propagates further into the tissue. The energy balance is given by:

$$I_0 = I_R + I_{b.s.} + I_r + I_{f.s.} + I_a + I_{rem.}$$

The equation above is approximate since it does not take into account the inelastic scattering of the laser light which may take place in the tissue; I_a describes not only the laser beam intensity absorbed along the main propagation line (which is mainly defined by the refracted beam direction) but also the absorption which takes place in all the tissue volume, scattered light included.

Out of the mentioned intensities, I_a is responsible for the excitation of the autofluorescence radiation. At the wavelengths used in these studies, water and hemoglobin (two important components of brain tissues) do not interfere with the fluorescence emission process. Water is practically nonabsorbing in the visible and the near-ultraviolet absorption does not lead to fluorescence emission by water molecules.

Hemoglobin does not absorb above 600 nm, and the strong absorption below 600 nm does not lead to significant fluorescence emission (hemoglobin fluoresces very weakly when excited below 300 nm, and the fluorescence lifetime is shorter than 25 ps). Even so, brain tissue samples not having blood within the structure (because they were abundantly washed with natural saline solution) were chosen for the study so that absorption of the laser beam due to hemoglobin in the samples was negligible. Autofluorescence of the tissue samples was excited at 337.1 nm and at longer wavelengths, up to 500 nm.

These wavelengths are also recommended for in vitro measurements for other reasons: the depth of laser beam penetration in the tissue is much lower (one-two orders of magnitude) below 337 nm, the radiation at 337.1 nm and above this wavelength is more intense (typically one order of magnitude higher) than in the case of beams (available for these studies) emitted below 300 nm; in vivo interaction of the brain tissues with radiation below

300 nm may lead to undesirable effects on the cells, such as cleavage of molecular bonds (Lin et al., 2001).

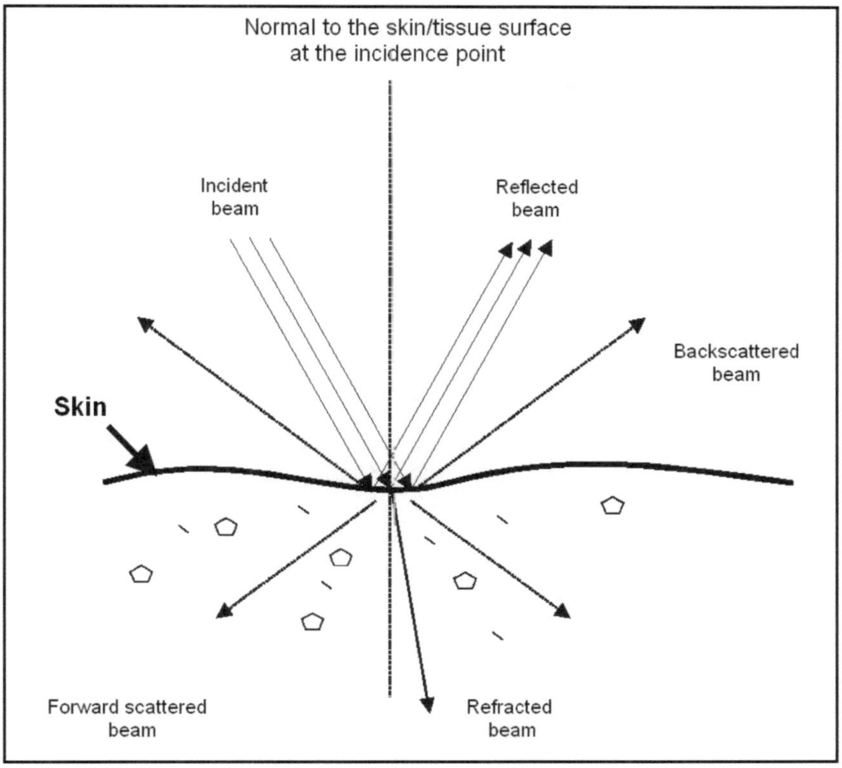

Fig. 13. Laser beam-tissue coupling processes

The excitation at the mentioned wavelengths allows to include contributions to the autofluorescence spectrum of all the fluorophores contained in the brain tissues (Drezek et al., 2001a,b; Trujillo et al., 1998). Since in vitro measurements were made in brain tissue samples extracted under anesthesia, the fluorescence properties of the utilized anesthetics were considered as well. The substances were sodium thiopental, fentanyl, pancuronium, suxamethonium, and sevoflurane. Following excitation, sodium thiopental, pancuronium, and fentanyl do not show fluorescence emission. Suxamethonium affects the tryptophan side-chain chromophores, and sevoflurane quenches tryptophan fluorescence and reversibly increases NADH fluorescence (Ramanujam et al., 1994; Utzinger et al., 1999). The anesthetics are distributed in both normal brain tissue and the tumor, so that their contribution to the autofluorescence spectrum may be detected in both cases. It might be that their concentration in the tumor is higher, in which case LIF signals would be stronger on the tumor side, so that the edge between the normal tissue and the tumor could be more precisely identified.

The tumor samples used for in vitro measurements were extracted by neurosurgical operations performed according to current medical procedures. The normal tissue samples were taken (using standard procedures) from zones around nonruptured aneurisms that had been operated to prevent accidental ruptures. The measurements were made in tissue samples extracted from different brain tumors. A set of tumors and their location in the brain as shown in the CT or MRI images are given in Figs. 14 - 17, which show the brain status before and after tumor extraction.

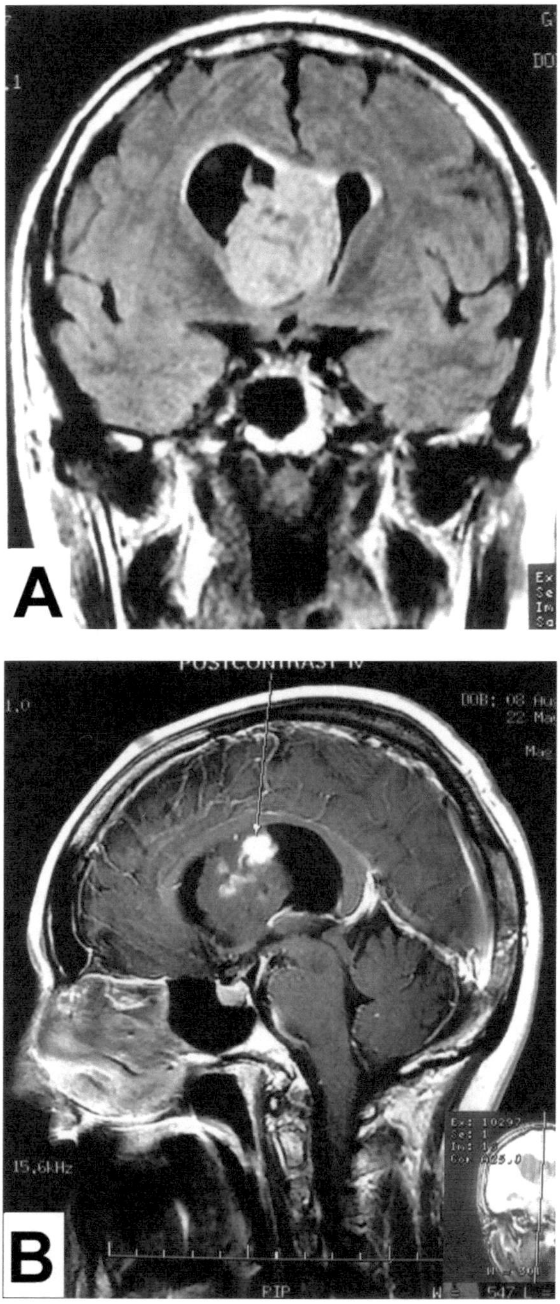

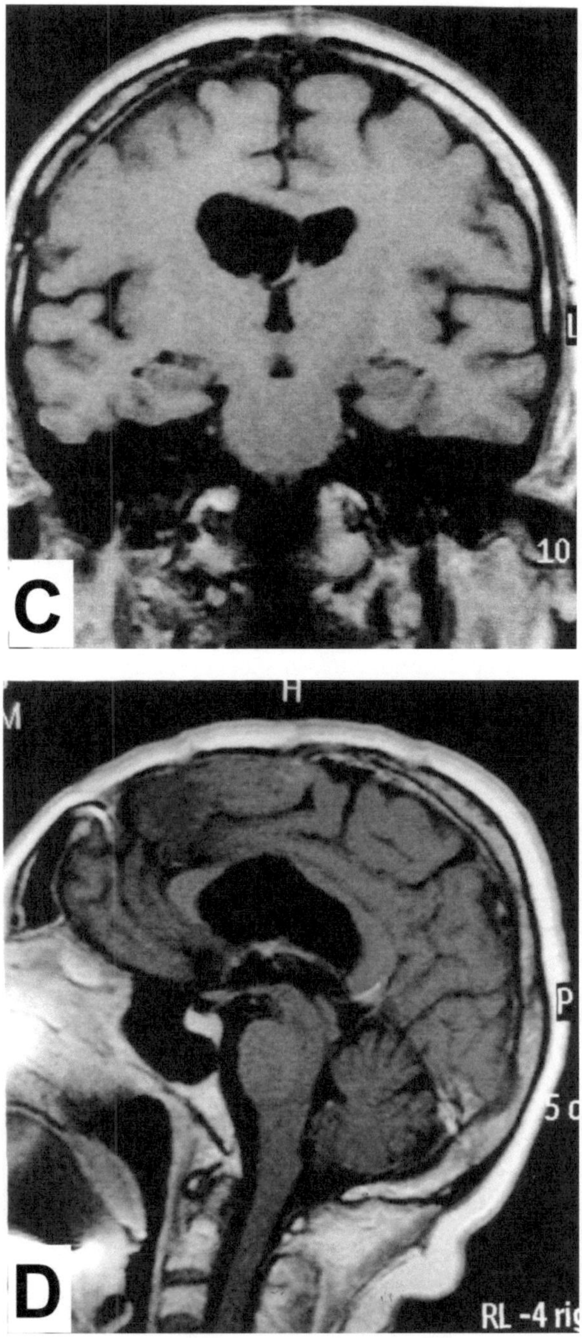

Fig. 14. A and B: Preoperative coronal and sagital T1-weight gadolinium-enhanced MRI, demonstrating of an anterior third ventricle tumor (astrocytoma); C and D: Images obtained after complete removal of the tumor making excision thorugh a midline transcallosal approach (surgeon Leon Danaila).

A typical autofluorescence curve for a normal tissue excited at 337.1 nm is shown in Fig. 18, measured under the conditions specified in paragraph 2.3.2; the emission peak is located at 460- 470 nm, and the curve shape shows a possible contribution of NADH, flavin, and porphyrin. Similar autofluorescence spectra were measured in different samples of normal brain tissue, excited at 337.1 nm. The curves are slightly different from each other, which show a relative variability and a low reproducibility of the autofluorescence signals from one patient to another. The differences may be due to the different optical properties of the tissues (the relative concentrations of the fluorophores in them, the pH, and the different homogeneity). The detailed studies of a large number of autofluorescence spectra of normal brain tissues excited in the visible and ultraviolet allow the conclusion that the autofluorescence of a brain tissue is not a mathematical sum of the contributions of the fluorophores existing in its structure, because (a) the autofluorescence peaks are quite broad, which makes it difficult to accurately estimate their wavelengths; (b) the different wavelengths to use for autofluorescence excitation (around 340 nm and particularly 337.1 nm) are most recommended due to relatively deeper penetration of the radiation in the tissues and at these wavelengths most fluorophores yield marked fluorescence signals; and (c) spectra differ, although not dramatically, from one brain zone to another and from one patient to another, even under strictly reproducible experimental conditions. These conclusions suggest that in order to use LIF for distinguishing between normal brain and (malignant) tumor tissues in real-time neurosurgical operations, "in situ" measurements for normal/tumor tissue pairs should be made. This could enable a correct evaluation of the tumor boundaries with respect to the normal tissues for each specific case.

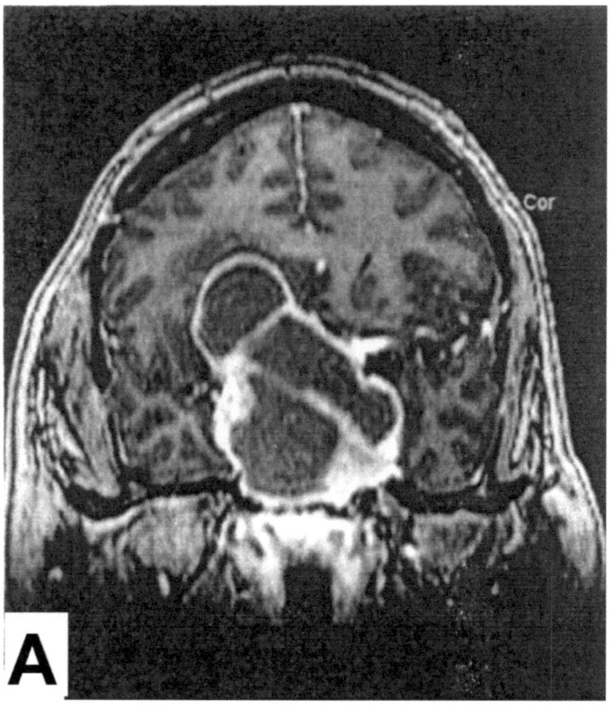

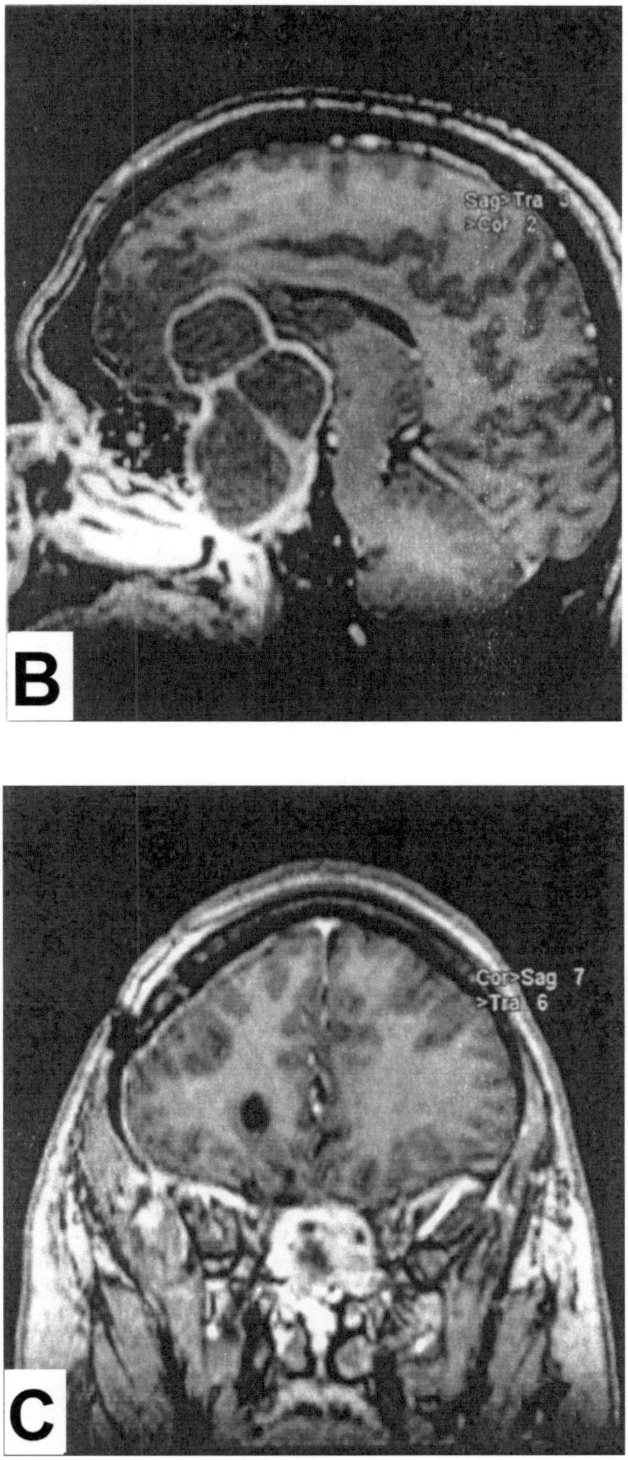
Sag>Tra 3
>Cor 2
B
Cor>Sag 7
>Tra 6
C

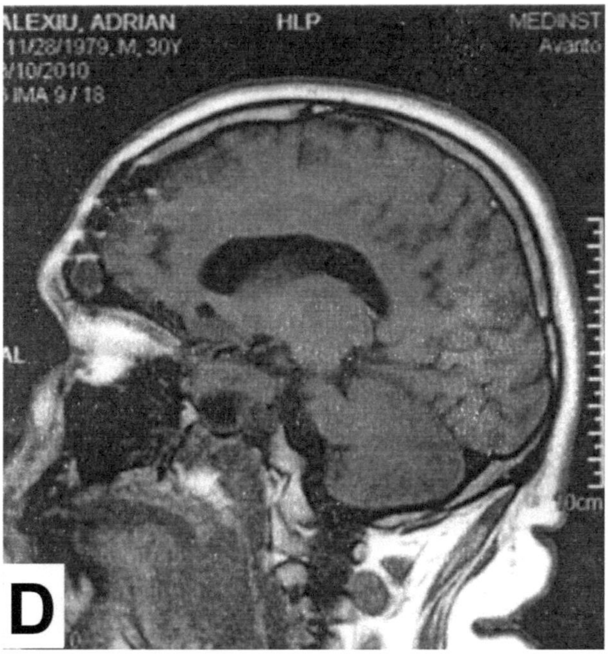

Fig. 15. A and B: Preoperative contrast -enhanced ,T1 -weighted, coronal and sagital MRI scan demonstrated hypointense sellar and suprasellar polycystic lesion a rim of cysts walls enhancement and a region of intracyst enhancement; C and D: T1-weighted coronal and surgical MRI after radical subfrontal resection (surgeon Leon Danaila).

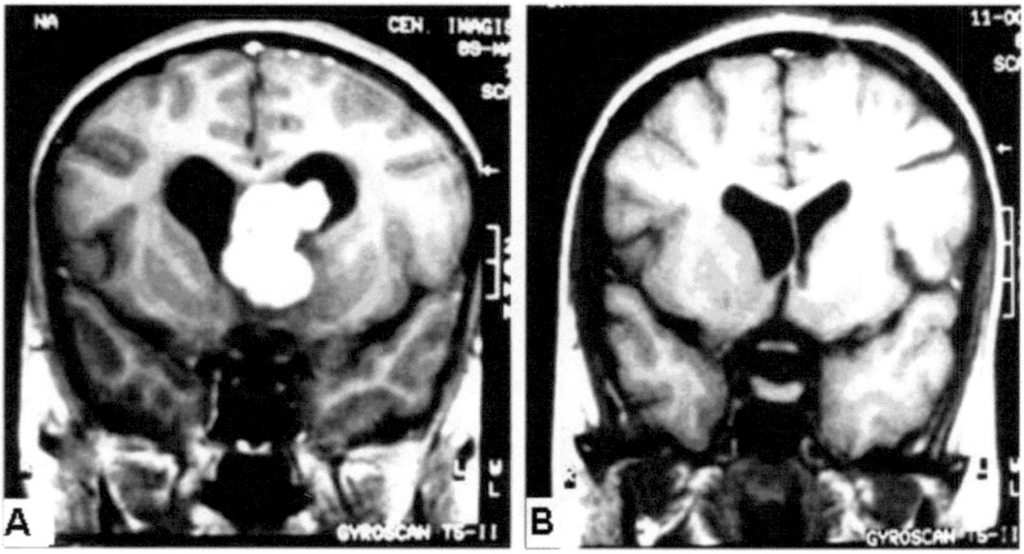

Fig. 16. Large left intraventricular astrocytoma. A: Preoperative contrass-enhanced coronal magnetic resonance imaging scan. B. Postoperative contrast-enhanced resonance imaging scan (surgeon Leon Danaila).

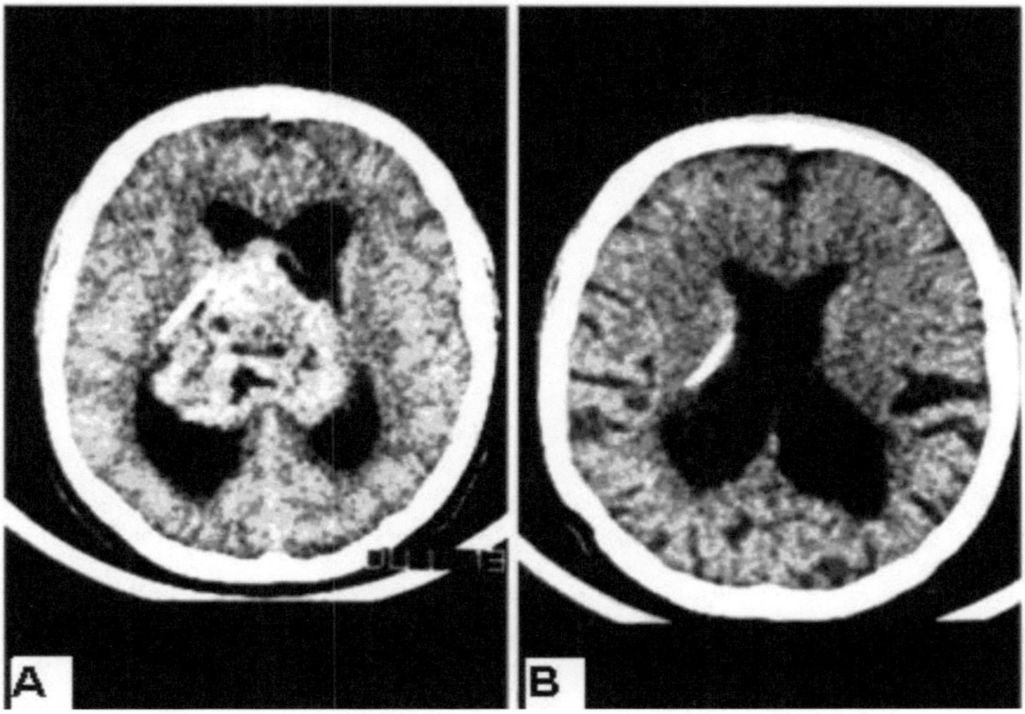

Fig. 17. Intraventricular astrocytoma. A: Preoperative contrast-enhanced axial CT scan demonstrates a heterogeneously enhancing tumor within the lateral ventricle. The patient underwent craniotomy and resection of this tumor through parieto-occipital approach. B: Postoperative CT scan demonstrates resection of the tumor (surgeon Leon Danaila).

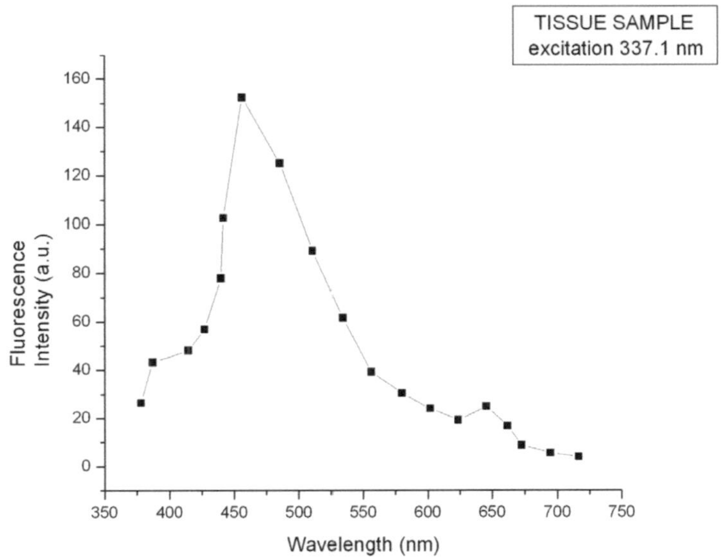

Fig. 18. The autofluorescence emission of a normal brain tissue excited at 337.1 nm.

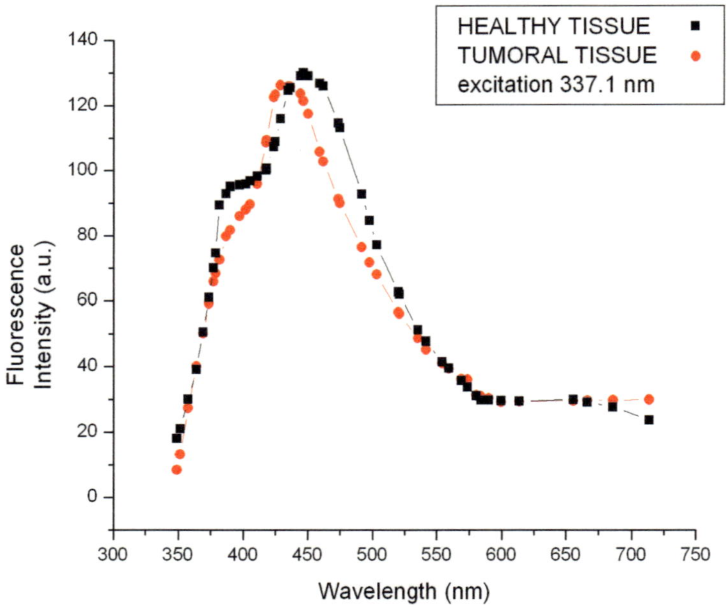

Fig. 19. The autofluorescence emission of a healthy brain tissue and of a barin malignant tumor tissue excited at 337.1 nm.

3.3 Autofluorescence of normal/tumor brain tissue pairs

Measurements were performed on several sample pairs (prepared as mentioned in the 2.3.2 paragraph), each pair consisting of tumor tissue and normal tissue extracted from the same patient. The normal tissue samples were prelevated to avoid zones of brain compression by the tumor. In collecting the samples, different kinds of tumor were chosen, so that the nature of the tumor was not a criterion in selecting the tissues to analyze. Given the fluorophores present in the structure of the brain tissues, and their autofluorescence properties, three wavelengths were selected to excite the autofluorescence: 337.1, 370, and 410 nm.

The measurements performed on homogenates showed that (a) the spectral distribution of the autofluorescence signals for a given homogenate is very close to that of the untreated sample and it is reproducible from one measurement to another; and (b) the autofluorescence spectra of the tumor samples are close to those of normal tissues, but the differences that do exist between them enable identification of the tumor and the normal tissue and consequently their differentiation. The main difference is that for each sample pair the peak autofluorescence spectrum for the normal tissue is shifted with respect to the tumor case. The overall intensity of the autofluorescence is also different for the components of the pair. As an example, Fig. 19 shows the autofluorescence of a normal sample excited at 337.1 nm and the spectrum obtained under the same conditions for the tumor sample. Comparison of the two curves illustrates that the autofluorescence peaks are shifted by 15 nm. The two autofluorescence peaks for the normal tissue are emitted at 390 and 450 nm, the intensity ratio being: $R_{337normal} = I_{450} / I_{390} = 1.44$; for the tumor sample, $R_{337tumor} = I_{450} / I_{390} = 1.31$. Another parameter measured to individualize the autofluorescence curves is the overall intensity, defined as $I_{overall} = \int I(\lambda)$. It is specific for each curve, and is a function of the pumping wavelength. For Fig. 19, $I_{337normal} = 18.298$, respectively, $I_{337tumor} = 12.852$. The above-mentioned quantities (the peak intensity walk-off, the ratio between the main fluorescence peaks, and the overall autofluorescence intensity) may be used as objective parameters to differentiate between normal and tumor brain tissues. For excitation of the samples at 337.1 nm, these parameters differ from the normal to the tumor tissue by 15 nm peak intensity walk-off, 10% variation of the ratio of the peak intensities, and about 40% difference in the overall autofluorescence intensity. The same kind of measurement is made for samples excited at 370 nm. Figure 20 shows the autofluorescence spectra for the normal and tumor samples. The peak intensity ratios for 470 and 525 nm are $R_{370normal} = I_{470} / I_{525} = 1.51$; $R_{370tumor} = I_{470} / I_{525} = 2.09$; the difference is about 40%. Thus, $I_{370normal} = 20.2$ and $I_{370tumor} = 16.4$, a difference of 23%. For the excitation at 410 nm, the obtained autofluorescence spectra are shown in Fig. 21; the respective parameters are $R_{410normal} = 1.45$ and $R_{410tumor} = 2.15$, the difference being 40%;

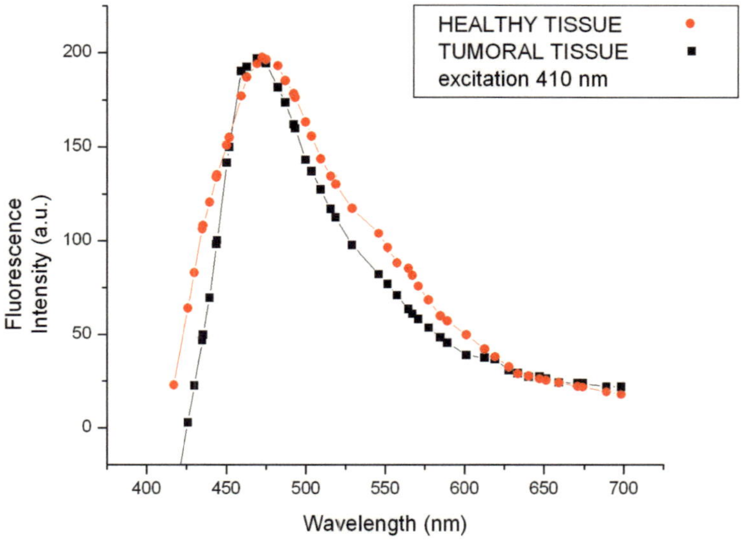

Fig. 20. The autofluorescence spectra for healthy and malignant tumor brain samples (excitation at 410 nm).

$I_{410normal} = 10.52$ and $I_{410tumor} = 16.125$, the difference being 27%.
Another parameter that may be used to distinguish between the normal and the tumor tissue is what we called the quality factor of the fluorescence curve, Q, defined as the ratio between the maximum fluorescence intensity I_{max} and the difference of the two wavelengths where the fluorescence intensity reaches half of its maximum value $\delta \lambda(I_{max}/2)$:

$$Q = I_{max} / \delta \lambda(I_{max}/2)$$

Calculating Q for the curves that represent the fluorescence emission of the two types of tissues at 337.1 nm excitation wavelength (Fig.19), the following values were respectively obtained: $Q_{337norm} = 0.99$ and $Q_{337tum} = 0.67$; these values of the quality factor for the two tissue homogenates differ by about 30%, which qualifies this parameter as a good candidate to describe the spectral differences between the two types of tissue - normal and tumor.

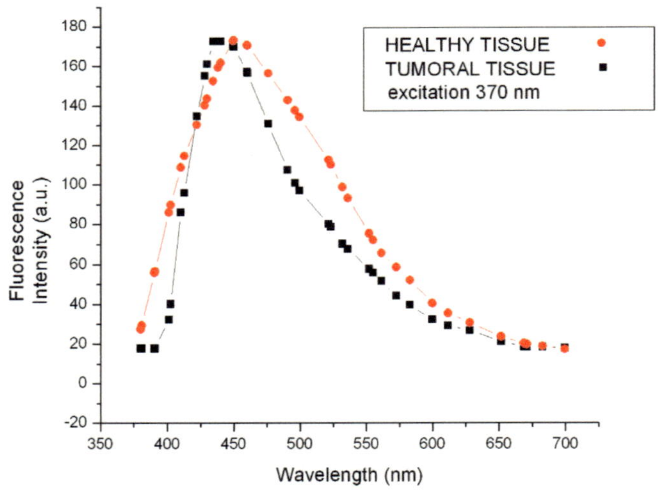

Fig. 21. The autofluorescence spectra for healthy and malignant tumor brain samples (excitation at 370 nm).

Given the fact that:

i. for measuring the pair of the two types of tissue homogenates precautions were taken to insure a reproducible measurement geometry, and

ii. a calibration of the measuring system was performed for each sample measurement the idea of direct subtraction of fluorescence intensity values of the two types of tissue at each wavelength is consistent and do not produce systematic errors.

The result of point by point subtraction of the two autofluorescence curves excited at 337.1 nm shown in Fig.19 is presented as the Figure 22.

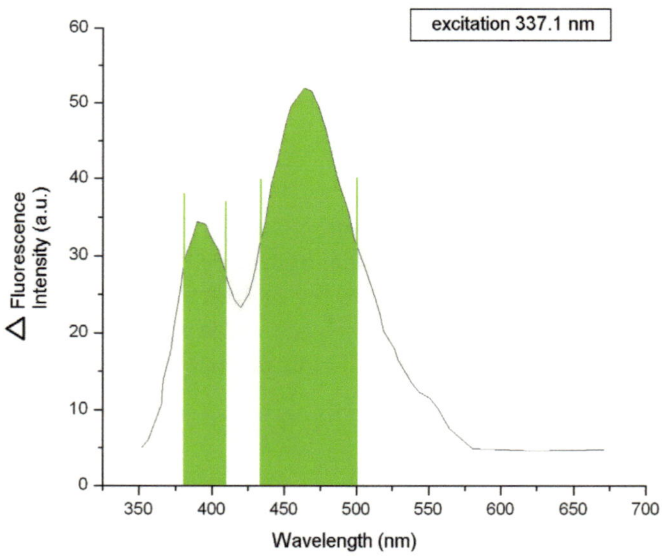

Fig. 22. Difference in autofluorescence spectra between tumor and normal tissue shown in Fig.19. ,Δ Fluorescence Intensity is given in arbitrary units and represents the difference between the autofluorescence signals for each wavelengths .

As results from the Fig. 22, there are two spectral ranges, namely 385 - 415 nm and 460 - 500 nm, within which the difference between the intensity of the fluorescence emitted by the two types of tissue is maximal. This shows the possibility to use this treatment procedure of the pairs of autofluorescence curves to spectrally evidence the difference between the normal and tumor tissue. The difference curve in Fig.22 shows two maxima, at 386 nm and 463 nm wavelengths, respectively. Moreover, at λ = 386 nm the difference of the two intensities is 26% out of the peak of the fluorescence intensity (Fig.19) , while at λ = 463 nm this difference reach even 41% (see Fig.19) , favoring this wavelength. Similar results are obtained from homogenates at excitation wavelengths 370 nm and 410 nm (data not shown).
A summary of all the parameters mentioned in this section (except the subtraction spectrum), computed from the autofluorescence curves obtained for the homogenates of the two types of tissue (normal and tumor) at each of the three excitation wavelengths used, is presented in Table 4.

Excitation Wavelength	Tissue type	Parameter			
		Ratio R	Quality factor Q	Overall intensity I	Walk off of the autofluorescence peak (nm)
337.1 nm	normal	1.44	0.99	18.298	
	tumor	1.31	0.67	12.852	15.0
370 nm	normal	1.51	1.26	20.2	
	tumor	2.09	1.69	16.4	13.0
410 nm	normal	1.45	1.59	10.52	
	tumor	2.15	1.60	16.125	3.0

Table 4. Summary of the parameters used to differentiate between the normal and tumor tissue samples on the base of autofluorescence spectra

In Table 4 are shown only the results obtained when the autofluorescence is excited, respectively, with 3 wavelengths: 337.1 nm (NPL), 370 nm (SHG starting form the fundamental beam at 540 nm) and 410 nm (POPOP). Of course, during the experiments and tests one may select other wavelengths, namely those that may provide the most important differences between the autofluorescence spectra excited for normal and corresponding tumor brain tissues. Although it appears that the type of tumor does not dramatically influence the measuring techniques, it remains that for each such type, a selection of the most suitable parameter to best monitor the differences is made.

4. Discussion

The reported data, correlated with literature reports (Hogan, 2008; Kremer et al., 2009) show that autofluorescence measurements may constitute a promising method to differentiate between brain tumor tissue and normal brain tissue in the same patient.
In this paper it was demonstrated that by comparing the autofluorescence spectra induced by laser radiation in the ultraviolet and visible, brain tumor and normal tissues can be identified and differentiated. The recommended measurements were not performed on tissue samples kept as they were extracted from the brain, but on homogenates to ensure the

best possible reproducibility of the results. It was concluded that the autofluorescence spectra of the tumor samples are close to those obtained for normal tissues, but there are differences between them that allow distinguishing the tumor from normal tissue.

One difference is that for each tumor/normal tissue sample pair the peak autofluorescence for the normal tissue is translated with respect to that for the tumor, typically between 10 and 20 nm; the overall autofluorescence intensity is different for the components of the same pair, the difference being 15–30%.

Another parameter that may be used is the variation of the ratio of some peaks of fluorescence intensity (which correspond to each other) between the normal and the tumor tissue samples. When this parameter can be measured, the variation range is usually between 10% and 40%.

A specific factor that may be used to differentiate between normal and tumor brain tissues is the quality factor of the autofluorescence curves which may vary in the range 1 to 2 for normal tissues and from 0.5 to 1.6 for tumor tissues, function of the laser beam wavelength used to excite the fluorescence.

As for the difference spectra obtained by subtracting the autoflorescence signals in the normal, respectively tumor case, the peaks which are obtained could be used to distinguish between to the types of tissues in real time; on the other hand, it remains to chose the most recommended wavelength to excite the fluorescence, so that the difference spectra exhibit the best resolution of the difference peaks.

Another conclusion is that in vitro experiments show that for the measurements, it is mandatory to use normal /tumor tissue sample pairs taken from the same patient. In our case, for ethical considerations, the samples used were extracted from the brain during medically justified neurosurgical operations, in agreement with operative standards. For studies on normal tissues only, the samples were extracted from normal tissues affected by nonruptured aneurisms in patients who were different from the patients exhibiting malignant brain tumors. The results show that the method may be adapted, after further experimental in vitro tests, to real-time intraoperative conditions by measuring the autofluorescence of the tumor and of the adjacent normal tissue; to do that, it is first necessary to consider the effect of tumor pressure on the molecular content and structure of the adjacent normal tissues. Because real-time investigation does not require tissue extraction, the method could be acceptable to the ethics bodies supervising neurosurgical operations; intraoperative fluorescence guidance for resection of malignant tumors is currently receiving more clinical interest both for imaging purposes (Kantelhardt et al., 2007) and for fast intraoperative diagnostics (Croce et al., 2003; Kremer et al., 2009). The results reported in this paper demonstrate that for neurosurgical clinical use of autofluorescence measurements, the following precautions should be taken: (a) the autofluorescence measurements, either in vitro or in vivo, should be made using tissue pairs: normal/malignant tumor; (b) the contribution of any anesthetic to the measured autofluorescence should always be evaluated, to avoid unexpected interference with the natural autofluorescence of the tissues and errors in data interpretation; the fluorescence emitted by exogenous fluorophores which might be present in the brain area submitted to autofluorescence screening should also be carefully evaluated; (c) in obtaining the autofluorescence spectra, the optimal intensity of the laser excitation beam should be chosen to prevent both damage to the brain tissues and the quadratic Stark broadening of the absorption and fluorescence bands; the latter might induce errors in the accurate measurement of the peak wavelengths and of the overall fluorescence bands.

5. Acknowledgements

The authors would thank Mr. Ionut Relu Andrei for help in processing the CT and MRI images. They acknowledge the funding of this work by VIASAN project No. 125/2001 and ANCS LAPLAS-3/2009 project.

6. References

Andersson-Engels, S.; Brun, A.; Kjellén, E.; Salford, L. G.; Strömblad, L. G.; Svanberg, K.; Svanberg, S. (1989). Identification of brain tumors in rats using laser-induced fluorescence and haematoporphyrin derivative, *Lasers in Medical Science*, Vol. 4, No. 4, pp.241-249.

Andersson-Engels, S.; Johansson, J.; Stenram, U.; Svanberg, K.; Svanberg, S. (1990a). Malignant tumor and atherosclerotic plaque diagnosis using laser-induced fluorescence, *IEEE J Quant. Electronics*, Vol.26, Iss 12, pp.2207-2217. doi: 10.1109/3.64357.

Andersson-Engels, S.; Johansson, J.; Stenramb, U.; Svanberg, K.; Svanberg, S. (1990b). Time-resolved laser-induced fluorescence spectroscopy for enhanced demarcation of human atherosclerotic plaques, *J. Photochem. Photobiol. B: Biology*, Vol. 4, Iss. 4, pp. 363-369. doi:10.1016/1011-1344(90)85015-O

Andersson-Engels, S.; Johansson, J.; Svanberg, S. (1994). Medical diagnostic system based on simultaneous multispectral fluorescence imaging, *Appl Opt*, Vol. 33, pp. 8022-8029. doi:10.1364/AO.33.008022.

Ankerst, J.; Montán, S.; Svanberg, K.; Svanberg, S. (1984). Laser-Induced Fluorescence Studies of Hematoporphyrin Derivative (HPD) in Normal and Tumor Tissue of Rat, *Appl. Spectrosc.* , Vol. 38, pp.890-896.

Bottiroli, G.; Croce, A.; Locatelli, D.; Nano, R.; Giombelli, E.; Messina, A.; Benericetti, E. (1998). Brain tissue autofluorescence: an aid for intraoperative delineation of tumor resection margins. *Cancer Detect Prev*, Vol. 22, No.4, pp. 330–339.

Brewer, M.; Utzinger, U.; Silva, E.; Gershenson, D.; Bast, R. C.; Follen, M.; Richards-Kortum, R. (2001). Fluorescence Spectroscopy for In Vivo Characterization of Ovarian Tissue *Lasers in Surgery and Medicine*, Vol. 29, pp.128-135.

Butte, P. V.; Fang, Q.; Jo, J. A.; Yong, W. H.; Pikul, B. K.; Black, K. L.; Marcu, L. (2010). Intraoperative delineation of primary brain tumors using time-resolved fluorescence spectroscopy, *J Biomed Opt* , Vol.15, pp. 027008. doi:10.1117/1.3374049.

Butte, P.V.; Mamelak, A.N.; Nuno M.; Bannykh S. I.; Black K.L.; Marcu L.(2011).Fluorescence lifetime spectroscopy for guided therapy of brain tumors, *NeuroImage*, Vol. 54, pp. S125–S135.

Croce, A. C.; Fiorani, S.; Locatelli, D.; Nano, R.; Ceroni, M.; Tancioni, F.; Giombelli, E. (2003). Diagnostic potential of autofluorescence for an assisted intraoperative delineation of glioblastoma resectionmargins, *Photochem Photobiol*, Vol. 77, pp.309–318.

Cubillos, S.; Obregon, F.; Vargas, M. F.; Salazar, L. A.; Lima, L. (2006). Taurine concentration in human gliomas and meningiomas: tumoral, peritumoral and extratumoral tissue, *Adv Exp Med Biol* , Vol. 583, pp. 419–422.

Danaila, L. & Pascu, M. L. (1999). Photodynamic therapy of the cerebral malignant tumors, *Rom J Biophys* , Vol. 10, pp.:145–152.

Danaila, L. & Pascu, M, L. (2001). Lasers in neurosurgery. Bucharest: Academia Romana. ISBN 973-27-0802-6.

Drezek, R.; Sokolov, K.; Utzinger, U.; Boiko, I.; Malpica, A.; Follen, M.; Richards-Kortum , R. (2001a). Understanding the contributions of NADH and collagen to cervical tissue fluorescence spectra: modeling, measurements, and implications. J *Biomed Opt* , Vol.6, pp.385–396.

Drezek, R.; Brookner, C.; Pavlova, I.; Boiko, I.; Malpica, A.; Lotan, R.; Follen, M.; Richards-Kortum ,R. (2001b). Autofluorescence microscopy of fresh cervical-tissue sections reveals alterations in tissue biochemistrywith dysplasia. *Photochem Photobiol* , Vol.73, pp.636–641.

Gebhart, S. C.; Majumder, S. K.; Mahadevan-Jansen, A. (2006). Spectral Imaging for Brain Tumor Margin Demarcation, in *Biomedical Optics*, Technical Digest (CD) (Optical Society of America, 2006), paper SG5.

Gong, J.; Yi, J.; Turzhitsky, V. M.; Muro, K.; Li, X. (2008). Characterization of malignant brain tumor using elastic light scattering spectroscopy, *Disease Markers* , Vol. 25, No.6, pp.303-312.

Hogan, H. (2008). Mapping molecular highways: second harmonic generation reveals polarity in neurons, *Biophoton Int* October, pp. 36–37.

Kantelhardt, S. R.; Leppert, J.; Krajewski,; Petkus, N.; Reusche, E.; Tronnier, V. M.; Hüttmann, G.; Giese, A. (2007). Imaging of brain and brain tumor specimens by time-resolved multiphoton excitation microscopy ex-vivo. *Neuro Oncol* , Vol.9, pp.103–112.

Kremer P.; Mahmoudreza, F.; Ding, R.; Pritsch, M.; Zouba, S.; Frei E. (2009). Intraoperative fluorescence staining of malignant brain tumors using 5-aminofluorescein-labelled albumin, *Oper Neurosurg* , Vol. 64, pp.53–61.

Lin, W.-C.; Toms, S. A.; Motamedi, M.; Jansen, E. D.; Mahadevan-Jansen, A. (2000). Brain tumor demarcation using spectroscopy: an in vitrostudy, *J Biomed Opt* , Vol.5, pp.214–220.

Lin, W.-C.; Toms, S. A.; Johnson, M.; Jansen, E. D.; Mahadevan-Jansen, A. (2001). In vivo brain tumor demarcation using optical spectroscopy, *Photochem Photobiol* , Vol.73, pp. 396–402.

Lin, W.-C.; Mahadevan-Jansen, A.; Jansen, E. D.; Toms, S. A.; Steven, A. (2002). Tumor demarcation using optical spectroscopy. *US Pat. 6,377,841.*

Marcu, L.; Jo, J. A.; Butte, P. V.; Yong, W. H.; Pikul, B. K.; Black, K. L.; Thompson ,R. C. (2007). Fluorescence Lifetime Spectroscopy of Glioblastoma Multiforme, *Photochem and Photobiol* , Vol.80, Iss.1, pp.98-103; doi: 10.1111/j.1751-1097.2004.tb00055.

Montán, S.; Svanberg, K.; Svanberg, S. (1985). Multicolor imaging and contrast enhancement in cancer-tumor localization using laser-induced fluorescence in hematoporphyrin-derivative-bearing tissue, *Optics Letters*, Vol. 10, Iss. 2, pp. 56-58. doi:10.1364/OL.10.000056.

Pascu, M. L. (2000). Laser physics. In: Simunovic Z, editor. *Lasers in medicine and dentistry*, Rijeka, Croatia: Vitagraaf d. o. o. ISBN 953-6059-30-4.

Pascu, A.; Romanitan, M. O.; Delgado, J. M.; Danaila, L.; Pascu, M. L. (2009). Laser-induced autofluorescence measurements on brain tissues, *Anatomical Record* , Vol.292, pp. 2013–2022.

Ramanujam, N.; Mitchell, M. F.; Mahadevan, A.; Warren, S.; Thomsen, S.; Silva, E.; Richards-Kortum, R. (1994). In vivo diagnosis of cervical intraepithelial neoplasia using 337-nm-excited laser-induced fluorescence, *Proc Natl Acad Sci USA*, Vol.91, pp.10193–10197.

Ramanujam, N. (2000). Fluorescence spectroscopy in vivo. In: Meyers RA, editor. *Encyclopedia of analytical chemistry*, Chichester: Wiley. pp. 20–56.

Sokolov, K.; Follen, M. M.; Richards-Kortum, R. (2002). Optical spectroscopy for detection of neoplasia, *Curr Opin Chem Biol* , Vol. 6, pp. 651–658.

Sun, Y.; Hatami, N.; Yee, M.; Phipps, J.; Elson, D. S.; Gorin, F.; Schrot, R. J.; Marcu, L. (2010). Fluorescence lifetime imaging microscopy for brain tumor image-guided surgery, *J Biomed Opt* , Vol. 15, pp. 056022. doi:10.1117/1.3486612.

Svanberg, K & Svanberg, S. (1983). Diagnostics and treatment of cancer tumors based on photoactivation of hematoporphyrin derivative (HpD) - A literature survey, Literature survey, Lund Institute of Technology, *Lund Reports on Atomic Physics* LRAP-23, Sweden.

Svanberg, K.; Kjellén, E.; Ankerst, J.; Montán, S.; Sjöholm, E.; Svanberg, S. (1986). Fluorescence studies of hematoporphyrin derivative (HpD) in normal and malignant rat tissue, *Cancer Res.* , Vol. 46, pp. 3803-3808.

Svanberg, S.(1987). Medical diagnostics using laser-induced fluorescence, *Physica Scripta,* Vol. T19, pp.469-475.

Toms, S. A.; Lin, W. C.; Weil, R. J.; Johnson, M. D.; Jansen, E. D.; Mahadevan-Jansen, A. (2005). Intraoperative Optical Spectroscopy Identifies Infiltrating Glioma Margins with High Sensitivity, *Neurosurgery* , Vol.57, Iss 4, pp. 382-391. doi: 10.1227/01.NEU.000176855.39826.2D.

Trujillo, E. V.; Sandison, D. R.; Utzinger, U.; Ramanujam, N.; Follen-Mitchell, M.; Richards-Kortum, R. (1998). Method to determine tissue fluorescence efficiency in vivo and predict signal-to-noise ratio for spectrometers, *Appl Spectrosc* , Vol. 52, pp. 943–951.

Utzinger, U.; Trujillo, E. V.; Atkinson, E. N.; Mitchell, M. F.; Cantor, S. B.; Richards-Kortum, R. (1999). Performance estimation of diagnostic tests for cervical precancer based on fluorescence spectroscopy: effects of tissue type, sample size, population, and signal-to-noise ratio, *IEEE Trans Biomed Eng*, Vol.46, pp. 1293–1303.

Valeur, B. (2001). Molecular fluorescence: principles and applications. Weinheim: Wiley.

Wu, T.; Qu, J. Y. ; Cheung, T.-H.; Lo, K. W.-K. (2003). Preliminary study of detecting neoplastic growths in vivo with real-time calibrated autofluorescence imaging, *Opt Exp* , Vol.11, pp. 291–298.

Yong, W.; Butte, P. V.; Pikul, B. K.; Jo, J. A.; Fang, Q.; Papaioannou, T.; Black, K. L.; Marcu, L. (2006). Distinction of brain tissue, low-grade and high-grade glioma with time-resolved fluorescence spectroscopy, *Front Biosci* , Vol. 11, pp. 1255–1263.

Zuluaga, A. F.; Utzinger, U.; Durkin, A.; Fuchs, H.; Gillenwater, A.; Jacob, R.; Kemp, B.; Fan, J.; Richards-Kortum, R. (1999). Fluorescence excitation emission matrices of human tissue: a system for in vivo measurement and method of data analysis, *Appl Spectrosc* , Vol. 53, pp. 302–311.

14

Brain Tumors Diagnostic by Tumor Imaging Agents

Masoud Sadeghzadeh and Fariba Johari Daha
Nuclear Science & Technology Research Institute
Iran

1. Introduction

Diagnostic nuclear medicine (NM) is among the imaging procedures (together with X-ray, computerized tomography, magnetic resonance, and echography) the clinicians can routinely adopt to image organs or tissues and related disorders. In this chapter, we will describe the role of nuclear medicine imaging in diagnosis of the brain tumors, application of metal complex-carbohydrates for this purpose and review how these imaging approaches can contribute to the diagnosis of disease. The chapter is organized into the following sections:

1. Background
2. Current state of nuclear medicine imaging for brain tumor imaging
3. Introduction another new compounds for brain tumor imaging

2. Background

2.1 Brain tumor

The brain tumor experience can be a journey into an unknown land filled with uncertainty. Brain tumors occurs when brain cells become abnormal and form cells in an uncontrolled manner. These extra brain cells form into a mass of tissue, also known as a tumor, which can be a classified as benign brain tumor, a mass of extra cells that are harmless and have distinct boundaries, or malignant, a mass of extra cells that are life-threatening and either cancerous or located in a vital brain area. For the most part, malignant brain tumors are indicative of cancer and the American Cancer Society estimate that malignant brain tumors will result in approximately 13,100 deaths (1.4% of all cancer deaths) in 2004. Although there are a number of different methods to classify brain tumors, the best way to distinguish between brain tumors is by classifying them as primary brain tumors and secondary brain tumors. A brain tumor diagnosis usually involves several steps, which can include a neurological examination, brain scan(s) and/or a biopsy and nuclear medicine imaging.

2.2 Brain tumor diagnosis methods

Identifying a brain tumor usually involves a neurological examination, brain scans, and/or an analysis of the brain tissue. Doctors use the diagnostic information to classify the tumor from the least aggressive (benign) to the most aggressive (malignant). In most cases, a brain tumor is named for the cell type of origin or its location in the brain. Identifying the type of tumor helps doctors determine the most appropriate course of treatment.

A *neurological examination* is a series of tests to measure the function of the patient nervous system and physical and mental alertness. If responses to the exam are not normal, the doctor may order a brain scan or refer the patient to a neurologist or neurosurgeon, who will then order a brain scan.

A *brain scan* is a picture of the internal structures in the brain. A specialized machine takes a scan in much the same way a digital camera takes a photograph. Using computer technology, a scan compiles an image of the brain by photographing it from various angles. Some types of scans use a contrast agent (or contrast dye), which helps the doctor see the difference between normal and abnormal brain tissue. The contrast agent is injected into a vein and flows into brain tissue. Abnormal or diseased brain tissue absorbs more dye than normal healthy tissue. The most common scans used for diagnosis are as follows:

a. *MRI (Magnetic Resonance Imaging)* is a scanning device that uses magnetic fields and computers to capture images of the brain on film.
b. *CT or CAT Scan (Computed Tomography)* combines sophisticated x-ray and computer technology. CT can show a combination of soft tissue, bone, and blood vessels. CT images can determine some types of tumors, as well as help detect swelling, bleeding, and bone and tissue calcification. Usually, iodine is the contrast agent used during a CT scan.
c. *Nuclear Medicine Imaging* provides a picture of the brains activity, rather than its structure. Nuclear medicine imaging non-invasively provides functional information at the molecular and cellular level that contributes to the determination of health status by measuring the uptake and turnover of target-specific radiotracers in tissue. These functional processes include tissue blood flow and metabolism, protein—protein interactions, expression of cell receptors in normal and abnormal cells, cell—cell interactions, neurotransmitter activity, cell trafficking and homing, tissue invasion, and programmed cell death. By providing information on these processes, nuclear medicine imaging offers a broad array of tools for probing normal and disease-related states of tissue function and response to treatment. The addition of anatomic imaging provided by computed tomography (CT) to functional imaging of positron emission tomography (PET) and single photon emission computed tomography (SPECT) has further expanded the utility and accuracy of nuclear medicine imaging (Committee on State of the Science of Nuclear Medicine, 2007).
d. *Molecular imaging* is expected to have a major impact on the treatment and management of brain tumors.

2.3 Diagnostic nuclear medicine and imaging techniques

Nuclear medicine is a highly multi-disciplinary specialty that develops and uses instrumentation and radiopharmaceuticals to study physiological processes and non-invasively diagnose, stage, and treat diseases. A radiopharmaceutical is either a radionuclide alone, such as iodine-131 (table1) or a radionuclide that is attached to a carrier molecule (a drug, protein, or peptide) or particle, which when introduced into the body by injection, swallowing, or inhalation accumulates in the organ or tissue of interest. In a nuclear medicine scan, a radiopharmaceutical is administered to the patient, and an imaging instrument that detects radiation is used to show biochemical changes in the body. Nuclear medicine imaging, in contrast to imaging techniques that mainly show anatomy (e.g., conventional ultrasound, computed tomography [CT], or magnetic resonance imaging [MRI]), can provide important quantitative functional information about normal tissues or disease conditions in living subjects. For treatment, highly targeted radiopharmaceuticals may be used to deposit lethal radiation at tumor sites (Committee on State of the Science of Nuclear Medicine, 2007).

Application	Radionuclide	Half-Life	Type of Radiation Emitted	Imaging Technique Used
Imaging	Carbon-11	20.33 min	Positron	PET
"	Nitrogen-13	9.97 min	"	"
"	Oxygen-15	2.04 min	"	"
"	Fluorine-18	109.75 min	"	"
"	Technetium-99m	6.02 hours	gamma	SPECT
"	Indium-111	2.8 days	"	"
"	Iodine-123	13 hours	"	"
"	Thallium-201	73 hours	"	"
Therapy	Iodine-131	8 days	beta	
"	Yttrium-90	2.7 days	"	

Table 1. Commonly used radionuclides for imaging and therapy

Diagnostic nuclear medicine (DNM) is among the imaging procedures (together with X-ray, computerized tomography, magnetic resonance, and echography) the clinicians can routinely adopt to image organs or tissues and related disorders. In spite of many advances in diagnosis and therapy, brain tumors still represent a serious challenge for clinicians. Today, contrast-enhanced CT or MRI is the first examination performed in a patient with symptoms typical of brain tumor (i.e. nausea, headache, seizure or focal neurological signs). Both MRI and CT allow exactly localizing brain neoplasia and defining the extension of the tumoral mass to the surrounding normal tissue. Nevertheless, these techniques present some limitations, especially regarding patients' follow-up after treatments when discrimination between tumor recurrence-persistence versus scar tissue is required. In such cases, nuclear functional imaging by PET (Positron Emission Tomography) and SPECT (Single Photon Emission Computed Tomography) was successfully proposed to obtain a metabolic characterization of the morphological lesions detected by MRI or CT scan. By using combined-modality PET/CT and SPECT/CT devices, functional processes can be localized within the body to an anatomically identified or, in some instances, as yet unidentifiable structural alteration. These devices have enhanced the accuracy with which disease can be detected, aided in the determination of the extent and severity of disease, enhanced the accuracy for identifying disease-related risk, and improved the ability to monitor patient response to therapy (Committee on State of the Science of Nuclear Medicine, 2007). In diagnostic nuclear medicine two techniques are used for imaging of tumors:

a. PET (Positron Emission Tomography)

One of the most important uses of Positron Emission Tomography (PET) technology is its use in diagnosing and treating brain tumors by measuring the rate at which a tumor absorbs glucose derivatives or amino acids. In cases where structural change has been detected through MRI or CT, a physician often uses PET imaging to determine the nature of the detected structural changes. The PET scan measures the brains activity and sends this information to a computer, which creates a live image. Doctors use PET scans to see the difference between scar tissue, recurring tumor cells, and necrosis (cells destroyed by radiation treatment). PET imaging is a non-invasive diagnostic imaging tool that has an advantage over anatomical imaging tools in that it is a metabolic imaging tool that is able to distinguish between benign and malignant tumors. It is often used to accurately determine the stage of the brain tumor. Brain tumor PET imaging involves the administration of a radioactive tracer that is a combination of a radioisotope (a radioactive compound such as ^{18}F or ^{11}C whose movements are detectable by a PET scanner) with a natural body compound. When used in brain tumor scanning, the radioactive tracer used in PET is Fluorodeoxyglucose (FDG), which combines the natural body compound glucose with the radioisotope Fluorine-18. This radioactive tracer, or radiopharmaceutical, is used in brain PET imaging as the radioactive compound that it uses has a short half-life that will disappear from the body within hours.

The routinely used PET radiotracer ^{18}F-fluorodeoxyglucose (FDG) proved useful to diagnose primary brain tumors and their recurrences; moreover, the entity of FDG uptake was found to correlate with brain tumor histology. Nevertheless, FDG is physiologically taken by normal brain tissue, so this radiotracer is less accurate in detecting very low grade gliomas due to their relatively low target to background uptake ratio. To overcome the drawbacks of FDG, ^{11}C-methionine was applied in brain tumors imaging. Its uptake is related to the increased amino acid transport and protein synthesis and it is accumulated in the neoplastic lesion and not in the normal parenchyma. Actually, ^{11}C-methionine proved useful to visualize low grade gliomas not detected by FDG (Filippi et al., 2005).

PET and Brain Tumor Follow-Up

Besides brain tumor staging, Positron Emission Tomography is a valuable tool in brain tumor treatment when it is used as a follow-up to brain tumor treatment. Brain tumors are a difficult to fully treat due to the sensitivity of its location. Therefore, brain tumor recurrence is often possible. Imaging tests such as magnetic resonance imaging (MRI) and computed tomography (CT) are able to be used to detail structural changes, such as tumor formation, in the brain. However, these imaging tests often detect structural changes caused by side effects from previous brain tumor treatments, such as surgery or radiation therapy.

b. SPECT (Single Photon Emission Computed Tomography)

Although PET technology is becoming more and more available in many institutions, its diffusion is still limited and it presents very high cost. Moreover, in the case of ^{11}C-methionine an in situ cyclotron should be available due to the short ^{11}C physical half-life. Because the production of ^{18}F requires a cyclotron and the isotope has a short (110 min) half-life, its utility is somewhat limited compared to that of single photon emission computed tomography (SPECT) in nuclear medicine. Although conventional scintigraphy (i.e. single photon emission tomography [SPECT] and planar images) presents lower spatial resolution when compared to PET, the high diffusion of Anger camera, the device used to perform conventional scintigraphy, has accounted for the search of γ-emitting radiotracers as brain tumors imaging agents. In terms of developing novel drugs for use in diagnostic and therapeutic brain tumor in nuclear medicine, it would be of great interest to label sugars (such as glucose and analogue derivatives) and amino acids with the transition metal isotopes (such as ^{99m}Tc, $^{186/188}Re$, ^{201}Tl, ^{123}I, *etc.*) to substitute the expensive but readily used ^{18}F-labeled 2-deoxyglucose (^{18}F-FDG) for localization of tumor and metastatic tissue. ^{201}Tallium was firstly used to detect cerebral neoplasia showing high sensitivity but relatively low specificity mainly due to its physical characteristics suboptimal for imaging with Anger camera (Filippi et al., 2005).

3. Current state of diagnostic nuclear medicine for brain tumor imaging

3.1 Anatomic imaging procedures (CT scan and MRI)

Anatomic imaging procedures (computed tomography [CT] and magnetic resonance imaging [MRI]) have become essential tools for brain tumor assessment. Serial MRI is routinely performed in these patients after primary treatment to detect tumor recurrence. However, conventional contrast-enhanced CT scans or MRI cannot reliably distinguish radiation necrosis from recurrent tumor. Both entities can cause extensive edema and blood–brain barrier disruption that result in mass effect and abnormal contrast enhancement.2,3 Radiation-induced necrosis often occurs within 2 years after radiation therapy, the same time frame during which tumor recurrence is most frequent. Differentiation between tumor progression and radiation necrosis carries obvious prognostic and therapeutic implications. To overcome this problem, several functional and physiological imaging techniques, such as MR spectroscopy (MRS), perfusion-weighted MRI, positron emission tomography (PET), and thallium-201 single-photon emission computed tomography (^{201}Tl-SPECT) have been examined for clinical use (Tie et al., 2008).

3.2 Functional imaging procedures (PET and SPECT)

Using anatomical imaging modalities, such as computed tomography (CT) or magnetic resonance imaging (MRI), it is difficult to differentiate tumor recurrence from necrosis induced by radiotherapy or other treatments. Functional imaging of the brain, in the form single photon emission computed tomography (SPECT) utilizing various "tumor seeking" tracers, is the most commonly performed investigation to differentiate recurrence from necrosis (Barai et al., 2005). Functional imaging procedures (positron emission tomography [PET] and singe-photon emission computed tomography [SPECT]) can provide additional information useful during the diagnostic workup to determine the degree of malignancy and as a substitute or guide for biopsy. After surgery and/or radiotherapy, nuclear medicine examinations are essential to assess persistence of tumor, to differentiate recurrence from radiation necrosis and gliosis, and to monitor the disease. The combination of functional images with anatomic ones is of the utmost importance for a full evaluation of these patients, which can be obtained by means of imaging fusion. Brain imaging is performed using radiopharmaceuticals by single photon emission computed tomography (SPECT) and positron emission tomography (PET). SPECT and PET radiopharmaceuticals are classified according to blood-brain-barrier permeability, cerebral perfusion and metabolism receptor-binding, and antigen-antibody binding.

3.2.1 PET radiopharmaceuticals

PET radiopharmaceuticals for brain imaging are commonly labeled with positron-emitters such as ^{11}C, ^{13}N, ^{15}O, and ^{18}F, although other radionuclides such as ^{82}Rb, ^{62}Cu and ^{68}Ga also were used. The brain uptake of [^{13}N]glutamate, [^{68}Ga]EDTA and [^{82}Rb]RbCl depends on the BBB permeability, but these are rarely used for brain imaging. Several cerebral perfusion agents have been introduced, of which [^{15}O]water, [^{13}N]ammonia, and [^{15}O]butanol have been used more frequently. Regional CBF has been quantitated by using these tracers in normal and different cerebral disease states. Other perfusion agents include [^{15}O]O_2, [^{11}C]CO, [^{11}C[CO_2, [^{18}F]fluoromethane, [^{15}O]O_2, [^{11}C]butanol, and [^{62}Cu]PTSM. Among the PET cerebral metabolic agents, [^{18}F]fluoro-deoxyglucose (FDG) is most commonly used to detect metabolic abnormalities in the brain. Various brain tumors have been graded by

[^{18}F]FDG PET. This technique was used to detect epileptic foci by showing increased uptake in the foci during the ictal period and decreased uptake in the interictal period. Differentiation between recurrent tumors and radiation necrosis and the detection of Alzheimer's disease have been made successfully by [^{18}F]FDG PET. Other PET metabolic agents such as [^{11}C]deoxyglucose, and [^{11}C]methylmethionine have drawn attention in the detection of brain tumors. [^{18}F]fluorodopa is a cerebral neurotransmitter agent, which has been found very useful in the detection of Parkinson disease that shows reduced uptake of the tracer in the striatum of the brain. The distribution of different receptors in the brain and their alteration in different disease states are assessed by using different receptor-binding PET radiotracers such as [^{11}C]methylspiperone, [^{18}F]fluoroethylspiperone, [^{18}fluoropropylspiperone, [^{11}C]carfentanil, [^{11}C]diprenorphine, [^{11}C]raclopride, [^{11}C]flumasenil, and so on (Saha et al., 1994).

3.2.2 SPECT radiopharmaceuticals

Despite the fast-growing diffusion of PET, in most cases of brain tumors, SPECT studies are adequate and provide results that parallel those obtained with PET. The main limitation of SPECT imaging with brain tumor-seeking radiopharmaceuticals is the lack of precise anatomic details; this drawback is overcome by the fusion with morphological studies that provide an anatomic map to scintigraphic data. In the past, software-based fusion of independently performed SPECT and CT or MRI demonstrated usefulness for brain tumor assessment, but this process is often time consuming and not practical for everyday nuclear medicine studies. The recent development of dual-modality integrated imaging systems, which allow the acquisition of SPECT and CT images in the same scanning session, and their coregistration by means of the hardware, has facilitated this process. In SPECT studies of brain tumors with various radiopharmaceuticals, fused images are helpful in providing the precise localization of neoplastic lesions, and in excluding the disease in sites of physiologic tracer uptake. This information is useful for optimizing diagnosis, therapy monitoring, and radiotherapy treatment planning, with a positive impact on patient management. Imaging Fusion of SPECT Studies (Schillaci et al., 2007):

1. ^{201}Tl
2. ^{99m}Tc Sestamibi
3. ^{99m}Tc Tetrofosmin
4. ^{123}I-Alpha-Methyl-Tyrosine
5. ^{111}In-Pentetreotide
6. Labeled Leukocytes

a. Clinical used radiopharmaceuticals

The blood-brain-barrier (BBB) SPECT agents, such as $^{99m}TcO_4^-$ [^{99m}Tc]DTPA, ^{201}Tl and [^{67}Ga]citrate are excluded by normal brain cells, but enter into tumor cells because of altered BBB. These agents were used in the earlier period for the detection of brain tumors. SPECT perfusion agents such as [^{123}I]IMP, [^{99m}Tc]HMPAO, [^{99m}Tc]ECD are lipophilic agents and therefore, diffuse into the normal brain. These tracers have been successfully used to detect various cerebrovascular diseases such as stroke, Parkinson disease, Huntington's disease, epilepsy, dementia, and psychiatric disorders. Xenon-133 and radiolabeled microspheres have been used for the measurement of cerebral blood flow (CBF). Important receptor-binding SPECT radiopharmaceuticals include [^{123}I]QNE, [^{123}I]IBZM, and [^{123}I]iomazenil. These tracers bind to specific receptors in the brain, thus displaying their distribution in various receptor-related cerebral diseases. Radioiodinated monoclonal antibodies were used for the detection of brain tumors.

A variety of radiolabeled amino acids have been developed as potential tumor imaging agents for positron emission tomography (PET) and single photon emission computerized tomography (SPECT). Many radiolabeled amino acids developed for tumor imaging enter cells via the A-type (sodium dependent) and/or the L-type (sodium independent) transport systems, which are upregulated in many neoplasms. The L-type substrate $[^{123}I]$IMT represents the most widely used amino acid for tumor imaging with SPECT (Yu et al., 2008).

MIBI and Tetrofosmin are technetium labeled compounds which were firstly introduced as imaging agent for myocardial scintigraphy. These two radiopharmaceuticals are passively accumulated in cells characterized by high metabolic activity so they have been successfully used also in oncology (i.e. lung, parathyroid, breast cancer). Regarding brain tumors imaging, MIBI was widely applied in diagnosis and follow-up, while few experiences were performed using Tetrofosmin. MIBI was proved useful to detect intracranial tumors before therapy with higher sensitivity and specificity for gliomas than for the other histologies (i.e. lymphomas). Moreover, the entity of MIBI uptake was found to be related to the grade of malignancy of gliomas. In patients' follow-up, MIBI scintigraphy showed great diagnostic accuracy to discriminate tumor recurrence versus scar tissue also when compared to CT scan. As MIBI is a substrate of Pgp, it was proposed to diagnose chemoresistance in brain tumors patients. Nevertheless, the preliminary experiences suggest that Pgp expression is inversely related to the grade of malignancy of gliomas so that Pgp seems not to be the main cause of chemoresistance in these tumors. Tetrofosmin scintigraphy presents similar characterisitics in sensitivity and specificity as MIBI, so it may represent a suitable tool to image brain tumors (Filippi et al., 2005).

b. New research radiopharmaceuticals

Flourine-18 (^{18}F) fluorodeoxyglucose (FDG) has been used to measure normal tissue and tumor glucose utilization rates. Although metabolic tumor imaging with $[^{18}F]$-FDG has been studied for more than two decades, the use of this examination in clinical practice is still limited by factors such as difficult access, limited availability, and high cost. In addition, positron emission tomography (PET) radiosynthesis must be performed rapidly because the half-life of ^{18}F is only 109 min. Thus, it would be very desirable to develop less costly imaging agents based on γ-emitter isotopes, especially for developing countries, where single photon emission computed tomography (SPECT) is still dominant. Technetium-99m (^{99m}Tc) has been mostly used for radiopharmaceuticals labeling due to its suitable physical and chemical characteristics and inexpensive isotope cost. Organometallic metal cores often exhibit advantages in terms of kinetic inertness, stability, and size and thus could lead to the development of more efficient and stable compounds compared to classical inorganic complexes. We elected to use the versatile low valent fac-$[^{99m}Tc(I)\text{-}(CO)_3]$ core, which its chemistry has recently been pioneered by Alberto and co-workers. The facially coordinated carbonyl ligands stabilize the Tc^{+1} oxidation state, obviating the elaborate, often macrocyclic, polydentate structures required to stabilize other intermediate oxidation states of Tc. In neutral complexes with simple N,O donors the fac-$[^{99m}Tc(I)\text{-}(CO)_3]$ core possesses intermediate lipophilicity, an advantage in living systems. Lots of ^{99m}Tc-labeled glucose derivatives have been synthesized in order to develop one subrogate in SPECT for $[^{18}F]$-FDG in PET recently. Developed by Yang, ^{99m}Tc-labeled ethylenedicysteine-deoxyglucose (EC-DG) showed similarities with $[^{18}F]$-FDG in tumor uptake. This suggests that there is feasibility for ^{99m}Tc-labeled deoxyglucose as a metabolic tumor imaging agent. However, [^{99m}Tc]-EC-DG still has some drawbacks such as slow cleanup from the blood, which would cause high background activity; and large molecular weight, which would limit its penetration through blood–brain barrier (BBB). Thus, it would be desirable to develop a smaller ^{99m}Tc based deoxyglucose derivative with rapid blood clearance and still maintaining its high tumor uptake. In terms of developing novel drugs for use in diagnostic nuclear medicine, it would be of great interest to label glucosamine derivatives with ^{99m}Tc to substitute the expensive but readily used ^{18}F-labeled 2-deoxy glucose (^{18}F-FDG) for localization of tumor and metastatic tissue. ^{99m}Tc Due to the ideal decay properties, low cost production is used the most frequently in nuclear medicine today. Reported by Sadeghzadeh, three glucosamine derivatives showed negligible to moderate brain uptake similar to ^{99m}Tc-EC (Johari et al., 2007). Compounds (1) and (2) were prepared in one step by reaction of glucosamine, ethylcholoroformate and 3-chloro-1,2-propandiol as starting materials (Scheme1).

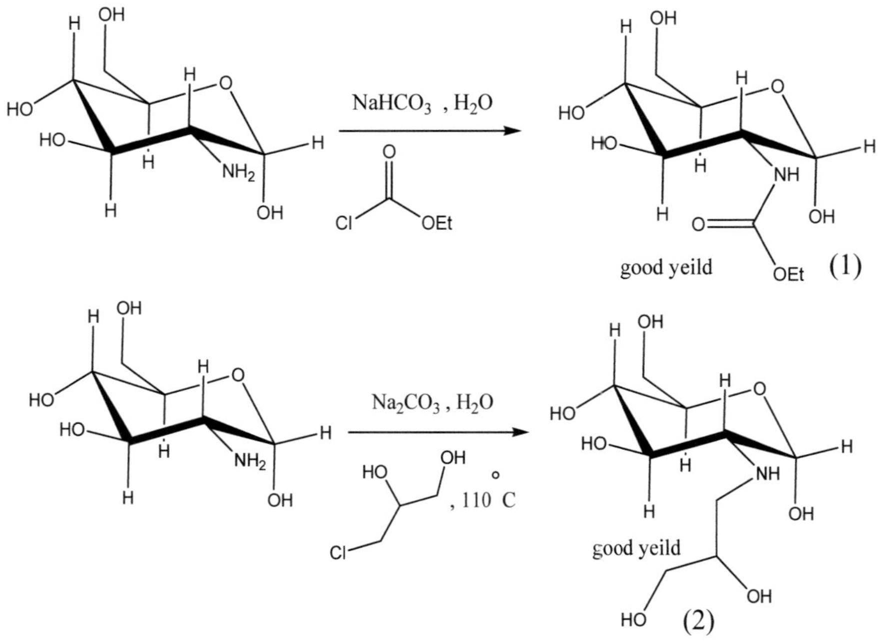

Scheme1. Syntesis of two glucosamine derivatives

The biodistribution of the [^{99m}Tc]-1 and [^{99m}Tc]-2 complexes were studied in normal mice (body mass 25–35 g) at 30 min and 1 h post-injection, according to a published procedure. These complexes showed moderate brain uptake (0.613%±0.03 ID) and (0.512%±0.03 ID) at 30 min post-injection, an efficient clearance from the blood, a rapid excretion to the urine and a low retention in the liver and kidneys. Planar SPECT imaging of the compound1 showed moderate uptake brain in mice after 2 hours administration (Figure 1).

At a same work, the proligand 3 is prepared by thioglycolic acid as a starting material (Scheme2). The biodistribution of the [^{99m}Tc]-(3) complex showed negligible brain uptake (0.13%±0.03 ID) at 30 min post-injection (Johari et al., 2007).

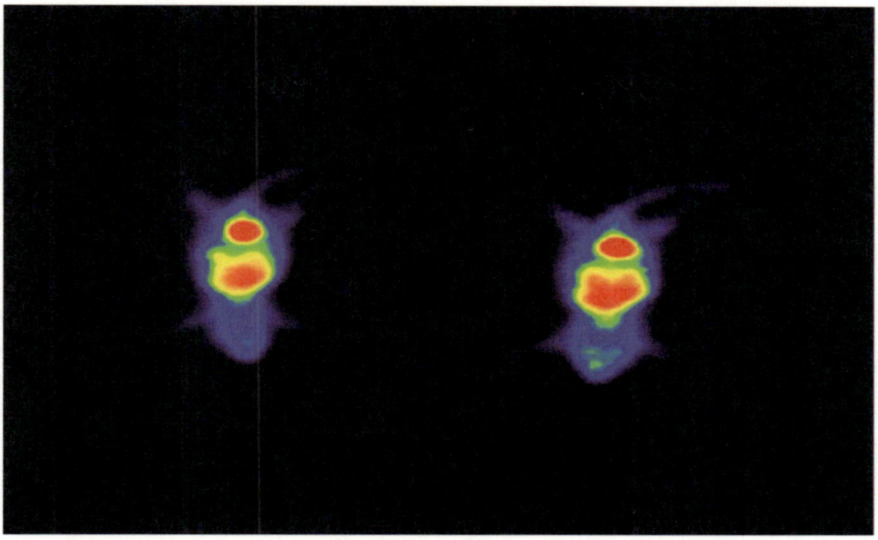

Fig. 1. Planar SPECT imaging of the compound1 after 2 hours administration.

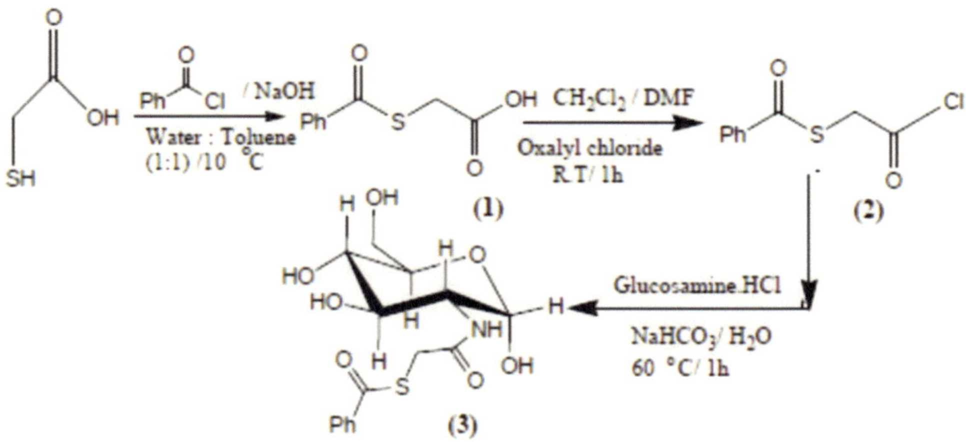

Scheme 2. Synthesis of 2-Amino-2-Deoxy(S-Benzoylthioacetyl)-D-Glucose (3)

4. New imaging agents for brain tumor diagnosis

4.1 Molecular imaging (Phosphatidylserine (PS) as a marker for brain tumor)

Noninvasive molecular-imaging technologies are playing a keyrole in drug discovery, development and delivery. Positron Emission Tomography (PET) is such a molecular imaging technology and a powerful tool for the observation of various diseases. Anionic phospholipids are largely absent from the surface of resting mammalian cells under normal conditions. PS, which is the most abundant anionic phospholipid of the plasma membrane, is tightly segregated to the internal leaflet of the plasma membrane in most cell types.

- Anionic phospholipid-targeting agent

PSVueTM reagents are a family of fluorescent probes containing a bis (Zn^{2+}-dipicolylamine) group (Zn-DPA), a motif that has been found to bind with high affinity to surfaces enriched with anionic phospholipids, especially phosphatidylserine (PS) exposed on cell membranes (Figure 2). The fluorescent part of the probe is a reporter element that provides a means of detecting the probe once it is bound to the membrane of interest. Key features of PSVueTM Probes are following: (I) Bind to a tumor cells which have negatively charged phospholipids exposed on their membranes. (II) Available in a range of detection wavelengths from long-UV to near infrared. (III) Suitable for in vitro and in vivo use. (IV) Suitable for high-throughput screening assays. PSVueTM binds to the same PS site as annexin-V (Qi et al., 2010). Location of PSVue794 in tumor bearing mice revealed by fluorescence imaging. Photon emission from tumors or tissues was detected, digitized and electronically displayed as a pseudocolor overlay onto a gray scale animal image. Luminescence and fluorescence imaging of excised brains was also performed using the IVIS-200 system (Figure 3).

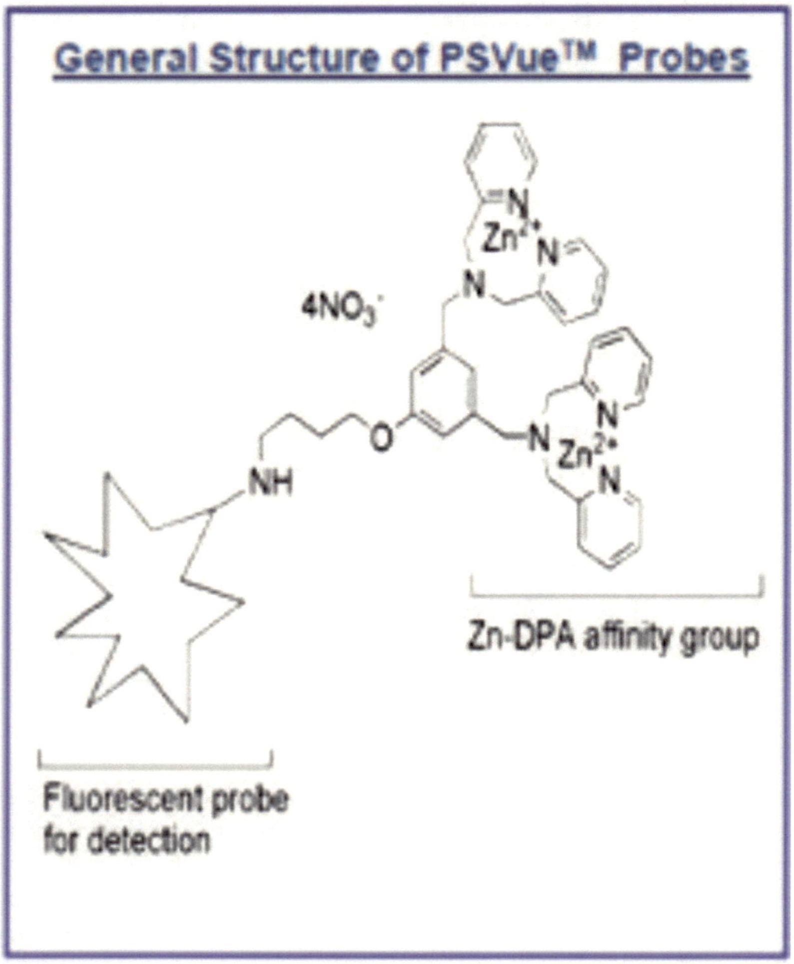

Fig. 2. General structure of PSVue™ Probes

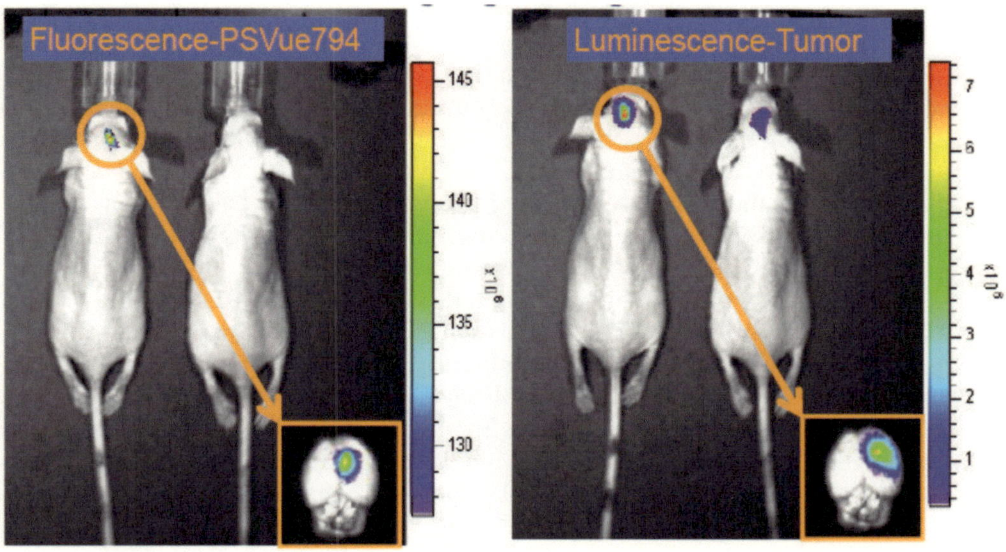

Fig. 3. Brian-Tumor Imaging using PSVue794

Dose-dependent imaging of brain tumor by tail vein injection of PSVue794 for 24 h (Figure 4). Left panel: fluorescence imaging with 1 sec imaging time, 745/840 filter set. Right panel Luminescnece imaging for tumors with 10 sec imaging time.

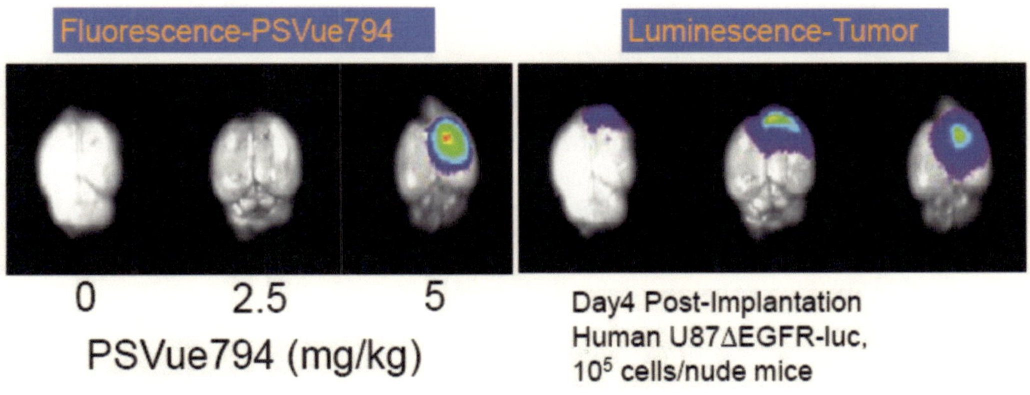

Fig. 4. Dose-Dependent Brain Tumor Imaging

4.2 Nanomedicine techniques

The field of nanomedicine is expected to have a major impact on the treatment and management of brain tumors. Over the past decade, significant efforts have been made in using nanoparticles for diagnosis and treatment of brain tumors. One class of nanoparticles, liposomes, have received considerable attention for use as nanocarriers for delivery of therapeutics and contrast agents.

5. References

Barai S., Rajkamal, Bandopadhayaya G. P., Pant G. S., Haloi A. K., Malhotra A. & Dhanpathi H. 2005. Thallium-201 versus ^{99m}Tc-glucoheptonate SPECT for evaluation of recurrent brain tumors: a within-subject comparison with pathological correlation, *Journal of Clinical Neuroscience,* Vol. 12, No. 1, pp. 27-31.

Committee on State of the Science of Nuclear Medicine, National Research Council. 2007. *Advancing Nuclear Medicine Through Innovation,* THE NATIONAL ACADEMIES PRESS, ISBN: 0-309-11068-8, U.S.A., Washington D.C.

Filippi L., Santoni R., Manni C., Danieli R., Floris R. & Schillaci O. 2005. Imaging Primary Brain Tumors by Single-Photon Emission Computerized Tomography (SPECT) with Technetium-99m Sestamibi (MIBI) and Tetrofosmin, *Current Medical Imaging Reviews,* Vol. 1, No. 1, pp. 61-66, 1573-4056/05.

Johari D. F., Sadeghzadeh M., Charkhlooie A., Ebrahimabadi K. H. & Saidi M. R. 2007. An Improved Synthesis and Preliminary Biodistribution Study of a Technetium-99m-labeled 2-amino-2-deoxy(thioacetyl)-D-glucose Complex ([^{99m}Tc]-TA-DG) As a Tumor Imaging Agent. *Iran J Nucl Med,* Vol. 15, No. 2, September 2007, pp. 43-48.

Qi X., Chu Z., Kaur B., Chiocca A., Gray B. D., Smith B. D. & Pak K. Y. 2010. Anionic Phospholipid-Targeting Agent for Brain Tumor Imaging, *2010 World Molecular Imaging Congress,* Kyoto, Japan, September 8-11.

Schillaci O., Filippi L., Manni C. & Santoni R. *Seminars in Nuclear Medicine,* Vol. 37(1), January 2007, 34-47.

Saha G. B., MacIntyre W. J. & Go R. T. *Seminars in Nuclear Medicine,* Vol. 4(4), October 1994, 324-349.

Tie J., Gunawardana D. H. & Rosenthal M. A. 2008. Differentiation of tumor recurrence from radiation necrosis in high-grade gliomas using ^{201}Tl-SPECT, *Journal of Clinical Neuroscience,* Vol. 15, pp. 1327-1334.

Yu W., Williams L., Malveaux E., Camp V. M., Olsonb J. J. & Goodman M. M. 2008. Synthesis and evaluation of [^{123}I] labeled iodovinyl amino acids syn-, anti-1-amino-3-[2-iodoethenyl]-cyclobutane-1-carboxylic acid, and 1-amino-3-iodomethylene-cyclobutane-1-carboxylic acid as potential SPECT brain tumor imaging agents, *Bioorganic & Medicinal Chemistry Letters, Vol. 18, pp.* 1264 –1268.

15

MR-Based Methods for pH Measurement in Brain Tumors: Current Status and Clinical Potential

Xiao-Fang Cheng[1] and Ren-Hua Wu[1,2]
[1]*Department of Medical Imaging, the 2nd Affiliated Hospital, Shantou University Medical College, Shantou,*
[2]*Provincial Key Laboratory of Medical Molecular Imaging, Guangdong Province, China*

1. Introduction

This study is supported in part by a grant from the National Natural Science Foundation of China (NSFC), key program 30930027. Corresponding to Wu RH.
Alteration in tissue pH is an indicator of many pathological processes. In tumors, the pH gradient exists between the intracellular (pHi) and extracellular (pHe) compartments. pHe is usually lower, and pHi could be higher or unchanging compared with normal tissue, which can be correlated with prognosis and response to treatment. In recent years, non-invasive MR-based methods have been developed to assess tissue pH in brain tumors. In addition to protons (^{1}H) and phosphorus (^{31}P), pH measurement approaches have been applied with other NMR nuclei such as fluorine (^{19}F) and carbon (^{13}C). By using hyperpolarized ^{13}C-labelled bicarbonate, the average tumor interstitial pH was found significantly lower than the surrounding tissue in mouse tumor model. Gd (3+)-based pH sensors and chemical exchange-dependent saturation transfer （CEST） and paramagnetic (PARACEST) agents are useful for further delineation of brain tumors. We use an optimized CEST technique to provide non-invasive pH information for human brain tumors. This article primarily focuses on the measurement of pH in brain tumors with MR-based methods and relevant clinical potential.

2. pH and tumours

As we know, intra- and extracellular pH are regulated in a dynamic steady state driven by metabolic acid production, export of H^+ from cells, and diffusion of these H^+ equivalents from the site of production to the blood, where they are buffered by an open and dynamic CO_2/HCO_3^- system[1]. However, although this balance is quite robust, many pathological states are associated with changes in tissue acid–base balance, including inflammation, ischaemia, renal disease, chronic lung disorders and intrauterine abnormalities [2-4] and tumors. In this review, we will focus on discussing pH alteration relevant to tumors.
Evidence accumulated over the past 50 years and more has shown that electrode-evaluated human tumor pH is on average, lower than the pH of normal tissues [5-6]. The increase in

hydrogen ion concentration is thought to be due to a combination of a more glycolytic phenotype, as well as reduced oxygen availability, leading to lactic acidosis from glycolysis [7].In addition, a poor and chaotic tumor vascularization leads to the inefficient washout of the acidic products and contributes further to development of the chronically acidic extracellular environment [8]. However, although most tumors had relatively acidic extracellular pH, there were some exceptions. Engin et al reported that tumour pHe was significantly different between different histological groups, the mean tumour pHe for the entire group of tumours was 7.06 +/- 0.05 (range 5.66-7.78) [9]. Prior to the application of ^{31}P-MRS to living tissue, it was not recognized that tissue pH is compartmentalized into an intracellular component (pHi) and an interstitial or extracellular component (pHe) [10]. To our knowledge, currently, there weren't concomitant measurements of pHi and pHe in spontaneous tumors. pH evaluated by electrodes primarily measures interstitial or extracellular tissue pH, whereas pH evaluated by^{31}P-MRS primarily reflects the aggregate pHi of tissue. pHi is similar in tumors and normal tissue. To date, the majority of pHi values have been obtained using ^{31}P-MRS. The measurement of pH by MRS is largely standardized, provides accuracy of$\pm$0.1 pH units [11]. The explaination is that the excess hydrogen ion is excreted from the cell by hydrogen ion pumps, in this way the intracellular environment is maintained at a more physiologically normal pH [5,12-13].

In recent years, there were some reports suggested that cellular uptake of chemotherapeutic drugs may depend on the pH gradient (pHi-pHe).The naturally occurring cell pH gradient difference between tumor and normal tissue is a major and exploitable determinant of the uptake of weak acids in the complex tumor microenvironment [14]. A low pHe enhances the uptake of weakly acidic drugs such as chlorambucil and 5-fluorouracil, whereas a low pHe reduces the uptake of mitoxantrone and the cytotoxicity of weakly basic drugs, such as doxorubicin [15-17]. By i.v.-injected glucose in a xenografted human tumor, Kozin [14] et al showed that the tumor-specific pH gradient may be exploited for the treatment of cancer by weak acid chemotherapeutics. Similarly, some efforts have been made to increase the intracellular acidity via disturbing the pH-regulating mechanisms, which therefore causing cell death at a sufficiently low pH [18-19]. To date, the majority of treatment-related studies conducted have focused on hyperthermia (combined with radiotherapy) due to the recognized importance of acidic pH as a thermal sensitizer. What surprised us for the results was that patients with a better response to hyperthermia radiotherapy have higher pH (as measured by electrode or ^{31}P MRS) prior to treatment [20].

3. pH measurement with ^{1}H-MRSI

With high inherent sensitivity of ^{1}H nucleus, many attempts have been made to produce pH-sensitive MRI contrast. Gillies et al[1] have employed an exogenously administered imidazole, IEPA, which has a pH-dependent chemical shift of the H-2 resonance in the 7-9 ppm range. This has been used for imaging pHe in orthotopic breast cancer by MR spectroscopic imaging (MRSI). Our colleagues [22] used conventional FSE sequence to study phantom (Histidine is included) and found there were some relationship between pH value and signal intensity on T2-weighted images, which enables the magnetic resonance pH imaging.

Currently, there were two major approaches for measuring pH, relaxation methods and magnetization transfer methods. Relaxation methods requires the injection of exogenous contrast agents (CAs). Actually, magnetic resonance spectroscopy with ^{31}P or ^{19}F probes can be attached to a contrast agent (CA). Nevertheless, although these probes can be effective, ^{1}H-based probes are preferred because they are intrinsically the most sensitive of MR-based probes. Current clinical CAs are small-molecule Gd3+ chelates that work by shortening the longitudinal and/or transverse relaxation times of the protons in their close proximity. These relaxation agents have a number of shortcomings. First, they do not target specific areas or disease regions, nor do they respond to cellular stimuli, but rather they matriculate throughout the body, confined to the circulatory system, prior to eventual elimination [23]. As a consequence, relatively large agent doses are required to reach clear contrast detection. Second, patients suffered gadolinium exposure have risk in with renal insufficiency [24]. The rapidly emerging field of molecular imaging seeks to develop CAs as molecular probes that respond to cellular processes or cellular markers in contrary [23]. To date, some recent prototype MRI CAs that respond to pH have been developed [25-28]. Gadolinium-based carbon nanostructures were poised to make a significant impact as advanced CAs for magnetic resonance imaging (MRI) in medicine. It was forecasted that gadonanotubes as synthons for the design of high-performance MRI CA probe with efficacies up to 100 times greater than current clinical CAs. These new materials will be useful for in vivo MRI applications as circulating drug nanocapsules because of their low toxicities, extremely high relaxivities, and potential for cellular targeting and induced cell death by magnetic hyperthermia [29]. In Hartman's [23] study, gadonanotubes have also been shown to maintain their integrity when challenged ex vivo by phosphate-buffered saline solution, serum, heat, and pH cycling. Nevertheless, although these relaxation-based agents are responsive to the state of their environment (e.g. pH, temperature, etc.), the measured effect is a function of both the environment and the agent concentration, which is usually unknown in vivo, leading to the difficulty of quantification of the environmental parameter of interest [30]. In addition, only one target per MRI exam can be obtained with targeted relaxation contrast agents [31]. Considering the limitations of relaxation-based agents mentioned above, a new class of contrast agents is required. It was reported that use of chemical-exchange-dependent saturation transfer (CEST) methods in combination with agents possessing a proton exchange site can provide a significant change in the magnitude of the water proton signal, potentially providing a non-metal-based contrast mechanism [32].

When selecting a suitable CEST contrast agent, two characteristics including chemical exchange rate and longitudinal relaxation time must be considered. For maximum CEST efficiency, the chemical system must be exchanging slowly on the NMR chemical shift time-scale. A good CEST contrast agent must, therefore, possess mobile protons that exchange with water as fast as possible before exchange broadening makes selective RF presaturation ineffective. Larger frequency separations permit shorter proton lifetimes and thus result in larger CEST effects [30].

Currently, there are two major CEST contrast agents. The first CEST agents were diamagnetic small molecules (DIACEST) reported by Ward et al in 2000 [32], which contains exchangeable -NH or -OH protons. The major disadvantage of DIACEST agents is their small chemical shift difference between -NH and -OH groups and bulk water(<5ppm), which results in an overlap between the CEST effects of exogenous contrast agents and strong endogenous MT effects, and the activation of these exchange groups by semi-selective pulses usually also results in partial saturation of bulk water protons. Another kind of CEST agents are PARACEST agents, of which chemical shift difference between two exchanging pools can be increased as much as possible. One example of PARACEST agents are Lanthanide complexes. They are stable enough for in vivo applications and have one water molecule coordinated directly to the metal ion [33], which exchanges with the bulk water molecules. The rate of water exchange is in direct relationship to the metal ion's requirement for electron density from the water molecule [33]. In more recent years, highly sensitive supramolecular and liposome-based CEST agents were developed by moving beyond the simple complex towards supramolecular structures. Two kinds of representative agents are ion-paired assemblies of poly-L-arginine and Tm^{3+}-DOTP proposed by Aime and co-workers [34] and dubbed LIPOCEST which involves the incorporation of a shift reagent, such as Tm^{3+}-DOTMA, inside a liposome [35]. To date, CEST agents present some challenges in terms of application to human studies. Although their theoretical detection limit may be lower than that of relaxation-based agents, their experimental detection limit remains higher, due to practical limitations [30].

Nowadays, there are some evdiences showing that it is possible to produce pH-sensitive MRI contrast by exploiting the exchange between the hydrogen atoms of water and the amide hydrogen atoms of endogenous mobile cellular proteins and peptides. It was reported that endogenous, low-concentration mobile proteins and peptides in tissue can be detected with amide proton transfer (APT) imaging technique via using a change in bulkwater intensity due to saturation transfer of the amide protons in the peptide bonds [36]. APT imaging is actually a variant of CEST imaging, of which the backbone is APT effect. To indicate the existence of APT effects, it was reported that there was a very small dip at frequency difference of 3.5 ppm from water, corresponding to about 8.3 ppm in the WEX spectra, where amide protons resonate [36]. Initial studies [37] have shown promise to distinguish tumor from surrounding brain in patients, but this data was hampered by magnetic field inhomogeneity and by low signal to noise ratio (SNR). Zhou [38] et al proposed a practical six-offset APT data acquisition scheme, together with a separately acquired CEST spectrum, which can provide B0-inhomogeneity corrected human brain APT images of sufficient SNR within a clinically relevant time frame.

CEST imaging, however, is also dependent on experimental parameters such as the power, duration, and waveform of the irradiation RF pulse, for which, its sensitivity and specificity for microenvironment properties such as pH is not optimal. Animal models are always used to acquire Z-spectrum, from which we can observe the offset frequency away from water resonance center, and obvious APT effect. The Z spectrum can provide good evidence for what offset frequency should be applied. However, there are still many problems about how to optimize pulse sequence for improving SNR and imaging contrast. Thus, in addition to search for better CAs, some researchers are working directly at improving pulse sequence technology. In Sun et al's study [39], they solved the dependence of CEST contrast on experimental parameters and proposed an iterative compensation algorithm that corrects the experimentally measured CEST contrast from the concomitant RF irradiation effects, thereby to accurately calibrate the chemical exchange rate.

In all, APT imaging could provide important biomarker for assessing many diseases. However, due to the low amide protons concentration (in the millimolar range), low signal-to-noise ratio, motional artifacts and so on, more efforts should be made to reach good APT imaging.

4. Measurement of pH with ^{31}P MRSI

It is reported that brain energy metabolism can be assessed by using 31P MRS to measure changes in the intracellular pH and relative concentrations of adenosinetriphosphate (ATP), phosphocreatine (PCr), and inorganic phosphate (Pi) [40-41]. By calculating from the difference in chemical shifts between Pi and PCr resonances, pH values can be obtained. As we know, although both the intracellular and extracellular compartments of tissue contain phosphate, they are different in the concentration, with 2-3 mM in intracellular compartment and 1.0 mM in extracellular compartment. Dimethyl methyl phosphate (DMMP) is a colorless liquid with chemical formula $C_3H_9O_3P$ or $CH_3PO(OCH_3)_2$. It distributed among all the water spaces. 3-aminopropylphosphonate (3-APP) has a pKa in the physiological range and accesses only the extracellular compartment. Both DMMP and 3-APP are chemically inert and non-toxic. With these materials as markers for total and extracellular water spaces respectively, non-invasively measuring the intra- and extracellular volume fraction can be accomplished [42]. For greater intracellular volume fraction and relative higher concentration of phosphate of intracellular volume, the chemical shift of the endogenous Pi resonance is generally assumed to reflect intracellular pH. Under physiological conditions, the change in intracellular pH produced by unit change in extracellular pH ranges from 0.4 to 0.8 [43-44].

In tumors, pHi of tumor cells in situ is neutral or slightly alkaline compared with that of normal tissues. Thus comparisons of intracellular pH values between systems are meaningless without knowledge of the extracellular pH [45]. Measurements of pHe in tumors have been made using an invasive microelectrodes technique. Some argument was that this invasive probe may change relative volume of cell and artifactually increase the extracellular pH. Some agents have been reported to be used as a ^{31}P-MRS indicator of extracellular pH, however, these have not also been fully developed for use in vivo [46-48]. pH indicators for in vivo use should meet some criteria which include no toxic or cytostatic effects, a pK, in the physiological range, a clearly separable signal, demonstrable localization, specificity to pH, and a large pH sensitivity [48]. An agent satisfies all these criteria is 3-APP. 3-APP is non-toxic and has a pKa in the physiological range, and in vitro results indicate that its resonant frequency is sensitive to pH and not significantly affected by temperature or ionic strength. Bioreactor experiments indicate that this compound is neither internalized nor metabolized by cells [45]. In additon, the clear separation of this signal from the cellular phosphate resonances allows extracellular pH to be measured more accurately than with extracellular Pi [45,48]. By intraperitoneally administering 3-APP , Gillies [45] et al carried out experiments in vivo which sucessfully demonstrated the use of 3-APP as a ^{31}P-MRS-based indicator of extracellular pH in cells and tissues.

5. Measruement of pH with hyperpolarized ^{13}C MRSI

^{13}C magnetic resonance spectroscopy (MRS) has long been used in the investigation of metabolic processes in vivo [49]. ^{13}C nuclear magnetic resonance (NMR) spectroscopy allows

observation of the backbone of organic compounds, yielding specific information about the identity and structure of biologically important compounds [50].With a broad chemical shift range for carbon (250ppm), which is much larger than that for proton (15 ppm), it allows for improved resolution of metabolites. However, ^{13}C MRS is limited by the low natural abundance of ^{13}C (1.1%) and its very low nuclear spin polarization (2.5×10-6 polarization at 3 T and 37°C) [51-52].

Several techniques have been used to overcome these limitations. One way to improve the sensitivity of ^{13}C spectroscopy is to perform a technique known as proton (^{1}H) decoupling. By eliminating these couplings, the signal-to-noise ratio of ^{13}C resonances can be significantly increased via irradiating the entire ^{1}H NMR absorption range, consequently collapsing ^{13}C resonances to singlets [50]. Another technique to improve the sensitivity of ^{13}C MRS is dynamic nuclear polarization (DNP), which introduces one or more ^{13}C molecules into a metabolic substrate [53]. DNP has emerged recently as a technique for radically increasing the sensitivity of solution-state ^{13}C MRS [54]. When DNP is performed in a strong magnetic field and at cryogenic temperatures, nearly 100% nuclear polarization for ^{1}H and 50% for ^{13}C can be achieved in various organic molecules. In addition, replacing the ^{12}C isotope (98.9% natural abundance) with the ^{13}C isotope at a specific carbon or carbons in a metabolic substrate does not affect the substrate's biochemistry [52]. There are four mechanisms accounted for in the DNP process: the overhauser effect, the solid effect, thermal mixing, and the cross effect or electronuclear crosspolarization [55]. In general, the DNP experiments are conducted at low temperatures, by which to attenuate competing spin-lattice relaxation processes and avoid loss of efficiency during the polarization transfer [56]. It was reported that the sensitivity in the ^{13}C MRS experiment can be increased by 10,000-fold or more by using DNP technique, which allows not only detection of ^{13}C-labeled substrates in vivo but imaging of their tissue distribution as well [57-59]. Preclinical model clearly demonstrated the feasibility of obtaining high-spatialresolution ^{13}C MRSI data with a high signal-to-noise ratio from tumor implanted mice injected by injecting the animals with hyperpolarized 1-[^{13}C] pyruvate [59].

A new application for DNP is for measuring extracellular tissue pH using hyperpolarized ^{13}C labelled bicarbonate. Gallagher et al [60-61] generated a non-toxic, pH-probe, hyperpolarized $H^{13}CO_3$- and exploited the pH in tumors. With measurement of the $H^{13}CO_3^-$ and $^{13}CO_2$ concentration ratio after administration of hyperpolarized $H^{13}CO_3^-$, tissue pH could be determined by using the Henderson-Hasselbalch equation [62]:

$$pH = pKa + \log_{10}([HCO3^-]/[CO2]) \quad (1)$$

(pKa is assumed to be known in vivo)

6. Measruement of pH with ^{19}F NMR

^{19}F NMR has several distinct strengths: a large chemical shift range, high gyromagnetic ratio, no background signal from tissues inherently 12.5 times the sensitivity of ^{31}P NMR [63]. Ojugo et al [64] compare the effect of pHe measurements made by the ^{31}P probe (3-APP) with those made by the ^{19}F probe, 3-[N-(4-fluor-2-trifluoromethylphenyl)-sulphamoyl]-propionic acid (ZK-150471). Result showed, with wide chemical shift range, improved signal-to-noise and absence of signal overlap, ^{19}F pH probe ZK-150471 allowed a more rapid and precise measurement of pHe compared to 3-APP. Development of exogenous NMR pH indicators opens the opportunity to exploit ^{19}F nuclei. There were some evidences showing Fluorinated vitamin B6 derivatives have been developed for ^{19}F NMR methods to study cellular pHi and pHe. 6-FPOL (29fluoro-5- hydroxy-6-methyl-3,4-

pyridinedimethanol, 6-fluoropyridoxol) is one example. pH values are calculated from the ^{19}F spectra on the basis of chemical shift of 6-FPOL (δ_{obs}) with respect to a NaTFA (sodium trifluoroacetate) standard. Substituting (δ_{obs}) into the Henderson-Hasselbalch equation with coefficients pk_a=8.2; δ_{acid}=-9.85; δ_{base}=-19.61 and the pH is estimated [65]:

$$pH=pK_a+\log_{10}[\delta_{obs}-\delta_{acid}/\delta_{base}-\delta_{obs}] \quad (2)$$ [66].

Mason et al [65] have demonstrated 6-FPOL readily enters cells and provides well resolved resonances reporting both intra- and extracellular simultaneously in whole blood), and the perfused rat heart. As mentioned above, the pKa of 6-FPOL is 8.2. It is appropriate for monitoring pH in the basic range, whereas it is not ideal for measurements under normal physiological conditions. There were some studies on modifications of vitamin B6 suggesting that the introduction of electron donating or withdrawing groups at the 4- and 5-positions of thepyridoxol ring could significantly alter the pKa of the 3-phenolic group, and the NMR properties at the 6-position [67]. He et al [68] have synthesized a series of novel fluorinated vitamin B6 analogues (6-fluoropyridoxol derivatives) as potential ^{19}F NMR pH indicators for use in vivo. The variation in chemical shift with respect to acid±base titration showed pKa values in the range 7.05±9.5 with a chemical shift sensitivity in the range 7.4±12 ppm. Among them, 6-Fluoropyridoxamine (6-FPAM) exhibits a pKa=7.05, which is closer to normal physiological pH than the parent molecule 6-FPOL (pKa=8.2), and should thus, be useful for precise and accurate measurements of pH in vivo [68].

7. Summary

Alteration in tissue pH is an indicator of many pathological processes, such as inflammation, ischaemia, renal disease, chronic lung disorders and intrauterine abnormalities and tumors. In tumors, the pH gradient exists between the intracellular (pHi) and extracellular (pHe) compartments. pHe is usually lower, and pHi could be higher or unchanging compared with normal tissue. Some evidences reaveal that cellular uptake of chemotherapeutic drugs may be depend on the pH gradient, which therefore, may help monitor tumour progression and evaluate drug treatment response. To date, pH measurement approaches have been applied with some NMR nuclei such as protons (^{1}H), phosphorus (^{31}P), fluorine (^{19}F) and carbon (^{13}C). ^{31}P-MRS has low spatial resolution (20-30ml) and is not available on standard clinical equipment, which is limited predominantly (99%) to proton (^{1}H) studies [36]. Currently, it is usually used as a control experiment when carrying ^{1}H or ^{13}C MRS study. The rapid development of contrast agents and improvement on technology attracts researchers to devote their effort on ^{1}H–MRSI for exploiting pH. As a variant of CEST imaging, APT imaging can detects endogenous, low-concentration mobile proteins and peptides in tissue using a change in bulkwater intensity due to saturation transfer of the amide protons in the peptide bonds with or without the need for exogenous contrast agents. DNP technique introduces one or more ^{13}C molecules into a metabolic substrate to improve the sensitivity of ^{13}C MRS. Based on this technology, a non-toxic, pH-probe is generated by intravenous injecting hyperpolarized $H^{13}CO_3^-$. Nevertheless, the current standard clinical MRI scanners can't perform ^{13}C MRS, the addition of the ability to detect nuclei other than ^{1}H represents an added cost, and the clinical motivation to date has not been adequately demonstrated [50]. To date, due to the low amide protons concentration (in the millimolar range), low signal-to-noise ratio, motional artifacts and so on, to reach a good APT imaging may require long stage of development.

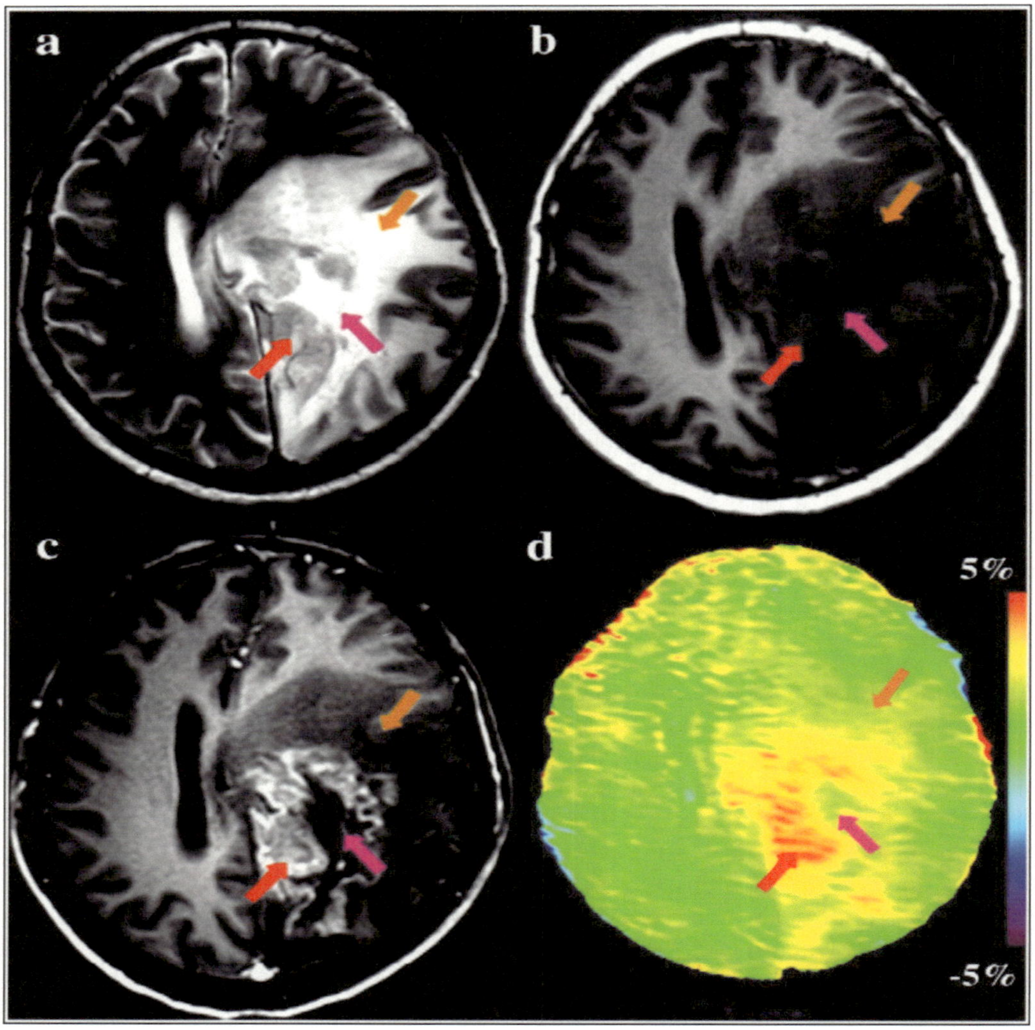

(Courtesy of Dr Jinyuan Zhou and Elsevier)

Fig. 1. MR images acquired on a Philips 3 T MRI scanner (Achieva 3.0 T; Philips Medical Systems, Best, The Netherlands) from a patient with recurrent astrocytoma (grade III), acquired four months after treatment. (a), (b) T2-weighted image and T1-weighted image show the recurrence of glioma with heterogeneous intensity in the left parietal lobe. The exact location of the tumor core is obscure. (c) Post-contrast T1-weighted image reveals a gadolinium-enhancing tumor core (red arrow) and a necrotic area (pink arrow). The recurrent tumor is associated with the surrounding edema and mass effect. (d) APT image shows an obvious increase in APT signal intensity in the tumor core. The regions of necrosis (pink arrow) and edema (orange arrow) are almost isointense on APT.

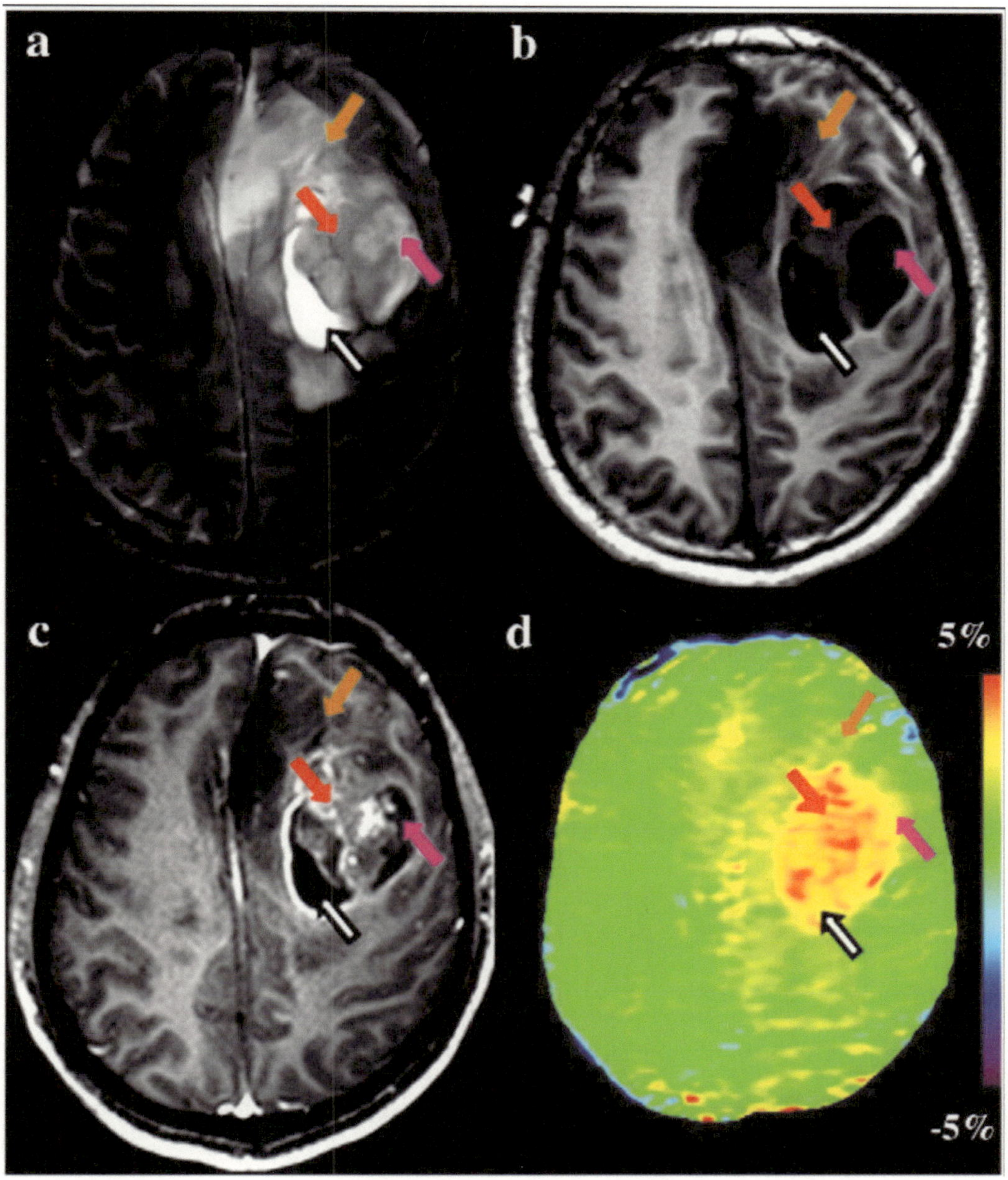

(Courtesy of Dr Jinyuan Zhou and Elsevier)

Fig. 2. MR images for another patient with glioblastoma multiforme. (a), (b) T2-weighted image T1-weighted image show a large tumor of abnormal signals in the left frontal lobe. (c) Gadolinium-enhanced T1-weighted image demonstrates an enhancing tumor core (red arrow) with non-enhancing necrotic areas. (d) APT image shows that both the gadolinium-enhancing tumor core (red arrow) and the cystic cavity (black arrow) have high APT signal intensities, while the necrotic regions (pink arrow) and edema areas (orange arrow) have low APT signal intensities.

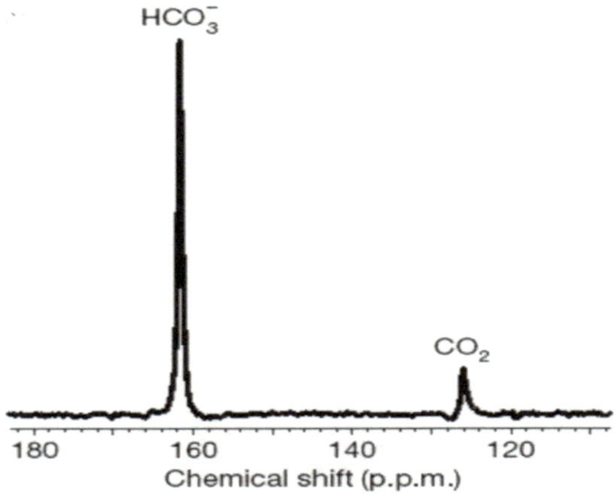

(Courtesy of Dr Kevin M. Brindle)

Fig. 3. 13C spectrum from a murine lymphoma (EL4) tumour in vivo, acquired 10 s after the intravenous injection of hyperpolarized H13CO3-, showing resonances from H13CO3- (at 161 p.p.m.) and 13CO2 (at 125 p.p.m.).

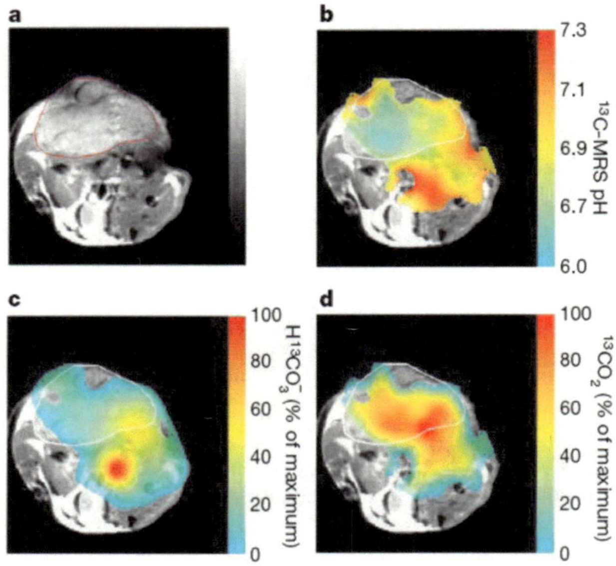

(Courtesy of Dr Kevin M. Brindle)

Fig. 4. The spatial distribution of 13CO2 and H13CO3- in a transverse slice was imaged using a gradient echo pulse sequence. A shows transverse proton magnetic resonance image of a mouse with a subcutaneously implanted EL4 tumour. Tumor is margined in red. B shows the pH map calculated from the ratio of the H13CO3- and 13CO2 voxel intensities ,which demonstrated a low intratumoral pH. C and d show the spatial distribution of H13CO3- and 13CO2, displayed as voxel intensities relative to their respective maxima, respectively. the highest concentration of 13CO2 was in the tumour and the H13CO3- signal was highest in the aorta and there was little difference in signal intensities between muscle and tumour. The tumour margin in b, c and d is outlined in white.

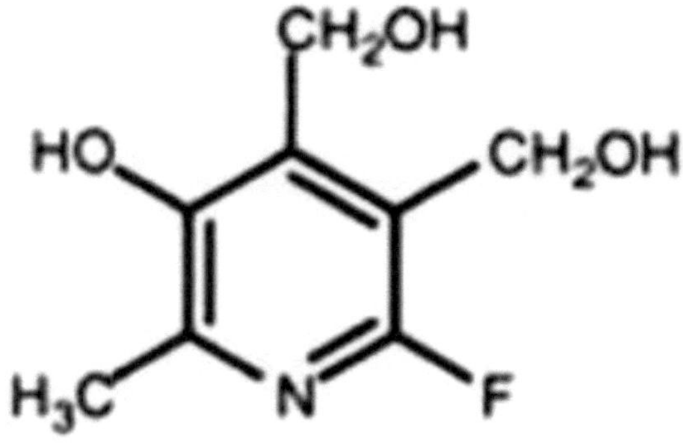

(Courtesy of Dr Ralph Mason)

Fig. 5. Struture of 6-FPOL(6-fluoropyridoxol)

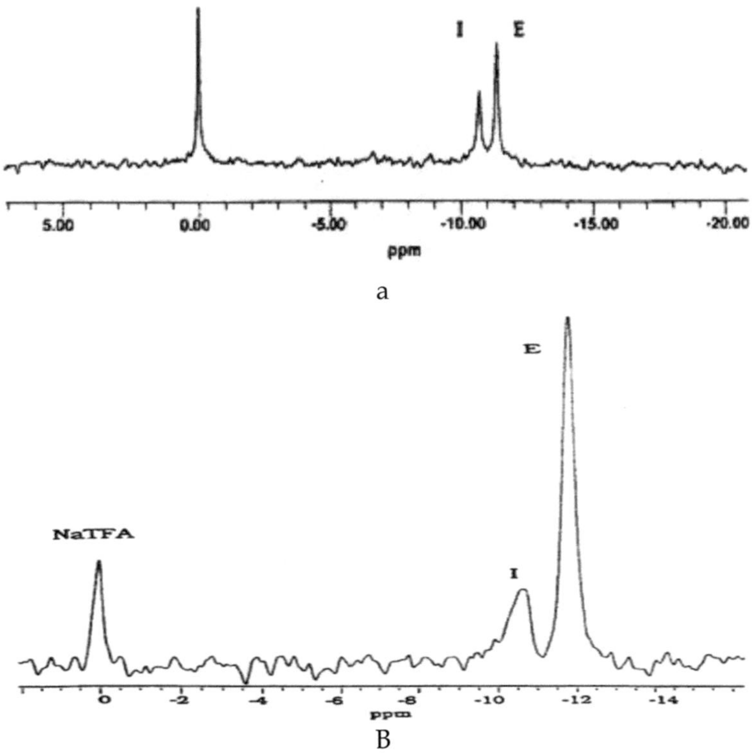

(Courtesy of Dr Ralph Mason)

Fig. 6. a 282MHz 19F NMR spectrum of 6-FPOL in whole unwashed rabbit blood:pHi=7.19(δ=-10.72ppm).pHe 7.45(δ=-11.34ppm). ΔpH=0.26(Δδ=0.62ppm) with respect to external NaTFA capillary standard. 6b 376MHz 19F NMR spectrum of 6-FPOL in a sanguinous perfused rat heart: pHi=7.16(δ=-10.60ppm).pHe 7.55(δ=-11.64ppm). ΔpH=0.39(Δδ=1.04ppm) with respect to external NaTFA in balloon in left ventricle.

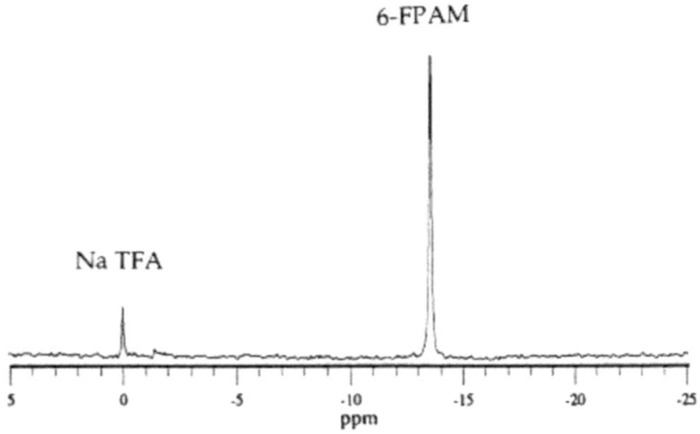

a

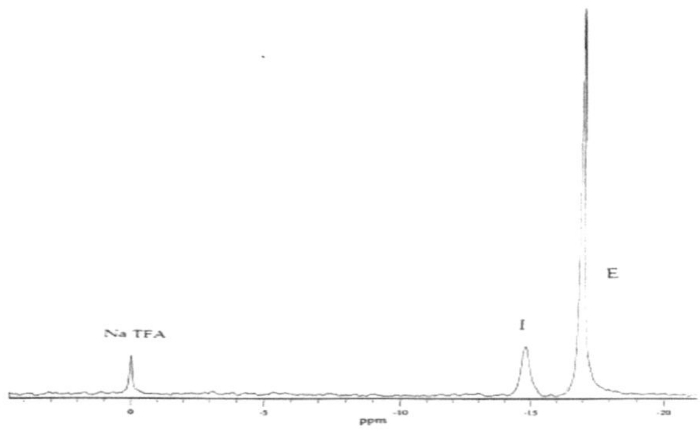

b

(Courtesy of Sha He and Elsevier)

Fig. 7. a 19F NMR spectrum of 6-FPAM in water at pH 6.9 (δ=-13.57 ppm). 7b Spectrum of 6-FPAM in whole rabbit blood. Two signals are observed for 6-FPAM attributed to intra (δ=-14.793 ppm) and extra (δ=-16.935 ppm) cellular compartments corresponding to pH 7.16 and 7.59, respectively. A capillary of sodium TFA served as external chemical shift reference.

8. References

[1] Gillies RJ, Raghunand N, Garcia-Martin ML, Gatenby RA. pH imaging. A review of pH measurement methods and applications in cancers. IEEE Eng Med Biol Mag. 2004; 23(5):57-64.

[2] Adrogue HJ, Madias NE. Management of life-threatening acid-base disorders. First of two parts. N. Engl. J. Med.1998, 338, 26–34

[3] Hohn-Berlage M, Okada Y, Kloiber O , Hossmann KA. Imaging of brain tissue pH and metabolites. A new approach for the validation of volume-selective NMR spectroscopy. NMR Biomed. 1989, 2, 240–245.

[4] Grinstein S, Swallow CJ, Rotstein OD. Regulation of cytoplasmic pH in phagocytic cell function and dysfunction. Clin. Biochem. 1991, 24, 241–247.

[5] Gerweck LE, Seetharaman K. Cellular pH gradient in tumor versus normal tissue: potential exploitation for the treatment of cancer. Cancer Res. 1996; 56(6):1194-8.
[6] Wike-Hooley JL, Haveman J, Reinhold HS. The relevance of tumour pH to the treatment of malignant disease. Radiother. Oncol, 1984, 2: 343-366,
[7] Gulledge CJ, Dewhirst MW. Tumor oxygenation: a matter of supply and demand. Anticancer Res, 1996, 16: 741–750.
[8] Prescott DM, Charles HC, Poulson JM, Page RL, Thrall DE, Vujaskovic Z, Dewhirst MW. The relationship between intracellular and extracellular pH in spontaneous canine tumors. Clin Cancer Res. 2000; 6(6):2501-5.
[9] Engin K, Leeper DB, Cater JR, Thistlethwaite AJ, Tupchong L, McFarlane JD. Extracellular pH distribution in human tumours. Int. J. Hyperthermia, 1995, 11: 211–216.
[10] Vaupel P, Kallinowski F, Okunieff P. Blood flow, oxygen and nutrient supply, and metabolic microenvironment of human tumors: a review. Cancer Res. 1989, 49:6449–6465,.
[11] Robert JRK, Wade-Jardetzsky N, Jardetzsky O. Intracellular pH measurements by ^{31}P-NMR. Influence of factors other than pH on f/P chemical shifts. Biochemistry. 1981, 20: 5389-5392.
[12] Gerweck LE, Vijayappa S, Kozin S. Tumor pH controls the in vivo efficacy of weak acid and base chemotherapeutics. Cancer Res.1996, 56: 1194–1198.
[13] Simon S, Roy D, and Schindler M. Intracellular pH and the control of multidrug resistance. Proc. Natl. Acad. Sci. USA, 1994, 91: 1128– 1132.
[14] Kozin SV, Shkarin P, Gerweck LE. The cell transmembrane pH gradient in tumors enhances cytotoxicity of specific weak acid chemotherapeutics. Cancer Res. 200; 61(12):4740-3.
[15] Atema A, Buurman KJ, Noteboom E, and Smets LA. Potentiation of DNA-adduct formation and cytotoxicity of platinumcontaining drugs by low pH. Int. J. Cancer, 1993, 54: 166–172.
[16]Vukovic V, Tannock IF. Influence of low pH on cytotoxicity of paclitaxel, mitoxantrone and topotecan. Br. J. Cancer, 1997, 75: 1167– 1172.
[17] Engin K, Leeper DB, ThistlethwaiteAJ, Tupchong L, McFarlane JD. Tumor extracellular pH as a prognostic factor in thermoradiotherapy. Int. J. Radiat. Oncol. Biol. Phys., 29: 125–132, 1994.
[18] Song, CW, Lyons JC, Luo Y. Intra- and extracellular pH in solid tumors: Influence on therapeutic response. In Drug Resistance in Oncology, B Teicher (ed), 1993b, pp. 25–51. Marcel Dekker: New York
[19] Newell KJ, Tannock IF. Reduction of intracellular pH as a possible mechanism for killing cells in acidic regions of solid tumors: effects of carbonylcyanide-3-chlorophenylhydrazone. Cancer Res. 1989, 49: 4477-4482.
[20] Evelhoch JL. pH and therapy of human cancers. Novartis Found Symp. 2001; 240:68-80.
[21] van Sluis R, Bhujwalla ZM, Raghunand N, Ballesteros P, Alvarez J, Cerdán S, Galons JP, Gillies RJ. In vivo imaging of extracellular pH using1H-MRSI, Magn Reson Med. 1999; 41(4):743-50 .
[22] Qiu QC,Wei MB,Shen ZW, Wu RH.T2-weighted magnetic resonance imaging based on the different pH values. Chinese Journal of Medical Physics, 2009, 26(5):1405-08.

[23] Hartman KB, Laus S, Bolskar RD, Muthupillai R, Helm L, Toth E, Merbach AE, Wilson LJ. Gadonanotubes as ultrasensitive pH-smart probes for magnetic resonance imaging. Nano Lett. 2008; 8(2):415-9.

[24] Broome DR. Nephrogenic systemic fibrosis associated with gadolinium based contrast agents: a summary of the medical literature reporting. Eur. J. Radiol. 2008, 66, 230–234.

[25] Woods M, Kiefer GE, Bott S, Castillo-Muzquiz A, Eshelbrenner C, Michaudet L, McMillan K, Mudigunda SD, Ogrin D, Tircsó G, Zhang S, Zhao P, Sherry AD. Synthesis, relaxometric and photophysical properties of a new pH-responsive MRI contrast agent: the effect of other ligating groups on dissociation of a p-nitrophenolic pendant arm. J Am Chem Soc. 2004; 126(30):9248-56.

[26] Zhang S, Wu K, Sherry AD. Gd3+ complexes with slowly exchanging bound-water molecules may offer advantages in the design of responsive MR agents. Invest Radiol. 2001; 36(2):82-6.

[27] Jebasingh B, Alexander V. Synthesis and relaxivity studies of a tetranuclear gadolinium(III) complex of DO3A as a contrast-enhancing agent for MRI. Inorg Chem. 2005; 44(25):9434-43.

[28] Lowe MP, Parker D, Reany O, Aime S, Botta M, Castellano G, Gianolio E, Pagliarin R. pH-dependent modulation of relaxivity and luminescence in macrocyclic gadolinium and europium complexes based on reversible intramolecular sulfonamide ligation. J Am Chem Soc. 2001; 123(31):7601-9.

[29] Sitharaman B, Wilson LJ. Gadonanotubes as new high-performance MRI contrast agents. Int J Nanomedicine. 2006; 1(3):291-5. protons.

[30] Hancu I, Dixon WT, Woods M, Vinogradov E, Sherry AD, Lenkinski RE. CEST and PARACEST MR contrast agents. Acta Radiol. 2010; 51(8):910-23.

[31] Huinink HP, Sanders HM, Erich SJ, Nicolay K, Strijkers GJ, Merkx M, et al. High-resolution NMR imaging of paramagnetic liposomes targeted to a functionalized surface. Magn Reson Med 2008; 59:1282–6

[32] Ward KM, Aletras AH, Balaban RS. A new class of contrast agents for MRI based on proton chemical exchange dependent saturation transfer (CEST). J Magn Reson 2000; 143:79–87.

[33] Merbach AE, Toth E, editors. The chemistry of contrast agents in medical magnetic resonance imaging. New York: Wiley; 2001.

[34] Aime S, Delli Castelli D, Terreno E. Supramolecular adducts between poly-L-arginine and [TmIIIdotp]: a route to sensitivity- enhanced magnetic resonance imaging-chemical exchange saturation transfer agents. Angew Chem Int Ed Engl 2003; 42:4527–9

[35] Aime S, Delli Castelli D, Terreno E. Highly sensitive MRI chemical exchange saturation transfer agents using liposomes. Angew Chem Int Ed Engl 2005; 44:5513–15.

[36] Zhou J, Payen JF, Wilson DA, Traystman RJ, van Zijl PC. Using the amide proton signals of intracellular proteins and peptides to detect pH effects in MRI. Nat Med. 2003; 9(8):1085-90.

[37] Wen Z, Hu S, Huang F, Wang X, Guo L, Quan X, Wang S, Zhou J. MR imaging of high-grade brain tumors using endogenous protein and peptide-based contrast.
Neuroimage. 2010; 51(2):616-22.

[38] Zhou J, Blakeley JO, Hua J, Kim M, Laterra J, Pomper MG, van Zijl PC. Practical data acquisition method for human brain tumor amide proton transfer (APT) imaging. Magn Reson Med. 2008; 60(4):842-9.

[39] Sun PZ, Sorensen AG.Imaging pH using the chemical exchange saturation transfer (CEST) MRI: Correction of concomitant RF irradiation effects to quantify CEST MRI for chemical exchange rate and pH. Magn Reson Med. 2008; 60(2):390-7.

[40] Wu RH, Poublanc J, Mandell D, et al. Evidence of brain mitochondrial activities after oxygen inhalation by 31P magnetic resonance spectroscopy at 3T. Conf Proc IEEE Eng Med Biol Soc, 2007, pp. 2899-2902.

[41] Wu RH, Liu WW, Chen YW, Wang H, Shen ZHW, Brugge KT and Mikulis DJ. Preliminary study of mapping brain ATP and brain pH using multivoxel ^{31}P MR spectroscopy. 13th International Conference on Biomedical Engineering IFMBE Proceedings, 2009, Volume 23, Track 1, 362-365, DOI: 10.1007/978-3-540-92841-6_89.

[42] Bhujwalla ZM, McCoy CL, Glickson JD, Gillies RJ, Stubbs M. Estimations of intra- and extracellular volume and pH by ^{31}P magnetic resonance spectroscopy: effect of therapy on RIF-1 tumours. Br J Cancer. 1998; 78(5):606-11

[43] Gillies RJ. Intracellular pH and growth control in eukaryoticcells. In: The Transformed Cell, edited by I. L. Cameron and T. B. Poole. New York: Academic, 1981, p. 347-395.

[44] Wilding T J, Boron W. pH regulation in adult rat carotid body glomus cells: importance of extracellular pH, sodium, and potassium. J. Gen. Physiol. 1992, 100: 593-608.

[45] Gillies RJ, Liu Z, Bhujwalla Z. ^{31}P-MRS measurements of extracellular pH of tumors using 3-aminopropylphosphonate. Am J Physiol. 1994; 267(1 Pt 1):C195-203.

[46] Fisher MJ, Dillon PF. Phenylphosphate: a ^{31}P-NMR indicator of extracellular pH and volume in the isolated perfused rabbit bladder. Circ. Res. 1987, 60: 472-477.

[47] Meyer R A, Brown TR, Kusmerick MJ. Phosphorus nuclear magnetic resonance of fast- and slow-twitch muscle. Am. J. Physiol. 1985, 248 (CeZZ Physiol. 17): C279-C287.

[48] Szwergold BS. NMR spectroscopy of cells. Annu. Rev. Physiol. 1992, 54:775-798,.

[49] Shulman RG, Brown TR, Ugurbil K, Ogawa S, Cohen SM and den Hollander JA. Cellular applications of ^{31}P and ^{13}C nuclear magnetic resonance. Science 1979, 205, 160–166

[50] Kurhanewicz J, Bok R, Nelson SJ, Vigneron DB. Current and potential applications of clinical 13C MR spectroscopy. J Nucl Med. 2008; 49(3):341-4.

[51] Rajesh A, Coakley FV, Kurhanewicz J. 3D MR spectroscopic imaging in the evaluation of prostate cancer. Clin Radiol 2007;62:921–929.

[52] Shan L. Hyperpolarized 13C-labeled bicarbonate (H13CO3 -) for in vivo pH measurement with 13C magnetic resonance spectroscopy. Molecular Imaging and Contrast Agent Database (MICAD) [Internet]. Bethesda (MD): National Center for Biotechnology Information (US); 2004-2010.

[53] Golman K, Olsson LE, Axelsson O, Mansson S, Karlsson M, Petersson JS. Molecular imaging using hyperpolarized ^{13}C. Br J Radiol 2003; 76 (Spec No 2):S118–27.

[54] Ardenkjaer-Larsen JH et al. Increase in signal-to-noise ratio of 10,000 times in liquid-state NMR. Proc. Natl Acad. Sci. USA 2003, 100, 10158–10163.

[55] Joo CG, Hu KN, Bryant JA. Griffin RG. In situ temperature jump high-frequency dynamic nuclear polarization experiments: enhanced sensitivity in liquid-state NMR spectroscopy. J Am Chem Soc 2006; 128(29):9428–32.

[56] Zhang H. Hyperpolarized sodium 1-[13C]pyruvate. Molecular Imaging and Contrast Agent Database (MICAD) [Internet]. Bethesda (MD): National Center for Biotechnology Information (US); 2004-2010.

[57] Golman K, Ardenkjaer-Larsen JH, Petersson JS, Mansson S, Leunbach I.Molecular imaging with endogenous substances. Proc. Natl. Acad. Sci. USA 2003, 100, 10435–10439.

[58] Golman K, Petersson, JS. Metabolic imaging and other applications of hyperpolarized 13C. Acad. Radiol. 2006, 13, 932–942.

[59] Golman K, Zandt RI, Lerche M, Pehrson R, Ardenkjaer-Larsen JH. Metabolic imaging by hyperpolarized 13C magnetic resonance imaging for in vivo tumor diagnosis. Cancer Res. 2006, 66, 10855–10860.

[60] Gallagher FA, Kettunen MI, Day SE, Hu DE, Ardenkjaer-Larsen JH, Zandt R, Jensen PR, Karlsson M, Golman K, Lerche MH, Brindle KM. Magnetic resonance imaging of pH in vivo using hyperpolarized 13C-labelled bicarbonate. Nature. 2008; 453(7197):940-3.

[61] Day SE, Kettunen MI, Gallagher FA, Hu DE, Lerche M, Wolber J, Golman K, Ardenkjaer-Larsen JH, Brindle KM. Detecting tumor response to treatment using hyperpolarized 13C magnetic resonance imaging and spectroscopy. Nat Med. 2007; 13(11):1382-7.

[62] White A, Handler P, Smith EL. Principles of Biochemistry (McGraw-Hill Kogakusha, New York, 1968). Stabenau EK, Heming TA. Determination of the constants of the Henderson- Hasselbalch equation, aCO2 and pKa, in sea turtle plasma. J. Exp. Biol. 1993, 180, 311–314.

[63] Gadian DG. NMR and its application to living systems; 2nd ed; OUP: Oxford,1995

[64] Ojugo AS, McSheehy PM, McIntyre DJ, McCoy C, Stubbs M, Leach MO, Judson IR, Griffiths JR. Measurement of the extracellular pH of solid tumours in mice by magnetic resonance spectroscopy: a comparison of exogenous (19) F and (31)P probes. NMR Biomed. 1999; 12(8):495-504.

[65] Mason RP. Transmembrane pH gradients in vivo: measurements using fluorinated vitamin B6 derivatives. Curr Med Chem. 1999; 6(6):481-99.

[66] Roos A, Boron WF. Intracellular pH. Physiol Rev 1981; 61:296-434

[67] Scott RD, Chang YC, Graves DJ, Metzler DE. Studies of 6-fluoropyridoxal and 6-fluoropyridoxamine 5′-phosphate in cytosolic aspartate aminotransferase. Biochemistry 1985, 24, 7668-7681

[68] He S, Mason RP, Hunjan S, Mehta VD, Arora V, Katipally R, Kulkarni PV, Antich PP. Development of novel 19F NMR pH indicators: synthesis and evaluation of a series of fluorinated vitamin B6 analogues. Bioorg Med Chem.1998; 6(9):1631-9.

16

Metabolic Imaging of Brain Tumor by ^{99m}Tc-Tetrofosmin Scintitomography

Spyridon Tsiouris, George Alexiou,
Athanasios Papadopoulos and Andreas Fotopoulos
University General Hospital of Ioannina
Greece

1. Introduction

Primary brain tumors have an annual incidence rate ranging between 7 and 19 new cases per 100,000 population. Metastatic tumors to the brain are more common, with more than 100,000 patients per year in the United States. Gliomas are the most common primary brain tumors (DeAngelis, 2001). Among them, astrocytomas account for more than half of all primary malignancies of the central nervous system (CNS). They are classified into 4 grades: Grades I and II are considered as low-grade; anaplastic tumors (Grade III) and glioblastoma multiforme (Grade IV) are considered high-grade tumors.

Glioblastoma multiforme (GBM) is the most common and most malignant of the glial tumors occurring in adults (Liu et al., 2010). Other types are oligodendrogliomas, ependymomas, meningiomas, pituitary adenomas, embryonal tumors and gangliogliomas. Among them meningiomas are the most common benign intracranial tumors, accounting for up to one fourth of all primary lesions (Whittle et al., 2004). The most common presenting symptoms of brain tumors are due to increased intracranial pressure (headache, nausea, vomiting), seizures, focal neurological deficits and possibly cognitive deterioration.

With regards to treatment, in low-grade lesions radical surgical removal will generally allow functional survival for many years. Adjuvant radiotherapy can halt disease progress for a time and probably increases survival. For high-grade tumors surgical resection is almost always followed by radiotherapy and adjuvant chemotherapy that are usually given concomitantly. Temozolomide is the mainstay of treatment administered in parallel with and post-radiotherapy, with benefits in overall survival (Stupp et al., 2005). Patients younger than 60 years, with good functional status and gross total tumor resection have a better prognosis (Scott et al., 1999).

Computed tomography (CT) and magnetic resonance imaging (MRI) are necessary to characterize gross tumor appearance, size and extension. Nevertheless, in patients with brain lesions it is not uncommon for radiomorphological modalities to provide non-specific information, even after infusion of iodine-based contrast media or gadolinium-based paramagnetic complexes. An enhancing lesion may represent a glioma, an abscess, a metastasis or even a primary CNS lymphoma.

To gain additional diagnostic information from that acquired by conventional radiology, functional metabolic imaging by nuclear medicine techniques has been introduced, aiming to provide information related to the metabolic status of brain tumors. These metabolic imaging modalities comprise single-photon emission computed tomography (SPECT) and positron emission tomography (PET). Although PET may be credited with providing the impetus for the new clinical interest in functional neuroimaging, SPECT has offered a credible alternative with the advantage of lower cost and wider availability.

Various single-photon emitting radiotracers have been used to date, thallium-201 (^{201}Tl) being among the first and mostly studied. Technetium-99m (^{99m}Tc)-labeled compounds have also been evaluated, including ^{99m}Tc-methionine, ^{99m}Tc-glucoheptonate and more extensively ^{99m}Tc-hexakis-2-methoxy isobutyl isonitrile (^{99m}Tc-sestamibi or ^{99m}Tc-MIBI). For a number of reasons including higher photon flux, better spatial resolution, less radiation burden to the patient and excellent availability, the use of ^{99m}Tc-based compounds has progressively prevailed over ^{201}Tl.

^{99m}Tc-tetrofosmin (^{99m}Tc-TF) is another ^{99m}Tc-based SPECT radiotracer that demonstrates certain similarities with ^{99m}Tc-MIBI. Both are routinely used for myocardial perfusion imaging, but also exhibit tumor-seeking properties. Whereas ^{99m}Tc-MIBI has been extensively evaluated in imaging brain tumors for nearly two decades, ^{99m}Tc-TF has been introduced in this field for a considerably shorter period of time.

2. The radiotracer and its cellular uptake mechanism

^{99m}Tc-TF is a lipophilic cationic diphosphine routinely used for myocardial perfusion imaging and has also been shown to exhibit certain tumor-seeking properties. These properties have been verified in various neoplasms including parathyroid adenoma and several carcinomas (e.g. of the breast, thyroid, nasopharynx and lung). Its uptake by intracranial tumors is under meticulous investigation during the past few years.

After intravenous administration, the tracer reaches the brain by the arterial blood flow. Despite being a lipophilic molecule, ^{99m}Tc-TF cannot cross the intact blood-brain barrier (BBB), which results in negligible tracer uptake in the healthy brain parenchyma. There is, however, some tracer accumulation normally occurring in the choroid plexuses and the pituitary gland, brain structures that lack BBB.

In order for ^{99m}Tc-TF to be taken up by the cells of a brain lesion, this has to disrupt the BBB. Its uptake mechanism depends on the blood flow to the lesion, as well as on the integrity of the membrane of the lesion cells, an indicator of their viability. The tracer enters viable cells mainly via passive transport, driven by the negative electric potential of the intact cell membrane, and it mostly localizes within the cytosol, with only a fraction passing into the mitochondria. In that sense, cellular ^{99m}Tc-TF uptake mainly reflects on the viability of lesion cells and their metabolic status.

As discussed in the following paragraphs, initial clinical evidence from *in vivo* studies suggests that there is a significant correlation between tracer uptake and cellular proliferation in both gliomas and meningiomas (Alexiou et al., 2008a, 2008b; Fotopoulos et al., 2008). Cellular proliferative activity may thus be regarded as a major driving force that leads to significant intracellular tracer accumulation and retention.

Other studies on human glioma cell lines *in vitro* and *in vivo* revealed that ^{99m}Tc-TF is influenced to a very small degree by the expression of P-glycoprotein (P-gp) (Le Jeune et al., 2005; Alexiou et al., 2011). P-gp is a membrane protein encoded by the multi-drug resistance (MDR) gene and acts as an ATP-dependent drug efflux pump, excreting anticancer pharmaceuticals and radiopharmaceutical imaging agents outside the tumor cell. Although both ^{99m}Tc-TF and ^{99m}Tc-MIBI have been found *in vitro* to be substrates of P-gp, the fact that

^{99m}Tc-TF uptake in glioma cells is not particularly influenced by the expression of their MDR protein genotype substantiates a plausible clinical superiority over ^{99m}Tc-MIBI, which is prone to extracellular excretion by P-gp.

3. Protocol of brain SPECT imaging

The radiopharmaceutical is prepared in the nuclear medicine department with the use of a commercially available powder kit (Myoview™, General Electric Healthcare Ltd., Buckinghamshire, UK), which is reconstituted with freshly eluted ^{99m}Tc pertechnetate ($^{99m}TcO_4^-$) sterile solution. Comparison of ^{99m}Tc-TF uptake in various types of lesions during imaging performed consecutively at 20, 40 and 120 min post-injection did not reveal any considerable fluctuations of relative tracer uptake over time (Soricelli et al., 1998). Hence, image acquisition at 20–30 min after radiotracer administration can be safely adopted as a convenient rule of thumb. The radiopharmaceutical is injected intravenously, at an administered activity of approximately 740-925 MBq (20-25 mCi).
All SPECT studies in our department are implemented on the same dual-head γ-camera (Millennium™ VG3, General Electric Medical Systems - Europe, Buc Cedex, France), equipped with a pair of low-energy, high-resolution, parallel-hole collimators. The matrix is set at 128 × 128 pixels; the photopeak is centered at 140 keV, allowing a symmetrical 10% window. The tomographic imaging parameters consist of a full-circle (360°) rotation angle, a 3°-step-and-shoot technique and an acquisition time of 30 sec per frame. Raw imaging data are reconstructed using the Butterworth-filtered back-projection algorithm (critical frequency [order]: 0.25; filter power: 5.0), generating tomographic views of the brain in the three planes (transverse, coronal and sagittal). In the case of γ-cameras with an integrated computed tomograph (hybrid SPECT/CT systems), data from a low-dose CT scan can be used for attenuation correction of the scintigraphic image. In non-hybrid modalities — currently comprising the vast majority— attenuation correction can be applied empirically during tomographic image reconstruction following the Chang method (attenuation factor: 0.11/cm).

3.1 Image analysis and interpretation

Radiotracer uptake in the brain is first assessed visually. ^{99m}Tc-TF cannot penetrate the intact BBB and does not accumulate in the normal brain parenchyma, so any abnormal uptake is readily identifiable against the negligible normal-brain background. Exceptions to this are the choroid plexuses and the pituitary, structures that lack BBB so they normally accumulate an amount of the tracer (Fig. 1). Space-occupying lesions adjacent to these structures could face obvious limitations in delineating their true scintigraphic margins and estimate the tracer uptake that is attributable to the lesion *per se*.
Semi-automated, semi-quantitative image analysis is a valuable adjunct to the objective visual image reading and adds subjectivity to the interpretation of the study. It is applied on the reconstructed SPECT images by calculating the lesion-to-normal (L/N) ratio of relative radiotracer uptake —hence the term 'semi-quantitative'. In our department the transversal SPECT slice in which lesion tracer uptake appears to be maximal is chosen manually — hence the term 'semi-automated'. This is performed in close reference to the corresponding CT/MRI transversal slices that serve as a reference guide of the lesion's topography.
After the selection of the slice with maximal lesion uptake, relative tracer concentration is calculated with the use of the Java-based, open-source image processing software *ImageJ*

(http://rsb.info.nih.gov/ij/index.html), developed by the National Institutes of Health. A region of interest (ROI) encircling the lesion is defined manually on the selected transversal slice and a second identical (mirror) region is drawn on the contra lateral normal side of the brain (Fig. 2). The L/N ratio is calculated by dividing the average counts in the lesion ROI by those in the contra lateral (background) ROI. The ROIs are independently evaluated for eligibility by two experienced nuclear medicine physicians and possible disagreements are resolved by consensus.

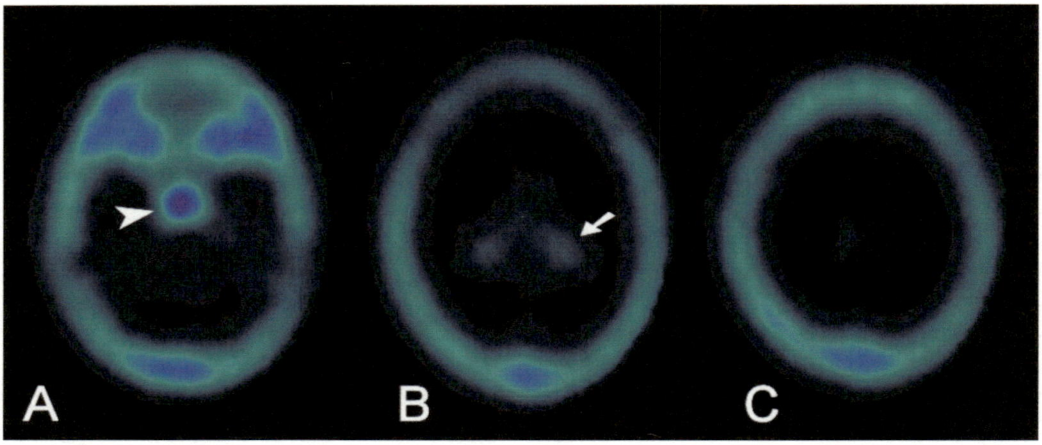

Fig. 1. A normal ^{99m}Tc-tetrofosmin brain SPECT study (transversal slicing in three different planes) displaying physiological tracer accumulation in the choroid plexuses (arrow), the pituitary (arrowhead) and the scalp.

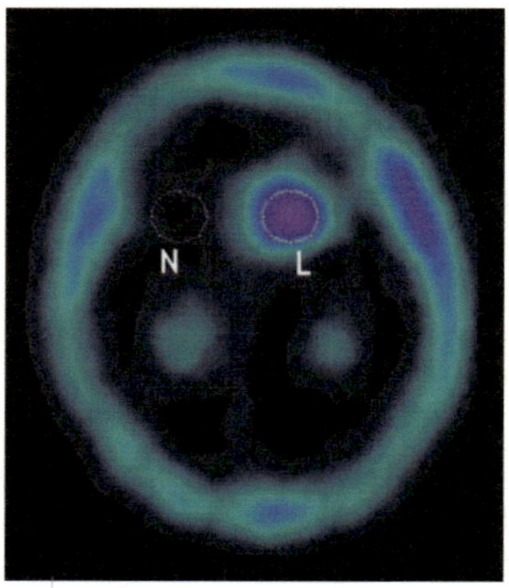

Fig. 2. ROI definition over the lesion (L) and over the normal brain parenchyma (N).

The application of the above methodology for L/N ratio calculation in everyday clinical practice is, in most cases, a straightforward process that provides reproducible results without significant deviations. Nevertheless, the location of the lesion within the brain and its morphology are critical factors for the application and effectiveness of the proposed technique. Lesion adjacency to anatomical structures with normal tracer uptake (choroid plexus, pituitary) increases the difficulty of reliable L/N calculation and the chances of its overestimation. In such cases, the operator has to make sure that the lesion ROI avoids normal structure uptake and encompasses only areas unquestionably pathologic, even if these do not appear to exhibit the maximum intensity of relative tracer uptake. Heterogeneity of tracer distribution within a lesion (e.g. due to local necrosis) may impose L/N calculation in more than one areas/SPECT slices. When large variations in tracer uptake intensity are apparent, a tight ROI around the highest uptake region may be more reliable than a looser one, which could lead to L/N underestimation. For lesions located around the midline there may not be a definite mirror area to draw the normal ROI; a nearby site could be safely selected in the majority of similar cases, since the level of the background activity is generally very low throughout.

4. Clinical applications

Our experience thus far with ^{99m}Tc-TF is based on its clinical use in SPECT imaging studies performed in nearly 200 cases of space-occupying brain lesions. Obtained results to date conform to the fact that ^{99m}Tc-TF brain SPECT can contribute substantial functional information to the structural data already obtained by CT and conventional MRI, thus helping to establish non-invasively an accurate diagnosis. Furthermore, based on observations in patients with high-grade gliomas, it looks like this radiotracer also carries a plausible prognostic role that merits further investigation.

In the following paragraphs the discussion will focus on the experience gained so far by the use of ^{99m}Tc-TF SPECT in the management of patients treated for brain tumor; the role of other SPECT and PET radiotracers and of other CNS imaging modalities such as conventional and functional MRI will also be mentioned.

4.1 Evaluation of intracranial space-occupying lesions: differentiation of high-grade from low-grade gliomas and non-neoplastic pathologies

Differentiating neoplastic from non-neoplastic intra-axial lesions is of paramount importance for patient management. Neoplastic and non-neoplastic pathologies may equally produce abnormal contrast enhancement, mass effects and perilesional edema on CT and classic MRI (Al-Okaili et al., 2007). Consequently, such clinical situations often constitute a diagnostic dilemma and it is not uncommon to seek the help of histological verification to establish a diagnosis.

The data of a prospectively implemented study comprising 106 patients hospitalized in the neurosurgery department of our institution over a 5-year period (between September 2004 and September 2009) were analyzed recently; all cases have been submitted to surgery due to an intracranial lesion suspicious of tumor on conventional radiological imaging. The patients underwent ^{99m}Tc-TF brain SPECT within a 7-10 day period after radiological diagnosis, with surgery following shortly after SPECT to establish histologically the final diagnosis. The only cases that did not receive surgery were among previously treated tumors resubmitted owning to suspected recurrence. These individuals were closely followed-up clinically and radiologically over a period of 6 months, to verify stability suggestive of radionecrosis, or on the other hand, disease progression consistent with tumor relapse.

Ninety patients suffered from neoplastic lesions and 16 harbored non-neoplastic pathologies (abscesses, non-malignant hemorrhages, radiation necroses). ^{99m}Tc-TF was taken up more avidly by high-grade gliomas (Fig. 3) than by low-grade lesions and could reliably distinguish them, with an L/N ratio of 2.8 providing the optimal discrimination threshold (Fotopoulos et al., 2011). Similar findings have also been reported by other authors (Choi et al., 2000). Furthermore, ^{99m}Tc-TF differentiated effectively high- and low-grade gliomas from non-neoplastic lesions. Nonetheless, differentiation between gliomas between gliomas – either low- or high-grade– and metastases was not feasible on the basis of scintigraphic (L/N) criteria.

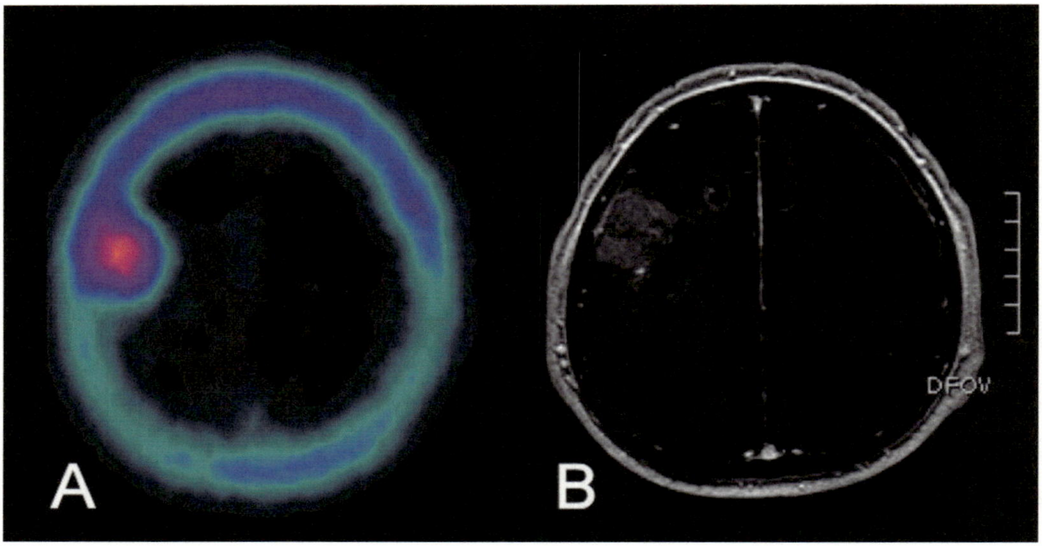

Fig. 3. High-grade glioma associated with significant tracer uptake (L/N=16).

Several other SPECT tracers have been used for the initial evaluation of brain lesions. ^{201}Tl was able to differentiate malignant tumors from poorly vascularized benign lesions, yet faced a limited ability to separate between the latter and low-grade astrocytomas, as well as tumors from abscesses (Staffen et al., 1998; Kinuya et al., 2002). ^{99m}Tc-MIBI has been evaluated in various brain pathologies. If performed within 5 days of symptom onset, it has been found capable of differentiating neoplastic from non-neoplastic intracerebral hematomas (Minutoli et al., 2005). Iodine-123-α-methyl tyrosine (^{123}I-IMT) was also among the SPECT tracers to provide encouraging results for imaging tumor recurrence (Samnick et al., 2002).

4.1.1 Discriminating recurrent disease from radiation necrosis in previously treated tumors

Treatment of brain gliomas depends on their localisation, cell type and grade of malignancy. It normally combines surgery, radiation therapy and chemotherapy. Radiotherapy –in the form of external beam radiation, brachytherapy, or stereotactic radiotherapy– consists the primary adjuvant treatment after surgical resection. Among the delayed side effects of radiation therapy, radionecrosis is the most prominent, primarily depending on the administered dose and rate of delivery and usually occurs within 6 months to 2 years, the same period during which disease recurrence is also rather frequent (Marks & Wong, 1985).

Radiation injury is usually localized around the tumor bed umor bed —where recurrent glioma is also typically located—, although occasional reports describe necrosis arising anywhere in the path of the irradiation beam. It is not uncommon for radiation injury and recurrent disease to coexist.

Since these two entities have diverse treatment approach and prognosis, differentiation between them is crucial and several imaging techniques have been evaluated towards this objective. Morphological depiction of the brain by classic MRI and CT can merely recognize edema and BBB disruption, so it is usually inconclusive and faces inherent limitations in discriminating viable tumor from post-irradiation change (Byrne, 1994).

Depiction of recurrent tumor was the first imaging challenge against which we evaluated ^{99m}Tc-TF brain SPECT accuracy a few years back (Alexiou et al., 2007). A prospective ongoing study enrolled 24 patients that had been previously treated surgically for brain tumor followed by external beam radiotherapy, while some had also received adjuvant chemotherapy. No residual tumor had been recognized on radiological imaging immediately after initial treatment. On follow-up they developed neurological symptomatology consistent with tumor recurrence, with radiological investigation verifying the presence of a contrast-enhancing lesion with edema and mass effects. In 5 cases surgical excision of the lesion was performed within a week after ^{99m}Tc-TF scintigraphy and a diagnosis was reached histologically. In the rest the diagnosis was based on clinical and neuromorphological follow-up, owning to various reasons (technically inoperable lesions, critical clinical condition, patient refusal to re-operate etc.). A 6-month 'wait-and-see' period is considered sufficient by most to reach a safe estimation of the diagnosis. This is because by that time glioma growth within the limited space of the cranial cavity will definitelly result in clinical deterioration and radiological progression, which may safely be considered as indicative of recurrence.

On tumor recurrence SPECT depicted increased ^{99m}Tc-TF uptake in the region of the brain that corresponded to the radiologically detected lesion, suggesting the presence of viable hypermetabolic tissue (Fig. 4). On the contrary, radionecrotic lesions tended to exhibit significantly fainter tracer uptake (Fig. 5). Receiver operating characteristic (ROC) curve statistical analysis returned a threshold L/N value of 4.8 as most accurately discriminating these two clinical entities. However, it must be kept in mind that, according to relevant reports, ^{99m}Tc-TF SPECT exhibits suboptimal sensitivity in detecting recurrence of tumors located subtentorially in the posterior fossa (Barai et al., 2003).

^{201}Tl was one of the first single-photon emitting radiotracers evaluated in the same clinical setting. Published data thus far suggest a wide range of sensitivity and specificity in detecting tumor recurrence in patients with previously treated supratentorial gliomas, partially owning to varying occurrence of false positives; still ^{201}Tl SPECT is reported to have an advantage over conventional MRI (Vos et al., 2007). ^{99m}Tc-MIBI has also been extensively evaluated with good reported results and a significant diagnostic advantage over contrast-enhanced MRI (Soler et al., 1998). Imaging protein synthesis using radiolabeled amino acids is another approach employed towards non-invasive revelation of tumor recurrence. Various natural amino acids have been labeled with radioactive isotopes —mostly PET— and are currently investigated. As regards SPECT, encouraging results were reported for ^{99m}Tc-methionine and ^{123}I-IMT (Barai et al., 2004; Samnick et al., 2002).

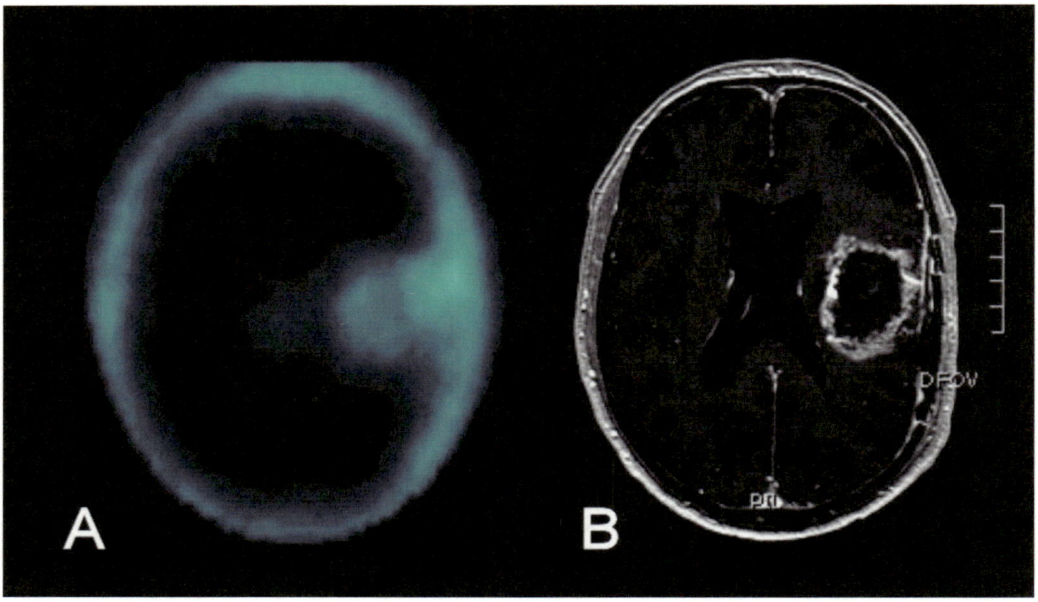

Fig. 4. Recurrent astrocytoma characterized by intense tracer uptake (L/N=8.7).

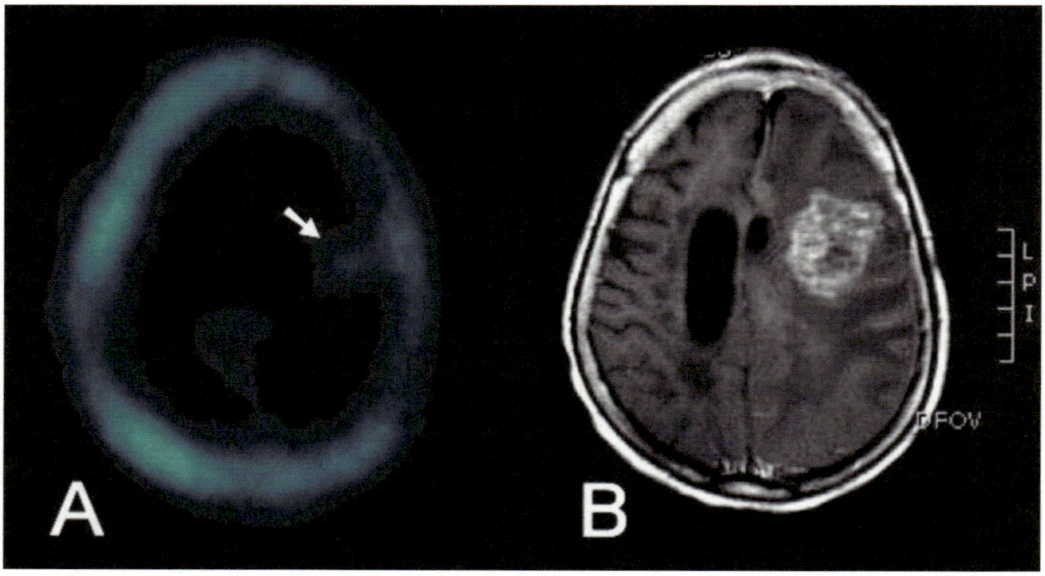

Fig. 5. Radiation necrosis exhibiting only mildly increased tracer uptake (L/N=2.9).

4.1.2 Spontaneous intracerebral hemorrhage: Masking an underlying neoplasm?

With reference to non-traumatic intracerebral hemorrhage (ICH), distinguishing a neoplastic from a non-neoplastic one constitutes a challenging task, since neoplasms can be hidden behind an intracerebral hematoma, while some non-neoplastic hemorrhages may mimic neoplasms on standard radiomorphological imaging. Bleeding deriving from a malignant brain lesion accounts for approximately 10% of all ICHs, with metastases displaying the highest susceptibility. The pre-operative diagnosis of a tumor as the underlying cause of an ICH is usually very difficult for CT and MRI, even for the modern functional MRI techniques. Hence diagnosis is based on evolution patterns of the hematoma in a series of sequential radiological studies over a period of several weeks, until the extravasated blood is absorbed so the tumor revealed.

^{99m}Tc-TF SPECT can play a role in differentiating neoplastic from non-neoplastic hemorrhages, since only the latter exhibit negligible to no radiotracer uptake (Alexiou et al., 2006) (Fig. 6). Our experience is based on an increasing series of patients with spontaneous ICH referred to our department, most of whom bear some kind of malignancy. Out of the 8 cases reviewed so far, in half the diagnosis was based on surgery and on a 'wait-and-see' clinical and morphologic follow-up in the rest. Although only two hemorrhages were finally proven to be of neoplastic origin, ^{99m}Tc-TF SPECT managed to accurately identify both (Fotopoulos et al., 2011).

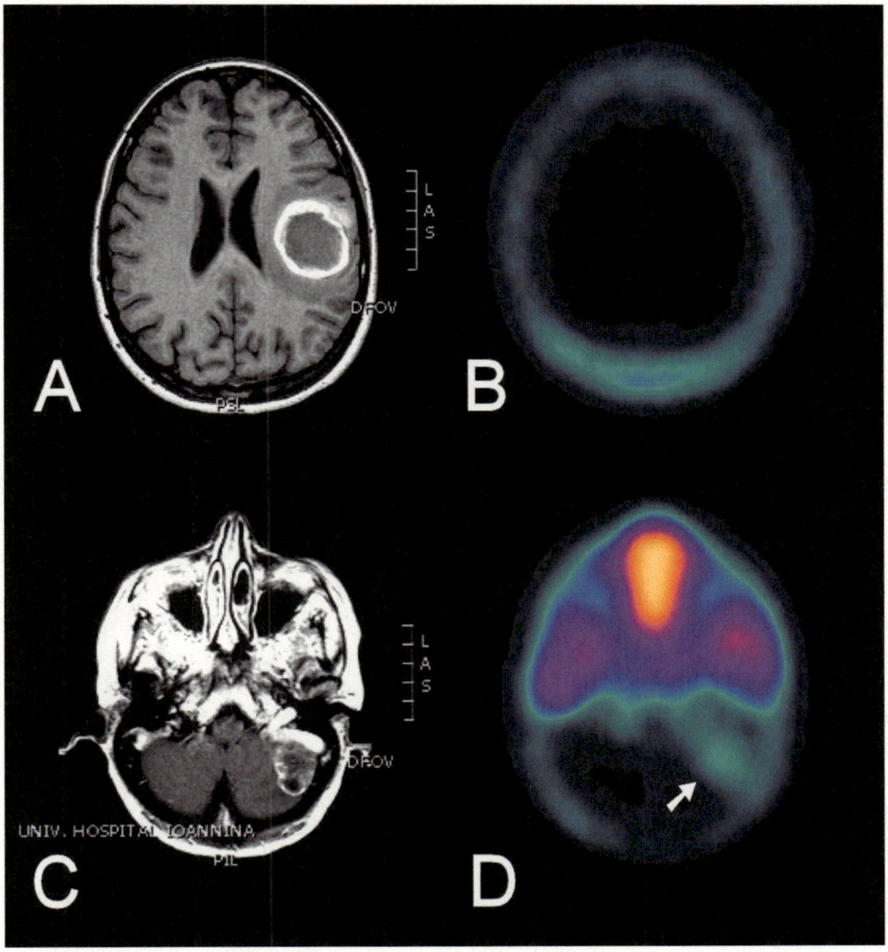

Fig. 6. Intracerebral hemorrhage without signs of tracer uptake, suggesting a benign origin (A, B). On the other hand, a cerebellar hemorrhage exhibits significant tracer uptake (arrow), strongly suggesting the presence of an underlying neoplasm (C, D).

4.2 Assessment of glioma aggressiveness

Assessing the proliferative potential of tumor cells is of paramount importance for predicting their biological behavior, response to therapy and prognosis. Proliferation is equally important in gliomas, since patients with the same histopathological profile that receive equivalent treatment may display diverse natural history and prognosis, owning to differences in the proliferative potential of their disease.

As a result, various methodologies and immunohistological markers have been developed to estimate proliferation in tissue samples. MIB-1 antibody immunostaining to the nuclear antigen Ki-67 is performed routinely and is considered as the most reliable proliferation index, since it is expressed in nearly all phases of the cell cycle, with the exception of phase G_0 (McKeever et al., 1997). Flow cytometry assessing DNA ploidy and S-phase fraction can also provide reliable clues on glioma aggressiveness (Garcia et al., 1997). Nevertheless, these methods require tissue sampling through biopsy or over the course of a surgical procedure. It is therefore equally important for functional imaging to develop radiolabeled tracers that can provide non-invasively an accurate *in vivo* estimate of glioma proliferation.

In a prospective pilot study we evaluated the relationship between glioma proliferation, as expressed by the Ki-67 immunohistological index, and ^{99m}Tc-TF uptake. Patients bearing space-occupying lesions suspicious of glioma on structural brain imaging were enrolled. Within a week after SPECT imaging the lesion was removed surgically and Ki-67 was assessed in the excised specimens. The diagnosed tumors were glioblastoma multiforme (6 cases), anaplastic astrocytoma (1), anaplastic oligodendroglioma (2), low-grade oligodendroglioma (1), and low-grade astrocytoma (1). Statistical analysis revealed a strong positive linear correlation between L/N tracer uptake ratio and Ki-67 expression (Alexiou et al., 2008a). These initial results were supported by another prospective study to follow, in which we sought for a possible correlation between ^{99m}Tc-TF uptake and glioma proliferative activity assessed by flow cytometry. Again, a significant positive linear correlation between radiotracer uptake and the fraction of tumor cells on the S-phase of the cell cycle was verified (Alexiou et al., 2008b).

As regards other SPECT radiotracers, ^{201}Tl was one of the first studied. Reports described a correlation with bromodeoxyuridine (BrdU) and proliferating cell nuclear antigen (PCNA) tissue labeling indices (Oriuchi et al., 1993; Ishibashi et al., 1995; Gungor et al., 2000). ^{99m}Tc-MIBI was found to display a positive correlation with glioma proliferation, as assessed by both flow cytometry and Ki-67, and this was stronger compared to ^{201}Tl (Ak et al., 2003; Nagamachi et al., 2001). With regards to labeled amino acid SPECT, ^{123}I-IMT was similarly reported to correlate with Ki-67 expression (Kuwert et al., 1997). Finally, pentavalent ^{99m}Tc-dimercapto-succinic acid (^{99m}Tc-[V]DMSA) is another tumor-seeking tracer whose proliferative imaging potential in gliomas has been suggested *in vitro* and sporadically reported *in vivo* (Denoyer et al., 2005; Tsiouris et al., 2007).

4.3 Assessment of meningiomas: differentiation between typical and anaplastic and estimation of aggressiveness

Meningiomas account for nearly 30% of all intracranial tumors and are usually diagnosed after the third decade of life, being twice more frequent in women. According to the World Health Organization (WHO) they are classified into benign (grade I), atypical (grade II) and anaplastic/malignant (grade III) (Lamszus, 2004). Although they usually have a relatively benign clinical course and only a 15% recurrence rate, atypical and malignant lesions are associated with high recurrence rates and poor outcome (Kayaselcuk et al., 2004). Their proliferative potential is essential for their biological characterization, which affects patient management and has prognostic implications. Hence, similarly to gliomas, their non-invasive metabolic characterization constitutes a major objective for CNS imaging.

As with gliomas, we investigated prospectively whether ^{99m}Tc-TF SPECT can provide useful clues for meningioma grade and cellular proliferative activity. After radiomorphological imaging revealed the lesion, scintigraphic imaging by ^{99m}Tc-TF was performed within a week before surgical excision and the surgical specimens were graded following the WHO criteria and stained for Ki-67. The intensity of tumoral radiotracer uptake ranged from restrained to prominent. Malignant lesions tended to exhibit a significantly higher uptake compared to lesions of low histological grade. ROC analysis provided an L/N ratio value of 9.6 as the optimal cut-off point thresholding the two groups. L/N tracer uptake analysis also revealed a significant linear correlation with both meningioma grade and Ki-67 expression (Fotopoulos et al., 2008). These findings pertaining to Ki-67 were sustained by another study, which aimed to correlate meningioma tracer uptake with its proliferative profile, as assessed by flow cytometry. Result analysis revealed a significant correlation of ^{99m}Tc-TF uptake with both the S-phase fraction and the level of DNA aneuploidy (Alexiou et al., 2008b).

^{201}Tl was among the first single-photon emitting radiotracers studied in meningioma. Its uptake pre-operatively has been proposed to differentiate meningiomas with different biological behaviors, while tracer retention by a lesion correlated with its malignant potential (Jinnouchi et al., 1993; Tedeschi et al., 1996). Nevertheless, later reports did not verify any correlation between ^{201}Tl uptake and PCNA labeling index in meningiomas, dissimilar to gliomas (Gungor et al., 2000).

4.4 Patient prognosis

Glioblastoma is the most common and most malignant of the glial tumors occurring in adults, with unfavorable prognosis. Even so, a subset of patients demonstrates long-term survival reaching or even exceeding three years. Since no reliable biomarker has been established for use in clinical practice, prognostic factors already proposed are age at diagnosis, the Karnofsky Performance Score (KPS) and extent of surgical resection, although these inadequately predict outcome (Scott et al., 1999; Lacroix et al., 2001). Identification of solid prognostic variables could recognize patients that may benefit from aggressive treatment schemes and allow for the selection of more homogenous populations in clinical trials.

The correlation between *in vivo* ^{99m}Tc-TF uptake and glioma proliferation, as assessed by the Ki-67 index and flow cytometry, has already been described (Alexiou et al., 2008a, 2008b). Due to the established prognostic value of Ki-67 in gliomas, investigating a possible association between pre-treatment tumoral tracer uptake and overall survival seemed as the next logical step. We followed-up 18 newly diagnosed GBM cases who had been submitted to ^{99m}Tc-TF SPECT prior to surgery. All patients received post-operative standard radiotherapy (6000 rads) with adjuvant temozolomide chemotherapy and then temozolomide up to a year after surgery, or until recurrence. Cases of tumor recurrence were treated by supportive care, with no additional surgery or chemotherapy. Patients bearing lesions with radiotracer L/N uptake 4.7 or less exhibited significantly better survival compared to those with a ratio exceeding 4.7. KPS exceeding 90 was also associated with a better course. Patients with near-total resection or aged under 60 displayed a longer survival trend, although not statistically significant. Multivariate analysis similarly proved

radiotracer uptake and KPS as the only variables with independent prognostic power (Alexiou et al., 2010).
The prognostic value of tumoral ^{201}Tl uptake has been evaluated in the same clinical context and was found associated with worse survival for lesions located supratentorially (Oriuchi et al., 1993). Post-treatment ^{99m}Tc-MIBI uptake has also been described to exhibit prognostic implications in high-grade gliomas and similar results were also reported for ^{123}I-IMT (Beauchesne et al., 2004; Weber et al., 2001).

5. Other metabolic imaging modalities: PET

Brain PET imaging is extensively evaluated towards the distinction between tumors and non-neoplastic brain lesions. Although initial results for fluorine-18 fluoro-deoxyglucose (^{18}F-FDG) PET were encouraging, later studies revealed considerable limitations and, for that reason, other positron-emitting radiotracers were put under perspective (Ricci et al., 1998). Carbon-11 methionine (^{11}C-MET) gave promising results, yet it suffers limited availability owning to the need of an on-site cyclotron to produce the short-lived ^{11}C (Galldiks et al., 2010). ^{18}F-fluoro-choline, O-(2-[^{18}F]fluoro-ethyl)-L-tyrosine (^{18}F-FET) and 3,4-dihydroxy-6-^{18}F-fluoro-L-phenylalanine (^{18}F-FDOPA) are PET tracers that have been proven superior to ^{18}F-FDG for brain tumor imaging (Kwee et al., 2007; Pauleit et al., 2009; Chen et al., 2006).
Diagnosis of brain tumor recurrence has been an imaging challenge also for PET. Although initial reports for ^{18}F-FDG were encouraging (Di Chiro et al., 1988), more recent studies questioned its diagnostic accuracy, which was found considerably inferior to that of ^{201}Tl SPECT in several series (Kahn et al., 1994; Gómez-Río et al., 2008). A significant disadvantage of ^{18}F-FDG derives from its physiological uptake in the glucose-metabolizing normal brain. For that reason other tumor-seeking positron-emitting radiotracers have been developed. ^{11}C-MET PET has given superior results compared to ^{18}F-FDG because of its sensitivity and clearer delineation of recurrence (Van Laere et al., 2005), yet suffers limited availability due to the need of an on-site cyclotron to produce ^{11}C and the same applies for ^{13}N-NH_3 (ammonia), which has also been tried (Xiangsong et al., 2006). Perhaps the most promising PET tracers to date are the labeled analogues of thymidine, 3'-deoxy-3'-^{18}F-fluoro-thymidine (^{18}F-FLT) and of tyrosine, ^{18}F-FET. Their greatest advantage compared to other PET tracers lies in their low uptake by normal brain parenchyma, thus providing a better contrast between tumor and normal brain. Initial experience gained from a series of studies suggests that these agents are superior to ^{18}F-FDG and to conventional MRI in distinguishing tumor recurrence from radiation-induced brain injury (Chen et al., 2005; Pöpperl et al., 2004).
PET has been widely utilized to evaluate glioma proliferation. The uptake kinetics of ^{18}F-FDG reflect glucose metabolism, whose modifications are only indirectly related to the proliferation status of the tumor. Moreover, the physiological high dependence of normal brain on glucose metabolism results in normally increased fluoro-deoxyglucose uptake, which accounts for the tracer's suboptimal diagnostic performance. Among radiolabeled amino acids, ^{11}C-MET is the most extensively studied with encouraging results, still the short-lived ^{11}C precludes its use in centers without a cyclotron on-site (Kim et al., 2005; Hatakeyama et al., 2008). ^{11}C-thymidine PET is of great interest, since thymidine is the native pyrimidine base used in DNA synthesis, yet suffers from rapid *in vivo* degradation and the limited availability issues of ^{11}C. To overcome these restrictions, ^{18}F-FLT has been

developed as an alternative estimator of the DNA synthesis rate and is currently proving a useful proliferation imaging tracer, correlating well with Ki-67 (Shields et al., 1996; Ullrich et al., 2008).

As in CNS gliomas, ^{18}F-FDG uptake kinetics in meningiomas reflect on glucose metabolism that is only indirectly related to proliferation. In a pilot PET study comprising ^{11}C-MET, tracer uptake succesfully predicted meningioma proliferation (Ki-67) (Iuchi et al., 1999). ^{18}F-FLT also holds plenty of theoretical advantages that remain to be proven in practice.

6. Functional MRI techniques

Conventional radiomorphological imaging —in the form of CT and classic MRI— may face significant limitations in discriminating benign from malignant intracranial space-occupying pathologies, since these modalities basically recognize BBB disruption, mass-effects and edema that can equally accompany both categories of lesions. An answer to these limitations towards the discrimination of neoplastic from non-neoplastic lesions has been attempted by the introduction of functional MRI techniques, namely perfusion MRI and MR spectroscopy (MRS).

Perfusion MRI estimates tumor neovascularity and capillary permeability *in vivo*, by measuring the relative cerebral blood volume (rCBV); higher vascularity usually corresponds to a more aggressive pathology. In the diagnosis between tumor recurrence and radiation injury, perfusion MR holds a role by measuring vascularity within the suspicious brain areas. Since vasculature adjusts perfusion to meet metabolic tissue demands, rich vascularity can be an indirect measure of increased tissue metabolism, with relapsing tumor generally being highly vascular as opposed to radionecrosis (Covarrubias et al., 2004).

Proton MRS is able to depict the metabolic composition of a tissue, by detecting the relative concentrations of several major metabolites such as choline (Cho), creatine (Cr), *N*-acetyl aspartate (NAA) and other macromolecules. NAA is predominantly localized in neurons, Cho is a marker of cell membrane metabolism and Cr reflects energy metabolism. Despite no tumor-specific metabolite has been identified to date, an increased level of Cho with decreased NAA and Cr were proven suggestive of brain tumor (Hollingworth et al., 2006). MRS has been evaluated by several investigators for the differentiation of neoplastic from non-neoplastic intra-axial lesions — such as brain abscess, demyelination, infarct and radiation necrosis — with good results. The Cho/Cr and Cho/NAA ratios tend to increase in cases of tumor reccurence and thus contribute to its differentiation from radiation injury (Ando et al., 2004). This modality has also been evaluated for the non-invasive assessment of glioma aggressiveness, with initial findings associating Cho/Cr and Cho/NAA ratios with proliferative activity (Shimizu et al., 2000; Tamiya et al., 2000).

Diffusion weighted imaging (DWI) and diffusion tensor imaging (DTI) constitute modern functional MR techniques, which reflect on the viability and structure of tissues at the cellular level. Their role in differentiating between tumor recurrence and radionecrosis is under study (Hein et al., 2004; Sundgren et al., 2006), while it also remains to be determined whether they can provide findings clearly linkable to glioma proliferative activity.

7. Advantages of ^{99m}Tc-TF for brain SPECT imaging

The ^{99m}Tc-labeled compounds ^{99m}Tc-TF and ^{99m}Tc-MIBI bear certain imaging characteristics that are proven advantageous over ^{201}Tl. The single-photon (γ-ray) emitted by ^{99m}Tc peaks at

140 keV, which is optimal for imaging in the γ-camera, while its higher photon flux results in improved spatial resolution and less radiation burden to the patient. Of note is the excellent availability of ^{99m}Tc in every nuclear medicine department.

^{99m}Tc-TF shares a similar cellular uptake mechanism with ^{99m}Tc-MIBI, yet it mostly localizes within the cytosol, whereas the latter accumulates predominantly in the mitochondria. *In vitro* studies in glioma cell lines substantiated a plausible clinical superiority of ^{99m}Tc-TF over ^{99m}Tc-MIBI in imaging gliomas and meningiomas, largely due to the considerably lesser reliance of its intracellular concentration on cellular MDR expression (P-gp) (Le Jeune et al., 2005). In a recent study we verified *in vivo* this non-dependence of ^{99m}Tc-TF uptake on the glioma MDR phenotype, suggesting that it constitutes an appropriate radiotracer for glioma imaging, although less ideal for identifying P-gp-avid lesions that are likely to respond poorly to chemotherapy (Alexiou et al., 2011).

8. Limitations of ^{99m}Tc-TF brain SPECT

The method's limitations derive mainly from the nature of ^{99m}Tc-TF kinetics in the brain. Although it does not cross the intact BBB, which drastically results in its negligible concentration in the normal brain parenchyma, it physiologically accumulates in the choroid plexuses and the pituitary gland, which are structures normally lacking BBB. Physiological tracer activity comes also from the scalp. This normal uptake may therefore hamper image processing by hindering precise ROI definition for lesions lying adjacently to these anatomical structures and this can prove elaborate even under CT/MRI guidance. In such cases, hybrid SPECT/CT modalities could partially overcome this limitation by providing better spatial tumor localization to co-register with SPECT and also by applying attenuation correction to SPECT image processing and L/N calculation.

Apart from the proximity to areas of normal tracer uptake, location also matters when it comes to lesions sited subtentorially. There are reports suggesting that tumors of the posterior fossa tend to exhibit a lower-than-anticipated tracer uptake that hinders diagnostic accuracy (Barai et al., 2003).

Inherent to the integrity of the BBB is also the fact that ^{99m}Tc-TF has limited ability to penetrate into and characterize metabolically those brain lesions that do not exhibit contrast-enhancement on radiological imaging. Non-enhancement is an indicator of a non-ruptured BBB and is usually observed in low-grade gliomas.

Limitations innate to SPECT instrumentation ought not to be ignored. Spatial resolution is confined to 7.0 mm on ideal situations. In practice this limit usually reaches larger values (8.0-1.0 cm) due to various reasons, which can significantly affect the modality's ability to depict small lesions sized close to that limit.

We should not disregard certain restrictions originating from study design and implementation. Our experience thus far derives from small-scale studies implemented on a single-institution basis and with relatively small numbers of cases. Possible limitations might also emerge from the lack of histological verification in subgroups of the enrolled patients, like in those studies aiming to distinguish tumor recurrence from radionecrosis. Although histology provides the definitive diagnosis, this cannot always be achieved, as in cases of patient denying surgery or when surgical access to the lesion is not feasible. In such instances, a 6-month clinical and radiomorphological close follow-up could provide an acceptable diagnostic alternative, as explained earlier.

9. Conclusion

Radiomorphological imaging of the brain by conventional MRI and CT is of paramount importance in identifying structural abnormalities secondary to the development of space-occupying lesions, especially when those pathologies disrupt the BBB and give rise to contrast enhancement, edema and mass effects. Nevertheless, the true nature of each visible lesion may lie well beyond gross structural patterns, down to the cellular and molecular level. This is where functional metabolic imaging by SPECT, PET and modern MRI techniques come into play and excel.

Histopathology, immunodiagnostic labeling assays to certain cellular antigens and other techniques like flow cytometry applied on excised tissue specimens are considered as the reference standard of diagnosis, of assessing aggressiveness and the likelihood of response to therapy, while also provide an estimate of prognosis. Yet tissue samples are obtained through surgical intervention, which is not always possible for numerous reasons already discussed. Furthermore, regional tissue heterogeneity within brain tumors may result in sampling errors. This underscores the importance of functional brain imaging in providing easily implemented, non-invasive diagnostic and prognostic alternative markers.

Novel MRI techniques like MRS, DWI and DTI, together with certain PET and SPECT radiotracers, show promising results in the non-invasive assessment of tumor grade, proliferative potential, response to therapy and prognostication. In healthcare units without a PET facility, brain SPECT by ^{99m}Tc-TF can render useful metabolic information for newly diagnosed intracranial lesions prior to surgical intervention. Whether pertaining to gliomas or meningiomas, the lesions' grade and proliferation can be efficaciously estimated and credible evaluations may be extracted for their prognosis. The method can also hold a role in the non-invasive diagnostic work-up of hemorrhagic intracerebral lesions, while it certainly has much to offer in differentiating radiation necrosis from brain tumor recurrence in patients previously treated by surgery and adjuvant radio-chemotherapy.

Overall, there is gathering evidence to substantiate the need for larger scale, well-designed, prospective comparative studies between functional MR techniques and PET/SPECT radiotracers like ^{99m}Tc-TF, aiming to increase diagnostic accuracy and establish their clinical role in optimizing treatment decisions and reliably contribute on assessing patient prognosis.

10. References

Ak, I.; Gulbas, Z.; Altinel, F. & Vardareli, E. (2003). Tc-99m MIBI uptake and its relation to the proliferative potential of brain tumors. *Clin Nucl Med*, Vol.28, No.1, (January 2003), pp.29-33, ISSN 03639762

Al-Okaili, R.N.; Krejza, J.; Woo, J.H.; Wolf, R.L.; O'Rourke, D.M.; Judy, K.D.; Poptani, H. & Melhem ER. (2007). Intraaxial brain masses: MR imaging based diagnostic strategy—initial experience. *Radiology*, Vol.243, No.2, (May 2007), pp.539–550, ISSN 0033-8419

Alexiou, G.A.; Bokharhii, J.A.; Kyritsis, A.P.; Polyzoidis, K.S. & Fotopoulos, A.D. (2006). Tc-99m Tetrofosmin SPECT for the differentiation of a cerebellar hemorrhage mimicking a brain metastasis from a renal cell carcinoma. *J Neurooncol*, Vol.78, No.2, (March 2006), pp.207-208, ISSN 0167-594X

Alexiou, G.A.; Fotopoulos, A.D., Papadopoulos, A.; Kyritsis, A.P.; Polyzoidis, K.S. & Tsiouris, S. (2007). Evaluation of brain tumor recurrence by (99m)Tc-tetrofosmin SPECT: a prospective pilot study. *Ann Nucl Med*, Vol.21, No.5, (July 2007), pp.293-298, ISSN 0914-7187

Alexiou, G.A.; Tsiouris, S.; Goussia, A.; Papadopoulos, A.; Kyritsis, A.P.; Polyzoidis, K.S. & Fotopoulos, A.D. (2008). Evaluation of glioma proliferation by ^{99m}Tc-Tetrofosmin. *NeuroOncol*, Vol.10, No.1, (February 2008), pp.104-105, ISSN 1522-8517

Alexiou, G.A.; Vartholomatos, G.; Tsiouris, S.; Papadopoulos, A.; Kyritsis, A.P.; Polyzoidis, K.S.; Voulgaris, S. & Fotopoulos, A.D. (2008). Evaluation of meningioma aggressiveness by (99m)Tc-Tetrofosmin SPECT. *Clin Neurol Neurosurg*, Vol.110, No.7, (July 2008), pp.645-648, ISSN 0303-8467

Alexiou, G.A.; Tsiouris, S.; Kyritsis, A.P.; Fotakopoulos, G. ; Goussia, A.; Voulgaris, S. & Fotopoulos, A.D. (2010). The Value of ^{99m}Tc-Tetrofosmin Brain SPECT in Predicting Survival in Patients with Glioblastoma Multiforme. *J Nucl Med*, Vol.51, No.12, (December 2010), pp.1923-1926, ISSN 0161-5505

Alexiou, G.A.; Goussia, A.; Kyritsis, A.P.; Tsiouris, S.; Ntoulia, A.; Malamou-Mitsi, V.; Voulgaris, S. & Fotopoulos, A.D. (2011). Influence of Glioma's Multidrug Resistance Phenotype on (99m)Tc-Tetrofosmin Uptake. *Mol Imaging Biol*, Vol.13, No.2, (April 2011), pp.348-351, ISSN 1536-1632

Ando, K.; Ishikura, R.; Nagami, Y.; Morikawa, T.; Takada, Y.; Ikeda, J.; Nakao, N.; Matsumoto, T. & Arita, N. (2004). Usefulness of Cho/Cr ratio in protonMR spectroscopy for differentiating residual/recurrent glioma from non-neoplastic lesions. *Nippon Igaku Hoshasen Gakkai Zasshi*, Vol.64, No.3, (March 2004), pp.121–126, ISSN 0048-0428

Barai, S.; Bandopadhayaya, G.P.; Julka, P.K.; Haloi, A.K.; Seith, A. & Malhotra A. (2003). Evaluation of single photon emission computerised tomography (SPECT) using Tc99m-tetrofosmin as a diagnostic modality for recurrent posterior fossa tumours. *J Postgrad Med*, Vol.49, No.4, (October-December 2003), pp.316-320, ISSN 0022-3859

Barai, S.; Bandopadhayaya, G.P.; Julka, P.K.; Kale, S.S.; Malhotra, A.; Haloi, A.K.; Seith, A. & Gopendro Sing, N. (2004). Evaluation of ^{99m}Tc-L-methionine brain SPECT for detection of recurrent brain tumor: a pilot study with radiological and pathological correlation. *Acta Radiol*, Vol.45, No.6, (October 2004), pp.649-657, ISSN 0284-1851

Beauchesne, P.; Pedeux, R.; Boniol, M. & Soler, C. (2004). ^{99m}Tc-sestamibi brain SPECT after chemoradiotherapy is prognostic of survival in patients with high-grade glioma. *J Nucl Med*, Vol.45, No.3, (March 2004), pp.409-413, ISSN 0161-5505

Byrne, T.N. (1994). Imaging of gliomas. *Semin Oncol*, Vol.21, No.2, (April 1994), pp.162-171, ISSN 0093-7754

Chen, W.; Cloughesy, T.; Kamdar, N.; Satyamurthy, N.; Bergsneider, M.; Liau, L.; Mischel, P.; Czernin, J.; Phelps, M.E. & Silverman, D.H. (2005). Imaging proliferation in brain tumors with ^{18}F-FLT PET: comparison with ^{18}F-FDG. *J Nucl Med*, Vol.46, No.6, (June 2005), pp.945-952, ISSN 0161-5505

Chen, W.; Silverman, D.H.; Delaloye, S.; Czernin, J.; Kamdar, N.; Pope, W.; Satyamurthy, N.; Schiepers, C. & Cloughesy, T. (2006). ^{18}F-FDOPA PET imaging of brain tumors: comparison study with ^{18}F-FDG PET and evaluation of diagnostic accuracy. *J Nucl Med*, Vol.47, No.6, (June 2006), pp.904-911, ISSN 0161-5505

Choi, J.Y.; Kim, S.E.; Shin, H.J.; Kim, B.T. & Kim, J.H. (2000). Brain tumor imaging with ^{99m}Tc-tetrofosmin: comparison with ^{201}Tl, ^{99m}Tc-MIBI, and ^{18}F-fluorodeoxyglucose. *J Neurooncol*, Vol.46, No.1, (January 2000), pp.63-70, ISSN 0167-594X

Covarrubias, D.J.; Rosen, B.R. & Lev, M.H. (2004). Dynamic magnetic resonance perfusion imaging of brain tumors. *Oncologist*, Vol.9, No.9, (May 2004), pp.528-537, ISSN 1083-7159

DeAngelis, L.M. (2001). Brain tumors. *N Engl J Med*, Vol.344, No.2, (January 2001), pp.114-123, ISSN 0028-4793

Denoyer, D.; Perek, N.; Le Jeune, N.; Cornillon, J. & Dubois, F. (2005). Correlation between ^{99m}Tc-(V)-DMSA uptake and constitutive level of phosphorylated focal adhesion kinase in an in vitro model of cancer cell lines. *Eur J Nucl Med Mol Imaging*, Vol.32, No.7, (July 2005), pp.820-827, ISSN 1619-7070

Di Chiro, G.; Oldfield, E.; Wright, D.C.; De Michele, D.; Katz, D.A.; Patronas, N.J.; Doppman, J.L.; Larson, S.M.; Ito, M. & Kufta, C.V. (1988). Cerebral necrosis after radiotherapy and/or intraarterial chemotherapy for brain tumors: PET and neuropathologic studies. *AJR Am J Roentgenol*, Vol.150, No.1, (January 1988), pp.189-197, ISSN 0361-803X

Fotopoulos, A.D., Alexiou, G.A.; Goussia, A.; Papadopoulos, A.; Kyritsis, A.P.; Polyzoidis, K.S.; Voulgaris, S. & Tsiouris, S. (2008). (99m)Tc-Tetrofosmin brain SPECT in the assessment of meningiomas - correlation with histological grade and proliferation index. *J Neurooncol*, Vol.89, No.2, (September 2008), pp.225-230, ISSN 0167-594X

Fotopoulos, A.D.; Kyritsis, A.P.; Tsiouris, S.; Al-Boucharali, J.; Papadopoulos, A.; Voulgaris, S. & Alexiou, G.A. (2011). Characterization of intracranial space-occupying lesions by ^{99}(m)Tc-Tetrofosmin SPECT. *J Neurooncol*, Vol.101, No.1, (January 2011), pp.83-89, ISSN 0167-594X

Galldiks, N.; Kracht, L.W.; Berthold, F.; Miletic, H.; Klein, J.C.; Herholz, K.; Jacobs, A.H. & Heiss, W.D. (2010). [(11)C]-L: -Methionine positron emission tomography in the management of children and young adults with brain tumors. *J Neurooncol*, Vol.96, No.2, (January 2010), pp.231-239, ISSN 0167-594X

Garcia, R.; Bueno, A. & Castanon, S. (1997). Study of the DNA content by flow cytometry and proliferation in 281 brain tumors. *Oncology*, Vol.54, No.2, (March-April 1997), pp.112-117, ISSN 0890-9091

Gómez-Río, M.; Rodríguez-Fernández, A.; Ramos-Font, C.; López-Ramírez, E. & Llamas-Elvira, J.M. (2008). Diagnostic accuracy of ^{201}Thallium-SPECT and ^{18}F-FDG-PET in the clinical assessment of glioma recurrence. *Eur J Nucl Med Mol Imaging*, Vol.35, No.5, (May 2008), pp.966-975, ISSN 16197070

Gungor, F.; Bezircioglu, H.; Guvenç, G.; Tezcan, M.; Yildiz, A.; Uluc, E. & Isisag, A. (2000). Correlation of thallium-201 uptake with proliferating cell nuclear antigen in brain tumours. *Nucl Med Commun*, Vol.21, No.9, (September 2000), pp.803-810, ISSN 01433636

Hatakeyama, T.; Kawai, N.; Nishiyama, Y.; Yamamoto, Y.; Sasakawa, Y.; Ichikawa, T. & Tamiya, T. (2008). ^{11}C-methionine (MET) and ^{18}F-fluorothymidine (FLT) PET in patients with newly diagnosed glioma. *Eur J Nucl Med Mol Imaging*, Vol.35, No.11, (November 2008), pp.2009-2017, ISSN 16197070

Hein, P.A.; Eskey, C.J.; Dunn, J.F. & Hug, E.B. (2004). Diffusion-weighted imaging in the follow-up of treated high-grade gliomas: tumor recurrence versus radiation injury. *AJNR Am J Neuroradiol*, Vol.25, No.2, (February 2004), pp.201-209, ISSN 01956108

Hollingworth, W.; Medina, S.; Lenkinski, R.E.; Shibata, D.K.; Bernal, B.; Zurakowski, D.; Comstock, B. & Jarvik, J.G. (2006). A Systematic Literature Review of Magnetic Resonance Spectroscopy for the Characterization of Brain Tumors. *AJNR Am J Neuroradiol*, Vol.27, No.7, (August 2006), pp.1404-1411, ISSN 01956108

Ishibashi, M.; Taguchi, A.; Sugita, Y.; Morita, S.; Kawamura, S.; Umezaki, N.; Shigemori, M. & Hayabuchi, N. (1995). Thallium-201 in brain tumors: relationship between tumor cell activity in astrocytic tumor and proliferating cell nuclear antigen. *J Nucl Med*, Vol.36, No.12, (December 1996), pp.2201-2206, ISSN 01615505

Iuchi, T.; Iwadate, Y.; Namba, H.; Osato, K.; Saeki, N.; Yamaura, A. & Uchida, Y. (1999). Glucose and methionine uptake and proliferative activity in meningiomas. *Neurol Res*, Vol.21, No.7, (October 1999), pp.640-644, ISSN 01616412

Jinnouchi, S.; Hoshi, H.; Ohnishi, T.; Futami, S.; Nagamachi, S.; Watanabe, K.; Ueda, T. & Wakisaka, S. (1993). Thallium-201 SPECT for predicting histological types of meningiomas. *J Nucl Med*, Vol.34, No.12, (December 1993), pp.2091-2094, ISSN 01615505

Kahn, D.; Follett, K.A.; Bushnell, D.L.; Nathan, M.A.; Piper, J.G.; Madsen, M. & Kirchner, P.T. (1994). Diagnosis of recurrent brain tumor: value of ^{201}Tl SPECT vs ^{18}F-fluorodeoxyglucose PET. *AJR Am J Roentgenol*, Vol.163, No.6, (Decenmber 1994), pp.1459-1465, ISSN 0361803X

Kayaselcuk, F.; Zorludemir, S.; Bal, N.; Erdogan, B.; Erdogan, S. & Erman, T. (2004). The expression of survivin and Ki-67 in meningiomas: correlation with grade and clinical outcome. *J Neurooncol*, Vol.67, No.1-2, (March-April 2004), pp.209-214, ISSN 0167594X

Kim, S.; Chung, J.K.; Im, S.H.; Jeong, J.M.; Lee, D.S.; Kim, D.G.; Jung, H.W. & Lee, M.C. (2005). ^{11}C-methionine PET as a prognostic marker in patients with glioma: comparison with ^{18}F-FDG PET. *Eur J Nucl Med Mol Imaging*, Vol.32, No.1, (January 2005), pp.52-59, ISSN 16197070

Kinuya, K.; Ohashi, M.; Itoh, S.; Yamamoto, K.; Sakai, S.; Kakuda, K.; Nobata, K.; Kato, N.; Terahara, S. & Taki, S. (2002). Differential diagnosis in patients with ring-like thallium-201 uptake in brain SPECT. *Ann Nucl Med*, Vol.16, No.6, (September 2002), pp.417-421, ISSN 09147187

Kuwert, T.; Probst-Cousin, S.; Woesler, B.; Morgenroth, C.; Lerch, H.; Matheja, P.; Palkovic, S.; Schäfers, M.; Wassmann, H.; Gullotta, F. & Schober, O. (1997). Iodine-123-alpha-methyl tyrosine in gliomas: correlation with cellular density and proliferative activity. *J Nucl Med*, Vol.38, No.10, (October 1997), pp.1551-1555, ISSN 01615505

Kwee, S.A.; Ko, J.P.; Jiang, C.S.; Watters, M.R. & Coel, M.N. (2007). Solitary brain lesions enhancing at MR imaging: evaluation with fluorine 18 fluorocholine PET. *Radiology*, Vol.244, No.2, (August 2007), pp.557-565, ISSN 00338419

Lacroix, M.; Abi-Said, D.; Fourney, D.R.; Gokaslan, Z.L.; Shi, W.; DeMonte. F.; Lang, F.F.; McCutcheon, I.E.; Hassenbusch, S.J.; Holland, E.; Hess, K.; Michael, C.; Miller, D. & Sawaya, R. (2001). A multivariate analysis of 416 patients with glioblastoma multiforme: prognosis, extent of resection, and survival. *J Neurosurg*, Vol.95, No.2, (August 2001), pp.190–198, ISSN 0022308

Lamszus, K. (2004). Meningioma pathology, genetics, and biology. *J Neuropathol Exp Neurol*, Vol.63, No.4, (April 2004), pp.275-286, ISSN 0022-3069

Le Jeune, N.; Perek, N.; Denoyer, D. & Dubois, F. (2005). Study of monoglutathionyl conjugates TC-99M-sestamibi and TC-99M-tetrofosmin transport mediated by the multidrug resistance-associated protein isoform 1 in glioma cells. *Cancer Biother Radiopharm*, Vol.20, No.3, (June 2005), pp.249-259, ISSN 10849785

Liu, Y.; Shete, S.; Etzel, C.J.; Scheurer, M.; Alexiou, G.; Armstrong, G.; Tsavachidis, S.; Liang, F.W.; Gilbert, M.; Aldape, K.; Armstrong, T.; Houlston, R.; Hosking, F.; Robertson, L.; Xiao, Y.; Wiencke, J.; Wrensch, M.; Andersson, U.; Melin, B.S. & Bondy, M. (2010). Polymorphisms of LIG4, BTBD2, HMGA2, and RTEL1 genes involved in the double-strand break repair pathway predict glioblastoma survival. *J Clin Oncol*, Vol.28, No.14, (May 2010), pp.2467-2474, ISSN 0732-183X

Marks, J.E. & Wong, J. (1985). The risk of cerebral radionecrosis in relation to dose, time and fractionation: a followup study. *Prog Exp Tumor Res*, Vol.29, No.1, (January 1985), pp.210–218, ISSN 00796263

McKeever, P.E.; Ross, D.A.; Strawderman, M.S.; Brunberg, J.A.; Greenberg, H.S. & Junck, L. (1997). A comparison of the predictive power for survival in gliomas provided by MIB-1, bromodeoxyuridine and proliferating cell nuclear antigen with histopathologic and clinical parameters. *J Neuropathol Exp Neurol*, Vol.56, No.7, (July 1997), pp.798–805, ISSN 00223069

Minutoli, F.; Angileri, F.F.; Conti, A.; Herberg, A.; Aricò, D.; Baldari, S.; Cardali, S.; de Divitiis, O.; Germanò, A. & Baldari, S. (2005). Timing of examination affects reliability of ^{99m}Tc-methoxyisobutylisonitrile SPECT in distinguishing neoplastic from nonneoplastic brain hematomas. *J Nucl Med*, Vol.46, No.4, (April 2005), pp.574-579, ISSN 01615505

Nagamachi, S.; Jinnouchi, S.; Nabeshima, K.; Nishii, R.; Flores, L. 2nd; Kodama, T.; Kawai, K.; Tamura, S.; Yokogami, K.; Samejima, T. & Wakisaka, S. (2001). The correlation between ^{99m}Tc-MIBI uptake and MIB-1 as a nuclear proliferation marker in glioma—a comparative study with ^{201}Tl. *Neuroradiology*, Vol.43, No.12, (December 2001), pp.1023-1030, ISSN 00283940

Oriuchi, N.; Tamura, M.; Shibazaki, T.; Ohye, C.; Watanabe, N.; Tateno, M.; Tomiyoshi, K.; Hirano, T.; Inoue, T. & Endo, K. (1993). Clinical evaluation of thallium-201 SPECT in supratentorial gliomas: relationship to histologic grade, prognosis and proliferative activities. *J Nucl Med*, Vol.34, No.12, (December 1993), pp.2085-2089, ISSN 01615505

Pauleit, D.; Stoffels, G.; Bachofner, A.; Floeth, F.W.; Sabel, M.; Herzog, H.; Tellmann, L.; Jansen, P.; Reifenberger, G.; Hamacher, K.; Coenen, H.H. & Langen, K.J. (2009). Comparison of (18)F-FET and (18)F-FDG PET in brain tumors. *Nucl Med Biol*, Vol.36, No.7, (October 2009), pp.779-787, ISSN 09698051

Pöpperl, G.; Götz, C.; Rachinger, W.; Gildehaus, F.J.; Tonn, J.C. & Tatsch, K. (2004). Value of O-(2-[^{18}F]fluoroethyl)- L-tyrosine PET for the diagnosis of recurrent glioma. *Eur J Nucl Med Mol Imaging*, Vol.31, No.11, (November 2004), pp.1464-1470, ISSN 16197070

Ricci, P.E.; Karis, J.P.; Heiserman, J.E.; Fram, E.K.; Bice, A.N. & Drayer, B.P. (1998). Differentiating recurrent tumor from radiation necrosis: time for re-evaluation of positron emission tomography? *AJNR Am J Neuroradiol*, Vol.19, No.3, (March 1998), pp.407-413, ISSN 01956108

Samnick, S.; Bader, J.B.; Hellwig, D.; Moringlane, J.R.; Alexander, C.; Romeike, B.F.; Feiden, W. & Kirsch, C.M. (2002). Clinical value of iodine-123-alpha-methyl-L-tyrosine single-photon emission tomography in the differential diagnosis of recurrent brain tumor in patients pretreated for glioma at follow-up. *J Clin Oncol*, Vol.20, No.15, (January 2002), pp.396-404, ISSN 0732183X

Scott, J.N.; Rewcastle, N.B.; Brasher, P.M.; Fulton, D.; MacKinnon, J.A.; Hamilton, M.; Cairncross, J.G. & Forsyth, P. (1999). Which glioblastoma multiforme patient will become a long-term survivor? A population-based study. *Ann Neurol*, Vol.46, No.2, (August 1999), pp.183-188, ISSN 03645134

Shields, A.F.; Grierson, J.R.; Kozawa, S.M. & Zheng, M. (1996). Development of labeled thymidine analogs for imaging tumor proliferation. *Nucl Med Biol*, Vol.23, No.1, (January 1996), pp.17–22, ISSN 09698051

Shimizu, H.; Kumabe, T.; Shirane, R. & Yoshimoto, T. (2000). Correlation between choline level measured by proton MR spectroscopy and Ki-67 labeling index in gliomas. *AJNR Am J Neuroradiol*, Vol.21, No.4, (April 2000), pp.659-665, ISSN 0195-6108

Soler, C.; Beauchesne, P.; Maatougui, K.; Schmitt, T.; Barral, F.G.; Michel, D.; Dubois, F. & Brunon, J. (1998). Technetium-99m sestamibi brain single-photon emission tomography for detection of recurrent gliomas after radiation therapy. *Eur J Nucl Med*, Vol.25, No.12, (December 1998), pp.1649-1657, ISSN 16197070

Soricelli, A.; Cuocolo, A.; Varrone, A.; Discepolo, A.; Tedeschi, E.; Mainenti, P.P.; Grivet-Fojaja, M.R.; Covelli, E.M.; Postiglione, A. & Salvatore, M. (1998). Technetium-99m-tetrofosmin uptake in brain tumors by SPECT: comparison with thallium-201 imaging. *J Nucl Med*, Vol.39, No.5, (May 1998), pp.802-806, ISSN 01615505

Staffen, W.; Hondl, N.; Trinka, E.; Iglseder, B.; Unterrainer, J. & Ladurner, G. (1998). Clinical relevance of ^{201}Tl-chloride SPET in the differential diagnosis of brain tumours. *Nucl Med Commun*, Vol.19, No.4, (April 1998), pp.335-340, ISSN 01433636

Stupp, R.; Mason, W.P.; van den Bent, M.J.; Weller, M.; Fisher, B.; Taphoorn, M.J.; Belanger, K.; Brandes, A.A.; Marosi, C.; Bogdahn, U.; Curschmann, J.; Janzer, R.C.; Ludwin, S.K.; Gorlia, T.; Allgeier, A.; Lacombe, D.; Cairncross, J.G.; Eisenhauer, E.; Mirimanoff, R.O.; European Organisation for Research and Treatment of Cancer Brain Tumor and Radiotherapy Groups & National Cancer Institute of Canada Clinical Trials Group. (2005). Radiotherapy plus concomitant and adjuvant temozolomide for glioblastoma. *New Engl J Med*, Vol.352, No.10, (March 2005), pp.987-996, ISSN 00284793

Sundgren, P.C.; Fan, X.; Weybright, P.; Welsh, R.C.; Carlos, R.C.; Petrou, M.; McKeever, P.E. & Chenevert, T.L. (2006). Differentiation of recurrent brain tumor versus radiation injury using diffusion tensor imaging in patients with new contrast-enhancing lesions. *Magn Reson Imaging*, Vol.24, No.9, (November 2006), pp.1131-1142, ISSN 0730-725X

Tamiya, T.; Kinoshita, K.; Ono, Y.; Matsumoto, K.; Furuta, T. & Ohmoto, T. (2000). Proton magnetic resonance spectroscopy reflects cellular proliferative activity in astrocytomas. *Neuroradiology*, Vol.42, No.5, (May 2000), pp.333-338, ISSN 00283940

Tedeschi, E.; Soricelli, A.; Brunetti, A.; Romano, M.; Bucciero, A.; Iaconetta, G.; Alfieri, A.; Postiglione, A. & Salvatore, M. (1996). Different thallium-201 single-photon emission tomographic patterns in benign and aggressive meningiomas. *Eur J Nucl Med*, Vol.23, No.11, (November 1996), pp.1478-1484, ISSN 16197070

Tsiouris, S.; Pirmettis, I.; Chatzipanagiotou, T.; Ptohis, N. & Papantoniou, V. (2007). Pentavalent technetium-99m dimercaptosuccinic acid [^{99m}Tc-(V)DMSA] brain scintitomography--a plausible non-invasive depicter of glioblastoma proliferation and therapy response. *J Neurooncol*, Vol.85, No.3, (December 2007), pp.291-295, ISSN 0167594X

Ullrich, R.; Backes, H.; Li, H.; Kracht, L.; Miletic, H.; Kesper, K.; Neumaier, B.; Heiss, W.D.; Wienhard, K. & Jacobs, A.H. (2008). Glioma proliferation as assessed by 3'-fluoro-3'-deoxy-L-thymidine positron emission tomography in patients with newly diagnosed high-grade glioma. *Clin Cancer Res*, Vol.14, No.7, (April 2008), pp.2049-2055, ISSN 1078-0432

Van Laere, K.; Ceyssens, S.; Van Calenbergh, F.; de Groot, T.; Menten, J.; Flamen, P.; Bormans, G. & Mortelmans, L. (2005). Direct comparison of ^{18}F-FDG and ^{11}C-methionine PET in suspected recurrence of glioma: sensitivity, inter-observer variability and prognostic value. *Eur J Nucl Med Mol Imaging*, Vol.32, No.1, (January 2005), pp.39-51, ISSN 16197070

Vos, M.J.; Tony, B.N.; Hoekstra, O.S.; Postma, T.J.; Heimans, J.J. & Hooft, L. (2007). Systematic review of the diagnostic accuracy of ^{201}Tl single photon emission computed tomography in the detection of recurrent glioma. *Nucl Med Commun*, Vol.28, No.6, (June 2007), pp.431-439, ISSN 01433636

Weber, W.A.; Dick, S.; Reidl, G.; Dzewas, B.; Busch, R.; Feldmann, H.J.; Molls, M.; Lumenta, C.B.; Schwaiger, M. & Grosu, A.L. (2001). Correlation between postoperative 3-[(123)I]iodo-L-alpha-methyltyrosine uptake and survival in patients with gliomas. *J Nucl Med*, Vol.42, No.8, (August 2001), pp.1144-1150, ISSN 01615505

Whittle, I.R.; Smith, C.; Navoo, P. & Collie, D. (2004). Meningiomas. *Lancet*, Vol.363, No. 9431, (May 2004), pp.1535-1543, ISSN 01406736

Xiangsong, Z.; Changhong, L.; Weian, C. & Dong, Z. (2006). PET Imaging of cerebral astrocytoma with ^{13}N-ammonia. *J Neurooncol*, Vol.78, No.2, (June 2006), pp.145-151, ISSN 0167594X

17

Immunolocalization of the Glioblastoma Cells by Nanoparticles Using Microscopy Tools

Lorena Favaro Pavon et al.*
[1]*Instituto do Cérebro - Instituto Israelita de Ensino e Pesquisa Albert Einstein - IIEPAE, São Paulo Brasil*

1. Introduction

According to World Health Organization (WHO 2007), tumors of the nervous system are classified into seven major groups including primary tumors (neuroepithelial, meningeal, cranial nerves, paraspinal nerves, germinal, region sellar and hematopoietic) and the secondary tumors or metastatic.

The primary tumors of the nervous systems are relatively rare. According to data from the Central Tumor Registry of the Central Nervous System from Unites States (CBTRUS 2011), it is estimates that about 64.530 new cases (approximately 22.020 of them malignant) diagnosed in 2010, representing 1.44% of all malignancies diagnosed in this country. Despite the low incidence, malignant primary tumors are highly lethal - responsible for about 13.140 deaths in the Unites States in 2010.

Gliomas are tumors that arise from glial cells and include astrocytomas, oligodendrogliomas, oligoastrocitomas (also called mixed gliomas) and ependymomas. Gliomas are among the group of neuroepithelial tumors and account for 31% of primary tumors and 80% of malignant tumors of the nervous system. The astrocytoma group represents 76% of all gliomas, and glioblastoma represents 53.7% of cases (CBTRUS 2011). Glioblastoma is the most frequent and malignant astrocytoma, and despite numerous advances in the diagnosis and treatment of these tumors, their prognosis remains limited (Brandes et al. 2008; Wen; Kesari, 2008).

---

* Luciana Cavalheiro Marti[2], Tatiana Tais Sibov[1], Suzana M.F. Malheiros[3], Daniela Mara Oliveira[4], Maria Izabel Camargo-Mathias[5], Edson Amaro Junior[1,6], Reynaldo Andre Brandt[7], Jorge Roberto Pagura[7], Marcos Augusto Stavale[7], Guilherme Carvalhal Ribas[7] and Lionel Fernel Gamarra[1]
[1] *Instituto do Cérebro - Instituto Israelita de Ensino e Pesquisa Albert Einstein - IIEPAE, São Paulo,*
[2] *Centro de Pesquisa Experimental - Instituto Israelita de Ensino e Pesquisa Albert Einstein - IIEPAE, São Paulo,*
[3] *Departamento de Neurologia e Neurocirurgia - Universidade Federal de São Paulo - UNIFESP, São Paulo,*
[4] *Universidade Federal de São João Del-Rei, São João Del Rei, MG*
[5] *Departamento de Biologia, Instituto de Biociências - Universidade Estadual Paulista - UNESP, Rio Claro, SP*
[6] *Departamento de Radiologia, Universidade de São Paulo - USP, São Paulo,*
[7] *Programa Integrado Neuro-Oncologia, Hospital Albert Einstein, São Paulo, SP*
Brasil

It is described that the glioma is the most common neoplasm of the human central nervous system (CBTRUS 2011), being difficult therapeutic approach, due to several factors: i) presenting infiltrative ii) possess tumor composed of cells with different morphofunctional characteristics that express a variety of neural markers, iii) be highly resistant to radiotherapy and chemotherapy procedures (Singh et al., 2003).

Glioblastoma cell lineages express a set of cell surface antigens also found in mesenchymal stem cells (MSC), such as CD29, CD44, CD73 (SH3, SH4), CD90 (Thy-1) and CD105 (SH2) (Sordi et al., 2005). In addition, a small population of cancer stem cells has been identified in brain (Singh et al., 2004). Some evidence suggests that CD133 is a marker for a subset of glioblastoma cancer stem cells. The MSC-like phenotype and CD133 positive cells isolated from human glioblastoma may play a role in tumorigenesis or tumor recurrence and could be a potential target for therapies for glioblastoma. The transcription factor Forkhead BoxM1 (FoxM1) also has been described as up-regulated in glioblastoma cells and may act as a malignancy marker.

Nanobiotechnologic technologies can offer excellent tools for evaluating and understanding tumorigenesis, tumor mapping and tumor behaviour. One example is the use of superparamagnetic iron oxide nanoparticles (SPIONS). Recently, SPIONs have attracted attention for their use in nanotechnology (Tartaj et al., 2003) and biomedical applications, including drug delivery (Voltairas et al., 2002), hyperthermia in cancer treatment (Jordan et al., 1997; Jordan et al., 1999) and as image contrast agents in magnetic resonance imaging (MRI) (Cheng et al., 2005; Kumar et al., 2007).

It was also used in this study, superparamagnetics iron oxide nanoparticles for cell separation process with MACS Technology. Applying the magnetic cell sorting (MACS) technology, we reported results of purifying the CD133 positive cells from the glioblastoma cells. In malignant brain tumors, CD133 has been suggested to be a cancer stem cell marker, since only CD133 positive cells from brain tumor biopsy material were able to initiate brain cancer in a mouse model (Singh et al., 2004). Prominin-1 (PROM-1), also called CD133, is a protein with several isoforms of unknown physiological or pathological function, and is localized both in the cytoplasm and at the cell surface (Miraglia, et al. 1997). It is expressed by human neural stem cells and has been proposed to have a function in central nervous system development.

Another possible nanobiotechnologic tool of great relevance are the Quantum Dots (QD). Semiconductor QDs are nanoparticles that have attracted widespread interest in biology and medicine due to their unique optical and electronic properties. These properties, especially their reduced tendency to photobleach and the dependence of their fluorescence wavelength on their size, make them suitable for fluorescent probing applications to detect cancer biomarkers *in vitro* and *in vivo* in cells. Thus, the QD act as probes which are detectable by the optical techniques of spectroscopy and magnetic resonance imaging (Lee et al., 2007) including the technique of transmission electronic microscopy (TEM), due to the nanoparticles' electrondensity (Nisman et al., 2004).

The present study analyzed the use of nanoparticles for labelling human glioblastoma cell lineages (U87MG/A172). For this purpose, we used SPIONs, as well as monoclonal antibodies (CD29, CD44, CD105) or FOXM1 conjoined to secondary antibodies linked to quantum dots. This strategy was based on complete glioblastoma immunophenotypic profile determined by flow cytometry. Then, the analysis was performed by transmission electron microscopy and immunofluorescence glioblastoma cells using superparamagnetic nanoparticles, SPIONs and QD. We also described the immunolocalization of CD133 epitopes in cells from primary cultures derived from human glioblastoma.

2. Material and methods

2.1 Culture and labelling human glioblastoma lineages with quantum dots (QD)

The cell lines of human glioblastoma (U87MG and A172) were maintained in a culture of DMEM-LG: Dulbeccos Modified Eagle Medium Low Glucose to 10% Fetal Bovine Serum and 1% Antibiotic-Antimycotic (100X) and 200nM L-Glutamine (100X).
Human glioblastoma cells were labeled in the culture after their expansion and adhesion to the culture plate according to the manufacturer's instructions (Invitrogen). Briefly, cells were incubated with primary antibodies, such as CD29, CD44 and CD105 followed by incubation with secondary antibodies (pure goat anti-mouse, IgG) linked to quantum dots (QD 565nm). The lineages were labeled for the transcription factor FOXM1 (Zimed - Invitrogen), which was conjoined in advance with quantum dots (QD 525nm) according to the directions of the QD Antibody Conjugate Kit (Invitrogen).
The labeled glioblastoma cells were maintained in a humidified incubator (Thermo Fisher Scientific Inc. 3110, Waltham, MA) with 5% CO_2 at 37°C for 24 hours and subsequently fixed in 1% glutaraldehyde for later analysis in TEM (Philips CM100).

2.2 SPIONs synthesis and glioblastoma lineages labelling

The colloidal suspensions based on SPIONs (Fe_3O_4) were previously synthesized by the sol-gel process. These syntheses included the rapid hydrolysis of Fe^{3+}, by the addition of ammonium hydroxide to the 0.2 M $FeCl_3H_2O$ aqueous solution in the presence of a surfactant (dextran). The dialysis of the precipitate permitted its peptizing leading to the formation of a colloidal suspension with SPIONs which have a diameter of 6 nm.
Thus, the tumor cells lineages were labeled in the culture with a concentration of 0.5% SPIONs and kept in a humidified incubator (Thermo Fisher Scientific Inc. 3110, Waltham, MA) with 5% CO_2 at 37°C for 24 hours. Subsequently, they were fixed in 4% paraformaldehyde and stained with 5% Prussian blue, viewed under a light microscope (OLYMPUS IX51), and fixed in 1% glutaraldehyde for later analysis under a TEM (Philips CM100).

2.3 The immunophenotyping of glioblastoma lineage cells by flow cytometry

The established glioblastoma lineage cells were analyzed for the cell-surface expression of typical mesenchymal stem cell protein markers. These experiments were conducted using monoclonal antibodies commercially available. The staining technique followed the manufacturer's instructions. Briefly, the samples in the 4th stage were harvested by a treatment with 0.25% Tryple Express (GIBCO-Invitrogen, Carlsbad, CA), washed with PBS (pH= 7.4) and stained with the selected monoclonal antibodies and incubated in the dark for 30 minutes at 4°C. Cells were then washed and fixed with 1% paraformaldehyde. The following human antibodies were used: CD14-FITC (clone: M5E2; BD Pharmingen - San Diego - CA), CD29-PE (clone: MAR4; BD Pharmingen - San Diego - CA), CD31-PE (clone: WM59; BD Pharmingen - San Diego - CA), CD34-PE (clone: 581; BD Pharmingen - San Diego - CA), CD44-PE (clone: 515; BD Pharmingen - San Diego - CA), CD45-PerCP-Cy5 (clone: 2D1; Biosciences - San Jose - CA), CD73-PE (clone: AD2; BD Pharmingen - San Diego - CA), CD90-APC (clone: 5E10; BD Pharmingen - San Diego - CA), CD106-FITC

(clone: 51-10C9; BD Pharmingen - San Diego - CA), CD166-PE (clone: 3A6; BD Pharmingen - San Diego - CA), HLA-DR-PerCP-Cy5 (clone: L243; Biosciences - San Jose - CA) and CD105-PE (clone: 8E11; Chemicon - Temecula - CA).
The data acquisition was carried out by FACSARIA flow cytometry equipment (BD Biosciences, San Jose, CA) and data analyses were performed using FACSDIVA software (BD Biosciences, San Jose, CA) or Flow Jo Software (TreeStar, Ashland, OR).

2.4 Culture of primary glioblastoma cells

Glioblastoma tumor cell samples were washed with 1%PBS and the enzymatic dissociation was performed in 0.3% collagenase. The obtained cells were them resuspended in Dulbecco's Modified Eagle's Medium (DMEM-Low Glucose) and plated at a density of $3x10^6$ live cells/60mm plate.

2.5 Magnetic cell separation using MACS (Miltenyi Biotec)

The culture of primary glioblastoma cells were purified following the separation protocol by MiniMACS microbeads affinity chromatography using anti-CD133 bound to magnetic beads (Miltenyi Biotec).
The cells were filtrated in 30μm nylon filters and the cell number was determined by an automatic cell counter (Coulter). Afterwards, the cells were centrifuged (400g for 5 minutes) and resuspended 300 μL of PBS solution containing 2 mM EDTA and 0.5% BSA (solution 1) for each 10^8 cells. The next step was the addition of 100 μL of FcR blocker and 100 μL of magnetic micro-spheres with $CD133^+$ antibodies, followed by the incubation at 6°C for 30 minutes.
After incubation, the labelled cells were centrifuged and resuspended in solution 1 to be separated in the chromatography column to isolate only the $CD133^+$ cells. The selected $CD133^+$ cells were subsequently fixed in 1% glutaraldehyde for later analysis in a TEM.

2.6 Immunocytochemical staining of primary culture glioblastoma

Glioblastoma tumor samples were washed 1% PBS and tumor cells were disaggregated in a solution containing 0.3% collagenase in 1% PBS buffer. Cells derived from the tumor were then resuspended in Dulbecco's Modified Eagle's Medium (DMEM -Low Glucose) and plated at a density of $3x10^6$ live cells/60mm plate. Cells were fixed with 4% paraformaldehyde and stained with antibody against CD133/1 (human monoclonal IgG1; 1:1000 dilution; Miltenyi Biotec). After washing, the cells were incubated with KIT Advanced ™HRP Dako (K4067) Advanced ™HRP Enzyme and followed by the application of the substrate-chromogen solution (DAB^+).

2.7 QD labelled primary culture glioblastoma by fluorescence microscopy:

Primary antibodies CD29 in conjunction with the secondary (anti-mouse IgG) linked to 565nm nanocrystals QD (Qtracker 565 Cell Labelling Kit, Invitrogen, Carlsbad, CA) were used to label of the primary culture glioblastoma according to the manufactory's instruction. The labelling of glioblastoma cells was detected by using a fluorescence microscopy (IX51 Olympus) with a filter for detection of the QDs (QD655-A-OMF-ZERO filter, Semrock, Rochester, NY).

2.8 Transmission electron microscopy:

Glioblastoma lineages (10^7 cells) were fixed in 1% glutaraldehyde and 0.2M cacodylate buffer for two hours at 4°C. Cells were washed in cacodylate buffer, 2 times for 15 minutes each. Post-fixation was performed in 1% osmium tetroxide for one hour at 4°C, followed by another two 15 minute washes in the same buffer. For contrast, the pellet was immersed in a solution of uranyl acetate in acetone for 30 minutes. After dehydration, the material was embedded in Epon resin diluted in acetone (1:1) and incubated at 4°C with agitation for 24 hours. The pellet was then transferred to pure Epon resin and incubated at 60° C for 72 hours, until completely polymerized. Semi and ultrathin sections were obtained with the aid of a Porter Blum ultramicrotome. The semithin sections were stained with azur II (1%) and methylene blue (1%). The ultrathin sections were placed on copper grids and stained with uranyl acetate and lead citrate. The grids were studied and photographed under a TEM (PHILIPS CM100).

3. Results

3.1 The immunophenotypic profile of glioblastoma lineage cells:

The glioblastoma lineage cells were analyzed by flow cytometry and gated according their granularity versus size, and then followed by the surface markers analysis. These cells were analyzed for the expression of cell membrane proteins and found to be positive for the expressions of CD29, CD44, CD73, CD90, CD105, which are generally considered as a marker set for mesenchymal stem cells (Figure 1).

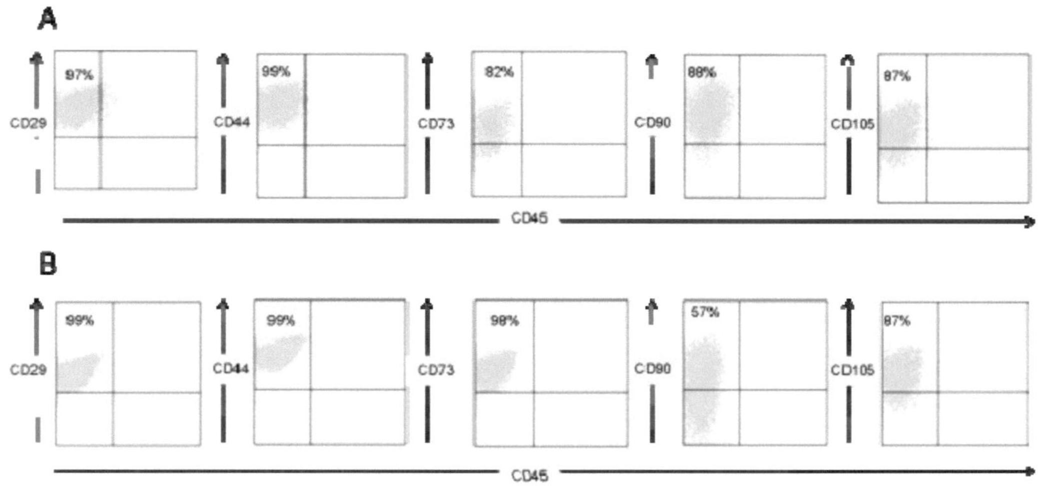

Fig. 1. Expression of mesenchymal markers as CD29, CD44, CD73, CD90 and CD105 on the cell of glioblastoma lineage A172 (A). Besides a variation on the percentage of CD73 and CD90, the same markers were found on the glioblastoma lineage U87MG (B).

3.2 Glioblastoma labelling by using monoclonal antibodies such as CD29, CD44, CD105 and the transcription factor FOxM1 conjugated to quantum dots (QD 565 nm and 525 nm)

The analysis of ultrastructural immunolocalization revealed the presence of electrondense clusters on the surface of tumor cells (Figure 2B), as well as scattered in the cytoplasm (Figures 2D; 4B, C) and in the interior of the vesicles (Figures 2E; 4B, D, F). This electrondensity demonstrates the presence of monoclonal antibodies linked to QD.

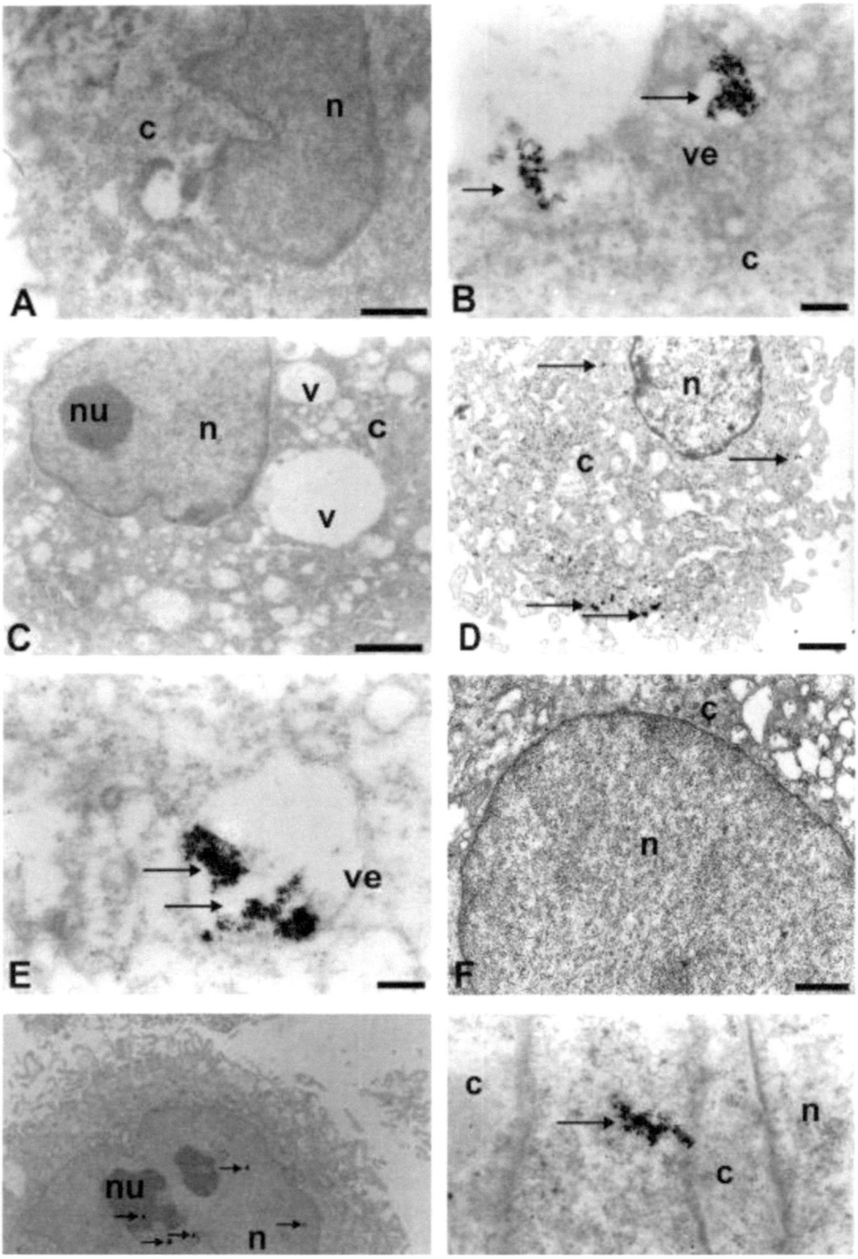

Fig. 2. Ultrastructural analysis of glioblastoma lineages marked with nanocrystal quantum dots (QDs) using TEM. B) QDs (565nm) conjoined with the CD29 monoclonal antibody. D, E) QDs (565nm) conjoined with the CD44 monoclonal antibody. G, H) QDs (525nm) conjoined with the FOxM1 transcription factor. A, C, F) Glioblastoma lineage cells of the control group. A, B, C, H) Scale: 0.25μm. D, E, G) Scale: 0.5μm. F) Scale: 2μm. n = nucleus; c = cytoplasm; nu = nucleolus; v = vacuole; ve = vesicle; arrow = electrondense nanoparticles (nanocrystals).

Figure 4B shows the presence of vesicles from the process of invagination of plasmic membrane.
Electrondense clusters were not observed in our control group U87MG and A172 lineage cells, which did not receive the QDs (Figures 2A, C, F; 4A). These QDs can also be associated with cytoplasmic organelles such as the rough endoplasmic reticulum (Figure 4E).
The transcription factor FOxM1 can also be evidenced by the QD electrondensity conjoined to this nuclear transcription factor. This compound can be observed by granules in various regions of the tumor cell nucleus (Figures 2G, H).
The figures 3A,B e C shows, by fluorescence microscopy, the glioblastoma cell membrane staining by both CD29 primary antibody and the secondary anti-mouse antibody and, as a control, the glioblastoma cells were stained with the secondary anti-mouse antibody only (Figure 3D). The analysis of ultrastructural revealed the presence of electrondense clusters on the surface of tumor cells (Figure 3E) staining by of the primary antibody CD29 and secondary anti-mouse polyclonal antibody. Electrondense clusters were not observed in control group (Figure 3F), depicts the glioblastoma cells stained with the secondary anti-mouse antibody only, showing no unspecific staining by this antibody in these experiments.

3.3 Primary culture glioblastoma marked with superparamagnetic nanoparticles using anti-CD133 bound to magnetic beads

The analysis of immunocytochemistry demonstrated CD133 expression in primary culture glioblastoma (Figure 5B). Under the electron microscopy, ultrastructural analysis highlighted the presence of electrondense granules in the glioblastoma cell surface. This demonstrates the presence of anti-CD133 monoclonal antibodies bound to superparamagnetic nanoparticles recognizing the CD133 membrane protein (Figures 5D, E). This does not occur in the cells of the control group ($CD133^-$) (Figure 5C). Electrondense signals related to superparamagnetic nanoparticles were also observed in the cell cytoplasm, suggesting their internalization through the process of the endocytosis of QD bound to the antibodies (Figures 5D, E). $CD133^+$ cells incorporated superparamagnetic nanoparticles through its small cytoplasmic projections forming the pinocytics vesicles, as shown in the figures 5E and 5F.

3.4 The glioblastoma lineage iron oxide superparamagnetic nanoparticles (SPIONs) markings

The analysis of light microscopy, with Prussian blue staining, revealed large amounts of iron oxide nanoparticles dispersed in the cytoplasm of tumor cells (Figure 6B), compared to cells from the control group (Figure 6A).
The ultrastructural SPIONs markings, using electrondensity resources, confirmed the presence of these nanoparticles, mainly in the interior of the vesicles (Figures 6D, E, F, G), that did not occur in the control group cells (Figure 6C). Figure 4D showed the process of internalization of the nanoparticles, as well as invaginations of the plasma membrane and subsequent vesicle formation.
Some cells showed intense cytoplasmic vacuolation (Figure 6G), loss of cell boundaries or disintegration of the plasmic membrane (Figure 6F), and the formation of concentric lamellae forming myelin figures (Figure 6H).

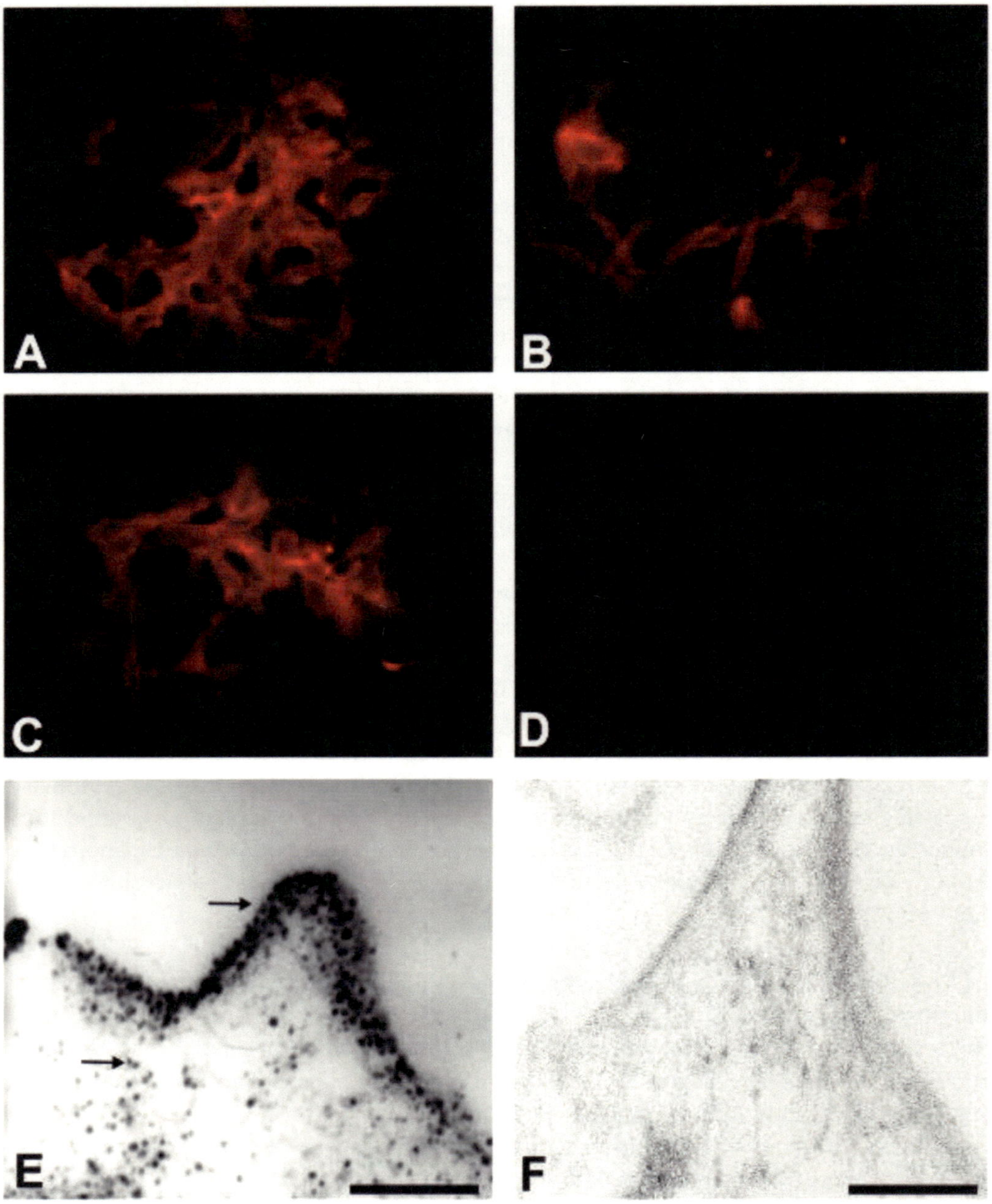

Fig. 3. Immunofluorescence and ultrastructural analysis of glioblastoma lineages marked with nanocrystal quantum dots (QDs). A, B, C, E) 565nm QDs conjoined with the CD44 monoclonal antibody. D, F) Glioblastoma cells with the secondary anti-mouse only. A, B, C, D) 600X. E, F) Scale: 0.25μm.

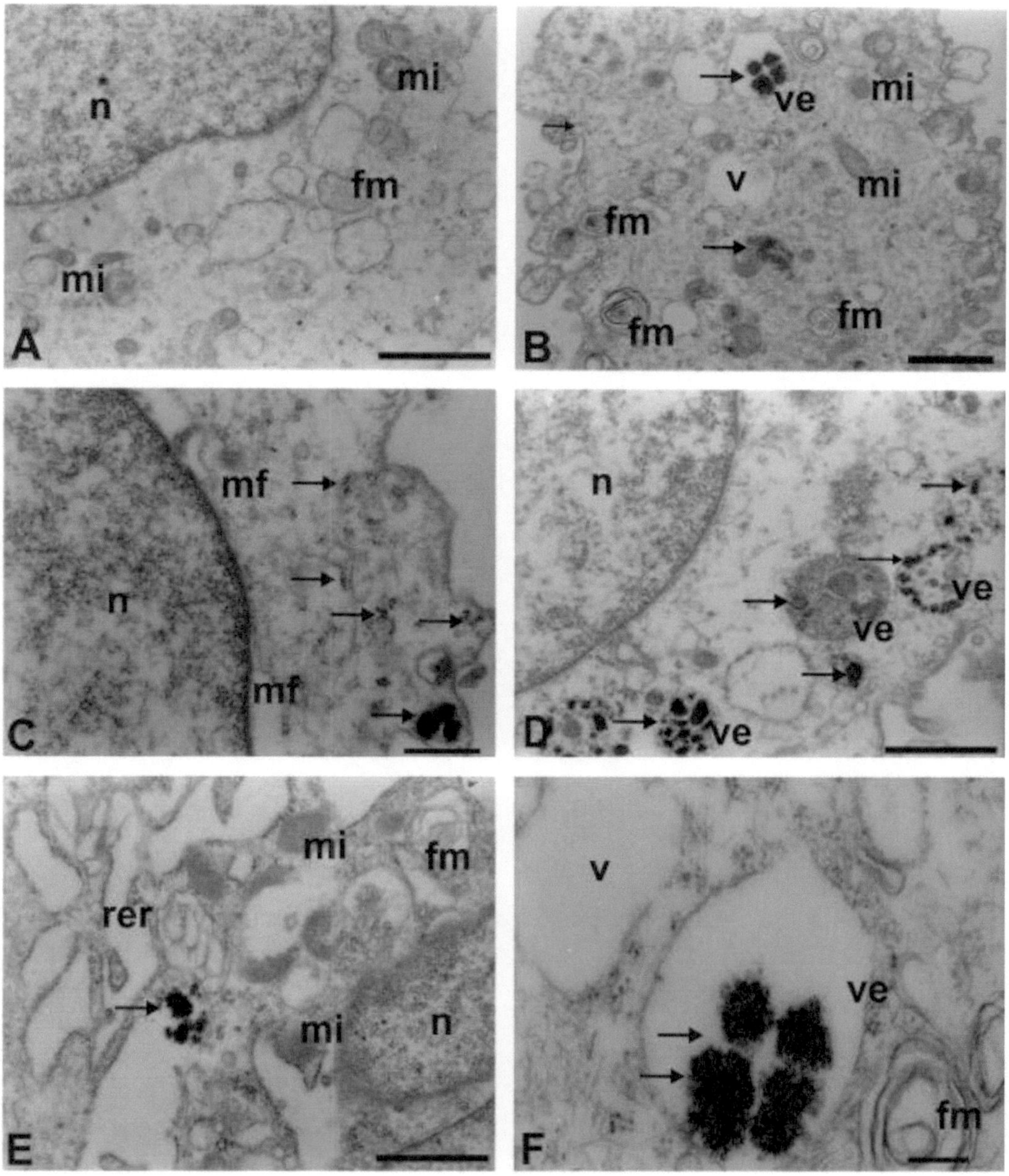

Fig. 4. B-F) Ultrastructural analysis of glioblastoma lineages marked with nanocrystal quantum dots (QD 565nm) conjoined with the CD105 monoclonal antibody. A) Glioblastoma lineage cells of the control group. A, C, D, E, F) Scale: 0.5μm. B) Scale: 1μm. n = nucleus; v = vacuole; mi = mitochondria; ve = vesicle; mf = microfilaments; fm = myelin figure; rer = rough endoplasmic reticule; arrow = electrondense nanoparticles (nanocrystals).

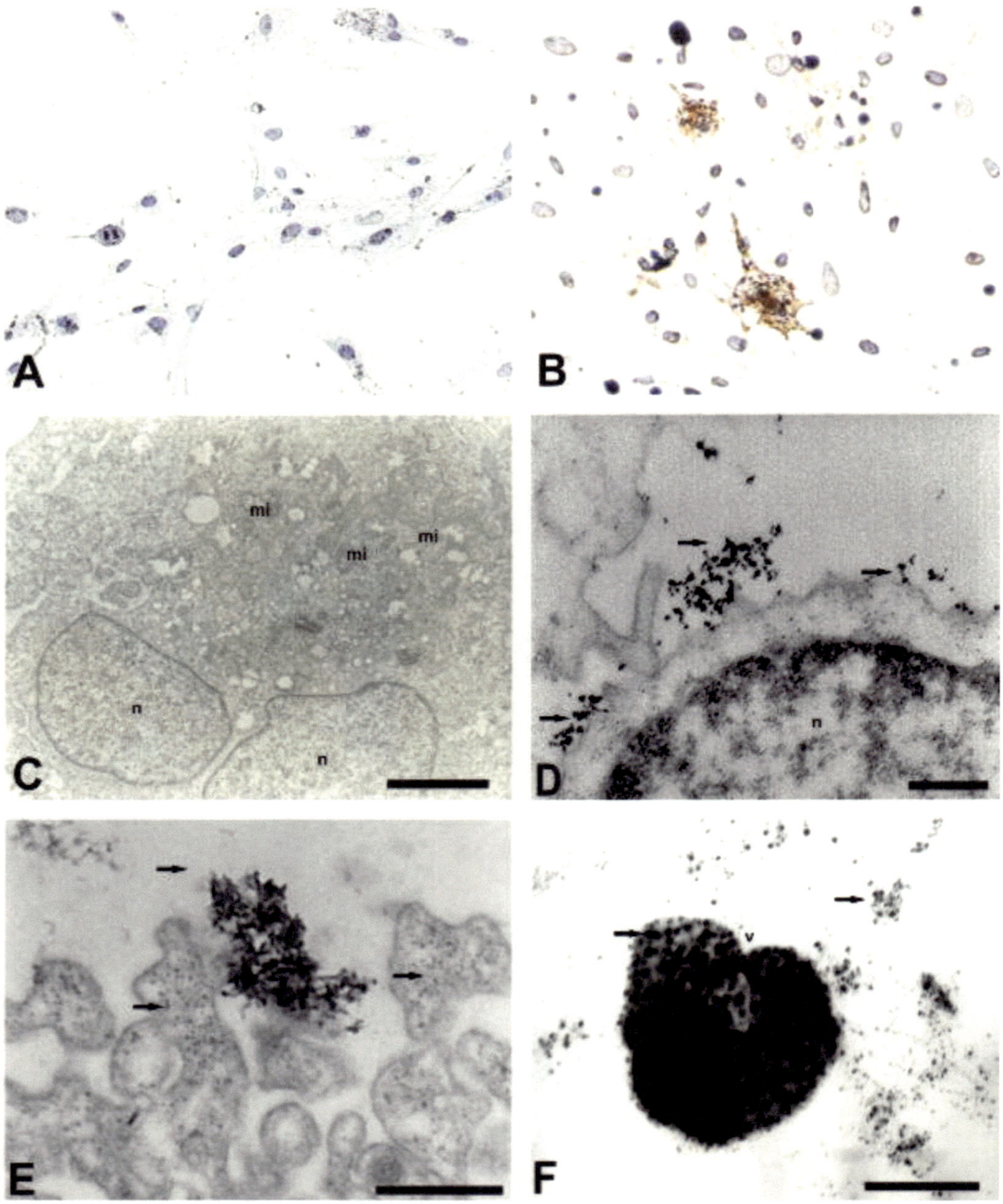

Fig. 5. Analysis of primary culture glioblastoma marked with microbeads CD133 by using immunocytochemical staining and transmission electron microscopy. (A, C) Primary culture glioblastoma of the control group. (B, D–F) Glioblastoma cells (CD133+). (A, B) 400. Scale bars: (C) 0.25 µm; (D, E) 0.5 µm; (F) 1 µm. n, nucleus; c, cytoplasm; mi, mitochondria. Arrows indicate electrondense nanoparticles.

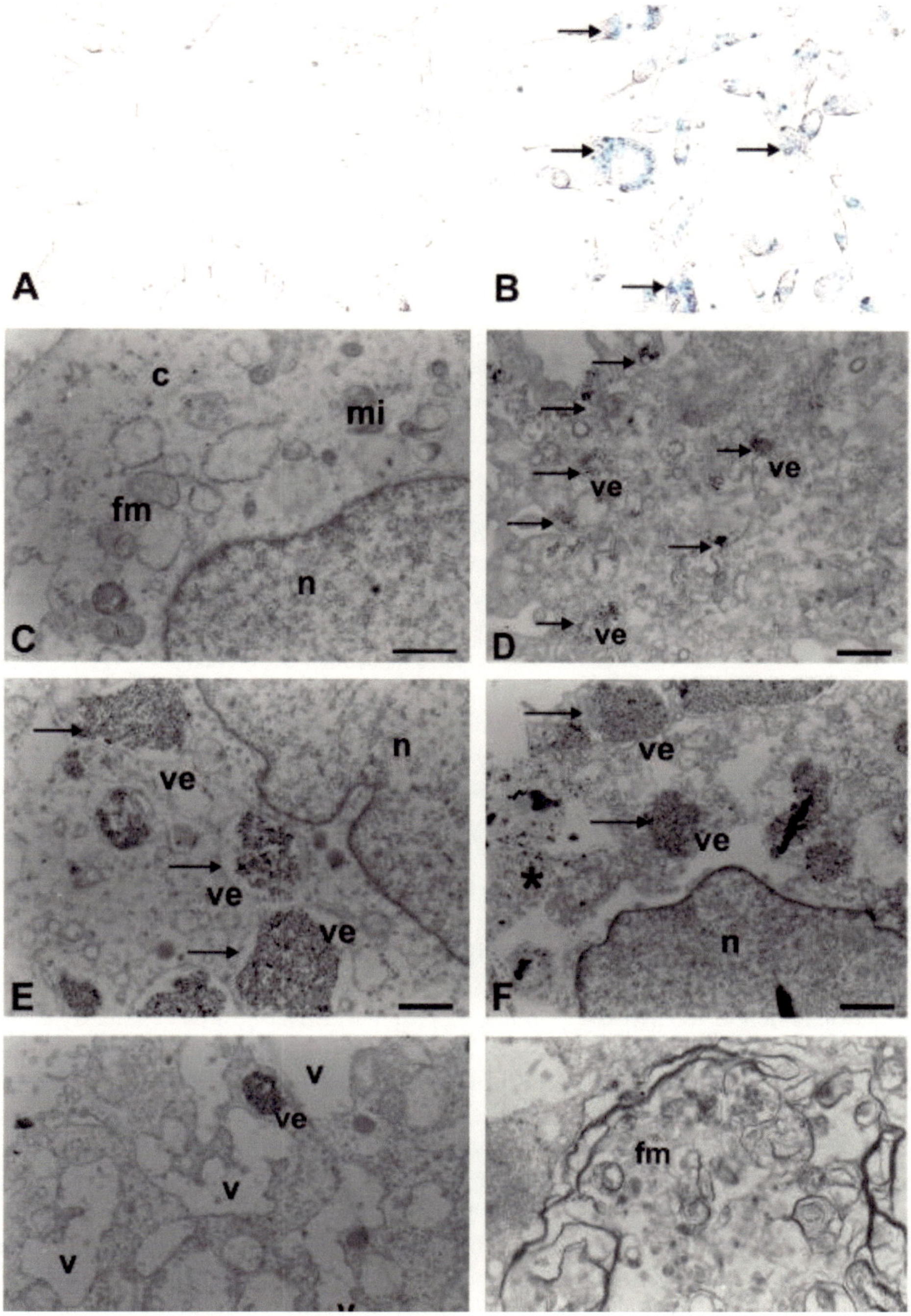

Fig. 6. Glioblastoma lineages marked with SPIONs. A, B) Light microscopy using Prussian blue staining. A, C) Glioblastoma lineage cells of the control group. A, B) 600X. C-H) Transmission electron microscopy. C-G) Scale: 1μm; H) Scale: 0.25μm. n = nucleus; v = vacuole; ve = vesicle; fm= myelin figure; mi = mitochondria; * = cell margin; arrow = electrondense nanoparticles.

4. Discussion

Glioblastoma is the most malignant brain tumor (Louis et al., 2007). Because of its invasive nature, it cannot be completely removed, reducing the success of chemo and/or radiotherapy procedures (Louis et al., 2007).

Some nanobiotechnology resources, using nanoparticles in the process of cell labelling, can be extended to areas of neuro-oncology trough the study of tumorigenic cells in the immunolocalization process (Simberg et al., 2007).

Our study suggests new approaches for the identification of the glioblastoma cells by ultrastructural examination using nanobiomarkers and it can contribute for further *in vivo* studies by understanding glioblastoma staining process.

Immunophenotypically, the glioblastoma lineages express a set of cell surface antigens also found in mesenchymal stem cells (MSC), such as CD29 (β1 integrin - receptor protein of extracellular matrix and a cell to cell interaction mediator), CD44 (hyaluronate receptor), CD73 (SH3, SH4), CD90 (Thy-1) and CD105 (SH2) (Sordi et al., 2005). These finding suggest that a subset of primary glioblastoma derives from transformed cells containing MSC-like properties with partial phenotypic aspects of the MSC.

Alternatively, glioblastomas cells could activate a series of pathways that result in the establishment of the cancer cells mesenchymal phenotype which may contributes to the tumor growth and malignant progression (Tso et al., 2006). Thus, MSC-like phenotype may play a role in tumorigenesis, invasive progression or tumor recurrence.

The analysis of ultrastructural immunolocalization of glioblastoma lineages showed the presence of monoclonal antibodies CD29, CD44 and CD105 linked to quantum dots, i.e., electrondense clusters on the surface of tumor cells and in vesicles.

The electronic micrographs described an important ultrastructural finding related to the presence of vesicles that internalize QD by the process of pinocytosis for all antibodies tested. We suggest that in our study the pynocytisis occur by receptor-mediated endocytosis. The endocytosis process happens after the antibody biding to the receptor, and then a depression arises on the cell membrane which is followed by the formation of the pinocytic vesicles. These pinocytic vesicles that are surrounded by the cytoplasmic proteins called clatrines are internalized.

Immunolocalization of the process by marking cells with CD29 primary antibody described control parameters for the study. This figure 6 shows, by microscopy fluorescence, the membrane staining by both CD29 primary antibody and the secondary anti-mouse antibody and, as a control, the cells were stained with the secondary anti-mouse antibody only. These results show that there is no unspecific reaction by the anti-mouse secondary polyclonal antibody in this experiment. The electronic micrographs also described the cells stained with the primary antibody CD29 and secondary anti-mouse polyclonal antibody, which the cells stained with the secondary anti-mouse antibody only, showing no unspecific staining by this antibody in these experiments.

The CD44 monoclonal antibody selected for this study is a transmembrane glycoprotein which acts primarily as a recipient of hyaluronana, and can bind to certain other ligands in an extracellular matrix. A correlation between the particular pattern of CD44 variants produced by strains of glioblastoma cells and tumor clinicopathological parameters, such as cell motility, invasive properties, potential for metastasis, and tumor cells survival could be established (Rudzki et al., 1997).

The CD105 monoclonal antibody, also included in this study, is intensely expressed in the tumor vascular system and can be an important indicator of prognosis of glioblastoma malignancy (Margaritescu et al., 2008).

Tumor growth and metastasis depend on the formation of new blood vessels. Tumor cells release a variety of compounds, which can act on endothelial progenitor cells activation, proliferation, and migration promoting neovascularization and consequent tumor angiogenesis (Reddy et al., 2006). Our study suggests the use of QD for tumor accumulation mechanism studies as well as targets for vascular mapping and consequent removal of tumorigenic glioblastoma cells.

Our study also proposes the use of a transcription factor called Forkhead Box M1 (FoxM1) previously conjoined with QD, as a glioblastoma marker, since this factor is described as up-regulated in glioblastoma cells (Liu et al., 2006). FoxM1 was ultrastructurally evident by the nanocrystal electrondensity conjoined to this nuclear transcription factor.

Reports showed that the level of protein expression in human gliomas tissues was directly related to the tumor grade or the glioblastoma cells tumorigenicity and may act as an index of tumor malignancy.

The electronic micrographs also demonstrated that glioblastoma cell lineages internalize the QD, expressing them ultrastructurally as electrondense structures that are located in different cellular regions, such as the cytoplasm or the rough endoplasmic reticulum.

The same process of tumor QD-marking was described by Jackson, et al. (2007) where the nanocrystals were phagocytised by macrophages and microglia, thus infiltrating experimental gliomas. Therefore, his study suggests the use of non-conjoined nanocrystals to assist the imaging system for surgical termination or glioblastoma tumor biopsies.

The analysis of immunocytochemistry demonstrated the CD133 expression in primary culture glioblastoma. Ultrastructural results showed anti-CD133 bound to the SPIONs by the presence of electrondense granules in cell membrane, as well as in the cytoplasm or forming vesicles.

CD133 localization in membrane protrusions suggests an involvement in the dynamic organization of membrane and therefore in the mechanisms influencing cell polarity, migration and interaction of stem cells with neighboring cells and/or extracellular matrix, but experimental data are currently lacking. In addition, it is not known whether CD133 has a role in self-renewal and differentiation of stem cells, witch has important implication in gliomagenesis (Singh et al., 2003; Beier et al., 2007; Zeppernick et al., 2008).

CD133 positive cells isolated from human brain tumours exhibit stem cells properties in *vitro* (Singh et al., 2003) and are able to initiate and drive tumor progression *in vivo* (Singh et al., 2004) strongly suggesting that CD133 positive cells might be the brain tumor initiating cells. This notion has been recently challenged by studies demonstrating that glioblastoma CD133 negative cells have also properties of stem cells and are tumorigenic when engrafted intracerebrally into nude mice (Beier et al., 2007).

Zeppernick, et al. (2008), for the first time, presented a direct link between the expression of a cancer stem cell antigen CD133 and patient survival in gliomas, giving support to the current cancer stem cell hypothesis. The authors demonstrated that the proportion of CD133 positive cells was an independent risk factor for tumor regrowth and time course of malignant progression in WHO grade 2 and 3 tumors. These data provide strong supportive evidence for image mapping the cancer stem cell structural model and the clinical relevance of the CD133 positive cell population in glioblastoma.

Iron oxide superparamagnetic nanoparticles (SPIONs) were also targets in the marking of glioblastoma cells. The SPIONs were enclosed by tumor cells through endocytosis and revealed by the Prussian blue cytochemical staining or the ultrastructural electrondensity resource within the vesicles.

Our work suggests the use of SPIONs as a contrast agent in magnetic resonance imaging techniques through the internalization of iron oxide by the endocytosis process (fluid phase - mediated receptor for transferrin linked to the oxide iron) (Daldrup-Link et al., 2003).

Transmission electron microscopy studies, using iron oxide-based markers, revealed no significant morphostructural changes in the tumor marked cells (Zeppernick et al., 2008). The results for the glioblastoma lineage markings by SPIONs describe, however, intense cytoplasmic vacuolation, loss of cell boundaries or disintegration of the plasma membrane and the formation of concentric lamellae forming myelin figures. Such indicators suggest ultrastructural signs of cell death probably derived from the process of marking, corroborating findings in the Alzheimer's disease studies using magnetic nanospheres (Hartig et al., 2003).

The ultrastructural findings of the tumorigenic glioblastoma cell labelling process using quantum dot and SPIONs suggest that these nanobiomarkers can play important role in cancer diagnosis and also help to understand tumor behavior, i.e., biomimetic amplification of tumoral "homing" revealing tumor invasive properties and its potential for metastasis, recognizing vascular targets for image mapping and treatment of brain tumors (Simberg et al., 2007), and describing the tumorigenicity of glioblastoma through therapeutic indicators of tumor malignancy (Voura et al., 2004; Simberg et al., 2007),

The process of tumor cell labelling *in vitro* by nanoparticles, using microscopic analysis, can successfully contribute in the future to the identification of the tumorigenic cells and consequently for better understanding glioblastoma genesis and recurrence. In addition, this method may help further studies in tumor imaging, prognostic markers detection, as well as to understand the selection process and isolation of the brain tumor stem cell ($CD133^+$)

5. Acknowledgements

This work was financed by Instituto Israelita de Ensino e Pesquisa Albert Einstein (IIEP/278-07). We are grateful to Laboratório de Microscopia Eletrônica, Departamento de Biologia - UNESP de Rio Claro, SP - Brasil and Antonio T. Yabuki and Monika Iamonte for the technical support.

6. References

Beier, D. et al. (2007). $CD133^+$ and $CD133^-$ glioblastoma-derived cancer stem cells show differential growth characteristics and molecular profiles. *Cancer Res.*, Vol. 67, N°.9, pp. 4010-4015.

Brandes, A.A. et al. (2008). Glioblastoma in adults Critical. Reviews in *Oncology/Hematology*, Vol.67, pp. 139–152.

Central Brain Tumor Registry of the US. http://www.cbtrus.org/reports//2007-2008/2007report.pdf

Cheng, F.Y. et al. (2005). Characterization of aqueous dispersions of Fe3O4 nanoparticles and their biomedical applications. *Biomaterials,* Vol.26, pp. 729-738.

Daldrup-Link, H.E. et al. (2003). Targeting of hematopoietic progenitor cells with MR contrast agents. *Radiology*, Vol.228, N°.3, pp. 760-767.

Hartig, W., et al. (2003). Electron microscopic analysis of nanoparticles, delivering thioflavin-T after intrahippocampal injection in mouse: implications for targeting β-amyloid in Alzheimer`s disease. *Neuroscience Letters*, Vol.338, pp.174-176.

Jackson, H. et al. (2007). Quantum dots are phagocytized by macrophages and colocalize with experimental gliomas. *Neurosurgery*, Vol.60, N°.3, pp. 524-529.

Jordan A., et al. (1997). Cellular uptake of magnetic fluid particles and their effects in AC magnetic fields on human adenocarcinoma cells in vitro. *Int. J. Hypertherm.*, Vol. 13, pp. 587–605.

Jordan A. et al. (1999). Endocytosis of dextran and silan-coated magnetite nanoparticles and the effect of intracellular hyperthermia on human mammary carcinoma cells in vitro. *J Magn. Magn. Mater*, Vol.194, pp. 185-96.

Kumar, C.S.S.R. (2007). Nanomaterials for Cancer Diagnosis (WILEY-VCH), Weinheim.

Lee, J.H. et al. (2007). Artificially engineered magnetic nanoparticles for ultra-sensitive molecular imaging. *Nature Medicine*, Vol. 13, N°.1, pp. 95-99.

Liu, M. et al. (2006). Fox M1B is overexpressed in human glioblstomas and critically regulates the tumorigenicity of glioma cells. *Clin. Cancer Res.* Vol. 66, N°.7, pp. 3593-3602.

Louis, D.N. et al. (2007). The 2007 WHO classification of tumours of the central nervous system. *Acta Neuropathol.*,Vol. pp. 114:197.

Margaritescu, C. et al. (2008). Endoglin (CD105) and microvessel density in oral squamous cell carcinoma. *Rom J Morphol Embryol.* Vol.49, N°.3, pp. 321-326.

Miraglia, S. et al. (1997). A novel five-transmembrane hematopoietic stem cell antigen: isolation, characterization, and molecular cloning. *Blood*. Vol. 90, pp. 5013–521.

Nisman, R. et al. (2004). Application of quantum dots as probes for correlative fluorescence, conventional, and energy-filtered transmission electron microscopy. *Journal of Histochemistry & Cytochemistry*, Vol.52, N°.1, pp. 13-18.

Reddy, G. R. et al. (2006). Vascular Targeted Nanoparticles for imaging and treatment of brain tumors. *Clin Cancer Res.*, Vol. 12, N°.22, pp. 6677-6686.

Rudzki, Z. & Jothy S. (1997). CD44 and the adhesion of neoplastic cells. *Mol. Pathol.*, Vol.50, pp. :57-71.

Simberg, D. et al. (2007). Biomimetic amplification of nanoparticle homing to tumors. *PNAS*, Vol. 104, N°.03, pp.932-936.

Singh, S.K. et al. (2003). Identification of a cancer stem cell in human brain tumors. *Cancer Res.*, Vol. 63, pp. 5821-5828.

Singh, S.K. et al. (2004). Identification of human brain tumour initiating cells. *Nature*, Vol.432, pp.396-401.

Sordi, V. et al. (2005). Bone marroe mesenchymal stem cell express a restricted set of sunctionally active chemokine receptors capacle of promoting migration to pancreatic islets. *Blood*, Vol.106, N°.2, pp. 419-427.

Tartaj, P. et al. (2003). Preparation, structural and magnetic characterization of synthetic anti ferromagnetic (SAF) nanoparticles. *Phys. D. Appl. Phy.*, Vol.36, pp. R182.

Tso, C. et al. (2006). Primary glioblastomas express mesenchymal stem-like properties. *Mol. Cancer Res.*, Vol.4, N°.9, pp. 607-619.

Voltairas, P. A. et al. (2002). Hydrodynamics of magnetic drug targeting. *J. Bioech.*,Vol. 35, pp. 813-821.

Voura, E.B. et al. (2004). Tracking metastatic tumor cell extravasation with quantum dot nanocrystals and fluorescence emission-scanning microscopy. *Nature Medicine*, Vol.10, N°.9, pp. 993-998.

Wen, P.Y. & Kesari, S. (2008). Malignant gliomas in adults. *N. Engl. J. Med.*, pp.359:492.

Zeppernick, F. et al. (2008). Stem cell marker CD133 affects clinical outcome in gliomas patients. *Clin. Cancer Res.*, Vol.14, N°.1, pp. 123-129.

18

Synchrotron Radiation: Applications in Diagnosis and Treatment of Malignant Brain Tumors

S. Kaiser Ali[1], Umashankar Das[2], Yanjie Lu[3],
Vijayanada Kundapur[4] and Tim May[5]
[1]College of Medicine, University of Saskatchewan, and Provincial Leader, Pediatric Oncology Program of Saskatchewan
[2]College of Pharmacy and Nutrition, University of Saskatchewan and Cancer Research Unit, Saskatchewan Cancer Agency
[3]Cancer Research Unit, Saskatchewan Cancer Agency
[4]College of Medicine, University of Saskatchewan, and Saskatoon Cancer Centre Saskatchewan Cancer Agency
[5]Canadian Light Source, University of Saskatchewan
Canada

1. Introduction

According to the reports published by the American Cancer Society, an estimated 22,020 cases of primary malignant tumors of brain and other central nervous system (CNS) sites were diagnosed in the United States in 2010 (Jemal et al. 2010, 277-300). During the same period, approximately 13,140 persons with these tumor types succumbed to their disease. Among adults, malignant brain tumors are estimated at 7.3 cases per 100,000 person-years, and in children 4.5 cases per 100,000 person-years (Maher and McKee 2010, 484-527). Malignant neoplasms of the brain and nervous system were estimated to have accounted for 1.5% of all new cancer cases and 2.3% of cancer deaths in the United States in 2008, as reported in the SEER Cancer Statistics Review (*Surveillance, Epidemiology, and End Results (SEER) Program,*
National Cancer Institute 1975-2005. www.seer.cancer.gov). Brain tumors aggregate in a bimodal age distribution pattern. The first occurs during infancy and early childhood between birth to 4 years of age, followed by a gradual rise in incidence after age 24, and a late second peak between 50–79 years of age. The Central Brain Tumor Registry of the United States reports that gliomas account for 36% of all primary brain tumors, and 81% of malignant tumors (*CBTRUS Statistical Report 2008: Primary brain tumors in the United States. Central brain tumor registry of the United States, Chicago. www. cbtrus.org)*. Among these, glioblastoma multiforme (GBM) is the most common (Raizer 2011, 152-157), accounting for at least 50% of cases. Glioblastoma multiforme remains an incurable disease, with a 5 year survival rate ranging from around 13% for patients aged 15-45 years to only 1% for those aged 75 years and older (*Surveillance, Epidemiology, and End Results (SEER) 2007, SEER* Stat software, version 6.3.5. www.seer.cancer.gov/seerstat/software*).

Obstacles to cure of brain tumors include, among others, the juxtaposition of tumor and vital centres of normal brain, "blood brain barrier"(Armulik et al. 2010, 557-561; Blanchette and Fortin 2011, 447-463; Kalra and Couldwell 2011, 179-180), limitations in achieving complete tumor resection, lack of concordance in tumor classification (Daumas-Duport and Varlet 2003, 622-636), and inherent resistance of untreated tumor to chemotherapy (Eimer et al. 2011, 1017-1027; Denysenko et al. 2010, 343-351; Luqmani 2005, 35-48), and radiation therapy (Friedman et al. 2009, 199-209). Newer approaches to investigating the biology of gliomas is the first step towards more precise identification of their dynamic evolution, which in turn should lead to development of more effective therapeutic strategies and improved long term survival.

2. Diagnosis of brain tumors

The World Health Organisation (WHO) Classification of Tumors of the CNS lists astrocytic tumors as the most common among tumors of neuroepithelial (or glial) tissue. The "gold standard" of this classification is a histopathological diagnosis based on light microscopy examination of hematoxylin and eosin (H&E) stained biopsy tissue sections. Slides are scanned to record gradation of tumor cell density, vascularisation, small-cell density and matrix loosening. Histologic grading of astrocytomas range from the most benign form (grade I - pilocytic astrocytomas) to the most malignant (grade IV - glioblastoma multiforme), based on the degree of anaplasia, mitotic index, degree of invasion into surrounding tissue, microvascular proliferation, and foci of necrosis (Kleihues et al. 2002, 215-25; Louis et al. 2007, 97-109). The term "multiforme" derives from the spectrum of different cell types and tissue heterogeneity observed within the tumor: astroblastic, oligodendroglial, and dedifferentiated cells in combination with anaplastic, gemistocytic, fibrillary, or pilocytic components (Iglesias-Rozas and Hopf 2005, 351-356).

However, subjectivity in interpretation and ambiguities in definitions and histologic criteria in the WHO classification (Tanaka et al. 2011; Reifenberger and Wesseling 2010, 549-551), such as multiple phenotypes within the same tumor at one or different points in time (Hassler et al. 2006, 46-55; Walker et al. 2003, 4841-4851) as well as newly-evolving tumor variants (Kozak and Moody 2009, 833-841; Valle-Folgueral et al. 2008, 343-349; Martinez et al. 2007, 26-34) and unclassifiable tumors (Cenacchi and Giangaspero 2004, 185-192) emphasize the limitations of histological classification.

Immunohistochemical stain panels provide more specific information regarding antigen expression associated with certain cell types, and also reflect patterns of genetic aberrations within tumors. These panels consist of a combination of immunoperoxidase stains and anti cellular-protein-specific monoclonal antibodies. Cytokeratins, vimentin, desmin, glial fibrillary acidic protein, and neurofilament protein stains serve to more accurately identify the cell lineage of tumors. In addition, immunocytochemical stains such as keratin, synaptophysin, S100, melanoma antigen recognized by T cells (MART-1), leukocyte common antigen (LCA), organic ion transporter 3/4 (OCT 3/4) and smooth muscle actin (SMA) provide a better definition in cases of less well-differentiated neoplasms (Wieczorek and Longtine 2010, 1-5). The advantage of these stains is that they can be used with paraffin-embedded stored tissue samples.

Increasingly, molecular biological and cytogenetic techniques are being used to investigate mechanisms of malignant transformation and to identify tumor markers predictive of behaviour and outcome (Martinez et al. 2007, 26-34; Krex et al. 2003, 1377-84). Aberrations within the tumor genome have been detected by such molecular genetic techniques as fluorescent in-situ hybridisation, comparative genomic hybridisation (Wiltshire et al. 2000, 164-173), spectral karyotyping (Zuber et al. 2002, 111-115) and gene expression profiling (Liang et al. 2005, 5814-5819). Newer variants of "classical" GBM including giant cell, small cell, epitheloid, and rhabdoid variants, as well as those containing PAS and trichrome stain-positive intracellular inclusions, continue to manifest (Kleinschmidt-DeMasters et al. 2006, 273-286). These evolutionary changes in the histopathological manifestations of GBM are reflected in the 2007 revision of the original 2002 WHO classification, where newer GBM variants such as GBM with an oligodendroglioma component have been recognized (Nakamura, Makino, and Kuratsu 2011). Tumor heterogeneity detected by the array of these diagnostic methods is a compelling reason for developing more refined and accurate recognition techniques.

3. Fourier Transform (FTIR) Infrared Spectroscopy

The challenges posed by heterogeneous (Bleau, Huse, and Holland 2009, 2936-2944) expressions of histological, cytogenetic, and oncogenetic mechanisms within brain tumors can be addressed by a relatively new biodiagnostic research tool, vibrational spectroscopy.

Fourier Transform Infrared (FTIR) vibrational spectromicroscopy combines light microscopy with infrared spectroscopy. It uses mid-infrared light obtained from a conventional thermal source as a probe to characterise qualitative and quantitative vibrational properties of biological specimens at a molecular level. FTIR spectroscopy is both a chemical and a molecular probe. The infrared (IR) spectra generated by biological tissues are a composite display of vibrational shifts in covalent bonds, derived from their biomolecular content (proteins, lipids, sugars, and nucleic acids).

The intensities of the spectra express quantitative information, while the frequencies at which they are displayed reflect qualitative information on the nature, composition, and relationships of their molecular structures. FTIR data can therefore be used as molecular "fingerprints" for correlation of spectral patterns with biological structure unique to normal tissues and their malignant counterparts. The technique of FTIR has the advantage of examining tissues "at the source" and not requiring any processing of the samples prior to testing. Scientists have capitalised on the finding that lipid, protein, carbohydrate and nucleic acid content of biological tissues can be precisely identified by specific spectral "signatures" generated when they are subjected to absorption spectroscopy using mid-infrared (mid-IR) light (wave numbers 4000-1000 cm^{-1}) (Marinkovic et al. 2002, 189-197). The amide I band (~1650 cm^{-1}) results mainly from the ν(C=O) stretching vibrations of protein amide bonds. The amide II band ~ 1549 cm^{-1} arises from the *d*(N–H) bending and ν(C–N) stretching vibrations of amide bonds. The ν(C=O) stretching of lipids is displayed ~ 1740 cm^{-1}, and the anti-symmetric ν ($PO2^{-}$) stretching of nucleic acids and phospholipids ~ 1225 cm^{-1}.

The precise frequency of absorption from a particular molecular bond or group is dependent on the environment in which it resides; specific changes within them characterise such conditions as skin cancer (McIntosh et al. 1999, 951-956). The commencement of transformation of normal tissues into a dysplastic state, and onwards to neoplasia, is most likely initiated at a subcellular level by molecular changes and subtle shifts in tissue components, amenable to detection by IR spectromicroscopy. The subtle changes in large numbers of spectra generated during biospectroscopy are prone to subjective error if interpreted by inspection alone. This problem can be overcome by means of multivariate statistical analyses performed by specific software programs designed for this purpose. FTIR spectromicroscopy is proving to be a useful complementary tool for purposes of enhanced diagnostic accuracy, improved tumor grading, developing treatment strategies, and monitoring responses to therapy.

3.1 Conventional FTIR - animal studies

In a study using FTIR imaging of C6 gliomas grown in the brains of Wistar rats, researchers were able to differentiate between normal brain structures and tumor tissue; altered patterns were detected in the intermediate zones. FTIR transmission spectroscopy confirmed decreased concentrations of lipids within tumors, which was correlated to the degree of myelination present. The spectroscopic findings correlated with light microcopy detection of myelin in healthy brain tissues using Luxol fast blue and Luxol fast blue-cresyl stains (Amharref et al. 2006, 892-899). Reflection/absorption IR spectromicroscopy studies were conducted on autopsied formalin-fixed de-paraffinised tumor tissue sections of rat C6 glioma allografted in Wistar rat brain. Spectral signatures from malignant tissue were compared with those of a normal control, and subjected to multivariate analyses. This allowed for generation of false-colour coded maps, comparing variations in lipoprotein composition. In contrast to the normal sample, tumor spectra displayed qualitative and quantitative variations in amide I and II bands pertaining to protein components (Bambery et al. 2006, 900-907). Another study with the same animal model and using transmission spectroscopy demonstrated several features of clinical relevance: i) spectral patterns of proteins and nucleic acids could be used to differentiate between normal, malignant, peri-tumoral and necrotic brain tissues, ii) the development of tumor was marked by a reduction in total lipid content (cholesterol, phosphatidyletanolamine, phosphatidyl-choline, and galactocerebroside), and iii) glioma tissues contained a high amount of sphingomyelin, nucleic acids, and oleic acids (Beljebbar et al. 2008, 8406-8415).

3.2 Conventional FTIR - human studies

A proof of concept diagnostic study using IR spectroscopy to classify biopsy specimens of 25 human brain tumors resulted in an overall 89% concordance with light microscopy re. WHO diagnosis and grading of astrocytic tumors (Steiner et al. 2003, 464-471). Researchers were able to identify changes within tumors in both the nature, and relative amounts, of brain lipids, including gangliosides and phospholipids. In view of the conundrum that conventional histological findings are not predictive of tumor behavior, correlation between histological diagnoses and FTIR spectroscopy was conducted in a few cases of human head and neck tumors (gingival squamous cell carcinoma and sarcomatoid carcinoma). In the former, high DNA, lipid and collagen components were detected; in the latter, similar findings also were documented, but in a heterogeneous distribution (Bruni et al. 2004, 19-26).

IR spectroscopy was used to differentiate normal brain from both *in vitro* glioblastoma cell lines as well as 56 tumor specimens from glioma patients. In normal control samples, molecular signatures demonstrated differences between white and grey matter, based on increased spectral endowments from lipids and cholesterol. As well, these researchers were able to demonstrate progressive decreases in brain lipids, inversely proportional to the degree of anaplasia (Krafft et al. 2004, 921-925). Characteristic IR spectral signatures of disparate tissue types from multiple tissue sections of two brain tumors were used to develop a multivariate classification model. The model was based on linear discriminant analysis (LDA) and used to classify single IR spectra from 51 patients. Results of analysis using the LDA model revealed 100% accuracy with normal brain tissue (5 samples), 80% accuracy for grade III astrocytomas (15 samples), and 74.2% accuracy for grade IV/GBM (31 samples) (Krafft et al. 2006, 301-305). Extension of this methodology to the macroscopic imaging mode of three tumor sections of GBM from one patient resulted in spectra that were almost identical. However, when a supervised classification model based on the LDA algorithm was applied to the data, gradation of tumor content was suggestive of tissue sections being derived from intra-tumor, tumor margin, and extra-tumor locations respectively (Krafft et al. 2007, 1669-1677).

Meningiomas comprise a group of brain tumors with significant risks of recurrence and unpredictable outcomes (Drummond, Zhu, and Black 2004, 113-130). We investigated, by means of mid-infrared reflectance spectromicroscopy, a number of meningiomas to determine their spectral signatures, and to more accurately differentiate tumor tissue from normal control (Ali et al. 2008, 297-301). Briefly, brain tumor samples were obtained at elective surgery from four patients with meningiomas. A sample derived from histologically proven normal brain tissue at the periphery of resected margins in one patient served as control. Paired tumor tissue sections 5 micrometres in thickness were cut in a cryostat at -20°C. The first section was placed on a glass slide for H&E stain, and the section immediately was transferred onto an IR-reflective slide for spectromicroscopy. Concordance of tumor-bearing areas was achieved by means of a novel technique developed in our lab. It requires superimposing a digital tractile grid over paired H&E and IR tissue section images of tumor bearing areas within the tissue section that are demarcated by a pathologist, and then transferring matching grid coordinates onto the overview image generated by the spectromicroscope in the preparation of mid-IR spectroscopy (**Figures 1a, 1b and 1c**) (Ali et al. 2010, 857-860).

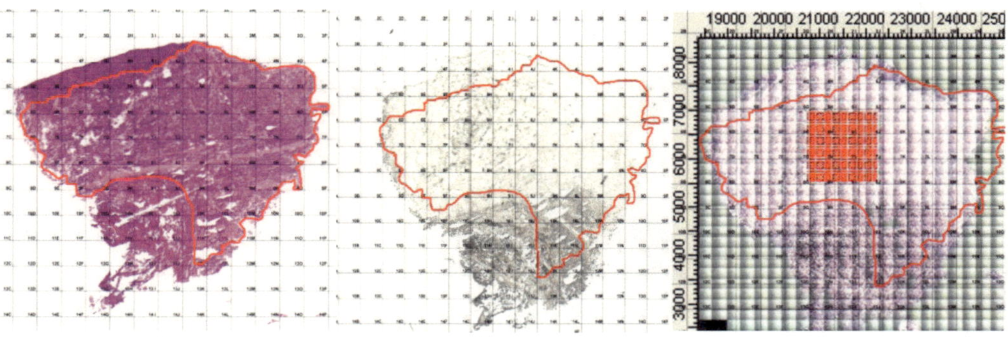

1a 1b 1c

Fig. 1. 1a. Equisized H&E stained tissue section with concordant grid and tumor-bearing area within digital boundaries (outlined in black). 1b. Equisized paired IR unstained tissue section showing tumor-bearing area (within red boundaries) with concordant grid and overlaid digital boundary map transferred from Figure 1a. Fig. 1c. Equisized spectromicroscopy overview image of tissue section with raster map (red square) outlined within tumor-bearing area (within red boundaries), in the preparation of mid-IR spectroscopy (note matched grid coordinates in all images).

Mid-IR microscopy data collection: Thin tumor section on the IR reflectance slide was raster scanned using Globar light-sourced spectromicroscopy at the Canadian Light Source (CLS) synchrotron facility. Spectromicroscopy was performed using an IFS 66v/S FTIR spectrometer with a conventional light source attached to a Hyperion IR microscope with a 15X Cassegrain objective and a single channel MCT detector. Raster scans were obtained in the mid-infrared range of 4000-900 cm^{-1} using a 50 micrometres x 50 micrometres aperture, 25 micrometres step size, 32 scans per step, and resolution of 4 cm^{-1}. Stage control, data collection and processing were done using OPUS software and analysed using CytoSpec, a software tool designed for FTIR image analysis. Visible images were obtained using a charged-couple device camera, which was linked to the infrared images.

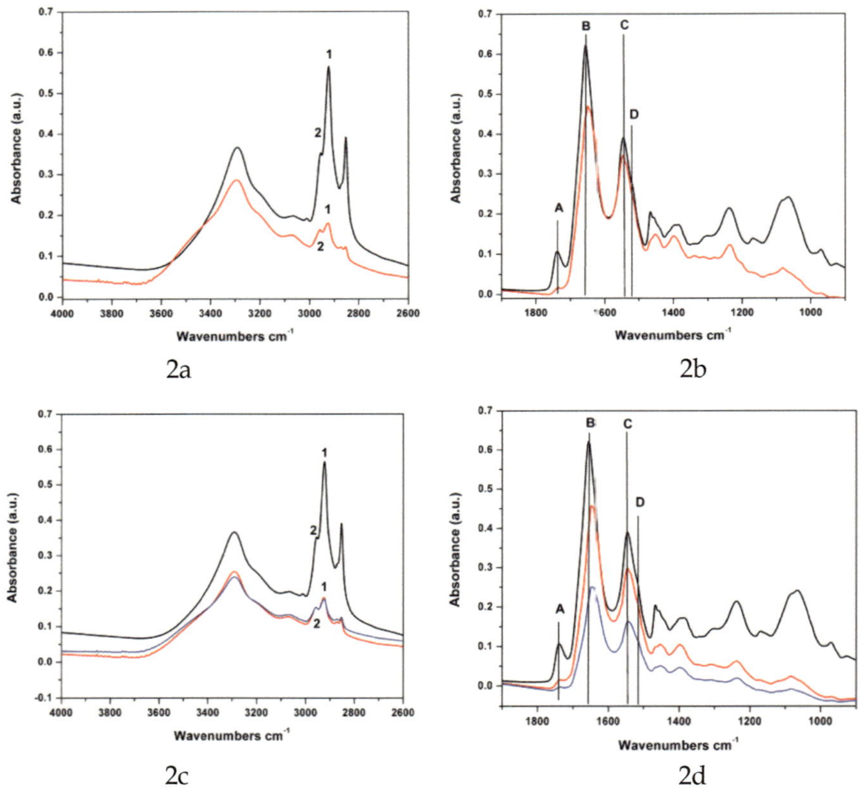

Fig. 2. Comparison of average mid-IR spectra of brain tissue samples, control and tumour in the spectral region of 4000-2600 cm^{-1} and 1900-900 cm^{-1}. 2a,b: Control spectrum (black) and a cluster from the tumour tissue (red). 2c,d: Control spectrum (black) and two clusters from the tumour tissue(red and blue). Despite similar spectra pattern in 2a-d, the following important points are noted. i) The relative CH_2 and CH_3 stretching intensities labeled as 1 and 2, respectively in 2a and 2c that represent lipid peaks are very different. ii) the peak A at 1735 cm^{-1} shows a large decrease in lipid concentrations in the tumour samples., iii) the peak B at 1655 cm^{-1} in 2c indicates the amide I peak in the tumour sample is largely unchanged from the control sample. This peak in 2d shifts towards 1631 cm^{-1}, iv) the peak C at 1548 cm^{-1} in 2c that represents protein amide II is largely unchanged from the control sample but this peak in 2d shifts slightly to 1544 cm^{-1}, and v) the peak D at 1515 cm^{-1} corresponds to tyrosine amidic linkage.

The average spectra shown in Figures **2a-d** compare two different brain tissue samples, control and tumor, each from a different patient.

The first, most striking difference occurs in the bands associated with lipids, particularly unsaturated fatty acids, demonstrating a marked decrease in all the clusters associated with tumor tissue. In particular, the bands at 3010, 2920, 2850, and 1735 cm^{-1} are all weaker than in the control spectra. More subtle differences are visible in the region between 1900-900 cm^{1}, particularly the among the protein bands. The amide I band of the control tissue shows a large proportion of undifferentiated proteins and a small contribution of α-helical proteins at 1655 cm^{-1}. The tumor tissue samples tend more towards undifferentiated proteins; however, some of the clusters show an increased beta-sheet band at 1631 cm^{-1}. A band associated with the amino acid tyrosine at 1515 cm^{-1} is generally more pronounced in the tumor samples than in the control samples. In the spectral region of 1500-900 cm^{-1}, the tumour samples shows very weak peak intensities compared to control.

The results to date indicate the presence of a unique signature that could help identify tumor tissue. The marked diminution of the bands associated with the lipids combined with subtle changes in the main protein bands seems to be an indicator that a sample tissue is derived from tumor. This fingerprint is similar for all the different samples studied to date, and it may be possible to refine this spectral fingerprint to detect to a specific tumour class. Comparable results were found in three other patients with meningiomas. One of the strengths of the study is that, in spite of small numbers, all four patients had the same type and grade of tumor confirmed by a pathologist. This avoided the potential problem arising from interpretation of disparate degrees of anaplasia within the same histological tumor type.

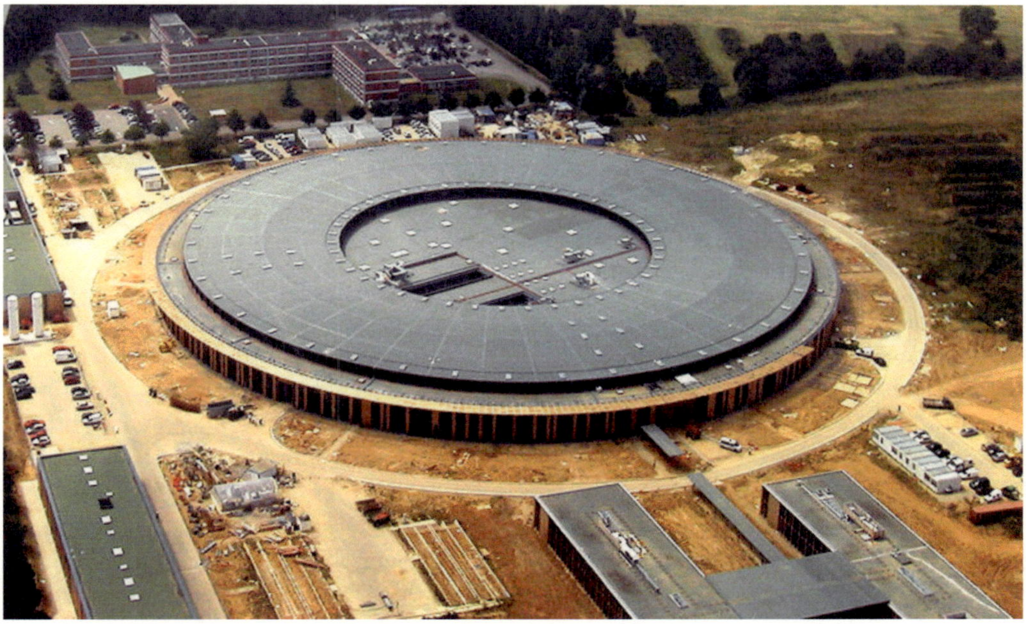

Fig. 3. SOLEIL synchrotron facility near Paris, France (Copyright © Synchrotron Soleil, reproduced with permission).

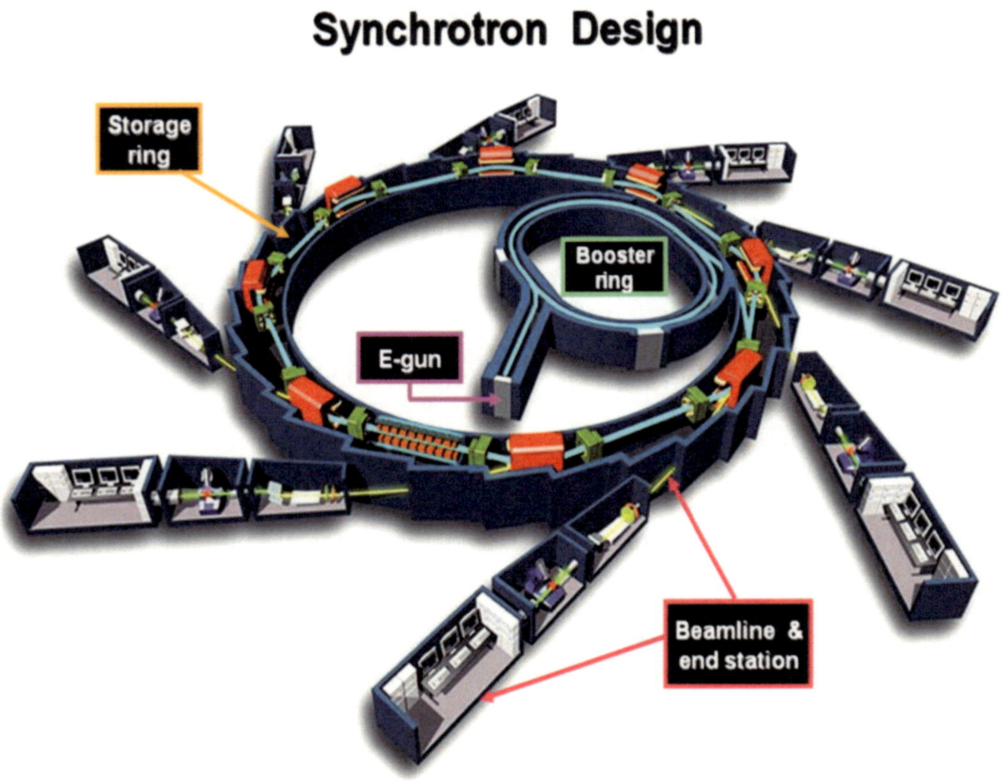

Fig. 4. Schematic diagram of Synchrotron Soleil. The circular ring is the synchrotron, a particle accelerator that brings electrons to very high speeds. The synchrotron emits "synchrotron radiation", especially X-rays; these are sent into the various beamlines (the straight lines branching out of the synchrotron). Each beamline contains scientific instruments, experiments etc. and receives an intense beam of radiation (Copyright © EPSIM 3D/JF Santarelli, Synchrotron Soleil, reproduced with permission).

4. Synchrotron

A synchrotron is a large ring-shaped particle accelerator into which electrons are fed from a smaller booster ring and a linear accelerator. The magnetic fields to turn the electrons, and electric fields to accelerate them within the main booster ring, are carefully synchronised with the electrons as they travel in a circular orbit at nearly the speed of light. The acceleration of electrons to this very high speed causes them to lose energy when they turn in magnetic fields. The energy is lost by emitting photons (light energy or electromagnetic radiation), which are then transported along tangential steel pipes called beamlines. The photon transport involves mirrors and devices for focusing and tuning the light for a particular use. The entire spectrum of electromagnetic radiation including, among others, (IR) Infrared light and monochromatic high energy x-ray beams, can be selectively extracted from photons within a given beamline and used for diagnostic and therapeutic applications **(Figure 5)**.

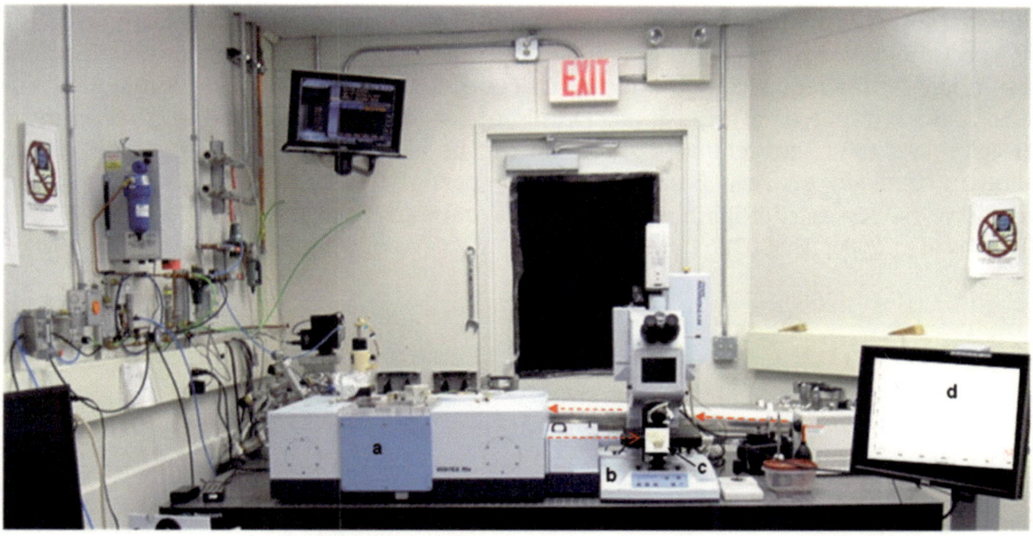

Fig. 5. Experimental hutch, 01B1-1 Mid-Infrared Spectromicroscopy beamline, Canadian Light Source, Saskatoon, Canada. Dotted arrows indicate pathway of synchrotron mid-IR beam entering spectrometer, passing through the tumour specimen, and generating the spectra. a. FTIR Spectrometer, b. spectromicroscope, c. unstained thin tumor section, d. spectra displayed on screen (author's files).

4.1 Synchrotron FTIR spectroscopy

Conventional thermal IR spectromicroscopy examination of biological tissues has limited spatial resolution, arising from low brightness diffraction or optical aberrations, including insufficient spatial resolution of only approximately 20-25 micrometres (Carr 2001, 1613). This problem is overcome by synchrotron IR light by virtue of its brightness, which is 100–1000 times greater than that from a conventional source (Miller and Dumas 2006, 846-857). Individual biological cells range from 5-30 micrometres in diameter, too small for probing by conventional IR sources. The much greater brightness of synchrotron-sourced light, however, permits intracellular imaging of molecular chemical structure and, compared to thermal IR light sources, provides greater spectroscopic detail and serves as a more refined diagnostic tool (Holman et al. 2002, 417-424) for a spectrum of malignant brain tumors, both in terms of differentiating tumor types as well as assessing degrees and patterns of anaplasia.

Figure 6 shows two absorbance spectra collected from 10 x 10 mm areas of the same region of a single tissue section. The upper trace was recorded using a synchrotron source, and the lower trace using a conventional thermal source. Each spectrum was collected for 1024 scans at 8 cm^{-1} spectral resolution. The advantage of the synchrotron as an infrared light source at high spatial resolution can clearly be seen in the difference between the spectra. The spectrum collected using the thermal source shows particularly high levels of "noise" in the fingerprint region below 1600 cm^{-1} (Tobin et al. 2004, 27-39).

It has become increasingly clear that synchrotron IR spectromicroscopy is an extremely valuable analytical tool when determining the chemical composition of biological and biomedical samples, at the diffraction-limited spatial resolution. Highly resolved IR spectromicroscopy, together with the high signal-to-noise level of recorded spectra, is essential in generating chemical and statistically-derived multivariate images. Synchrotron IR spectromicroscopy is very useful because of the achievable diffraction-limited spatial resolution, for the high signal-to-noise spectra obtained even with a diffraction-limited spot size, and for rapid data acquisition. Details of the secondary (alpha-helix) structure of proteins and their intracellular distribution can be identified with much greater clarity, allowing detailed analysis because of good spectral quality. The synchrotron source provides the necessary brightness to fulfill this requirement in the case of individual cells (Dumas et al. 2004, 289-302).

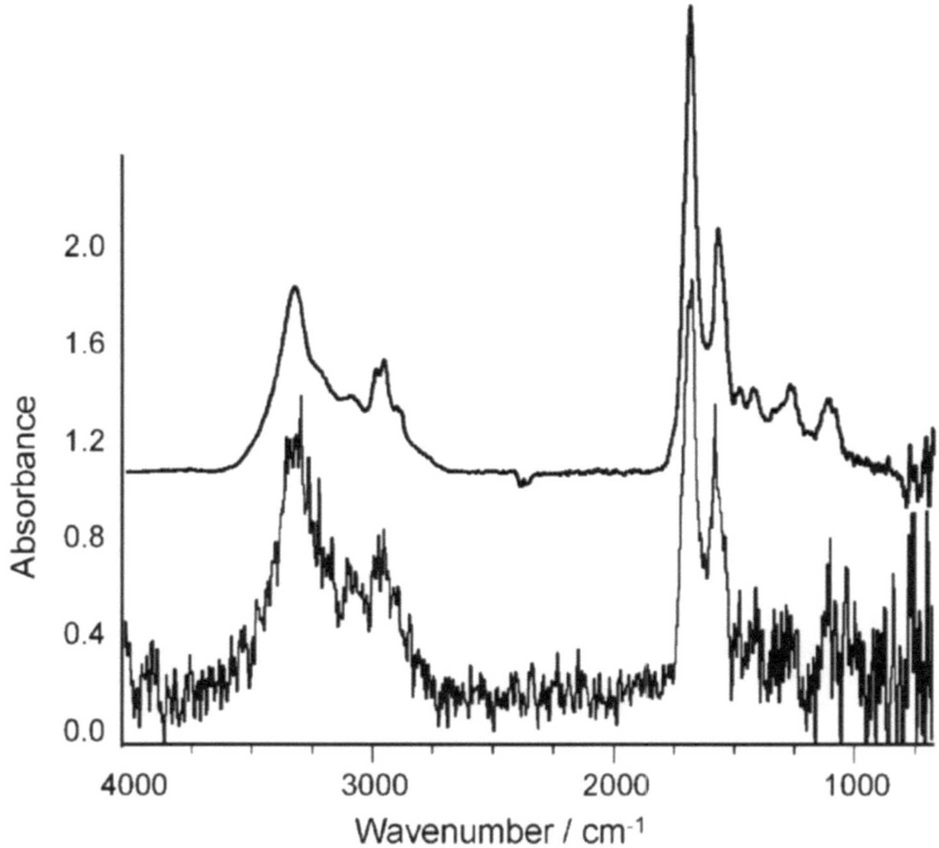

Fig. 6. Absorption spectra of tissue sample recorded under identical collection conditions using a thermal infrared source (lower trace) and synchrotron radiation (upper trace). (Copyright © The Royal Society of Chemistry, reproduced with permission)

Our diagnostic experiments progressed from using thermal light-sourced mid-IR reflectance spectromicroscopy to synchrotron light-sourced transmission spectromicroscopy to study human GBM tumor samples (Ali et al. 2010, 11-16). Tumor tissue was obtained from six patients with GBM and control samples from two other non-malignant patients. Experimental procedures were the same as for the meningioma study described earlier, with the following changes: The second of thin, paired tissue sections was mounted onto a CaF_2 slide for mid-IR transmission spectromicroscopy at the 01B1-1 beamline, Canadian Light

Source (CLS). Transmission spectromicroscopy was performed using a 36X Cassegrain objective and a single channel MCT detector. Raster scans were obtained in the range of 4000-900 cm^{-1} using a 10 x 10 micrometres aperture, 10 micrometres step size, 32 scans per step, and resolution of 4 cm^{-1}. A multivariate statistical analysis was performed after converting all spectra to their second derivative and subjecting them to hierarchical cluster analysis (HCA). Pseudo-color maps based on cluster analysis were then created by assigning a color to each spectral cluster.

A total of 16 raster maps of GBM tumour tissue specimens from 6 patients were obtained and the results compared with 7 maps of control brain tissue specimens from resection margins of two patients, one with craniopharyngioma and the other with astrocytic gliosis. A study pathologist confirmed normal brain tissue on histopathological examination of the two control samples. The average spectra of GBM and normal control tissues were generated using synchrotron-sourced mid-IR beamline at CLS (Figure 7)

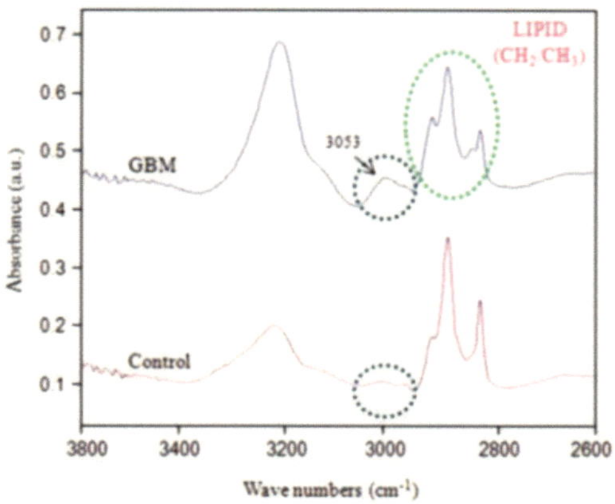

7a

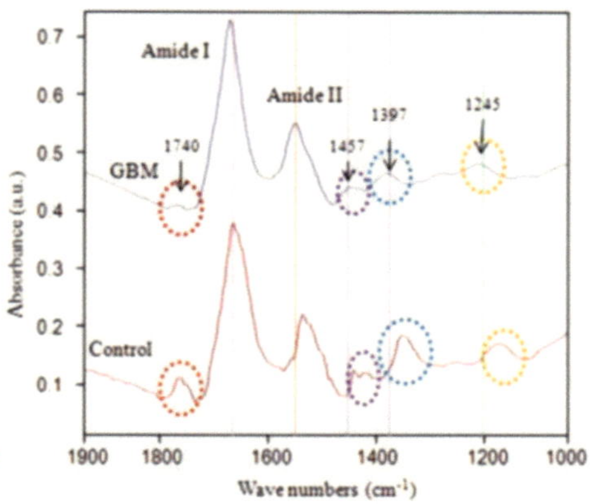

7b

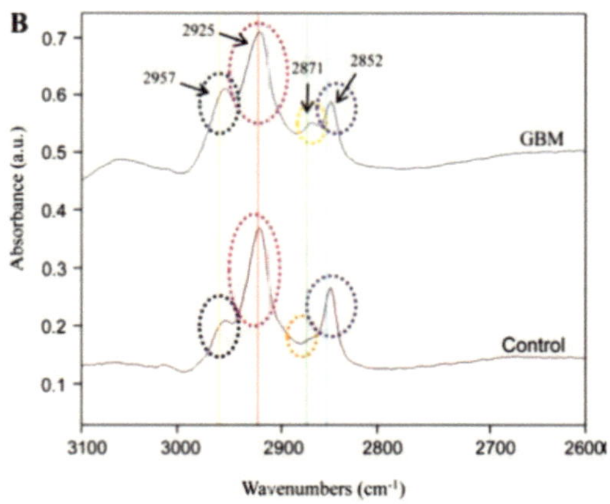

7c

Fig. 7. Comparison of average mid-IR spectra of GBM and control sample in the region of 3,800-2,600 (7a) and 1,900-900 cm^{-1} representing acyl vibrations fatty acids, peptide linkages of proteins, phosphodioxy groups of nucleic acids (7b) and the figure 7c depicts striking differences in the average spectra of GBM tumour and normal tissue in the spectral range of 3,100-2,600 cm^{-1}, representing lipid CH_2 and CH_3 stretching intensities.

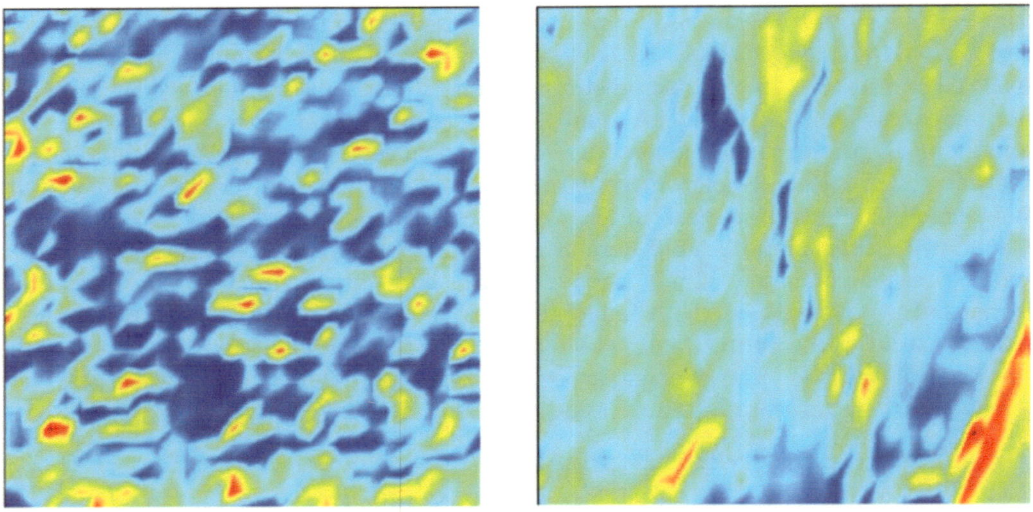

8a 8b

Fig. 8. Spectromicroscopic infrared mapping of tissue sections. False color codes represent varying tissue composition. 8a. Control, specimen displays four different clusters of spectra representing different tissue components. Blue and green pixels represent lipid and protein respectively; yellow & red pixels indicate nucleic acid components. 8b. GBM, displays marked reduction in lipid component.

The coloured cluster map representing control tissue (**Figure 8a**) clearly reflects four groupings of chemical moieties in normal brain tissue, including lipids, proteins, and nucleic acids. Blue pixels indicating lipid predominate; green and red pixel clusters indicate protein and DNA respectively. By contrast, in a GBM tumor sample (**Figure 8b**); lipid content is reduced drastically while protein content comprises the major portion of the image.

Data obtained from spectral comparisons of tumor and control samples graphically display spatial distribution of cluster groups representing different tissue components. **Figure 9** demonstrates false colour images displaying the spatial distribution of clusters from our experiments. Five clusters were considered for both control and tumour tissues. Each cluster was assigned a false color code for comparison purposes. The images in **Figures 9a and 9b**, representing control and GBM specimens respectively, clearly differentiate between the spatial distribution of the various clusters identified by the hierarchical cluster analysis (HCA) algorithm (Ward's algorithm). In GBM tumour samples, the cluster representing red pixels, most likely lipid, has been significantly reduced, while clusters identified by green pixels predominate, compared to control sample. These false colour cluster images demonstrate the sensitivity of these HCA method techniques in displaying subtle differences not obvious on visual inspection alone. A number of significant differences in the mid-IR spectral patterns of have been identified in GBM tumours compared to normal brain tissue. These differences could serve as diagnostic molecular spectral "signatures" in identifying residual GBM within tumour resection margins. A further study with larger number of patient samples for precise identification of a molecular signature unique to GBM has corroborated the spectral signatures identified in our pilot study (manuscript in preparation).

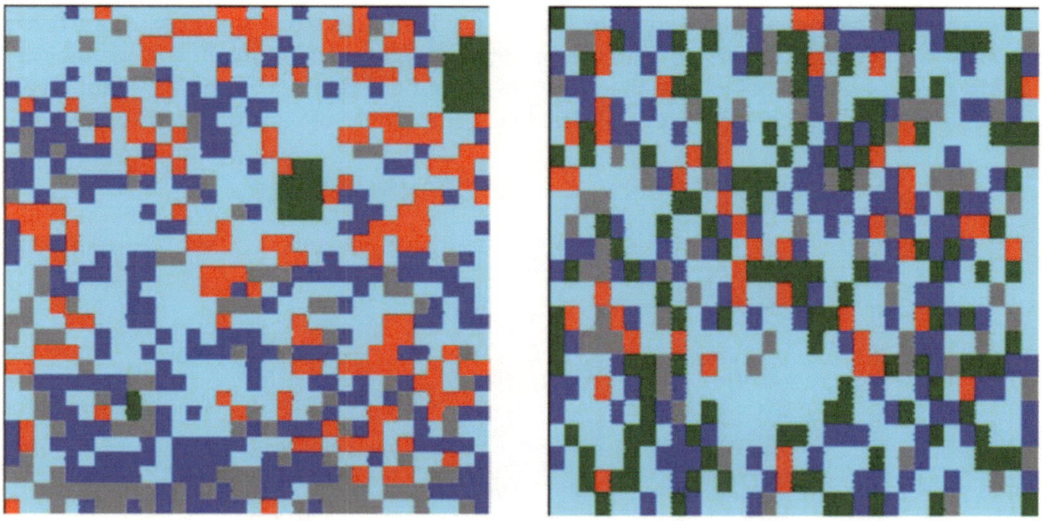

9a 9b

Fig. 9. Hierarchical (HCA) cluster analysis of (9a) control specimen and (9b) GBM tumor specimen. HCA false color image of 5 clusters displaying diversity in tissue composition of tumor tissue compared to control (see below).

4.2 Synchrotron Microbeam Radiation Therapy (MRT)

Curative management of human brain tumors is dependent upon accuracy of histological diagnosis and grading, achieving tumor-free margins during surgical removal, and inclusion of residual macroscopic and microscopic tumor within radiation therapy fields (Mason et al. 2007, 110-117) (Brem et al. 2011, 352-400). Obstacles to cure of a highly anaplastic tumor like GBM include inability to achieve complete tumor resection because of its rapid growth and invasive properties, migration of GBM cells several centimeters away from the primary tumor and even into the contralateral cerebral hemisphere (Lefranc, Brotchi, and Kiss 2005, 2411-2422), and its inherent resistance to radiation therapy and chemotherapy (Kemper et al. 2004, 415-423). Newer, innovative, and more precisely-targeted treatment approaches are required to positively impact on survival.

One of the limiting factors in delivery of curative radiation therapy to cancer patients is the dose-limiting tolerance of normal tissues (Deman et al. 2010, 586-589). There are several promising treatment approaches (Clarke, Butowski, and Chang 2010, 279-283) aimed at increasing the survival rate for patients with GBM tumors. One such therapy is microbeam radiation therapy (MRT), which has been designed for the specific purpose of maximising tumoricidal dose delivery while sparing surrounding normal tissues (Regnard et al. 2008, 861-878; Dilmanian et al. 2006, 9709-9714; Nettelbeck et al. 2009, 447-456; Serduc et al. 2009, 6711-6724; Prezado et al. 2009, 4897-4902).

Synchrotron-generated parallel, planar, micrometre-wide X-ray beams (microbeams) have been shown to safely deliver significantly higher than normal doses to the cerebella of weaning piglets without obvious neurological deficit one year later (Figure 10) (Laissue et al. 2007, 577-581). Histopathological examination at autopsy revealed preservation of normal cerebellar architecture except for thin, white horizontal parallel stripes approximately 20-30 micrometres in width, corresponding to the path of the microbeams. Degenerative changes in neurons and astroglial cells were noted only along the tracks of the microbeams; no tissue necrosis, hemorrhage or demyelination were noted by light microscopy. This leads the way for MRT as a potential tool to treat brain tumors in young children, whose CNS is still in the developmental stages and therefore vulnerable to compromise of neurocognitive functions.

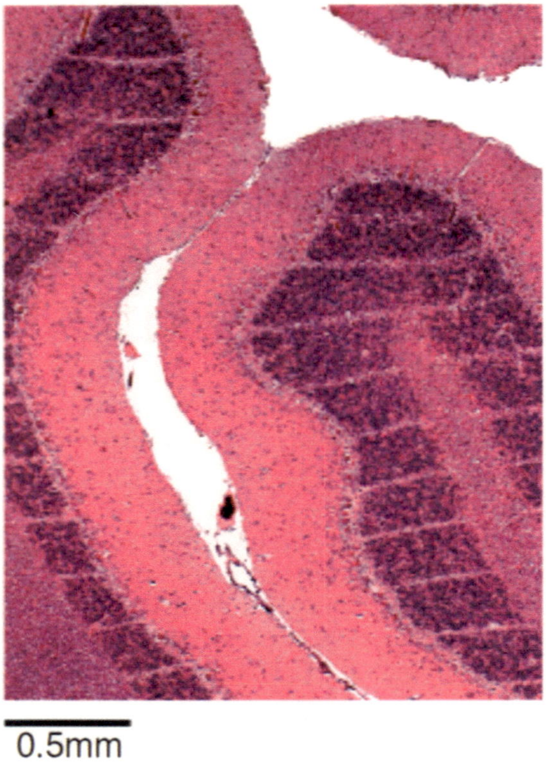

Fig. 10. Cerebellum of a piglet about 15 months after irradiation (skin entrance dose 300 Gy); hematoxylin/eosin-stained horizontal tissue section. Tissue has maintained its normal architecture. This white horizontal parallel stripes, clearly visible in inset, correspond to paths of approximately 27 μM-wide microbeam; beam spacing was about 210 μM (Copyright © Developmental Medicine & Child Neurology, reproduced with permission)

The concept of MRT is similar to GRID therapy (Tenzel 1952, 399-408; Huhn et al. 2006, 607-612; Mohiuddin et al. 1999, 721-727) in that healthy tissue is spared by applying discretely spaced beams as opposed to a continuous solid beam over the same volume. With MRT, several narrow beams tens of micrometres in width, spaced hundreds of micrometres apart, are delivered through the tumor. With high dose rates, these beams have been shown to preferentially kill glioblastoma tumors while better sparing the healthy brain tissues (Deman et al. 2010, 586-589; Sheleg et al. 2002, 53-59; Miura et al. 2006, 71-75; Dilmanian et al. 2003, 632-641). Although the mechanism of action of MRT remains to be elucidated, there are indications that the vasculature damaged by MRT is more readily repaired in healthy tissue than in glioblastoma tumors. This purported repair mechanism is felt to be dependent on differential regenerative activity of capillary endothelial cells in spared tissues in between the microbeams. Until now, MRT research has been carried out primarily at a limited number of international synchrotron facilities. The main advantage of a synchrotron-derived radiation source is a very high dose rate, at least several hundred Gy per second, which allows for near instantaneous treatment times. This is important when dealing with micrometre-sized beams. If treatment times are drawn out, the energy deposited by the microbeams is spread out due to vascular pulsations and organ motion. Another advantage of a synchrotron source is that it is essentially nondivergent. This allows for the production of very flat minibeam profiles with little offaxis fall off. Nondivergent beams also yield a sharper penumbra on the individual minibeams, which in turn yields lower valley doses. While awaiting validation of proven safety and efficacy, synchrotron MRT treatment studies to date have been restricted to *in vitro* and *in vivo* pre-clinical experiments, mostly with brain tumors grown in small animals.

In preparation for synchrotron MRT experiments, we designed and created a minibeam collimator for minibeam radiation therapy studies in rodents using a 250 kVp clinical X-ray machine as a simulated synchrotron source (Babcock et al. 2011, 2192-2197). Our research has been designed to lead up to pre-clinical studies using synchrotron MRT. We have established an animal model of GBM xenografts grown in brains of immunocompromised nude mice, and plan to commence studies at the Biomedical Imaging and Therapy (BMIT) beamline 05B1-1 at the Canadian Light Source (CLS). The CLS is Canada's national synchrotron facility, located on campus at the University of Saskatchewan (Wysokinski et al. 2007, 73-76).

A treatment strategy designed to overcome limitations in tissue radiation tolerance was studied in a rat F98 glioma model. Test animals with implanted brain tumor were treated with a synergistic combination of single dose beam synchroton radiation, simultaneous with an infusion of an iodinated contrast agent. The results were compared with two other control groups: untreated tumor-bearing rats, and those treated with synchrotron radiation therapy alone. A 20% and 44% increase in life spans were noted in the rats irradiated without or with iodine, respectively, albeit a modest one in terms of days of prolongation of life (median survival times of 12.5, 15 and 18 days for untreated controls, irradiated without iodine, or with iodine respectively)(Adam et al. 2003, 1413-1426). The research group developed a strategy aimed at disrupting the blood-brain barrier to increase delivery of iodinated contrast agent into F98 rat gliomas.

The blood-brain barrier (BBB) is an integrated physiological system composed of interdigitating endothelial cells supported by pericytes, astrocytes and extracellular matrix, as well as enzymes, and transporters, working in concert to maintain homeostasis of the extracellular milieu. In so doing, it impedes the transport of chemotherapeutic agents across the vascular compartment into the CNS matrix. Osmotic disruption of the BBB is achieved by administration of hypertonic solutions such as mannitol, which induce crenation of the endothelial cells, disruption of their tight interdigitations, and enhanced diffusion of drugs across the BBB (Kemper et al. 2004a, 415-423). In principle, osmotic disruption of the BBB should allow for increased deposition of radiosensitising agents within tumor, thereby increasing the total lethal dose of intra-tumoral irradiation following external beam radiation treatment.

In the next series of experiments in F98 glioma-bearing rats were treated with synchrotron stereotactic radiotherapy (SSR) in a single dose fraction, simultaneous with intravascular infusion (intra-arterial or intravenous) of a combination of iodinated contrast agent and mannitol. The latter drug was added to induce temporary BBB disruption and thereby allow greater deposition of photoactive contrast within the tumor while it was being irradiated.

Percentage increase in life span (ILS) was most significant (169%) in rats who received both SSR and combined drugs via intra-arterial (i.e., intra-carotid) administration for X-ray doses ≤ 15 Gy. Administration via the intravenous route of the same drug combination concomitant with SSR resulted in 116% ILS, while no benefit was noted (91% ILS) in the group treated with SSR only. Of interest is the fact that at 25 Gy dose, survival advantage was greatest in the group that was treated with SSR alone (Adam et al. 2006, 603-611).

Furthering the above studies, a platinum derivative, *cis*-Platinum (CDDP), was chosen to explore the synergistic effect of platinum compounds reported in human studies. Interestingly, this pioneering study (Biston et al. 2004, 2317-2323) showed more than twice the amount of double-strand breaks (DSB's) when mouse models were treated with a combination of CDDP and synchrotron beam radiation with energy in the vicinity of platinum K-edge. The study also correlated survival benefit compared to other energy beams.

Realisation that modulation of energy of electromagnetic beams given in combination with compounds that achieve supra-additive tumor ablation (De Stasio et al. 2006, 206-213), while sparing normal tissues, creates possibilities for ambitious research undertakings. Further understanding of this as yet unchartered territory will pave the way for developing novel treatment methods resulting in enduring control of these tumors.

5. Conclusions

Histological grading of tumors delineates a continuum from least to most malignant (grade I-IV, respectively). Gradations of malignancy, as well as variations in tumor type, may be identified in a single tissue section. The challenge for the pathologist lies in accurately identifying the tumor and assessing the degree of anaplasia in order to guide the clinician with information to optimise treatment strategy and obtain a favourable outcome.

Malignant tumors can be considered reverse versions of their tissues of origin, endowed with the ability to continually evolve their cellular structure and extracellular matrix in response to changes in their microenvironment. Diagnostic light microscopy examination and immunohistochemical stains identify events "frozen" at one point in time, i.e., when the tumor is biopsied or excised. As we begin to consider and understand tumors more as dynamic entities, our approach to studying their biologic behavior by conventional static diagnostic methodologies is increasingly being supplemented by biochemical, molecular genetic, and cell signaling probes. IR spectroscopy serves as a light probe, penetrating tissues and cells at a molecular level, in real time, to provide a composite display of the chemical composition and molecular structural relationships of tissues and individual cells.

The brilliant intensity of synchrotron-generated light energy, a form of electromagnetic radiation, reveals nuances of tumor tissue activity at a subcellular or molecular level. It "illumines" our minds to the understanding that tissues, normal and malignant, even when completely severed from the body, can still dance to a rhythm of inherent vibrations that identifies them as unique. Another form of synchrotron-sourced electromagnetic radiation, microbeam radiations, proves a tool for improved eradication of malignant tumors, which are themselves none other than condensed forms of electromagnetic radiations. Thus, in the domain of brain tumors, the synchrotron serves a triple purpose as a diagnostic, treating, and teaching tool.

6. Acknowledgement

Our research work described in this paper was funded by a peer-reviewed grant from the Saskatchewan Cancer Agency, and by a grant from office of the Vice-President, Research, College of Medicine, University of Saskatchewan. Research described in this paper was performed at the Canadian Light Source, which is supported by the Natural Sciences and Engineering Research Council of Canada, the National Research Council Canada, the Canadian Institutes of Health Research, the Province of Saskatchewan, Western Economic Diversification Canada, and the University of Saskatchewan.
http://www.lightsource.ca/uso/publications.php

7. References

Adam, J. F., H. Elleaume, A. Joubert, M. C. Biston, A. M. Charvet, J. Balosso, J. F. Le Bas, and F. Esteve. 2003. Synchrotron radiation therapy of malignant brain glioma loaded with an iodinated contrast agent: First trial on rats bearing F98 gliomas. *International Journal of Radiation Oncology, Biology, Physics* 57 (5) (Dec 1): 1413-26.

Adam, J. F., A. Joubert, M. C. Biston, A. M. Charvet, M. Peoc'h, J. F. Le Bas, J. Balosso, F. Esteve, and H. Elleaume. 2006. Prolonged survival of fischer rats bearing F98 glioma after iodine-enhanced synchrotron stereotactic radiotherapy. *International Journal of Radiation Oncology, Biology, Physics* 64 (2) (Feb 1): 603-11.

Ali, K., Y. Lu, C. Christensen, T. May, C. Hyett, R. Griebel, D. Fourney, K. Meguro, L. Resch, and R. K. Sharma. 2008. Fourier transform infrared spectromicroscopy and hierarchical cluster analysis of human meningiomas. *International Journal of Molecular Medicine* 21 (3) (Mar): 297-301.

Ali, K., Y. Lu, U. Das, R. K. Sharma, S. Wiebe, K. Meguro, V. Sadanand, et al. 2010. Biomolecular diagnosis of human glioblastoma multiforme using synchrotron mid-infrared spectromicroscopy. *International Journal of Molecular Medicine* 26 (1) (Jul): 11-6.

Ali, K., T. Reichert, D. Gomez, Y. Lu, A. Jan, and C. Christensen. 2010. A new approach to concordance in mid-infrared spectromicroscopy mapping of malignant tumors. *Oncology Reports* 24 (4) (Oct): 857-60.

Amharref, N., A. Beljebbar, S. Dukic, L. Venteo, L. Schneider, M. Pluot, R. Vistelle, and M. Manfait. 2006. Brain tissue characterisation by infrared imaging in a rat glioma model. *Biochimica Et Biophysica Acta* 1758 (7) (Jul): 892-9.

Armulik, A., G. Genove, M. Mae, M. H. Nisancioglu, E. Wallgard, C. Niaudet, L. He, et al. 2010. Pericytes regulate the blood-brain barrier. *Nature* 468 (7323) (Nov 25): 557-61.

Babcock, K., N. Sidhu, V. Kundapur, and K. Ali. 2011. Collimator design for experimental minibeam radiation therapy. *Medical Physics* 38 (4) (Apr): 2192-7.

Bambery, K. R., E. Schultke, B. R. Wood, S. T. Rigley MacDonald, K. Ataelmannan, R. W. Griebel, B. H. Juurlink, and D. McNaughton. 2006. A fourier transform infrared microspectroscopic imaging investigation into an animal model exhibiting glioblastoma multiforme. *Biochimica Et Biophysica Acta* 1758 (7) (Jul): 900-7.

Beljebbar, A., N. Amharref, A. Leveques, S. Dukic, L. Venteo, L. Schneider, M. Pluot, and M. Manfait. 2008. Modeling and quantifying biochemical changes in C6 tumor gliomas by fourier transform infrared imaging. *Analytical Chemistry* 80 (22) (Nov 15): 8406-15.

Biston, M. C., A. Joubert, J. F. Adam, H. Elleaume, S. Bohic, A. M. Charvet, F. Esteve, N. Foray, and J. Balosso. 2004. Cure of fisher rats bearing radioresistant F98 glioma treated with cis-platinum and irradiated with monochromatic synchrotron X-rays. *Cancer Research* 64 (7) (Apr 1): 2317-23.

Blanchette, M., and D. Fortin. 2011. Blood-brain barrier disruption in the treatment of brain tumors. *Methods in Molecular Biology (Clifton, N.J.)* 686 : 447-63.

Bleau, A. M., J. T. Huse, and E. C. Holland. 2009. The ABCG2 resistance network of glioblastoma. *Cell Cycle (Georgetown, Tex.)* 8 (18) (Sep 15): 2936-44.

Brem, S. S., P. J. Bierman, H. Brem, N. Butowski, M. C. Chamberlain, E. A. Chiocca, L. M. Deangelis, et al. 2011. Central nervous system cancers. *Journal of the National Comprehensive Cancer Network : JNCCN* 9 (4) (Apr): 352-400.

Bruni, P., C. Conti, E. Giorgini, M. Pisani, C. Rubini, and G. Tosi. 2004. Histological and microscopy FT-IR imaging study on the proliferative activity and angiogenesis in head and neck tumours. *Faraday Discussions* 126: 19-26.

Carr, GL. 2001. Resolution limits for infrared microspectroscopy explored with synchrotron radiation. *Review of Scientific Instruments* 72 : 1613-9.

Cenacchi, G., and F. Giangaspero. 2004. Emerging tumor entities and variants of CNS neoplasms. *Journal of Neuropathology and Experimental Neurology* 63 (3) (Mar): 185-92.

Clarke, J., N. Butowski, and S. Chang. 2010. Recent advances in therapy for glioblastoma. *Archives of Neurology* 67 (3) (Mar): 279-83.

Daumas-Duport, C., and P. Varlet. 2003. Dysembryoplastic neuroepithelial tumors. *Revue Neurologique* 159 (6-7 Pt 1) (Jul): 622-36.

De Stasio, G., D. Rajesh, J. M. Ford, M. J. Daniels, R. J. Erhardt, B. H. Frazer, T. Tyliszczak, et al. 2006. Motexafin-gadolinium taken up in vitro by at least 90% of glioblastoma cell nuclei. *Clinical Cancer Research : An official Journal of the American Association for Cancer Research* 12 (1) (Jan 1): 206-13.

Deman, P., M. Edouard, S. Besse, M. Vautrin, H. Elleaume, J. F. Adam, and F. Esteve. 2010. Synchroton radiotherapy (*La Revue De Medecine Interne)* 31 (8) (Aug): 586-9.

Denysenko, T., L. Gennero, M. A. Roos, A. Melcarne, C. Juenemann, G. Faccani, I. Morra, et al. 2010. Glioblastoma cancer stem cells: Heterogeneity, microenvironment and related therapeutic strategies. *Cell Biochemistry and Function* 28 (5) (Jul): 343-51.

Dilmanian, F. A., G. M. Morris, N. Zhong, T. Bacarian, J. F. Hainfeld, J. Kalef-Ezra, L. J. Brewington, J. Tammam, and E. M. Rosen. 2003. Murine EMT-6 carcinoma: High therapeutic efficacy of microbeam radiation therapy. *Radiation Research* 159 (5) (May): 632-41.

Dilmanian, F. A., Z. Zhong, T. Bacarian, H. Benveniste, P. Romanelli, R. Wang, J. Welwart, T. Yuasa, E. M. Rosen, and D. J. Anschel. 2006. Interlaced x-ray microplanar beams: A radiosurgery approach with clinical potential. *Proceedings of the National Academy of Sciences of the United States of America* 103 (25) (Jun 20): 9709-14.

Drummond, K. J., J. J. Zhu, and P. M. Black. 2004. Meningiomas: Updating basic science, management, and outcome. *The Neurologist* 10 (3) (May): 113-30.

Dumas, P., N. Jamin, J. L. Teillaud, L. M. Miller, and B. Beccard. 2004. Imaging capabilities of synchrotron infrared microspectroscopy. *Faraday Discussions* 126: 289-302.

Eimer, S., M. A. Belaud-Rotureau, K. Airiau, M. Jeanneteau, E. Laharanne, N. Veron, A. Vital, H. Loiseau, J. P. Merlio, and F. Belloc. 2011. Autophagy inhibition cooperates with erlotinib to induce glioblastoma cell death. *Cancer Biology & Therapy* 11 (12) (Jun 15): 1017-27.

Friedman, G. K., C. P. Langford, J. M. Coleman, K. A. Cassady, J. N. Parker, J. M. Markert, and G. Yancey Gillespie. 2009. Engineered herpes simplex viruses efficiently infect and kill CD133+ human glioma xenograft cells that express CD111. *Journal of Neuro-Oncology* 95 (2) (Nov): 199-209.

Hassler, M., S. Seidl, B. Fazeny-Doerner, M. Preusser, J. Hainfellner, K. Rossler, D. Prayer, and C. Marosi. 2006. Diversity of cytogenetic and pathohistologic profiles in glioblastoma. *Cancer Genetics and Cytogenetics* 166 (1) (Apr 1): 46-55.

Holman, H. Y., K. A. Bjornstad, M. P. McNamara, M. C. Martin, W. R. McKinney, and E. A. Blakely. 2002. Synchrotron infrared spectromicroscopy as a novel bioanalytical microprobe for individual living cells: Cytotoxicity considerations. *Journal of Biomedical Optics* 7 (3) (Jul): 417-24.

Huhn, J. L., W. F. Regine, J. P. Valentino, A. S. Meigooni, M. Kudrimoti, and M. Mohiuddin. 2006. Spatially fractionated GRID radiation treatment of advanced neck disease associated with head and neck cancer. *Technology in Cancer Research & Treatment* 5 (6) (Dec): 607-12.

Iglesias-Rozas, J. R., and N. Hopf. 2005. Histological heterogeneity of human glioblastomas investigated with an unsupervised neural network (SOM). *Histology and Histopathology* 20 (2) (Apr): 351-6.

Jemal, A., R. Siegel, J. Xu, and E. Ward. 2010. Cancer statistics, 2010. *CA: A Cancer Journal for Clinicians* 60 (5) (Sep-Oct): 277-300.

Kalra, R., and W. T. Couldwell. 2011. Regulation of the blood-brain barrier: New treatments for central nervous system neoplasms. *World Neurosurgery* 75 (2) (Feb): 179-80.

Kemper, E. M., W. Boogerd, I. Thuis, J. H. Beijnen, and O. van Tellingen. 2004a. Modulation of the blood-brain barrier in oncology: Therapeutic opportunities for the treatment of brain tumours? *Cancer Treatment Reviews* 30 (5) (Aug): 415-23.

Kleihues, P., D. N. Louis, B. W. Scheithauer, L. B. Rorke, G. Reifenberger, P. C. Burger, and W. K. Cavenee. 2002. The WHO classification of tumors of the nervous system. *Journal of Neuropathology and Experimental Neurology* 61 (3) (Mar): 215-25.

Kleinschmidt-DeMasters, B. K., L. Meltesen, L. McGavran, and K. O. Lillehei. 2006. Characterization of glioblastomas in young adults. *Brain Pathology (Zurich, Switzerland)* 16 (4) (Oct): 273-86.

Kozak, K. R., and J. S. Moody. 2009. Giant cell glioblastoma: A glioblastoma subtype with distinct epidemiology and superior prognosis. *Neuro-Oncology* 11 (6) (Dec): 833-41.

Krafft, C., S. B. Sobottka, K. D. Geiger, G. Schackert, and R. Salzer. 2007. Classification of malignant gliomas by infrared spectroscopic imaging and linear discriminant analysis. *Analytical and Bioanalytical Chemistry* 387 (5) (Mar): 1669-77.

Krafft, C., S. B. Sobottka, G. Schackert, and R. Salzer. 2004. Analysis of human brain tissue, brain tumors and tumor cells by infrared spectroscopic mapping. *The Analyst* 129 (10) (Oct): 921-5.

Krafft, C., K. Thummler, S. B. Sobottka, G. Schackert, and R. Salzer. 2006. Classification of malignant gliomas by infrared spectroscopy and linear discriminant analysis. *Biopolymers* 82 (4) (Jul): 301-5.

Krex, D., B. Mohr, H. Appelt, H. K. Schackert, and G. Schackert. 2003. Genetic analysis of a multifocal glioblastoma multiforme: A suitable tool to gain new aspects in glioma development. *Neurosurgery* 53 (6) (Dec): 1377-84.

Laissue, J. A., H. Blattmann, H. P. Wagner, M. A. Grotzer, and D. N. Slatkin. 2007. Prospects for microbeam radiation therapy of brain tumours in children to reduce neurological sequelae. *Developmental Medicine and Child Neurology* 49 (8) (Aug): 577-81.

Lefranc, F., J. Brotchi, and R. Kiss. 2005. Possible future issues in the treatment of glioblastomas: Special emphasis on cell migration and the resistance of migrating glioblastoma cells to apoptosis. *Journal of Clinical Oncology : Official Journal of the American Society of Clinical Oncology* 23 (10) (Apr 1): 2411-22.

Liang, Y., M. Diehn, N. Watson, A. W. Bollen, K. D. Aldape, M. K. Nicholas, K. R. Lamborn, et al. 2005. Gene expression profiling reveals molecularly and clinically distinct subtypes of glioblastoma multiforme. *Proceedings of the National Academy of Sciences of the United States of America* 102 (16) (Apr 19): 5814-9.

Louis, D. N., H. Ohgaki, O. D. Wiestler, W. K. Cavenee, P. C. Burger, A. Jouvet, B. W. Scheithauer, and P. Kleihues. 2007. The 2007 WHO classification of tumours of the central nervous system. *Acta Neuropathologica* 114 (2) (Aug): 97-109.

Luqmani, Y. A. 2005. Mechanisms of drug resistance in cancer chemotherapy. *Medical Principles and Practice : International Journal of the Kuwait University, Health Science Centre* 14 Suppl 1 : 35-48.

Maher, E. A., and A. C. McKee. 2010. Neoplasms of the central nervous system. in: Skarin AT, canellos GP, eds. atlas of diagnostic oncology, 3rd edition. london, united kingdom: Elsevier science ltd publishers. In , eds. A. T. Skarin, G. P. Canellos. 3rd ed., 484-527. London, United Kingdom: Elsevier Science Ltd.

Marinkovic, N. S., R. Huang, P. Bromberg, M. Sullivan, J. Toomey, L. M. Miller, E. Sperber, et al. 2002. Center for synchrotron biosciences' U2B beamline: An international resource for biological infrared spectroscopy. *Journal of Synchrotron Radiation* 9 (Pt 4) (Jul 1): 189-97.

Martinez, R., W. Roggendorf, G. Baretton, R. Klein, G. Toedt, P. Lichter, G. Schackert, and S. Joos. 2007. Cytogenetic and molecular genetic analyses of giant cell glioblastoma multiforme reveal distinct profiles in giant cell and non-giant cell subpopulations. *Cancer Genetics and Cytogenetics* 175 (1) (May): 26-34.

Mason, W. P., R. D. Maestro, D. Eisenstat, P. Forsyth, D. Fulton, N. Laperriere, D. Macdonald, J. Perry, B. Thiessen, and Canadian GBM Recommendations Committee. 2007. Canadian recommendations for the treatment of glioblastoma multiforme. *Current Oncology (Toronto, Ont.)* 14 (3) (Jun): 110-7.

McIntosh, L. M., M. Jackson, H. H. Mantsch, M. F. Stranc, D. Pilavdzic, and A. N. Crowson. 1999. Infrared spectra of basal cell carcinomas are distinct from non-tumor-bearing skin components. *The Journal of Investigative Dermatology* 112 (6) (Jun): 951-6.

Miller, L. M., and P. Dumas. 2006. Chemical imaging of biological tissue with synchrotron infrared light. *Biochimica Et Biophysica Acta* 1758 (7) (Jul): 846-57.

Miura, M., H. Blattmann, E. Brauer-Krisch, A. Bravin, A. L. Hanson, M. M. Nawrocky, P. L. Micca, D. N. Slatkin, and J. A. Laissue. 2006. Radiosurgical palliation of aggressive murine SCCVII squamous cell carcinomas using synchrotron-generated X-ray microbeams. *The British Journal of Radiology* 79 (937) (Jan): 71-5.

Mohiuddin, M., M. Fujita, W. F. Regine, A. S. Megooni, G. S. Ibbott, and M. M. Ahmed. 1999. High-dose spatially-fractionated radiation (GRID): A new paradigm in the management of advanced cancers. *International Journal of Radiation Oncology, Biology, Physics* 45 (3) (Oct 1): 721-7.

Nakamura, H., K. Makino, and J. I. Kuratsu. 2011. Molecular and clinical analysis of glioblastoma with an oligodendroglial component (GBMO). *Brain Tumor Pathology* (Jun 1).

Nettelbeck, H., G. J. Takacs, M. L. Lerch, and A. B. Rosenfeld. 2009. Microbeam radiation therapy: A monte carlo study of the influence of the source, multislit collimator, and beam divergence on microbeams. *Medical Physics* 36 (2) (Feb): 447-56.

Prezado, Y., S. Thengumpallil, M. Renier, and A. Bravin. 2009. X-ray energy optimization in minibeam radiation therapy. *Medical Physics* 36 (11) (Nov): 4897-902.

Raizer, J. 2011. Issues in developing drugs for primary brain tumors: Barriers and toxicities. *Toxicologic Pathology* 39 (1): 152-7.

Regnard, P., G. Le Duc, E. Brauer-Krisch, I. Tropres, E. A. Siegbahn, A. Kusak, C. Clair, et al. 2008. Irradiation of intracerebral 9L gliosarcoma by a single array of microplanar x-ray beams from a synchrotron: Balance between curing and sparing. *Physics in Medicine and Biology* 53 (4) (Feb 21): 861-78.

Reifenberger, G., and P. Wesseling. 2010. Molecular diagnostics of brain tumors. *Acta Neuropathologica* 120 (5) (Nov): 549-51.

Serduc, R., A. Bouchet, E. Brauer-Krisch, J. A. Laissue, J. Spiga, S. Sarun, A. Bravin, et al. 2009. Synchrotron microbeam radiation therapy for rat brain tumor palliation-influence of the microbeam width at constant valley dose. *Physics in Medicine and Biology* 54 (21) (Nov 7): 6711-24.

Sheleg, S. V., E. A. Korotkevich, E. A. Zhavrid, G. V. Muravskaya, A. F. Smeyanovich, Y. G. Shanko, T. L. Yurkshtovich, P. B. Bychkovsky, and S. A. Belyaev. 2002. Local chemotherapy with cisplatin-depot for glioblastoma multiforme. *Journal of Neuro-Oncology* 60 (1) (Oct): 53-9.

Steiner, G., A. Shaw, L. P. Choo-Smith, M. H. Abuid, G. Schackert, S. Sobottka, W. Steller, R. Salzer, and H. H. Mantsch. 2003. Distinguishing and grading human gliomas by IR spectroscopy. *Biopolymers* 72 (6): 464-71.

Tanaka, G., Y. Nakazato, T. Irie, T. Okada, and M. Abe. 2011. Indeterminacy in the WHO classification of tumors: An example of the histopathological diagnosis of brain tumors. *Brain Tumor Pathology* (Mar 11)[Epub ahead of print].

Tenzel, W. V. 1952. Experience with grid therapy. *Radiology* 59 (3) (Sep): 399-408.

Tobin, M. J., M. A. Chesters, J. M. Chalmers, F. J. Rutten, S. E. Fisher, I. M. Symonds, A. Hitchcock, R. Allibone, and S. Dias-Gunasekara. 2004. Infrared microscopy of epithelial cancer cells in whole tissues and in tissue culture, using synchrotron radiation. *Faraday Discussions* 126 : 27-39.

Valle-Folgueral, J. M., L. Mascarenhas, J. A. Costa, F. Vieira, J. Soares-Fernandes, P. Beleza, and C. Alegria. 2008. Giant cell glioblastoma: Review of the literature and illustrated case. *Neurocirugia (Asturias, Spain)* 19 (4) (Aug): 343-9.

Walker, C., D. G. du Plessis, K. A. Joyce, Y. Machell, J. Thomson-Hehir, S. A. Al Haddad, J. C. Broome, and P. C. Warnke. 2003. Phenotype versus genotype in gliomas displaying inter- or intratumoral histological heterogeneity. *Clinical Cancer Research*

:An Official Journal of the American Association for Cancer Research 9 (13) (Oct 15): 4841-51.

Wieczorek, T., and J. A. Longtine. 2010. The role of molecular probes and other markers in the diagnosis of malignancy. atlas of diagnostic oncology. In , eds. A. T. Skarin, G. P. Canellos. 4th ed., 1-5Mosby Elsevier Publishers.

Wiltshire, R. N., B. K. Rasheed, H. S. Friedman, A. H. Friedman, and S. H. Bigner. 2000. Comparative genetic patterns of glioblastoma multiforme: Potential diagnostic tool for tumor classification. *Neuro-Oncology* 2 (3) (Jul): 164-73.

Wysokinski, T. W., D. Chapman, G. Adams, M. Renier, P. Suortti, and W. Thomlinson. 2007. Beamlines of the biomedical imaging and therapy facility at the canadian light source--part 1. *Nuclear Instruments and Methods in Physics Research Section A: Accelerators, Spectrometers, Detectors and Associated Equipment* 582 (1): 73-6.

Zuber, M. A., W. Krupp, H. Holland, and U. G. Froster. 2002. Characterization of chromosomal aberrations in a case of glioblastoma multiforme combining cytogenetic and molecular cytogenetic techniques. *Cancer Genetics and Cytogenetics* 138 (2) (Oct 15): 111-5.

Part 2

Neurosurgical Approaches for Treating Brain Tumors

19

Anesthetic Considerations of Brain Tumor Surgery

Hala Goma
Cairo University
Egypt

1. Introduction

Anesthesia has a great responsibility in brain tumor surgery; it may be in some times the longest role in brain tumor team. Preparative role in form of preparation of the patient, intraoperative management, post operative care. The great price and challenge when the patient is systemically and neuro surgically stable, and leaving the hospital happy.

2. Mortality risk for elective brain tumor surgery

2.1 Impairment of general health by disease, or requiring surgery.

2.2 Ischemic heart disease.

2.3 Chronic lower Respiratory tract Infection.

2.4 Cardiac failure.

2.5 Obesity Impaired renal function.

2.6 Diabetes.

3. Preoperative evaluation

3.1 Aim of preoperative evaluation

To obtain pertinent information about the patient's medical history and physical and mental Conditions, in order to determine which tests and consultations are needed.
Guided by patient choices and the risk factors uncovered by the medical history, to choose the care plans to be followed.
To obtain informed consent.
To educate the patient about anesthesia, perioperative care, and pain treatments in the hope of reducing anxiety and facilitating recovery.
To make perioperative care more efficient and less expensive.
To utilize the operative experience to motivate the patient to more optimal health and thereby improve perioperative and/or long-term outcome.

3.2 Table 1. Medical problems discovered on pre anesthetic evaluation that could prompt a change in patient management

History Point	Concern/Area to Evaluate	Anesthesia Plans That May Require Extra Time
Airway perceived	Head, eyes, ears, nose, throat,	Obtain fiber optic equipment; obtain skilled
as difficult to intubate .	airway; prior anesthesia outcomes.	Help.
Asthma	Pulmonary disease	Optimize therapy; use bronchodilators; possibly extubate during deep anesthesia.
Diabetes, insulin dependent .-	Endocrine, metabolic, diabetes	Discuss insulin management with patient and primary care doctor; monitor blood glucose intra operatively; determine presence of autonomic neuropathy and plan management appropriately, such as administration of metoclopramide and PACU or ICU stay.
Drug abuse	Social history	Consider HIV testing; prescribe medications to avoid withdrawal symptoms in perioperative period.
Gastroesophageal	Gastrointestinal disease: hiatus	Administer H2 antagonists or oral antacids and
reflux or hiatus hernia.	Hernia.	use rapid-sequence induction of anesthesia; or use awake intubation techniques and obtain appropriate equipment .
Heart disease:	Antibiotic prophylaxis.	Arrange for antibiotic administration 1 h prior
valve disease,		to surgery.

History Point	Concern/Area to Evaluate	Anesthesia Plans That May Require Extra Time
risk of subacute bacterial Endocarditis.		
Malignant hyperthermia history, family history, or suspected potential history	Prior anesthetic/surgical history	Obtain clean anesthesia machine; use appropriate technique and precautions; have agents to treat malignant hyperthermia available.
Monoamine oxidase inhibitors.	CNS: psychiatric/medication	Discontinue therapy preoperatively if patient is not suicidal; plan for perioperative pain therapy.
Pacemaker or automatic implantable cardiac defibrillator.	Cardiovascular disease: Electrocardiogram.	Evaluate cause of pacemaker implementation; obtain repolarizing equipment or magnet; use electrocautery with altered position; use bipolar electrocautery .
Peripheral motor Neuropathy.	CNS disease: neurologic deficit	Avoid depolarizing muscle relaxants.
Pregnancy or uncertain Pregnancy status.	Genitourinary: pregnancy	Monitor fetal heart rate; use oral antacids; adjust induction of anesthesia; determine status of pregnancy.
Pulmonary Tuberculosis.	Pulmonary disease: Tuberculosis.	Use disposable breathing circuit or clean equipment; ensure adequate treatment of pulmonary TB.

3.3 Physical examination

Determination of arterial blood pressure in both arms, and in at least one arm 2 minutes after the patient assumes the upright position after lying down. (Third and fourth heart sounds).

Examination of the carotid and jugular pulses.

Examination of the chest and auscultation of the bases of the heart for subtle rales suggestive of congestive heart failure, or for rhonchi, wheezes, and other sounds indicative of lung disease. (Although history-taking may detect these symptoms that point to lung disease as accurately as auscultation.

Observation of the patient's walk for signs of neurologic disease and to assess back mobility and general health.

Examination of the eyes for abnormal movement and, along with the skin, for signs of jaundice, cyanosis, nutritional abnormalities, and dehydration.

The fingers are checked for clubbing.

Examination of the airway and mouth for neck mobility, tongue size, oral lesions, and ease of intubation.

Examination of the legs for bruising, edema, clubbing, mobility, sensation.

3.4 Preoperative surgical evaluation

The level of consciousness, neurological deficits and occurrence of seizures need to be noted. The existence of intracranial space occupation and raised ICP (persistent headache, vomiting, papilloedema) must be evaluated.

Posterior fossa tumors may cause bulbar palsy and the lower cranial nerves should be examined for impairment of swallowing or laryngeal palsy. A history of repeated aspiration of stomach contents, perhaps with nocturnal bronchospasm, reveals laryngeal incompetence.

The assessment of supratentorial lesions is made considerably easier by the improvement in imaging techniques, CT scanning and MRI. These allow early, precise location of lesions and give some idea of the probable histological diagnosis. The scans should be examined to give information on:

- Size of mass;
- Ventricular distortion or CSF obstruction;
- Midline shift;
- Amount of edema;
- Degree of contrast enhancement;
- Proximity to venous sinus.
    - The size of the mass depends partly on whether the tumor is developing in a silent or an eloquent area of the brain. Tumors in a silent area may grow so large before they present that they cause a very considerable compromise of intracranial dynamics.
    - Assessment of the degree of intracranial space occupation is important; if there is more than 10 mm shift of the midline structures, for example, volatile agents should be used with care. The amount of edema may turn a relatively small lesion into a more serious problem.
    - The degree of enhancement with intravenous radiographic contrast shows the degree of abnormal or damaged. Blood-brain barrier (BBB) in the lesion and it is through this damaged BBB that the contrast penetrated to the stroma of the tumor.

- A vascular tumor may have a low vascular resistance and frequently in angiography cerebral veins draining the tumor fill early, during the arterial or capillary phases of the angiogram, reflecting the fast flow. Such a tumor, especially if it is near one of theVenous sinuses, has the potential for causing major blood loss as resection is undertaken.
- The increasing availability of metabolic imaging such as PET, MR spectroscopy and single photon emission tomography (using thallium-201 which is specifically taken up by tumor cells but not by necrotic areas) will offer more precise information on the size and location of the tumor. Patients suspected of having an astrocytoma should undergo stereotactic biopsy prior to craniotomy to confirm the histological diagnosis.

3.5 Preoperative investigation

- **Electrocardiogram (ECG).**

ECG Abnormality.

T wave ,ST segment ,Arrhythmias ,SVT or PVC ,PAC ,QRS ,Q wave.

Ventricular conduction defects AV block ,AV, atrioventricular; ECG, electrocardiogram; LVH, Left ventricular hypertrophy; PAC, premature atrial contractions; PVC, premature ventricular contractions; SVT, supraventricular tachycardia.

- **Chest Radiographs.**

Tracheal deviation or compression; mediastinal masses; pulmonary nodules; a solitary lung mass; aortic aneurysm; pulmonary edema; pneumonia; atelectasis; new fractures of the vertebrae, ribs, and clavicles; dextrocardia; and cardiomegaly. However, a chest radiograph probably would not detect the degree of chronic lung disease requiring a change in anesthetic technique any better than would the history or physical examination.

- **Echocardiography is indicated in ischemic, valvular ,and pronged hypertension and diabetes.**
  - *Labaratory investigation:*

Hemoglobin, Hematocrit, and White Blood Cell Counts.

Blood Chemistries, Urinalysis, and Clotting Studies,fasting blood glucose, renal, hepatic functions, BUN, hepatitis markers for A and C for medico legal risk posed by post anesthetic ,jaundice .

- **Preparation of blood transfusion:**

A large meningioma can be associated with heavy blood loss but for most craniotomies 2–4 units of blood are sufficient.

3.6 Preoperative medication

Normal medication, especially anticonvulsants and antihypertensive drugs, should be continued until just before surgery. Sedative premedication may be desirable in order to allay anxiety. Respiratory depression with subsequent hypercarbia should be avoided, especially in the presence of raised ICP. For this reason we avoid opiates and usually prescribe 10–20 mg of temazepam or 10–15 mg, diazepam, with 10 mg metoclopramide orally 90 min preoperatively.

4. Monitoring

4.1 Standard monitoring

Heart rate and rhythm (electrocardiogram), noninvasive and direct arterial blood pressure measurement, pulse oximetry, end-tidal CO_2, body temperature, urinary output, CVP, and neuromuscular blockade. Arterial blood gases, hematocrit, electrolytes, glucose, and serum osmolarity should be measured periodically.

4.2 Monitoring for air embolism

Detection of venous air embolism by Doppler ultrasound should be considered for surgical procedures in which veins in the operative site are above the level of the heart.

4.3 Brain monitoring

Electroencephalogram, evoked potentials, jugular venous bulb oxygen saturation (Sjo_2), flow velocity measured by transcranial Doppler (TCD), brain tissue Po_2 ($btPo_2$), and ICP may be used.

- The Sjo_2 provides continuous information about the balance between global cerebral oxygen supply and demand. A Sjo_2 of <50% for >15 minutes is a poor prognostic sign and is often associated with a poor neurologic outcome. The decrease in Sjo_2 could be caused by excessive hyperventilation, decreased CPP, cerebral vasospasm, or a combination.
- Flow velocity of basal cerebral arteries as measured by the TCD technique is helpful in assessing the cerebral circulatory state at the bedside. However, it does not provide an absolute value for the CBF.
- Near-infrared spectroscopy, currently available in clinical practice, provides relative information about changes of oxy- and deoxyhemoglobin and the cytochrome oxidase redox status in the brain tissue of interest in a noninvasive and continuous fashion.
- ICP the association between severity of ICP elevation and poor outcome is well known. Monitoring ICP is useful, therefore, not only as a guide to therapy, but also for assessing.

5. Intraoperative management

The major goals of anesthetic management are to (a) optimize cerebral perfusion and oxygenation, (b)) provide adequate surgical conditions for the neurosurgeons with a slack brain and low intracranial pressure (ICP). When a patient has an intracranial space-occupying lesion (SOL), the achievement of a low ICP during surgery demands a careful choice of the most appropriate anesthetic and an attention to detail. A badly administered or inappropriate anaesthetic may add to the intracranial problems generated by the space occupation, increasing ICP. General anesthesia is recommended to facilitate control of respiratory and circulatory function.

5.1 Factors that influence cerebral blood flow

PaO2.

PaCO2.

Cerebral metabolic rate.

- Arousal/pain.
- Seizures.
- Temperature.
- Anesthetics.

Blood pressure/status of autoregulation.

- Vasoactive agents.

- Anesthetics.
- Pressors.
- Inotropes

5.2 The effects of anesthetics on intracranial and cerebral perfusion pressures

- Intravenous anesthetics:

Barbiturates. Thiopental and pentobarbital decrease CBF, cerebral blood volume (CBV), and ICP. The reduction in ICP with these drugs is related to the reduction in CBF and CBV coupled with metabolic depression. These drugs will also have these effects in patients who have impaired CO_2 response.

Etomidate. As with barbiturates, etomidate reduces CBF, $CMRo_2$, and ICP. Systemic hypotension occurs less frequently than with barbiturates. Prolonged use of etomidate may suppress the adrenocortical response to stress.

Propofol. The cerebral hemodynamic and metabolic effects of propofol are similar to those of barbiturates. Propofol might be useful in patients who have intracranial pathology if hypotension is avoided. Because the context-sensitive half-life is short, emergence from anesthesia is rapid, even after prolonged administration. This may offer an advantage over other intravenous anesthetics in providing the opportunity for early postoperative neurologic evaluation. Because of propofol's potent circulatory depressant effect, recent studies have shown a reduction in jugular bulb oxygen saturation during propofol anesthesia. Propofol can also reduce CBF more than $CMRo_2$, producing ischemia under certain conditions. Therefore, care should be taken when hyperventilating patients during propofol anesthesia.

Benzodiazepines. Diazepam and midazolam may be useful either for sedating patients or inducting anesthesia because these drugs have minimal hemodynamic effects and are less likely to impair cerebral circulation. Diazepam, 0.1 to 0.2 mg/kg, may be administered for inducting anesthesia and repeated, if necessary, up to a total dose of 0.3 to 0.6 mg/kg. Midazolam, 0.2 mg/kg, can be used for induction and repeated as necessary.

Narcotics.in clinical doses, narcotics produce a minimal to moderate decrease in CBF and $CMRo_2$. When ventilation is adequately maintained, narcotics probably have minimal effects on ICP. Despite its small ICP-elevating effect, fentanyl provides satisfactory analgesia and permits the use of lower concentrations of inhalational anesthetics. When these drugs are used, measures to maintain systemic blood pressure need to be implemented.

- Inhalational anesthetics:

Isoflurane has less effect on CBF and ICP than halothane has. Because isoflurane depresses cerebral metabolism, it may have a cerebral protective effect when the ischemic insult is not severe. Data favor the use of isoflurane over either halothane or enflurane. Isoflurane in concentrations of >1 minimum alveolar concentration should be avoided, however, because it can cause substantial increases in ICP.

Sevoflurane. Clinical studies have demonstrated, however, that sevoflurane's effect on cerebral hemodynamics is either similar to or milder than that of isoflurane. The disadvantage of sevoflurane is that its biodegraded metabolite may be toxic in high concentrations. There is no evidence of an adverse effect at clinically used concentrations, however, unless sevoflurane is administered in a low-flow circuit for prolonged periods. Rapid emergence from anesthesia with sevoflurane may be an advantage because it facilitates early postoperative neurologic evaluation.

Desflurane. Desflurane at high concentrations appears to increase ICP.
Nitrous oxide (N_2O). N_2O dilates cerebral vessels, thereby increasing ICP. Patients who have intracranial hypertension or a decrease in intracranial compliance should, therefore, not receive this drug.
Local anesthetic. The infiltration of either lidocaine 1% or bupivacaine 0.25%, with or without epinephrine, in the skin around the scalp incision and the insertion sites for the pin head holder is helpful in preventing systemic and intracranial hypertension in response to these stimuli and avoiding the unnecessary use of deep anesthesia.

- Muscle relaxants. Adequate muscle relaxation facilitates appropriate mechanical ventilation and reduces ICP. Coughing and straining are avoided because both can produce cerebral venous engorgement.

Vecuronium appears to have minimal or no effect on ICP, blood pressure, or heart rate and would be effective in patients with head injuries. This drug is given as an initial dose of 0.08 to 0.1 mg/kg followed by infusion at a rate of 1 to 1.7 mcg /kg /minute.
Pancuronium does not produce an increase in ICP but can cause hypertension and tachycardia because of its vagolytic effect, thereby increasing the patient's risk.
Atracurium has no effect on ICP. Because of its rapid onset and short duration of action, a bolus dose of 0.5 to 0.6 mg/kg followed by a continuous infusion at a rate of 4 to 10 mcg/kg/minute is administered with monitoring of neuromuscular blockade.
Rocuronium is useful for intubation because of its rapid onset of action and lack of effect on intracranial dynamics. For maintenance, drugs with longer durations of action are recommended.

5.3 Induction

- Adequate preoperative anxiolysis in the anesthetic room
- Electrocardiogram, capnometer, pulse oximeter, noninvasive blood pressure
- Venous, arterial lines: insert under LA
- Furosemide 1 mg/kg
- Preoxygenation.
- fentanyl, 1-2 mcg/kg, (alfentanil,,sufentanil,remifentanil),Propofol, 1.25-2.5 mg/kg, or thiopental, 3-6 mg/kg, then non depolarizing myo-relaxant
- Control ventilation ($Paco_2 \sim 35$ mm Hg)
- Intubation. The airway should be secured with an armoured endotracheal tube, taped on the contra lateral side to operation It may be desirable to secure the tube further using a throat pack. Careful taping is required to prevent both extubation and venous congestion.

5.4 Intraoperative respiratory management

5.5 Mechanical ventilation

Ventilation of the lungs is arranged so that there is a slow rate, with a long expiratory pause; PEEP is normally not applied. A naso gastric tube should be considered for long operations. Mechanical ventilation is adjusted to maintain a $Paco_2$ of around 35 mm Hg. The fraction of inspired oxygen (Fio_2) is adjusted to maintain a Pao_2 of >100 mm Hg.

5.6 Deliberate hypoventilation

Hypoventilation also increases cerebral blood flow and cerebral blood volume, which may impair surgical exposure. Until the benefits of hypoventilation are confirmed, mild hyperventilation is the more common practice.

5.7 Position

Operations may last several hours so the patient should be carefully positioned with bony points padded, eyes protected with tape or gel and care taken to ensure tubing is not pressed against the patient's skin. Patients may be positioned supine or slightly rotated, with one shoulder raised, or they may be placed in a lateral position. A head-up tilt of the table of about 15° is essential to aid cerebral venous drainage. Pinealomas may be approached with the patient either prone or sitting.
A urinary catheter is necessary to assess fluid status. The patient's head position on the operating table is fixed either on a horseshoe type head rest or by the insertion of skull pins. The application of the pins represents another stimulus causing an increase in blood pressure response, and great care should be taken to ensure that the patient is adequately anaesthetized before the pins are applied.

5.8 Maintenance of anesthesia

The ideal drug for maintenance of anesthesia should reduce ICP, maintain adequate oxygen supply to the brain tissue, and protect the brain against ischemic-metabolic insult. The selection of anesthetic drugs is based on a consideration of the intracranial pathology as well as systemic conditions such as cardiopulmonary disturbances.
There are different regimens can be used,
Isoflurane 1-2% versus sevoflurane 0.5-1.5%- fentanyl 150 mcg/kg/min, or desflurane 3-"6%, propofol infusion- fentanyl, propofol - remifentanil infusion, alfentanil, and sufentanil. Neuromuscular blockade maintained using peripheral nerve stimulation.

5.9 Intraoperative hemodynamic management

CPP (cerebral perfusion pressure) should be maintained between 60 and 110 mm Hg. The transducer for direct monitoring of arterial blood pressure is zeroed at the level of mastoids to reflect the cerebral circulation.

5.10 Intravenous fluids

Intravenous fluids should be chosen with care; over transfusion will lead to a high CVP and therefore predispose to high ICP and use of solutions of glucose in water worsen cerebral edema. Patients with severe intracranial hypertension may have been drowsy or vomiting preoperatively and therefore may be hypovolemic. If mannitol has been used, fluids should be given to replace the deficit produced by diuresis. Mannitol may also produce hyponatraemia and hypokalaemia. Normal saline or Hartmann's solution is indicated for fluid therapy during the procedure and should be given to replace fluid losses and controlled by the CVP to avoid over transfusion. Colloid solutions, such as modified gelatin (Gelofusine), may be given and blood loss over 1 liter should be replaced as appropriate.

5.11 Intra operative blood loss

Vascular tumors (notably meningiomas) can be associated with very fast blood loss and if the tumor is on the convexity of a cerebral hemisphere, the blood loss may occur during the cutting of the bone flap, when the surgeon may not be in a position to stop the bleeding. The anesthetist thus needs to have everything needed for rapid transfusion ready at the start of a craniotomy for a vascular tumor. Cross matched blood needs to be in the theatre suite and there must be a large-bore venous cannula in place, together with arterial and CVP measurement. A blood warmer needs to be set up and acid-base estimations available quickly. Further significant and persistent blood loss may occur during the subsequent resection of a meningioma, so it is important that the initial blood loss is replaced. The cerebral vasoconstriction that occurs with hemorrhage reduces CBF significantly, especially in the junctional areas between the major cerebral vessels.

5.12 Management intraoperative hypotension

Adequate oxygenation, ventilation, and fluid replacement, careful elevation of the blood pressure with a continuous infusion of an inotrope or vasopressor may be necessary. Phenylephrine, 0.1 to 0.5 mcg/kg/minute, and dopamine, 1 to 10 mcg /kg/minute, are appropriate drugs in this setting. A bolus dose of vasopressor must be used cautiously because abrupt increases in blood pressure can elevate ICP to dangerous levels, especially in patients who have disordered auto regulation. Balance between maintenance of CPP to areas of brain rendered ischemic due to compression by hematoma, and the risk of more vasogenic brain edema or bleeding. Jugular venous bulb oxygen saturation monitoring may help assess adequacy of global.

5.13 Management intraoperative hypertension

Hypertension is treated cautiously because the elevation in blood pressure may reflect compensatory hyperactivity of the sympathetic nervous system in response to elevated ICP and compression of the brain stem (Cushing's reflex). Adequate oxygenation, ventilation, volume replacement, and analgesia should be first assessed and corrected. (i.e., opioids) and/or depth of anesthesia (propofol, barbiturates, etomidate) before an antihypertensive drug, such as either labetalol or esmolol, which has minimal cerebral vasodilating effects, should be administered. When treating hypertension, maintenance of CPP is a major concern.

5.14 Induced hypotension

Hypotension to a MAP of 60-70 mmHg, which will provide a surgical field with reduced oozing, Before hypotension is used, the patient's physical state should be carefully assessed, particularly looking for signs of ischemia in the cerebral or coronary circulations or a history of hypertension. Hypotension should not normally be applied until the dura is open, and the length of hypotension should be kept as short as possible. Hypovolemia should not be allowed to coexist with induced hypotension; blood replacement must parallel blood loss. CBF is maintained constant as long as the MAP is between 60 and 160 mmHg, may be of value.

Monitoring must be extensive and reliable; as well as the monitoring mentioned, jugular venous oxygen content measurements are valuable, as are transcranial Doppler measurements of flow velocity. The use of propofol infusion with opioid analgesics and moderate hyperventilation provides a satisfactory surgical field for most neurosurgical operations but occasionally the resection of a large vascular tumor may still require hypotension. Hypotension is most easily induced by the combination of labetalol (10-20 mg) followed by sodium nitroprusside infusion (0.01%). The infusion is best given along the central venous line, so that the time lag between changing the infusion rate and observing the effect on blood pressure is kept to a minimum.

Sodium nitroprusside causes cerebral vasodilatation but the effect can be overcome by ensuring that the arterial pressure is lowered to at least 70% of the control value. If the anesthetic has been so arranged that the patient's cardiovascular system is stable and not responding to painful stimuli, hypotension should be easily achieved with such small doses of propofol that toxicity is not invoked. If the patient develops a tachycardia or is resistant to sodium nitroprusside, it is better to supplement the action of sodium nitroprusside by another drug, such as labetalol or propranolol to control heart rate, or to increase the infusion of propofol or the inhaled concentration of isoflurane, rather than using excessive infusion rates of sodium nitroprusside. Other hypotensive agents are available, such as trimetaphan and trinitroglycerine (GTN). GTN, like sodium nitroprusside, causes an increase in ICP and also a marked tachycardia. Trimetaphan is a less effective drug than either but does not because a rise in ICP, unless the patient is suffering from extreme degrees of intracranial space occupation, in which case the ganglionic blockade may produce an increase in CBF by blocking the sympathetic supply to the cerebral vessels. When induced hypotension is being used, it is important that the surgeon knows this and that, after the tumor is resected, blood pressure is returned to normal before the dura is closed. This is essential so that the bleeding points can be visualized and sealed.

6. Tight brain (increased intracranial tension ICT)

6.1 Prevention

Preoperative: adequate anxiolysis and analgesia.
Pre induction: hyperventilate on demand, head-up position; head straight, no jugular vein compression.
Avoid over hydration.
Osmotic diuretics, as (mannitol, hypertonic saline); and steroids.
Loop diuretics (furosemide).
Optimize hemodynamics: MAP, central venous pressure, pulmonary capillary wedge pressure, and heart rate; use beta-blockers, clonidine, or lidocaine if necessary.
Ventilation: Pao_2 >100; $Paco_2$ ~ 35 mm Hg, low intra thoracic pressure.
Induction, and maintenance by use of intravenous anesthetics.

6.2 Treatment

Cerebrospinal fluid drainage (lumbar catheter or ventricle)
Osmotic diuretics.
Hyperventilation.
Augment depth of anesthesia using intravenous anesthetics (propofol, thiopental, etomidate) .
Muscle relaxation.
Improve cerebral venous drainage: head up, no positive end-expiratory pressure, reduce inspiratory time.
Mild controlled hypertension, if cerebral autoregulation intact (MAP ~ 100 mm).

7. Emergence from general anesthesia

The closure of a craniotomy may take a little time. Following surgery for a space-occupying lesion, some postoperative brains welling is likely and great care should be taken to ensure that the end of the anesthetic is smooth, without undue hypertension, coughing or straining.

- Much movement of the head may take place then and the patient should not cough or strain. Normally, however, During the closure period, the propofol and relaxant infusions can be reduced, the aim being to ensure that the patient is awake at the end of the procedure, but reversal of the muscle relaxant must be left until after any dressings or head bandages have been applied.
- Avoiding of coughing and straining is essential. In order to avoid hypertension on extubation, removal of the endotracheal tube and suctioning of the pharynx may be covered with IV lignocaine 1.5 mg/kg 90 s before extubation. Labetalol can also be given to obtund these responses.
- Anesthetic technique should be so judged as to produce an awake, responding patient in the recovery area, so that neurological monitoring to detect the postoperative complications of hematoma formation may be started. 20% of elective craniotomy patients develop raised ICP in the early postoperative period. Systemic hypertension is frequent and has been associated with an increased risk of postoperative intracranial hemorrhage.
- Oxygen consumption is increased (up to 5 times) by re warming (shivering/ non shivering thermo genesis) and pain.
- Remifentanil can be used to control blood pressure during emergence of anesthesia after craniotomy for brain tumors. It has higher rapid recovery score than esmolol and other narcotics. In addition, it can be used when esmolol is contraindicated such as in cardiac patients, asthmatics, chronic obstructive pulmonary disease, or during pregnancy. Also, it decreases the need for postoperative analgesia and allows sedation if the infusion is continued as surgical patients are admitted to the ICU

7.1 Indications of postoperative intensive care unit after brain tumor surgery

1. Patients in whom a tight brain was present during surgery.
2. Excessive blood loss.
3. Edema spread is marked should be considered for postoperative pressure ventilation in an intensive care unit.
4. Obtunded consciousness
5. Inadequate airway control preoperatively;
6. Intraoperative catastrophe
7. Deranged intra cerebral hemo- or homeostasis postoperatively.
8. Long operation (>6 hours).
9. Repeated surgery,
10. Surgery involving or close to vital brain areas.
11. Surgery associated with significant brain ischemia (e.g., long vascular clipping times, extensive retractor pressure).

7.2 Differential diagnosis of unplanned delayed emergence

After 10 to 20 minutes of cessation of pharmacologically adequate anesthesia with short-acting agents, the patient should be awake enough to obey simple verbal commands.

1. Opioid overhang (fentanyl or sufentanil): try carefully titrated antagonization with small doses of naloxone or naltrexone
2. Nonanesthetic causes (seizure, cerebral edema, intracranial hematoma, pneumocephalus, vessel occlusion/ischemia, metabolic or electrolyte disturbances).

8. Specific anesthetic considerations

8.1 Posterior fossa tumors

8.2 Positioning

- **Prone postion:**

This position offers good access to midline structures but bleeding can obscure the surgical field. Head-up tilt is employed to reduce hemorrhage but this increases the risk of air embolism. The head is fixed in clamps in preference to a horseshoe in order to minimize pressure on the face and eyes.

- **Lateral position:**

This is suitable for approaches to lesions not in the midline, particularly the cerebellopontine angle. A pad should be placed under the body in the axilla to minimize weight on the lower arm and shoulder.

- **Sitting position:**

This was widely used for posterior fossa surgery in the past.

Advantages of sitting position:

It provides good surgical access to midline structures,
Improves surgical orientation
It allows good Drains of blood, and CSF.

Complications of sitting position:

Cord compression.
Pneumocephalus. Following a craniotomy, an air-filled space between the dura ,and arachnoids remains after CSF has leaked away during surgery ,and brain bulk is reduced. In the recovery period brain bulk increases again as cerebral edema develops, arterial carbon dioxide concentrations increase and CSF re accumulates. The trapped air then comes under increasing pressure. N2O will worsen the situation. Pneumocephalus presents as delayed recovery or deteriorating neurological state and should always be considered if this occurs. Pneumocephalus can be reduced by discontinuing nitrous oxide 15 minutes before surgery finishes and by allowing the PaCO2 to rise towards the end of surgery.

Venous air embolism.

The incidence of VAE during posterior fossa procedures in the sitting position is 40% to 45%. For seated cervical laminectomy or surgery in the prone or lateral positions, VAE occurs in approximately 10% to 15% of cases.
VAE can occur whenever pressure within an open vessel is sub atmospheric. Clinically significant VAE is unusual unless the surgical site is >20 cm above the level of the heart.
When open vessels cannot collapse, which is the case with major venous sinuses as well as bridging and epidural veins, the risk of VAE increases substantially.
Massive air embolism produces abrupt and catastrophic hemodynamic changes. Fortunately, this type of VAE is rare.
More commonly, air entrainment occurs slowly over a longer period of time and may produce little or no respiratory or hemodynamic compromise.

8.3 Monitoring for VAE

Hemodynamic changes. Monitoring of hemodynamics may not provide sufficient advanced warning in the case of massive air embolism because the hemodynamic changes are abrupt and catastrophic.

Doppler and $ETco_2$ monitoring are considered the acceptable minimum.
Precordial Doppler
This device can detect 1 mL of air or less, which makes it more sensitive than any other monitor except trans esophageal echocardiography (TEE). The Doppler is not quantitative, however, and it requires experience to recognize which of the various sounds it emits is indicative of air.
End-tidal gas monitoring VAE is associated with a decreasing $ETco_2$ and the presence of end-tidal nitrogen (ETn_2).
The CVP can help in positioning the Doppler. Also, the aspiration of air both confirms the diagnosis of VAE and serves as a treatment.
PA pressures rise with significant VAE, the PA catheter can be useful for both diagnosis and therapy.
Trans esophageal echocardiography (TEE) is more sensitive than Doppler ultrasound and is specific because the air bubbles are visualized directly.

8.4 Prevention of VAE

Positive end-expiratory pressure (PEEP)

- The use of PEEP to prevent VAE in the sitting position is controversial. High levels of PEEP (>10 cm H_2O) are needed to increase venous pressure at the head, and studies are inconsistent as to whether PEEP decreases the incidence of VAE. PEEP can, however, reduce venous return, cardiac output, and mean arterial blood pressure, which may be detrimental.

Volume loading

- Although hypovolemia has been proposed as a predisposing factor for VAE.
- Deliberate hypoventilation
    - While some studies suggest that moderate hypoventilation may reduce the risk of VAE, hypoventilation also increases cerebral blood flow and cerebral blood volume, which may impair surgical exposure.

9. Intraoperative anesthetic considerations of posterior fossa tumors

The conduct of anesthesia is similar to supratentorial surgery.
Muscle relaxation is best provided by continuous infusion (e.g. atracurium).This helps ventilation and prevents movement in a relatively lightly anesthetized patient. If motor nerve function is monitored, such as the facial nerve during acoustic neuroma surgery, muscle relaxation must be discontinued, and sufficient depth of anesthesia must be provided. A remifentanil infusion is ideal in this situation. Hypotensive techniques increase the risks of ischemic damage specially in sitting position, and when the head is up position.
Hemodynamic instability occurs if the brainstem is manipulated.
Bradycardia can occur when the peri ventricular grey matter and the reticular formation are stimulated. Most arrhythmias occur during surgery near the pons, and the roots of nerves V, IX and X.
Severe hypertension can result from stimulation of the trigeminal nerve.

9.1 Intraoperative brain stem monitoring

Monitoring techniques include somatosensory evoked potentials (SSEPs), brain stem auditory evoked potentials (BAEPs), and the spontaneous and evoked electromyogram (EMG). This monitoring can be a challenge for the anesthesiologist because muscle relaxants complicate interpretation of the EMG, and N_2O and high-dose inhalation anesthesia may interfere with SSEPs.

Extubation should be delayed if there are concerns of brainstem or cranial nerve injury.

10. Post operative special considerations after posterior fossa surgery

10.1 Ventilation/airway abnormalities

Because of disease- or surgery-induced dysfunction of cranial sensory or motor nerves, patients may have difficulty swallowing, vocalizing, or protecting the airway. In addition, damage to or edema of the respiratory centers from intraoperative manipulation can result in hypoventilation or erratic respiratory patterns. Therefore, longer-term ventilation and airway protection might be required in some patients.

Severe tongue and facial edema can occur owing to position-induced venous or lymphatic obstruction. The endotracheal tube should be left in place until the edema resolves.

Pulmonary edema may result from large VAE. Although pulmonary edema is usually responsive to conservative measures such as supplemental oxygen (O_2) and diuretics, continued postoperative ventilation may be appropriate until evaluation is completed.

10.2 Cardiovascular complications

Hypertension is common after posterior fossa surgery and may contribute to edema formation and intracranial hemorrhage. Hence, one should be prepared to control postoperative hypertension.

10.3 Neurologic complications

A variety of untoward neurologic complications can occur after posterior fossa operations. These include altered levels of consciousness, varying degrees of paresis, and specific cranial nerve deficits (e.g., visual disturbances, facial nerve paresis, impaired swallowing or phonation).

Treatment is supportive, but evaluation of delayed emergence should proceed lest a treatable non anesthetic cause go unrecognized. If cerebral paradoxical air embolism is suspected, hyperbaric oxygen therapy may be warranted.

Extreme neck flexion can cause mid cervical quadriplegia.

Peripheral nerve damage can result from faulty positioning. The brachial plexus, ulnar nerve and common peroneal nerve are most vulnerable.

10.4 Pneumocephalus

Air is retained in the cranial cavity after all craniotomies regardless of position. When the patient is in the sitting position, cerebrospinal fluid drains easily, and a larger amount of air may be trapped when the wound is closed. In most cases, the air is reabsorbed uneventfully over several days ,and no treatment is necessary. There is little evidence that anesthetic technique influences either the incidence or the volume of pneumocephalus.

Tension pneumocephalus can occur when the brain re-expands and compresses the air. This situation is difficult to diagnose but should be suspected if emergence is delayed after an otherwise uneventful operation or if either cardiovascular collapse or neurologic deterioration occurs postoperatively. In such rare circumstances, surgical evacuation may be indicated

11. Trans sphenoidal hypophysectomy

The Trans sphenoidal approach to the pituitary is used for the excision of tumors that lie within the
Sella or that has extension to the immediate supra sellar area.

11.1 Preoperative evaluation

Secreting lesions:

Prolactin Galactorrhea, a Cushing's disease (hypercortisolim, centripetal obesity, Diabetes mellitus, friable tissues .Acromegaly/gigantism, glucose intolerance, thick skin (difficult cannulation).

Non Secreting lesions:

Suprasellar Nonsecretory Panhypopituitarism, patients will commonly receive adrenal hormone supplementation at least temporarily. However, profound hypocortisolism with associated hyponatremia should be corrected preoperatively.in fact uncommon for thyroid deficiency to occur. However, hypothyroidism should be sought and corrected preoperatively because hypothyroid patients have a diminished tolerance to the cardiovascular depressant effects of anesthetics. SIADH (syndrome of inappropriate antidiuretic hormone secretion), visual (optic chiasm) symptoms, Hydrocephalus may occur.

Monitoring:

Many practitioners place an arterial catheter, but it is not absolutely necessary. Access for blood sampling is a valuable adjunct to postoperative care if diabetes insipidus develops. Blood loss is usually modest.

11.2 Anesthetic technique

The procedure is performed in a supine position, usually with some degree of head-up posture to avoid venous engorgement.

A pharyngeal pack will prevent an accumulation of blood in the stomach (which causes vomiting) or in the glottis (which contributes to coughing at extubation).

A RAE-type tube secured to the lower jaw at the corner of the mouth opposite the surgeon's dominant hand (e.g., the left corner of the mouth for a right-handed surgeon) is suitable.

A small esophageal stethoscope and temperature probe can lie with the endotracheal tube. Covering the entire bundle with a towel drape (a plastic sheet with an adhesive edge) placed just below the lower lip so that it hangs from the lower jaw like a veil will protect it from the preparation solutions.

The procedure requires a C-arm image intensifier (lateral views), and the head and arms are relatively inaccessible once the patient is draped. It is appropriate to establish the nerve stimulator at a lower extremity site.

The surgical approach is through the nasal cavity by means of an incision made under the upper lip. During the approach, the mucosal surfaces within the nose are infiltrated with a local anesthetic and epinephrine solution, and the patient should be observed for the occurrence of dysrhythmias.

Surgical preferences for CO2 management will vary. In some instances, hypocapania will be requested to reduce brain volume and thereby minimize the degree to which the arachnoid bulges into the sella.

Avoidance, when possible, of opening the arachnoid membrane. Postoperative CSF leaks can be persistent and are associated with a considerable risk of meningitis.

By contrast, in tumors with suprasellar extension, normal or increased CO2 will help deliver the lesion into the sella for excision. As an alternative method, some surgeons have resorted to "pumping" saline or air into the lumbar CSF space.

DI (Diabetes insipidus) usually develops 4 to 12 hours postoperatively and very rarely arises intraoperatively. The clinical picture is one of polyuria in association with a rising serum osmolality. The diagnosis is made by comparison of the osmolality of urine and serum. Hypoosmolar urine in the face of an elevated and rising serum osmolality strongly supports the diagnosis. Desmopressin (DDAVP) is usually administered. In general, the patient is losing fluid that is hypoosmolar and relatively low in sodium. Half-normal saline and 5% dextrose in water (D5 W) are commonly used as replacement fluids.

12. Awake craniotomy

Awake craniotomies are performed when tumors or epileptic foci lie close to the cortical areas required for either speech or motor function or close to the mesial temporal structures critical to short-term memory.

12.1 Pr anesthetic Evaluation/Preparation

At the preoperative interview, the patient should be educated about the nature and duration of the procedure and the limitations on movement. One should obtain a description of both the aura and the seizures to facilitate recognition of them. One should a scertain whether the patient is subject to grandmal convulsions.

If intraoperative electrocorticography to identify seizure foci is intended, it is common to discontinue or reduce the anticonvulsant dose by half according to the perceived risk of uncontrolled seizures.

Premedication drugs with an anticonvulsant effect, such as the benzodiazepines, should not be used because they may interfere with intraoperative EEG localization

12.2 The objectives of the anesthetic technique are to

Minimize patient discomfort associated with the potentially painful portions of the procedure, and with the prolonged restriction of movement.

Ensure patient responsiveness and compliance during the phases of the procedure that require assessment of either speech or motor/sensory responses to cortical stimulation.

Select anesthetic techniques that produce minimal inhibition of spontaneous seizure activity.

There are probably many ways of providing sedation that are consistent with the mentioned objectives, and many techniques are in active use. They range from minimal sedation approaches, through deep sedation during which intermittent unresponsiveness is achieved with spontaneous ventilation and an unprotected airway, to asleep-awake-asleep techniques with intermittent airway management with an LMA(laryngeal mask air way), sometimes with positive-pressure ventilation.

12.3 Anesthetic techniques

An awake craniotomy is the surgeon's local anesthetic technique. "Sedation" cannot compensate for inadequate anesthesia of the scalp, as accomplished with pin site infiltration and nerve blocks.

Typically, this procedure is performed as (a monitored anesthesia care) "MAC," although small doses of induction anesthetic, most often propofol, are usually required at the time of stimulation of the periosteum at the base of the skull by the needle.

After placement of the relevant electrodes, the patient's seizure medication is discontinued and the patient remains in an observation unit with EEG and patient behavior recorded continuously. In this manner, the EEG events associated with the clinically significant seizure events and their anatomic origin can be identified.

Several centers have used a droperidol/synthetic narcotic combination (e.g., droperidol, 2.5 to 7.5 mg; alfentanil, 5- to 10-mg/kg load, 0.5- to 1.0-mg/kg/min infusion; Fentanyl, 0.7-mg/kg load, 0.7- mg/kg/hr infusion).

Others use principally propofol by either physician- or patient-controlled infusion.

Care should be taken when administering additional sedative agents, especially narcotics, whose respiratory depressant effects might be synergistic with propofol. This consideration is especially relevant when pin fixation is used. Pin fixation severely restricts the Anesthesiologist's capacity to intervene quickly in the event of excessive respiratory depression or loss of patency of the airway.

Propofol, if used, should be discontinued at least 15 minutes before EEG recording. In spite of prompt awakening, propofol leaves a residual EEG "footprint" characterized by high-frequency, high-amplitude beta activity that can obscure the abnormal activity that is being sought in the cortical surface EEG. Various groups have reported use of the LMA, commonly with narcotic-propofol sedation and spontaneous ventilation during the craniotomy; administration of the sedative is discontinued and the LMA is removed once the brain surface is exposed.

Infusion of remifentanil and propofol and positive-pressure ventilation.

More recently, the α2 -agonist dexmedetomidine at low dose (0.1 to 0.3 mg/kg/hr) has been used by some, both with and without intermittent use of the LMA.

12.4 Monitoring during awake craniotomy

Routine, noninvasive monitors are almost always sufficient. Reliable capnography to provide breath by-breath confirmation of airway patency and respiratory drive is an essential component of the technique if deep sedation is intended for any portion of the procedure. These procedures are often lengthy, and attention to the details of patient comfort (warming blankets, a sheepskin, and room temperature) will improve patient tolerance.

13. References

[1] Nicolas J. Bruder ,Patrick A. Ravussin.Anesthesia for Supratentorial Tumors, Handbook of Neuroanesthesia, 4th Edition, 2007 Lippincott Williams & Wilkins.

[2] Patterson JT, Hanbali F, Franklin RL, Nauta HJW. Neurosurgey. In: Townsend CM, Beauchamp RD, Evers BM, Mattox KL, eds. *Sabiston Textbook of Surgery.* 18th ed. Philadelphia, Pa: Saunders Elsevier; 2007:chap 72.

[3] Michael F. Roizen; Preoperative Evaluation ,: Miller's Anesthesia, 6th ed., Copyright © 2005 ELSEVIER CHURCHILL LIVINGSTONE.

[4] John C. Drummond,Piyush M. Patel Neurosurgical Anesthesia Miller's Anesthesia, 6th ed., Copyright © 2005 ELSEVIER CHURCHILL LIVINGSTONE.

[5] Richard A, Girard F, Girard DC, et al. Cisatracurium-induced neuromuscular blockade is affected by chronic phenytoin or carbamazepine treatment in neurosurgical patients. Anesth Analg 2005;100:538â€"544.

[6] Petersen KD, Landsfeldt L, Cold GE, et al: Intracranial pressure and cerebral hemodynamics in patients with cerebral tumors: A randomized prospective study of patients subjected to craniotomy in propofol-fentanyl, isoflurane-fentanyl, or sevoflurane-fentanyl anesthesia. Anesthesiology 98:329, 2003.

[7] Hernandez-Palazon J, Martinez-Lage JF, Rosa-Carrillo VN, et al: Anesthetic technique and development of pneumocephalus after posterior fossa surgery in the sitting position. Neurocirurgia 14:216, 2003.

[8] Kaisti KK, Langsjo JW, Aalto S, et al. Effects of sevoflurane, propofol, and adjunct nitrous oxide on regional cerebral blood flow, oxygen consumption, and blood volume in humans. Anesthesiology 2003;99:603-613.

[9] Goma HM, Ali MZ Control of emergence hypertension after craniotomy for brain tumor surgery. Neurosciences (Riyadh). 2009 Apr;14(2):167-71.

[10] Yoshimitsu K, Suzuki T, Muragaki Y, Chernov MIseki H. Development of modified Intraoperative Examination Monitor for Awake Surgery (IEMAS) system for awake craniotomy during brain tumor resection. Conf Proc IEEE Eng Med Biol Soc. 2010;1:6050-3.

[11] Tsuruta S, Yamada M, Shimizu T, Satsumae T, Tanaka M, Mizutani T. Airway management using i-gel in two patients for awake craniotomy. Masui. 2010 Nov;59(11):1411-4.

[12] Andersen JH, Olsen KS .Anaesthesia for awake craniotomy is safe and well-tolerated. Dan Med Bull. 2010 Oct;57(10):A4194.

[13] Wu CT, Chen LC, Kuo CP, Ju DT, Borel CO, Cherng CH, Wong CS.A comparison of 3% hypertonic saline and mannitol for brain relaxation during elective supratentorial brain tumor surgery. Anesth Analg. 2010 Mar 1;110(3): 903-7.

[14] Sharma D, Ellenbogen RG, Vavilala MSUse of transcranial Doppler ultrasonography and jugular oximetry to optimize hemodynamics during pediatric posterior fossa craniotomy. J Clin Neurosci. 2010 Dec;17(12):1583-4. Epub 2010 Aug 25.

[15] Kassebaum N, Hairr J, Goldsmith W, Barwise J, Pandharipande PDiabetes insipidus associated with propofol anesthesia. . Clin Anesth. 2008 Sep;20(6):466-8.

20

Strategies in Glioma-Surgery

Sven R. Kantelhardt and Alf Giese
Dept. of Neurosurgery, Johannes-Gutenberg-University Mainz
Germany

1. Introduction

1.1 Epidemiology and classification of gliomas

Malignant glioma is one of the most feared diseases in the industrialized nations. About 77% of all malignant tumors within the central nervous system are gliomas. There are about 18.000 newly diagnosed cases annually within the USA (9/100.000 inhabitants per year) and the disease causes about 13.000 deaths each year. Statistically this is a higher loss of life-time than all other tumor-entities together (Schwartzbaum et al., 2006).

About 45-50% of these gliomas are histologically classified as gliobalstoma multiforme (GBM) the most aggressive type of glioma which is classified as WHO grade IV (following the classification of Kleihues et al., 2000). 20-30% are so called anaplastic astrocytoma and the rarer anaplastic oligodendroglioma (WHO grade III), while about 16-8% are classified as low-grade gliomas (WHO grade I and II). Generally they show a less aggressive behaviour and a comparatively well differentiated appearance.

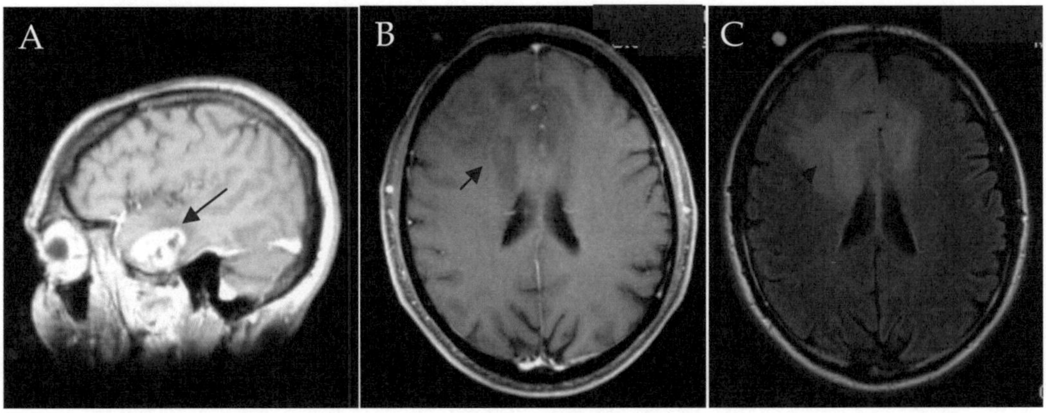

Fig. 1. A shows a sagittal gadolinium enhanced MRI scan of a Glioblastoma multiforme (WHO grade IV) with typical gadolinium enhancement of the tumor (arrow). Panel B shows a transversal gadolinium enhanced MRI scan of an Astrocytoma (WHO grade II). No contrast enhancement is noted (arrow). C shows the same tumor as FLAIR weighted image.

Among these are 10% differentiated astrocytoma, differentiated oligodendrogliomas and the mixed glioma (oligoastrocytoma) account for about 4-6%, 3-4% are so called ependymomas, and about 2% are pilocytic astrocytoma which is considered the only benign glioma (WHO grade I) (Wrench et al., 2002).

Astrocytic gliomas (anaplastic, differentiated and pilocytic astrocytoma) are believed to arise from astrocytic progenitor cells (type-I-astrocytes) whereas oligodendroglial tumors and mixed gliomas (oligoastrocytoma) arise from O-2-A progenitor cells. Ependymomas are derived from the ependyme of the ventricles (Schlegel et al. 2001)

1.2 Standard therapy and prognosis

Standard therapy of high-grade gliomas (WHO grade III and IV) includes gross total resection, concomitant radio-chemo-therapy with 60Gy and Temozolomide, followed by 6 cycles of Temozolomide, the so called Stupp-protocol (Stupp et al., 2005). The medium survival time for WHO grade IV tumors is about 15-18 months if this standard protocol is followed (Choi et al., 2008; Stupp et al., 2005). Before introduction of concomitant radio-chemo-therapy the survival time was about 12 months only with a 5-year survival rate of 3-4% (Davis et al., 1999; Barnholtz-Sloan et al., 2003). Following these authors the prognosis of WHO grade III tumors was better with a 5-years survival rate of 30-31% (Davis et al., 1999 und Barnholtz-Sloan et al., 2003). Recent studies (level I and II evidence) highlighted the role of the extend of surgical resection is an important predictor of progression-free and overall survival in the presence of high-grade glioma (WHO grade III and IV). More extensive surgery resulted generally in better outcome (Lacroix et al. 2001, Stummer et al. 2008, McGirt et al. 2009).

The less aggressive low-grade gliomas show generally a better prognosis of about 7-8 years survival after diagnosis, which however depends on the exact histological type (astrocytoma, oligodendroglioma; Schlegel et al., 2003). For these tumors no generally accepted standard-therapy protocol exists.

Pilocytic astrocytomas (WHO°I) show the best prognosis. They can be cured by complete resection. If this is not achievable patients should be followed closely and re-resection considered in case of progression (Bowers et al., 2001). Other treatment options include PCV chemotherapy and Radiotherapy. However, if a complete resection is achieved radiotherapy is generally not regarded as an option (Fisher et al., 2001; Karim et al., 1996).

More diffusely infiltrating low-grade gliomas like the differentiated astrocytoma (WHO°II), differentiated oligodendrogliomas (WHO°II) and oligoastrocytomas (WHO°II) show a significantly worse prognosis with a median survival of 3.2-7.7 years, depending on additional factors like age at diagnosis, largest tumor diameter, tumor crossing midline, histological type and neurological deficits at diagnosis (Pignatti et al., 2002). Although no level I evidence exists, several recent studies favour early surgery (soon after diagnosis versus surgery after progression or onset of symptoms) (Lang et al., 2006). Concerning the extend of resection the more recent evidence, mainly from retrospective case-series (evidence level V), supports a radical resection of diffuse low-grade gliomas if achievable at an adequate risk (Lang et al., 2006; McGirt et al., 2008; Schomas et al., 2009; Pouratian et al., 2010).

Radiotherapy can be applied, but again there remains controversy concerning the optimal timing (directly after surgery or if the tumor shows signs of progression) (Lang et al., 2006). Besides the comparatively long survival time after radiotheray leads to considerable side-effects by the neurotoxicity of the radiation (Klein et al., 2002; Olson et al., 2000; Laack et al., 2005).This supports later radiotherapy, whereas the authors of a mayor trial (EORTC 22845) favour early radiotherapy (van den Bent et al., 2005).

Chemotherapeutic options include adjuvant PCV after radiation and recent studies show some success of the treatment with Temozolomide, however larger studies are needed to assess the real benefits and risks (Baumert et al., 2008; Tosoni et al., 2008).

1.3 Factors limiting the surgical treatment of gliomas

Unfortunately, it remains clear that in spite of all these therapeutic efforts survival times of glioma patients are quite bad. So what is the reason for that?

A closer look on glioma-morphology and on historical treatment concepts might help to understand the problems of malignant glioma:

One issue is that gliomas are believed to arise from glial cells which are part of the normal brain histoarchitecture (astrocytic progenitor cells/type-I-astrocytes and O-2-A progenitor cells). Depending on the degree of mutation and degeneration these cells still closely resemble their normal progenitors and neighbouring cells. If a surgical resection of a glioma is encountered it can therefore be extremely difficult for the surgeon to identify the tumor-margin and to define the optimal extend of resection.

Another, even more problematic property of malignant gliomas is that they migrate along fiber tracts and vessels into the surrounding (often still functionally intact) brain tissue. In 1990 Kelly and colleagues could show by serial stereotactic biopsies that individual glioma cells can be found at a certain distance from the tumor, beyond the region of the tumor-oedema and even in the contra lateral hemisphere (Kelly et al., 1990). These cells are small and far distributed, they cannot be resected, because they are surrounded by functional brain tissue which should not be damaged and even the most sensitive imaging modalities (MRI and PET) are presently unable to detect most of them.

Therefore beside surgical resection other treatment modalities like radio- or chemotherapy which reach beyond the surgically resectable tumor margin are indispensible.

2. Surgical therapy of gliomas

2.1 Development of surgical techniques

The first intracerebral tumor was targeted surgically in 1884; the physician Alexander Hughes Bennett (1848-1901) indicated this surgery, while the operation was performed by the surgeon Rickman John Godlee (1849-1925). Although the patient died only a month after this procedure of meningitis this extensively discussed and well documented case marks the beginning of the surgical treatment of intracerebral tumors. Glioma surgery has gone a long way and seen many technical innovations since. In the following years the surgeons Williams Cushing (1869-1939), Fedor Krause (1859-1937) and Victor Horsley (1857-1916) paved the way for neurosurgery as an independent discipline in their countries (USA, UK and Germany). The problems of pain and infections were sufficiently solved by anaesthesia and antisepsis, yet the location of the concerned lesions in the scull remained problematic.

The discovery of x-rays by Wilhelm Konrad Röntgen (1845-1923) enabled a range of new diagnostic inventions. Further milestones were the development of cerebral angiography by Egas Antonio Aaetano de Moniz (1874-1955), computerized tomography by Johann Radon (1887-1956), Allen McLeod Cormack (1924-1998) and Godrey Newbold Hounsfield (1919-2004) and magnetic resonance imaging by Felix Block (1905-1983) and Edward Purcell (1912-1997)(Del Maestro et al., 2006; Eckart, 1990).

However surgeons soon discovered that the simple excision of glial tumors frequently led to recurrence of gliomas. In the 1960s this observation led to the development of super-radical resections. In some cases the complete hemispherectomy of the tumor bearing hemisphere was performed. Although these operations have shown some limited success they were unable to finally cure glioma (Giese et al., 2003). This is in accordance to Kelly´s above described observations who found glioma cells far beyond the margins of the solid tumor and even in the contra lateral hemisphere (Kelly et al., 1990).

Nevertheless, even though surgery was found unable to cure glioma it did improve symptoms and survival. Furthermore most recurrent glioma arise at its primary resection site or in a distance of no more than 2-3cm there off (Giese et al., 2003). Accordingly larger recent pro- and retrospective studies could show that the extend of the surgical resection is an important predictor of progression-free and overall survival for the patients suffering from malignant glioma as already stated above (Lacroix et al., 2001, Stummer et al., 2008, McGirt et al., 2009).

Unfortunately tumors are generally surrounded by still functional brain tissue often even in the direct neighbourhood of functionally important centres in the brain such as speech-areas or motor cortical areas (53,9% of newly diagnosed Glioblastoma multiforme are located within or close to such centres; Duffau et al., 2004). In these locations the consequences of an over-radical resection can be severe neurological deficits, while the consequence of an incomplete resection is an impaired prognosis.

Neurosurgeons around the world have therefore focused their research to optimize the intraoperative visualization of glioma cells and to monitor brain function. A first important step was the introduction of microsurgical techniques by M. Gazi Yaşargil and others by application of the operating microscope (Yaşargil, 2010).

Conventional operating microscopes have a magnification of about 5-80x and furthermore offer optimal illumination of the operating field. Using these operating microscopes, experienced neurosurgeons can distinguish characteristic features of the brain tumors as different shades of colour, thrombotic blood vessels or necrotic areas. Besides the consistency of the tissue features valuable information for the discrimination of tumor and adjacent brain tissue.

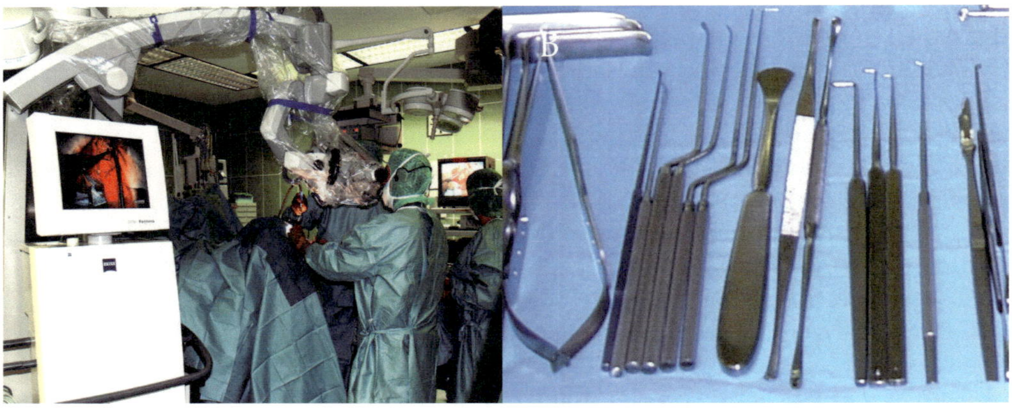

Fig. 2. Operating microscope (A), cerebral cortex during surgery and microsurgical instruments (B).

2.2 Optimizing the extend of resection

2.2.1 Image-guidance and macroscopic imaging

Further important steps were introduction of image-guidance, which allows the surgeon to exactly locate an area of interest on the preoperatively acuised CT or MR images.

Disadvantages of this technical milestone are at one hand the restricted resolution which does not allow the identification of very small tumor residues. The resolution of image guidance can obviously not exceed the resolution of the imaging modality applied for guidance which is about 0.6mm^3 for state of the art CT scans or 1mm^3 for modern MR tomographs (Foroglou et al., 2009) . The other important disadvantage is the fact that image-guidance refers to the anatomical situation at the time of acquisition of the images.

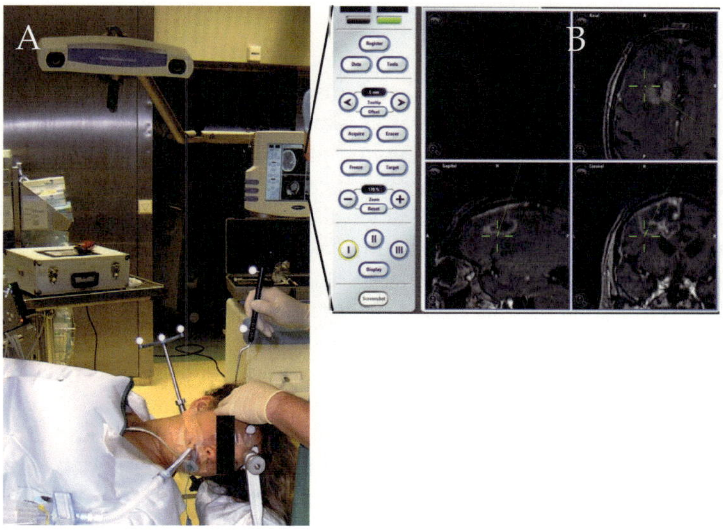

Fig. 3. Image-guiding system (A) and Screenshot of intraoperative image-guidance (B)

Unfortunately after craniotomy (opening of the skull) cerebrospinal fluid drains out and the intracranial pressure changes which results in gradual dislocation of the anatomical structures, an effect called brain-shift. Depending on the size of the craniotomy and the present intracranial pressure and the time after craniotomy this brain-shift can completely distort the neuronavigation.

Intraoperative imaging by ultrasound (Rygh et al., 2008) or intraoperative MR imaging (Foroglou et al., 2009) were introduced in order to counteract these problems and likewise optimize the extend of resection. However, the resolution of ultrasound imaging is even far lower than that of a CT or MRI scan and the procedure of an intraoperative MRI is expensive and time consuming.

Another imaging modality which can help to determine the real tumor size, especially if recurrent glioma and scar tissue formation have be discriminated, is the so called positron emission tomography (PET; Langleben et al., 2000). This technique uses radioactive marked variants of substrates of the cancer cells metabolism. These marked substrates (for example ^{18}F-desoxyglucose/FDG or ^{11}C-methylmethionin/MET) accumulate in the tumor with its high metabolic rate and the resulting in characteristic hot spots on the resulting images (Bénard et al., 2003; de Witte et al., 2001).

2.2.2 Neurophysiological monitoring

Besides resection control by image-guidance the integrity of some neurological functions of the tumor surrounding brain can be monitored directly.

By electric stimulation of motor areas and fiber tracts belonging to these areas the effector organ (muscle) can be activated. If these motor areas are stimulated during surgery, either transcranial or, if the concerned functional area is surgically exposed, by direct cortical stimulation, the induced activity of the effector organs (muscles) can be recorded by electromyography. A disturbance of motor cortical areas or corresponding fiber tracts leads directly to a disturbance of the measured activity in the effector organs and tell the surgeon that a further resection in the concerned area can be expected to result in neurological dysfunctions.

If surgery is performed near the sensory cortex or corresponding fiber tracts the same principle can be applied. The corresponding sensory organs (ears, eyes, perception sensors in the skin of a certain area etc.) can be stimmulated and the effect on the cerebral cortex is monitored by electro encephalograms or evoked potentials (Duffau, 2007).

More complex functions, like the human speech cannot be monitored by simple stimulation in the narcotized patient, as they involve several distinct functional areas within the brain. These tasks can however be monitored during awake operations (Duffau et al., 2009). For these awake operations nowadays most centres perform the craniotomy under general anaesthesia, after which the patient wakes up for the preparation of the brain tumor and is again sedated for wound closure (sleep/awake/sleep). By these means the patient can speak to the surgeon or an accompanying neuropsychologist during surgery and an impairment of the cortical areas responsible for speech production becomes directly apparent by dysfunctions of the normal speech. Normally the awake patient is asked to perform certain tasks like naming objects shown to him/her on a computer screen. Such awake procedures are less problematic than most people would expect, because the brain itself does not percept pain and the more painful craniotomy and wound closure can be nevertheless performed under general anaesthesia.

2.2.3 Intraoperative microscopy and fluorescent imaging

A further approach for to optimize the extend of resection is the staining of glioma tissue and optimization of the operating microscopes for enhanced intraoperative imaging. The most widely used technique is the staining of high-grade glioma tissue by 5-amino laevolinic acid (5-ALA; Hebeda et al., 1998; Stummer et al., 1998; Stummer et al., 2006). 5-AlA naturally occurs as an intermediate of the heame biosynthesis (Uehlinger et al., 2000) and external substitution of 5-ALA leads to accumulation of its fluorescent metabolite protoporphyrine-IX (PpIX) in many tumor cells including most high-grade gliomas. PpIX has a maximum absorption around 400nm (UV light excitation) and the resulting fluorescence (emission) is visible to the human eye and can likewise be visualized by modified operating microscopes (Hebeda et al., 1998; Stummer et al., 1998). Stummer and colleagues could show in their study, already cited above, that not only a more radical resection leads to prolonged progression free survival times of patients suffering from high-grade glioma, but that the application of intraoperative fluorescent guidance with 5-ALA could enhanced the rate of complete resections (as defined by an early postoperative contrast enhanced MR-scan) from 36 to 65% (Stummer et al., 2006).

In an ongoing project optical coherence tomography (OCT) has been used experimentally and in vivo to detect residual glioma tissue in the resection cavity (Boehringer et al., 2009).

Newer, yet experimental developments include the application of high performance fluorescent microscopes like confocal or multiphoton microscopes. which allow the identification of glioma cells down to the single cell level (Kantelhardt et al., 2009) and even gathering of functional information by time resolved fluorescent multiphoton microscopy

(Kantelhardt et al., 2007). Other techniques include infrared spectroscopic imaging (Steiner et al., 2008), or the staining of glioma cells by targeting the matrix metalloproteinases (MMP) which is present on the surfaces of high-grade glioblastoma cells (as on many tumor types) for the development of both drugs and MRI probes (Veiseh et al., 2007; Veiseh et al., 2009). Recently, the group of Tsien proposed using the MMP activity of tumor cells to incorporate dyes, nanoparticles and also drugs into tumor cells by unmasking a cell penetrating peptide sequence for guiding surgical resection and chemo therapy (Nguyen et al., 2010; Olson et al., 2010).
By the development of fluorescent nanoparticles (Quantum-dots) specifically targeting EGF-receptors, PDGF-receptors or other molecules believed to be specific for glioma cells within the brain, staining of living high- and low-grade glioma tissue was achieved in vitro (Kantelhardt et al., 2010). This is an important step, as the present gold-standard of intraoperative fluorescence imaging in gliomas 5-ALA does not stain low-grade gliomas.

2.3 Local chemotherapy

The second issue, remaining glioma cells beyond the margin of the tumor, was likewise a focus of neurosurgical research. The underlying idea is to deliver chemotherapeutics or radioactive substances directly into the tumor and, to the remaining glioma cells beyond the margin of the resection cavity. Several pass ways have been explored to reach this goal.

2.3.1 Intra-arterial delivery

Conventional administration of tumorocidic agents via vein or orally leads to a more or less equal concentration of the drug within the whole blood volume. Depending on the chemical and pharmacological specifities of the drugs penetration into different organs differs. Hydrophilic agents tend to stay in the blood stream, lipophilic ones generally penetrate much better into the different tissues. Likewise smaller molecules penetrate better than bigger ones. In case of a localized neoplasm a more specific administration of the tumorocidal agents is desirably. Malignant brain tumors rarely spread outside the central nervous system. The reason for this is not yet completely known. The fast progress of the disease for once limits the metastatic spread by limiting the survival time of the diseased patients. This might change when therapy regimes are available which prolong the survival times in highly malignant gliomas to several years. However most likely this is not the only reason, because other tumors, as malignant melanoma metastases much faster. The blood-brain barrier probably plays a major role in the restriction of the spread of malignant gliomas, either by hindering the migration of malignant tumor cells in the blood stream or by modulating the immune response in some way.
However, in order to minimize side effects and to enhance the concentration of chemotherapeutic agents in the tumor volume the local application of the drugs to an only locally growing tumor is an obvious idea. Every growing cell in the human organism needs sufficient supply of oxygen and nutrition, which are generally transported by the bloodstream. This is especially true for the fast growing and infiltrating tumor cells with their specific high metabolic turnover. As malignant glioma cells are derived from regular gill cells, or tumor stem cells which are themselves derived from regular stem cells as more recent theories go, they share a lot of specifities with normal glial cells in the brain. The higher consumption of substrates of the fast growing cells is one of the most striking differences. By administering tumorocidal agents via the bloodstream the antitumoral effects are multiplied due to the fact that the hyperperfused areas of the tumor, respectively

the metabolically most active or fastest growing areas in the tumor, get more of the tumorocidic agents than regularly perfused brain. The intra-arterial delivery of chemotherapeutics seems therefore a promising way to reach the most aggressive tumor cells. As many tumorocidal agents are furthermore eliminated in the liver it is desirable to bypass this organ. By intravenous or oral application a large amount of the tumoricidal agents may be cleared out of the circulation before even reaching the tumor, the so called first-pass effect. Intra-arterial administration in an artery directly leading to the tumor avoids this effect, therefore it is especially indicated for agents with a high systemic clearance-rate.

The chemotherapeutics are administered by an intra-arterial catheter in the carotid and/or the vertebral artery depending on the exact location of the tumor. If there are any doubts which vessel perfuses the tumor, an angiography can be performed prior to the administration of the tumorocidal agent. For the procedure (angiography and intra-arterial administration of the tumorocidic agent) the patient is punctated in the right femoral artery using the Seldinger technique (first punctation of the vessel with an canulae than a small wire is pushed through the lumen of the canula and than the catheter is placed guided by the wire). Than the administration-catheter is carefully maneuvered under radiographic control until it reaches the concerned artery and the tumorocidal agent is given via this catheter.

Preclinical studies in animal models and laboratory experiments were performed using different concentrations and combinations of chemotherapeutics. Furthermore intra-arterial treatment regimes were combined with intravenously or orally applicated drugs and radiotherapy. Some of the results were encouraging, so several pilot studies and phase I/II trials have been performed for low and high-grade gliomas, germ-cell tumors, primary CNS lymphoma, or primitive neuroectodermal tumor and brain metastasis (Doolittle et al., 2000). Among the substances used for intra-arterial administration are carboplatin, carmustine and other nitrosoureas, cisplatin, etoposide and methotrexate (Newton, 2005). Some authors described median survival rates for glioblastoma patients treated with intraarterial cisplatin and etoposide combined with radiotherapy to be dramatically longer than in patients treated with standard radio- and chemotherapies (Madajewicz et al., 2000; Osztie et al., 2001). However, limitations of the technique arise from the blood-brain-barrier and potentially significant complications such as neurologic toxicity like leukoencepalopathy, ototoxicity, seizures, visual loss; vascular complications like strokes or haematological complications like leukocytopenia or thrombocytopenia.

Osmotic blood-brain barrier disruption using isoflurane or propofol anesthesia showed some remarkable effects in the experimental setting as well as in a recent phase II study (Fortin et al., 2005; Hall et al., 2006). Unfortunately the disruption can also enhanced neurotoxic side effects. Especially an intraarterial administration of etoposide after osmotic disruption of the blood-brain-barrier showed unexpected severe complications (Fortin et al., 2000). Etoposide was thereafter administered before application of the blood-brain-barrier disrupting anaesthetics or it was given intravenously (Newton et al., 2002). Newer results suggest that the toxicities of carboplatin and tethotrexate based intraarterial administration regimes is comparatively low and well tolerated (Newton et al., 2005).

The safety of intra-arterial administration as a way to applicate some tumorocidal agents seems to be out of question by now. Yet no phase III study could demonstrate a survival benefit for patients treated with intraarterial chemotherapy compared to those receiving intravenous treatments.

2.3.2 Intratumoral injection

Another way of reaching high concentrations of antitumoral agents in malignant gliomas is to bypass the blood brain barrier instead of disrupting it. For this purpose tumoricidal agents are injected directly in the brain tumor tissue. In most cases, in the animal model as well as for the therapy of patients suffering from malignant gliomas, local injections are placed steriotactically to ensure the correct positioning of the agents. One or several bolus injections are placed on the same spot. The stereotactical technique allows the exact positioning of the needle in the lesion within the scull without the necessity to perform a large craniotomy. Prior to the procedure the exact position of the tumor within the scull has to be located. Therefore the skull is fixed in a rigid frame, than a CT-scan or MRI-scan is performed. By integrating the image data the exact location of the lesion within the frame is obtained. Now it is possible to calculate the angel and depth in which the tumor can be punctated. In the case of open surgery the injection can be placed under direct visualization. The systemic side effects of such an intratumoral or interstitial chemotherapy should be minimized respectively the tolerated dose of the tumoricidal agents in the tumor can be elevated without further damage to other organs, because only a small portion of the substance will end in the blood vessels. In theory this locally enhanced concentration of the injected substances will be present for a prolonged period, because the distribution via osmosis in the interstitial space will take much longer than the systemic clearance-rate of most substances allows the agent to stay in the bloodstream. Laboratory studies have been undertaken to prove this hypothesis. The concentration of a tumoricidal substance as for example DTI-015/BCNU in ethanol in the tumor tissue was found to be up to 100-1000 fold higher if injected directly into the tumor compared to the intravenous administration (Hamstra et al., 2005). Furthermore substances not passing the blood-brain barrier can be used. Among the tumoricidal agents applied for intratumoral injections were not only the classical chemotherapeutics as BCNU, but also immunoactive substances as beta interferon (Rainov et al., 2004), vaccine candidates or modified viruses (Rainov et al., 2006) or radioactive agents as the beta emitter 201Tl-chloride (Ljunggren et al., 2004). However in many cases the effects in preliminary animal studies seem more dramatic than expected by the specific mechanism of the concerned drug. Patient based studies are still very rare. A possible explanation for the astonishing good results may be local toxicity or chemical alteration of the tissue surrounding the injection site (for example pH mediated), as optimal doses for the interstitial therapy are often not yet established. Nevertheless the approach is still an interesting alternative to systemic administration. Considering the promising results from laboratory studies it takes no wonder that the technique has already been used for the treatment of patients. Data from a phase I/II trial for local injection of DTI-015 in recurrent malignant glioma has been published already in 2003 (Hassenbusch et al., 2003). These results suggested that the stereotactic injection of BCNU is well tolerated and a feasible alternative for the treatment of inoperable recurrent Glioblastomas.

2.3.3 Convection enhanced delivery

The fact that the efficacy of a treatment could be elevated by multiple injections leads to the problem of multiple punctations. Voulgaris and colleagues (Voulgaris et al., 2002) therefore used an omaya reservoir to administer Doxorubicin in recurrent high grade gliomas on 10 days. Many others used infusions instead of injections in order to administer a bigger amount of antitumoral agents over a prolonged time. These techniques portend a novel technique: The convection enhanced delivery (CED). The term convection enhanced delivery describes the interstitial application over a prolonged period via one or several previously implanted catheters by micropumps or sometimes gravity dependent infusion. Most researchers and physicians working on interstitial chemotherapy changed from single injections to this mode of delivery. They argued that the advantages of an interstitial therapy, higher dosage and lower systemic side effects, could be optimized by this technique. The catheters can either be placed under direct visualization following craniotomy or stereotactically, as described in the previous passage. A number of studies in animal models as well as in patients suffering from recurrent malignant gliomas have been performed to compare the dose distribution and safety of single or multiple bolus injections to CED. The first trials were performed in a nude mice flank tumor model of human malignant glioma. The in vivo effectiveness of CED was thus demonstrated. Further investigations on nude athymic mice using IL13 cytotoxin could show that the applied agent was distributed over a larger area by multiple injections compared to convection enhanced delivery, whereas the continuous infusion reached higher local concentrations in the target volume (Kawakami et al., 2004). Following this several phase I/II and III trials CED were initiated (Debinski et al., 2009). Nearly all antitumoral substances have been tested for intratumoral application. ACNU (nimustine) was administered in recurrent glioma and could induce necrosis and inhibit growth of the tumor (Wakabajashi et al., 2001). BCNU was administered in patients with recurrent glioma (Hassenbusch et al., 2003; Hamstra et al., 2005). Others were carboplatin or gemcitabine (Degen et al., 2003), several monoclonal antibodies (Wersall et al., 1997; Sampson et al. 2006), TP-38 a recombinant chimerical protein containing Pseudomonas exotoxin fused to transforming growth factor (TGF)-alpha (Sampson et al. 2005), a chimerical protein consisting of IL4 and Pseudomonas exotoxin or the IL13 cytotoxin (Rand et al., 2000) to name just some of the drugs. Likewise radioactive substances were locally applied as intracerebral brachy-therapy (gliasite^R, Chino et al. 2008). However although these trials could show some oncological effectivity severe problems were observed. The concerns mainly centered on ineffective tissue distribution and local adverse events due backflow and malpositioning of catheters or local infections (Bidros et al., 2010; Bonerba et al., 2010).

2.3.4 Local chemotherapy with implantable wafers

The problems with backflow and wound healing experienced in convection enhanced delivery of antitumoral agents resulted finally in the development of BCNU-wafers for implantation in the surgical resection cavity (gliadelR). A phase III study from 2003 showed that the intent-to-treat group showed a significantly better median survival of 13.9 to 11.6 months (Westphal et al. 2003). These BCNU wafers are presently the only intratumoral chemotherapy which got an approval from the FDA (Bonerba et al., 2010). Meanwhile the implantation of BCNU-wafers has been combined with the current standard therapy, the so called Stupp-protocol showing again favourable results (McGirt et al., 2009; Affronti et al., 2009). However others have reported about adverse events such as brain oedema, (transient) hydrocephalus, wound healing disorders (Bock et al., 2010; Giese et al., 2010).

Because of this the technique should be used after critical evaluation of the individual situation of the patient only.

Future developments might include a targeted local chemotherapy by chemotherapeutical agents coupled to specifically targeting nanoparticles or biomolecules and other upcoming substances.

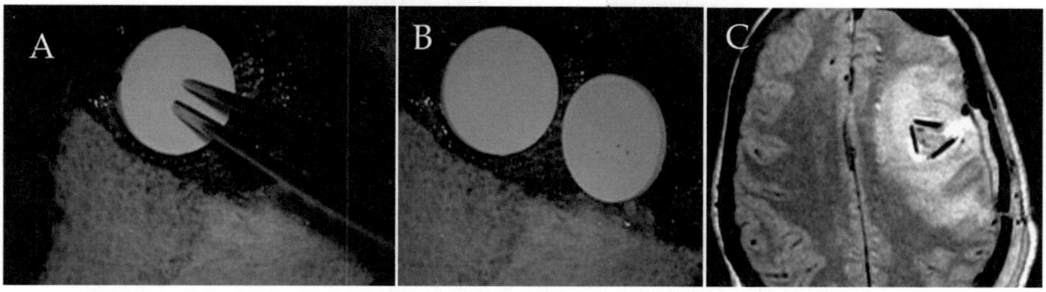

Fig. 4. A shows the implantation of an Gliadel[R] wafer. Two wafers in place (B) and a postoperative MRI scan showing 3 Gliadel[R] wafers in situ.

3. Conclusion

With about 9/100.000 newly diagnosed cases per year malignant glioma is one of most devasting diseases in the industrialized nations. Following the WHO grading system gliomas are classified from WHO grade IV (highly aggressive) to I (benign). Grade IV and III are called high-grade, while the less aggressive grade II is called low-grade gliomas.
The standard therapy of high-grade gliomas includes gross total resection, which has shown to improve the prognosis in recent phase III trials, concomitant radio-chemo-therapy with 60Gy and Temozolomide, followed by 6 cycles of Temozolomide, the so called Stupp-protocol. The medium survival time for WHO grade IV tumors is about 15-18 months if this standard protocol is followed, while the prognosis of WHO grade III tumors is slightly better (5-years survival rate of about 30%).
Low-grade gliomas show a better prognosis of about 7-8 years, and no standard-therapy protocol exists. All treatment modalities applied in high-grade glioma (surgery, radiotherapy, radio-chemotherapy, chemotherapy) are feasible and therapy is based on an individual decision. Recent case series however advocate early and complete surgery.
Nevertheless the prognosis of malignant brain tumors is generally still poor. The main reason for this is the ability of glioma cells to infiltrate the still functioning brain tissue beyond the margin of the solid tumor.
In order to further improve the prognosis many neurosurgeons have focused their research on optimization of the extend of resection. This goal is compromised by the fact that gliomas arise from glial progenitor cells which are part of the normal brain histoarchitecture. Depending on the degree of mutation and degeneration these cells still closely resemble their neighbouring (still functional) brain cells. CT- and MRI based image-guidance, intraoperative ultrasonography and MRI scanning were developed in order to guide the surgeon during resection. The accuracy of this image-guidance is restricted by the maximum resolution of the applied imaging modality (CT, MR, ultrasonography) and the accuracy of image-guidance is decreasing during the ongoing resection as the brain-shift alters the anatomy.
Another approach is the application of electrophysiological measurements and awake operations in order to control the integrity of neurological functions intraoperatievly. This is presently routineously applied if the glioma is in or close to a functionally important cortex areas like speech or motor areas.

Besides neurosurgeons have investigated novel optical technologies and dyes in order to differentiate glioma- and adjacent brain tissue. The staining of high-grade glioma tissue using 5-ALA is already in wide clinical use and recently the staining of living low-grade glioma tissue was achieved in vitro by specifically targeted nanoparticels. However further research is required before this can be introduced into clinical practice.

A completely different approach is the application of local chemo- or radio therapeutics.

Different modes for the local application of chemo- and radiotherapeutical agents were developed. The first approach was an arterial injection of chemotherapeutics with and without prior disruption of the blood brain barrier. Several studies could show that the therapy is generally well tolerated and safe, however it was not yet proven to be more effective than the conventional treatment. Therefore the blood-brain barrier was bypassed by direct injection into the tumors. This could be done once or repeatedly by stereotactic injection or under direct visualization at the end of an surgical procedure. In order to obtain even better results convection-enhanced delivery was developed, where the concerned chemotherapeutic is injected over a prolonged period of time by a pump or infusion. However results have yet likewise been suboptimal, most likely due to backflow and ineffective tissue distribution. The only local chemotherapy for malignant gliomas now in clinical use is the implantation of BCNU loaded wafers into the resection cavity at the end of surgical resection. This treatment option has recently been combined with the standard therapy (Stupp-protocol) for high-grade gliomas. Several studies could show its effectivity but likewise pointed out some dangers as the development of brain oedema, transient hydrocephalus or wound healing disorders. In future specifically targeted local chemotherapeutic agents could be developed to overcome these problems.

4. References

Affronti, M.L.; Heery, C.R.; Herndon, J.E., 2nd; Rich, J.N.; Reardon, D.A.; Desjardins, A.; Vredenburgh, J.J.; Friedman, A.H.; Bigner, D.D. & Friedman, H.S. (2009). Overall survival of newly diagnosed glioblastoma patients receiving carmustine wafers followed by radiation and concurrent temozolomide plus rotational multiagent chemotherapy. *Cancer,* Vol. 115, No. 15, (Aug 1), pp. 3501-3511, ISSN 0008-543X

Barnholtz-Sloan, J.S.; Sloan, A.E. & Schwartz, A.G. (2003). Relative survival rates and patterns of diagnosis analyzed by time period for individuals with primary malignant brain tumor, 1973-1997. *J Neurosurg,* Vol. 99, No. 3, (Sep), pp. 458-466, ISSN 0022-3085

Baumert, B.G. & Stupp, R. (2008). Low-grade glioma: a challenge in therapeutic options: the role of radiotherapy. *Ann Oncol,* Vol. 19 Suppl 7, No. (Sep), pp. vii217-222, ISSN 1569-8041

Benard, F.; Romsa, J. & Hustinx, R. (2003). Imaging gliomas with positron emission tomography and single-photon emission computed tomography. *Semin Nucl Med,* Vol. 33, No. 2, (Apr), pp. 148-162, ISSN 0001-2998

Bidros, D.S.; Liu, J.K. & Vogelbaum, M.A. Future of convection-enhanced delivery in the treatment of brain tumors. *Future Oncol,* Vol. 6, No. 1, (Jan), pp. 117-125, ISSN 1744-8301

Bock, H.C.; Puchner, M.J.; Lohmann, F.; Schutze, M.; Koll, S.; Ketter, R.; Buchalla, R.; Rainov, N.; Kantelhardt, S.R.; Rohde, V. & Giese, A. First-line treatment of malignant glioma with carmustine implants followed by concomitant radiochemotherapy: a multicenter experience. *Neurosurg Rev,* Vol. 33, No. 4, (Oct), pp. 441-449, ISSN 1437-

Bohringer, H.J.; Lankenau, E.; Stellmacher, F.; Reusche, E.; Huttmann, G. & Giese, A. (2009). Imaging of human brain tumor tissue by near-infrared laser coherence tomography. *Acta Neurochir (Wien),* Vol. 151, No. 5, (May), pp. 507-517; discussion 517, ISSN 0942-0940

Bowers, D.C.; Krause, T.P.; Aronson, L.J.; Barzi, A.; Burger, P.C.; Carson, B.S.; Weingart, J.D.; Wharam, M.D.; Melhem, E.R. & Cohen, K.J. (2001). Second surgery for recurrent pilocytic astrocytoma in children. *Pediatr Neurosurg,* Vol. 34, No. 5, (May), pp. 229-234, ISSN 1016-2291

Buonerba, C.; Di Lorenzo, G.; Marinelli, A.; Federico, P.; Palmieri, G.; Imbimbo, M.; Conti, P.; Peluso, G.; De Placido, S. & Sampson, J.H. A comprehensive outlook on intracerebral therapy of malignant gliomas. *Crit Rev Oncol Hematol,* Vol. No. (Sep 29), pp. 1879-0461, ISSN 1040-8428

Chino, K.; Silvain, D.; Grace, A.; Stubbs, J. & Stea, B. (2008). Feasibility and safety of outpatient brachytherapy in 37 patients with brain tumors using the GliaSite Radiation Therapy System. *Med Phys,* Vol. 35, No. 7, (Jul), pp. 3383-3388, ISSN 0094-2405

Choi, J.W.; Lee, M.M.; Kim, I.A.; Kim, J.H.; Choe, G. & Kim, C.Y. (2008). The outcomes of concomitant chemoradiotherapy followed by adjuvant chemotherapy with temozolomide for newly diagnosed high grade gliomas : the preliminary results of single center prospective study. *J Korean Neurosurg Soc,* Vol. 44, No. 4, (Oct), pp. 222-227, ISSN 2005-3711

Dahlborg, S.A.; Petrillo, A.; Crossen, J.R.; Roman-Goldstein, S.; Doolittle, N.D.; Fuller, K.H. & Neuwelt, E.A. (1998). The potential for complete and durable response in nonglial primary brain tumors in children and young adults with enhanced chemotherapy delivery. *Cancer J Sci Am,* Vol. 4, No. 2, (Mar-Apr), pp. 110-124, ISSN 1081-4442

Davis, F.G.; McCarthy, B.J.; Freels, S.; Kupelian, V. & Bondy, M.L. (1999). The conditional probability of survival of patients with primary malignant brain tumors: surveillance, epidemiology, and end results (SEER) data. *Cancer,* Vol. 85, No. 2, (Jan 15), pp. 485-491, ISSN 0008-543X

De Witte, O.; Goldberg, I.; Wikler, D.; Rorive, S.; Damhaut, P.; Monclus, M.; Salmon, I.; Brotchi, J. & Goldman, S. (2001). Positron emission tomography with injection of methionine as a prognostic factor in glioma. *J Neurosurg,* Vol. 95, No. 5, (Nov), pp. 746-750, ISSN 0022-3085

Debinski, W. & Tatter, S.B. (2009). Convection-enhanced delivery for the treatment of brain tumors. *Expert Rev Neurother,* Vol. 9, No. 10, (Oct), pp. 1519-1527, ISSN 1744-8360

Degen, J.W.; Walbridge, S.; Vortmeyer, A.O.; Oldfield, E.H. & Lonser, R.R. (2003). Safety and efficacy of convection-enhanced delivery of gemcitabine or carboplatin in a malignant glioma model in rats. *J Neurosurg,* Vol. 99, No. 5, (Nov), pp. 893-898, ISSN 0022-3085

Doolittle, N.D.; Miner, M.E.; Hall, W.A.; Siegal, T.; Jerome, E.; Osztie, E.; McAllister, L.D.; Bubalo, J.S.; Kraemer, D.F.; Fortin, D.; Nixon, R.; Muldoon, L.L. & Neuwelt, E.A. (2000). Safety and efficacy of a multicenter study using intraarterial chemotherapy in conjunction with osmotic opening of the blood-brain barrier for the treatment of patients with malignant brain tumors. *Cancer,* Vol. 88, No. 3, (Feb 1), pp. 637-647, ISSN 0008-543X

Duffau, H. (2007). Contribution of cortical and subcortical electrostimulation in brain glioma surgery: methodological and functional considerations. *Neurophysiol Clin,* Vol. 37, No. 6, (Dec), pp. 373-382, ISSN 0987-7053

Duffau, H. (2009). Surgery of low-grade gliomas: towards a 'functional neurooncology'. *Curr Opin Oncol,* Vol. 21, No. 6, (Nov), pp. 543-549, ISSN 1531-703X

Duffau, H. & Capelle, L. (2004). Preferential brain locations of low-grade gliomas. *Cancer,* Vol. 100, No. 12, (Jun 15), pp. 2622-2626, ISSN 0008-543X

Eckart, W. (1990).*Geschichte der Medizin,* Springer Verlag, ISBN 3540214429, Berlin, Germany

Fisher, B.J.; Leighton, C.C.; Vujovic, O.; Macdonald, D.R. & Stitt, L. (2001). Results of a policy of surveillance alone after surgical management of pediatric low grade gliomas. *Int J Radiat Oncol Biol Phys,* Vol. 51, No. 3, (Nov 1), pp. 704-710, ISSN 0360-3016

Foroglou, N.; Zamani, A. & Black, P. (2009). Intra-operative MRI (iop-MR) for brain tumour surgery. *Br J Neurosurg,* Vol. 23, No. 1, (Feb), pp. 14-22, ISSN 1360-046X

Fortin, D.; Desjardins, A.; Benko, A.; Niyonsega, T. & Boudrias, M. (2005). Enhanced chemotherapy delivery by intraarterial infusion and blood-brain barrier disruption in malignant brain tumors: the Sherbrooke experience. *Cancer,* Vol. 103, No. 12, (Jun 15), pp. 2606-2615, ISSN 0008-543X

Fortin, D.; McCormick, C.I.; Remsen, L.G.; Nixon, R. & Neuwelt, E.A. (2000). Unexpected neurotoxicity of etoposide phosphate administered in combination with other chemotherapeutic agents after blood-brain barrier modification to enhance delivery, using propofol for general anesthesia, in a rat model. *Neurosurgery,* Vol. 47, No. 1, (Jul), pp. 199-207, ISSN 0148-396X

Giese, A.; Bjerkvig, R.; Berens, M.E. & Westphal, M. (2003). Cost of migration: invasion of malignant gliomas and implications for treatment. *J Clin Oncol,* Vol. 21, No. 8, (Apr 15), pp. 1624-1636, ISSN 0732-183X

Giese, A.; Bock, H.C.; Kantelhardt, S.R. & Rohde, V. Risk management in the treatment of malignant gliomas with BCNU wafer implants. *Cen Eur Neurosurg,* Vol. 71, No. 4, (Nov), pp. 199-206, ISSN 1868-4912

Hall, W.A.; Doolittle, N.D.; Daman, M.; Bruns, P.K.; Muldoon, L.; Fortin, D. & Neuwelt, E.A. (2006). Osmotic blood-brain barrier disruption chemotherapy for diffuse pontine gliomas. *J Neurooncol,* Vol. 77, No. 3, (May), pp. 279-284, ISSN 0167-594X

Hamstra, D.A.; Moffat, B.A.; Hall, D.E.; Young, J.M.; Desmond, T.J.; Carter, J.; Pietronigro, D.; Frey, K.A.; Rehemtulla, A. & Ross, B.D. (2005). Intratumoral injection of BCNU in ethanol (DTI-015) results in enhanced delivery to tumor--a pharmacokinetic study. *J Neurooncol,* Vol. 73, No. 3, (Jul), pp. 225-238, ISSN 0167-594X

Hassenbusch, S.J.; Nardone, E.M.; Levin, V.A.; Leeds, N. & Pietronigro, D. (2003). Stereotactic injection of DTI-015 into recurrent malignant gliomas: phase I/II trial. *Neoplasia,* Vol. 5, No. 1, (Jan-Feb), pp. 9-16, ISSN 1522-8002

Hebeda, K.M.; Saarnak, A.E.; Olivo, M.; Sterenborg, H.J. & Wolbers, J.G. (1998). 5-Aminolevulinic acid induced endogenous porphyrin fluorescence in 9L and C6 brain tumours and in the normal rat brain. *Acta Neurochir (Wien),* Vol. 140, No. 5, pp. 503-512; discussion 512-503, ISSN 0001-6268

Kantelhardt, S.R.; Caarls, W.; de Vries, A.H.; Hagen, G.M.; Jovin, T.M.; Schulz-Schaeffer, W.; Rohde, V.; Giese, A. & Arndt-Jovin, D.J. Specific visualization of glioma cells in living low-grade tumor tissue. *PLoS One,* Vol. 5, No. 6, pp. e11323, ISSN 1932-6203

Kantelhardt, S.R.; Leppert, J.; Kantelhardt, J.W.; Reusche, E.; Huttmann, G. & Giese, A. (2009). Multi-photon excitation fluorescence microscopy of brain-tumour tissue and analysis of cell density. *Acta Neurochir (Wien),* Vol. 151, No. 3, (Mar), pp. 253-262; discussion 262, ISSN 0942-0940

Kantelhardt, S.R.; Leppert, J.; Krajewski, J.; Petkus, N.; Reusche, E.; Tronnier, V.M.; Huttmann, G. & Giese, A. (2007). Imaging of brain and brain tumor specimens by time-resolved multiphoton excitation microscopy ex vivo. *Neuro Oncol,* Vol. 9, No. 2, (Apr), pp. 103-112, ISSN 1522-8517

Karim, A.B.; Maat, B.; Hatlevoll, R.; Menten, J.; Rutten, E.H.; Thomas, D.G.; Mascarenhas, F.; Horiot, J.C.; Parvinen, L.M.; van Reijn, M.; Jager, J.J.; Fabrini, M.G.; van Alphen, A.M.; Hamers, H.P.; Gaspar, L.; Noordman, E.; Pierart, M. & van Glabbeke, M. (1996). A randomized trial on dose-response in radiation therapy of low-grade cerebral glioma: European Organization for Research and Treatment of Cancer (EORTC) Study 22844. *Int J Radiat Oncol Biol Phys,* Vol. 36, No. 3, (Oct 1), pp. 549-556, ISSN 0360-3016

Kawakami, K.; Kawakami, M.; Kioi, M.; Husain, S.R. & Puri, R.K. (2004). Distribution kinetics of targeted cytotoxin in glioma by bolus or convection-enhanced delivery in a murine model. *J Neurosurg,* Vol. 101, No. 6, (Dec), pp. 1004-1011, ISSN 0022-3085

Kelly, P.J.; Daumas-Duport, C.; Kispert, D.B.; Kall, B.A.; Scheithauer, B.W. & Illig, J.J. (1987). Imaging-based stereotaxic serial biopsies in untreated intracranial glial neoplasms. *J Neurosurg,* Vol. 66, No. 6, (Jun), pp. 865-874, ISSN 0022-3085

Kleihues P, C.W. (2000).*World Health Organization Classification of Tumours. Pathology Genetics. Tumours of the Nervous System.*, IARC Press, ISBN 9283224094, Lyon, France

Klein, M.; Heimans, J.J.; Aaronson, N.K.; van der Ploeg, H.M.; Grit, J.; Muller, M.; Postma, T.J.; Mooij, J.J.; Boerman, R.H.; Beute, G.N.; Ossenkoppele, G.J.; van Imhoff, G.W.; Dekker, A.W.; Jolles, J.; Slotman, B.J.; Struikmans, H. & Taphoorn, M.J. (2002). Effect of radiotherapy and other treatment-related factors on mid-term to long-term cognitive sequelae in low-grade gliomas: a comparative study. *Lancet,* Vol. 360, No. 9343, (Nov 2), pp. 1361-1368, ISSN 0140-6736

Laack, N.N.; Brown, P.D.; Ivnik, R.J.; Furth, A.F.; Ballman, K.V.; Hammack, J.E.; Arusell, R.M.; Shaw, E.G. & Buckner, J.C. (2005). Cognitive function after radiotherapy for supratentorial low-grade glioma: a North Central Cancer Treatment Group prospective study. *Int J Radiat Oncol Biol Phys,* Vol. 63, No. 4, (Nov 15), pp. 1175-1183, ISSN 0360-3016

Lacroix, M.; Abi-Said, D.; Fourney, D.R.; Gokaslan, Z.L.; Shi, W.; DeMonte, F.; Lang, F.F.; McCutcheon, I.E.; Hassenbusch, S.J.; Holland, E.; Hess, K.; Michael, C.; Miller, D. & Sawaya, R. (2001). A multivariate analysis of 416 patients with glioblastoma multiforme: prognosis, extent of resection, and survival. *J Neurosurg,* Vol. 95, No. 2, (Aug), pp. 190-198, ISSN 0022-3085

Lang, F.F. & Gilbert, M.R. (2006). Diffusely infiltrative low-grade gliomas in adults. *J Clin Oncol,* Vol. 24, No. 8, (Mar 10), pp. 1236-1245, ISSN 1527-7755

Langleben, D.D. & Segall, G.M. (2000). PET in differentiation of recurrent brain tumor from radiation injury. *J Nucl Med,* Vol. 41, No. 11, (Nov), pp. 1861-1867, ISSN 0161-5505

Ljunggren, K.; Liu, X.; Erlandsson, K.; Ljungberg, M.; Salford, L. & Strand, S.E. (2004). Absorbed dose distribution in glioma tumors in rat brain after therapeutic intratumoral injection of 201Tl-chloride. *Cancer Biother Radiopharm,* Vol. 19, No. 5, (Oct), pp. 562-569, ISSN 1084-9785

Madajewicz, S.; Chowhan, N.; Tfayli, A.; Roque, C.; Meek, A.; Davis, R.; Wolf, W.; Cabahug, C.; Roche, P.; Manzione, J.; Iliya, A.; Shady, M.; Hentschel, P.; Atkins, H. & Braun, A. (2000). Therapy for patients with high grade astrocytoma using intraarterial chemotherapy and radiation therapy. *Cancer,* Vol. 88, No. 10, (May 15), pp. 2350-2356, ISSN 0008-543X

Maestro, R.F.D. (2006).*A History of Neuro-Oncology,* DW Medical Consulting Inc., ISBN 0771706359, Montreal, Canada

McGirt, M.J.; Chaichana, K.L.; Gathinji, M.; Attenello, F.J.; Than, K.; Olivi, A.; Weingart, J.D.; Brem, H. & Quinones-Hinojosa, A.R. (2009). Independent association of extent of resection with survival in patients with malignant brain astrocytoma. *J Neurosurg,* Vol. 110, No. 1, (Jan), pp. 156-162, ISSN 0022-3085

McGirt, M.J.; Goldstein, I.M.; Chaichana, K.L.; Tobias, M.E.; Kothbauer, K.F. & Jallo, G.I. (2008). Extent of surgical resection of malignant astrocytomas of the spinal cord: outcome analysis of 35 patients. *Neurosurgery,* Vol. 63, No. 1, (Jul), pp. 55-60; discussion 60-51, ISSN 1524-4040

McGirt, M.J.; Than, K.D.; Weingart, J.D.; Chaichana, K.L.; Attenello, F.J.; Olivi, A.; Laterra, J.; Kleinberg, L.R.; Grossman, S.A.; Brem, H. & Quinones-Hinojosa, A. (2009). Gliadel (BCNU) wafer plus concomitant temozolomide therapy after primary resection of glioblastoma multiforme. *J Neurosurg,* Vol. 110, No. 3, (Mar), pp. 583-588, ISSN 0022-3085

Newton, H.B. (2005). Intra-arterial chemotherapy of primary brain tumors. *Curr Treat Options Oncol,* Vol. 6, No. 6, (Nov), pp. 519-530, ISSN 1527-2729

Newton, H.B.; Slivka, M.A.; Stevens, C.L.; Bourekas, E.C.; Christoforidis, G.A.; Baujan, M.A. & Chakeres, D.W. (2002). Intra-arterial carboplatin and intravenous etoposide for the treatment of recurrent and progressive non-GBM gliomas. *J Neurooncol,* Vol. 56, No. 1, (Jan), pp. 79-86, ISSN 0167-594X

Nguyen, Q.T.; Olson, E.S.; Aguilera, T.A.; Jiang, T.; Scadeng, M.; Ellies, L.G. & Tsien, R.Y. Surgery with molecular fluorescence imaging using activatable cell-penetrating peptides decreases residual cancer and improves survival. *Proc Natl Acad Sci U S A,* Vol. 107, No. 9, (Mar 2), pp. 4317-4322, ISSN 1091-6490

Olson, E.S.; Jiang, T.; Aguilera, T.A.; Nguyen, Q.T.; Ellies, L.G.; Scadeng, M. & Tsien, R.Y. Activatable cell penetrating peptides linked to nanoparticles as dual probes for in vivo fluorescence and MR imaging of proteases. *Proc Natl Acad Sci U S A,* Vol. 107, No. 9, (Mar 2), pp. 4311-4316, ISSN 1091-6490

Olson, J.D.; Riedel, E. & DeAngelis, L.M. (2000). Long-term outcome of low-grade oligodendroglioma and mixed glioma. *Neurology,* Vol. 54, No. 7, (Apr 11), pp. 1442-1448, ISSN 0028-3878

Osztie, E.; Varallyay, P.; Doolittle, N.D.; Lacy, C.; Jones, G.; Nickolson, H.S. & Neuwelt, E.A. (2001). Combined intraarterial carboplatin, intraarterial etoposide phosphate, and IV Cytoxan chemotherapy for progressive optic-hypothalamic gliomas in young children. *AJNR Am J Neuroradiol,* Vol. 22, No. 5, (May), pp. 818-823, ISSN 0195-6108

Pignatti, F.; van den Bent, M.; Curran, D.; Debruyne, C.; Sylvester, R.; Therasse, P.; Afra, D.; Cornu, P.; Bolla, M.; Vecht, C. & Karim, A.B. (2002). Prognostic factors for survival in adult patients with cerebral low-grade glioma. *J Clin Oncol,* Vol. 20, No. 8, (Apr 15), pp. 2076-2084, ISSN 0732-183X

Pouratian, N. & Schiff, D. Management of low-grade glioma. *Curr Neurol Neurosci Rep,* Vol. 10, No. 3, (May), pp. 224-231, ISSN 1534-6293

Rainov, N.G. & Heidecke, V. (2004). Long term survival in a patient with recurrent malignant glioma treated with intratumoral infusion of an IL4-targeted toxin (NBI-3001). *J Neurooncol,* Vol. 66, No. 1-2, (Jan), pp. 197-201, ISSN 0167-594X

Rainov, N.G.; Soling, A. & Heidecke, V. (2006). Novel therapies for malignant gliomas: a local affair? *Neurosurg Focus,* Vol. 20, No. 4, pp. E9, ISSN 1092-0684

Rand, R.W.; Kreitman, R.J.; Patronas, N.; Varricchio, F.; Pastan, I. & Puri, R.K. (2000). Intratumoral administration of recombinant circularly permuted interleukin-4-Pseudomonas exotoxin in patients with high-grade glioma. *Clin Cancer Res,* Vol. 6, No. 6, (Jun), pp. 2157-2165, ISSN 1078-0432

Remsen, L.G.; McCormick, C.I.; Sexton, G.; Pearse, H.D.; Garcia, R.; Mass, M.; Roman-Goldstein, S. & Neuwelt, E.A. (1997). Long-term toxicity and neuropathology associated with the sequencing of cranial irradiation and enhanced chemotherapy delivery. *Neurosurgery,* Vol. 40, No. 5, (May), pp. 1034-1040; discussion 1040-1032, ISSN 0148-396X

Remsen, L.G.; McCormick, C.I.; Sexton, G.; Pearse, H.D.; Garcia, R. & Neuwelt, E.A. (1995). Decreased delivery and acute toxicity of cranial irradiation and chemotherapy given with osmotic blood-brain barrier disruption in a rodent model: the issue of sequence. *Clin Cancer Res,* Vol. 1, No. 7, (Jul), pp. 731-739, ISSN 1078-0432

Rygh, O.M.; Selbekk, T.; Torp, S.H.; Lydersen, S.; Hernes, T.A. & Unsgaard, G. (2008). Comparison of navigated 3D ultrasound findings with histopathology in subsequent phases of glioblastoma resection. *Acta Neurochir (Wien),* Vol. 150, No. 10, (Oct), pp. 1033-1041; discussion 1042, ISSN 0942-0940

Sampson, J.H.; Akabani, G.; Friedman, A.H.; Bigner, D.; Kunwar, S.; Berger, M.S. & Bankiewicz, K.S. (2006). Comparison of intratumoral bolus injection and convection-enhanced delivery of radiolabeled antitenascin monoclonal antibodies. *Neurosurg Focus,* Vol. 20, No. 4, pp. E14, ISSN 1092-0684

Sampson, J.H.; Reardon, D.A.; Friedman, A.H.; Friedman, H.S.; Coleman, R.E.; McLendon, R.E.; Pastan, I. & Bigner, D.D. (2005). Sustained radiographic and clinical response in patient with bifrontal recurrent glioblastoma multiforme with intracerebral infusion of the recombinant targeted toxin TP-38: case study. *Neuro Oncol,* Vol. 7, No. 1, (Jan), pp. 90-96, ISSN 1522-8517

Schlegel U, W.M., Westphal M. (2003).*Neuroonkologie,* Thieme Verlag, ISBN 3-1310-9062-6, Stuttgart, Germany

Schomas, D.A.; Laack, N.N.; Rao, R.D.; Meyer, F.B.; Shaw, E.G.; O'Neill, B.P.; Giannini, C. & Brown, P.D. (2009). Intracranial low-grade gliomas in adults: 30-year experience with long-term follow-up at Mayo Clinic. *Neuro Oncol,* Vol. 11, No. 4, (Aug), pp. 437-445, ISSN 1522-8517

Schwartzbaum, J.A.; Fisher, J.L.; Aldape, K.D. & Wrensch, M. (2006). Epidemiology and molecular pathology of glioma. *Nat Clin Pract Neurol,* Vol. 2, No. 9, (Sep), pp. 494-503; quiz 491 p following 516, ISSN 1745-834X

Steiner, G.; Kuchler, S.; Hermann, A.; Koch, E.; Salzer, R.; Schackert, G. & Kirsch, M. (2008). Rapid and label-free classification of human glioma cells by infrared spectroscopic imaging. *Cytometry A,* Vol. 73A, No. 12, (Dec), pp. 1158-1164, ISSN 1552-4930

Stummer, W.; Pichlmeier, U.; Meinel, T.; Wiestler, O.D.; Zanella, F. & Reulen, H.J. (2006). Fluorescence-guided surgery with 5-aminolevulinic acid for resection of malignant glioma: a randomised controlled multicentre phase III trial. *Lancet Oncol,* Vol. 7, No. 5, (May), pp. 392-401, ISSN 1470-2045

Stummer, W.; Reulen, H.J.; Meinel, T.; Pichlmeier, U.; Schumacher, W.; Tonn, J.C.; Rohde, V.; Oppel, F.; Turowski, B.; Woiciechowsky, C.; Franz, K. & Pietsch, T. (2008). Extent of resection and survival in glioblastoma multiforme: identification of and adjustment for bias. *Neurosurgery,* Vol. 62, No. 3, (Mar), pp. 564-576; discussion 564-576, ISSN 1524-4040

Stummer, W.; Stocker, S.; Wagner, S.; Stepp, H.; Fritsch, C.; Goetz, C.; Goetz, A.E.; Kiefmann, R. & Reulen, H.J. (1998). Intraoperative detection of malignant gliomas by 5-aminolevulinic acid-induced porphyrin fluorescence. *Neurosurgery,* Vol. 42, No. 3, (Mar), pp. 518-525; discussion 525-516, ISSN 0148-396X

Stupp, R.; Mason, W.P.; van den Bent, M.J.; Weller, M.; Fisher, B.; Taphoorn, M.J.; Belanger, K.; Brandes, A.A.; Marosi, C.; Bogdahn, U.; Curschmann, J.; Janzer, R.C.; Ludwin, S.K.; Gorlia, T.; Allgeier, A.; Lacombe, D.; Cairncross, J.G.; Eisenhauer, E. & Mirimanoff, R.O. (2005). Radiotherapy plus concomitant and adjuvant temozolomide for glioblastoma. *N Engl J Med,* Vol. 352, No. 10, (Mar 10), pp. 987-996, ISSN 1533-4406

Tosoni, A.; Franceschi, E.; Ermani, M.; Bertorelle, R.; Bonaldi, L.; Blatt, V. & Brandes, A.A. (2008). Temozolomide three weeks on and one week off as first line therapy for patients with recurrent or progressive low grade gliomas. *J Neurooncol,* Vol. 89, No. 2, (Sep), pp. 179-185, ISSN 0167-594X

Uehlinger, P.; Zellweger, M.; Wagnieres, G.; Juillerat-Jeanneret, L.; van den Bergh, H. & Lange, N. (2000). 5-Aminolevulinic acid and its derivatives: physical chemical properties and protoporphyrin IX formation in cultured cells. *J Photochem Photobiol B,* Vol. 54, No. 1, (Jan), pp. 72-80, ISSN 1011-1344

van den Bent, M.J.; Afra, D.; de Witte, O.; Ben Hassel, M.; Schraub, S.; Hoang-Xuan, K.; Malmstrom, P.O.; Collette, L.; Pierart, M.; Mirimanoff, R. & Karim, A.B. (2005). Long-term efficacy of early versus delayed radiotherapy for low-grade astrocytoma and oligodendroglioma in adults: the EORTC 22845 randomised trial. *Lancet,* Vol. 366, No. 9490, (Sep 17-23), pp. 985-990, ISSN 1474-547X

Veiseh, M.; Gabikian, P.; Bahrami, S.B.; Veiseh, O.; Zhang, M.; Hackman, R.C.; Ravanpay, A.C.; Stroud, M.R.; Kusuma, Y.; Hansen, S.J.; Kwok, D.; Munoz, N.M.; Sze, R.W.; Grady, W.M.; Greenberg, N.M.; Ellenbogen, R.G. & Olson, J.M. (2007). Tumor paint: a chlorotoxin:Cy5.5 bioconjugate for intraoperative visualization of cancer foci. *Cancer Res,* Vol. 67, No. 14, (Jul 15), pp. 6882-6888, ISSN 0008-5472

Veiseh, O.; Sun, C.; Fang, C.; Bhattarai, N.; Gunn, J.; Kievit, F.; Du, K.; Pullar, B.; Lee, D.; Ellenbogen, R.G.; Olson, J. & Zhang, M. (2009). Specific targeting of brain tumors with an optical/magnetic resonance imaging nanoprobe across the blood-brain barrier. *Cancer Res,* Vol. 69, No. 15, (Aug 1), pp. 6200-6207, ISSN 1538-7445

Voulgaris, S.; Partheni, M.; Karamouzis, M.; Dimopoulos, P.; Papadakis, N. & Kalofonos, H.P. (2002). Intratumoral doxorubicin in patients with malignant brain gliomas. *Am J Clin Oncol,* Vol. 25, No. 1, (Feb), pp. 60-64, ISSN 0277-3732

Wakabayashi, T.; Yoshida, J.; Mizuno, M. & Kajita, Y. (2001). Intratumoral microinfusion of nimustine (ACNU) for recurrent glioma. *Brain Tumor Pathol,* Vol. 18, No. 1, pp. 23-28, ISSN 1433-7398

Wersall, P.; Ohlsson, I.; Biberfeld, P.; Collins, V.P.; von Krusenstjerna, S.; Larsson, S.; Mellstedt, H. & Boethius, J. (1997). Intratumoral infusion of the monoclonal antibody, mAb 425, against the epidermal-growth-factor receptor in patients with advanced malignant glioma. *Cancer Immunol Immunother,* Vol. 44, No. 3, (May), pp. 157-164, ISSN 0340-7004

Westphal, M.; Hilt, D.C.; Bortey, E.; Delavault, P.; Olivares, R.; Warnke, P.C.; Whittle, I.R.; Jaaskelainen, J. & Ram, Z. (2003). A phase 3 trial of local chemotherapy with biodegradable carmustine (BCNU) wafers (Gliadel wafers) in patients with primary malignant glioma. *Neuro Oncol,* Vol. 5, No. 2, (Apr), pp. 79-88, ISSN 1522-8517

Wrensch, M.; Minn, Y.; Chew, T.; Bondy, M. & Berger, M.S. (2002). Epidemiology of primary brain tumors: current concepts and review of the literature. *Neuro Oncol,* Vol. 4, No. 4, (Oct), pp. 278-299, ISSN 1522-8517

Yasargil, M.G. Editorial. Personal considerations on the history of microneurosurgery. *J Neurosurg,* Vol. 112, No. 6, (Jun), pp. 1347, ISSN 1933-0693

21

Neurosurgical Management of Gliomas

Melissa C Werndle, Timothy L Jones and Marios C Papadopoulos
Academic Neurosurgery Unit, St. George's Hospital, London
United Kingdom

1. Introduction

Gliomas are the commonest brain tumours. They are tumours derived from the three most common glial cells, the astrocytes, oligodendrocytes and ependymal cells, with each cell type giving rise to its named tumour i.e. astrocytoma, oligodendroglioma and ependymoma. Other less abundant glial cells give rise to rarer tumours e.g. subependymal astrocytes leading to subependymoma. Table 1 summarises the different gliomas, their incidences and subtypes (Bigner et al, 1996; Han et al, 2010, Kozak & Moody, 2009; Louis et al, 2007). The grading depends on the number of histological features of malignancy such as cellular atypia, presence of mitoses, endothelial proliferation, and necrosis and is known as the World Health Organisation grade (WHO). For the astrocytomas, grade I has none, grade II has one feature, grade III (anaplastic astrocytoma) has two and grade IV (glioblastoma) has three or four. The majority of gliomas arise in the brain, with only a minority in the spinal cord.

Surgery for brain tumours is very different from surgery for peripheral tumours. The major difference is that brain tumours directly affect mental function. The effect on quality of life is therefore more pronounced than a peripheral tumour causing a physical disability in isolation. Unlike other major cancers such as breast, lung and colon where large advances have been made over the last twenty years (Office for National Statistics, 2010), little advance has been made with brain tumours. As a result, the mortality of patients with glioblastoma (grade IV astrocytoma) has not improved much over this period (Cancer Research UK, 2010; Erridge et al, 2011).

In this chapter we will consider surgery for gliomas. Surgery has a role to play in virtually all gliomas at some stage or another. The extent of surgery varies from a simple biopsy, to establish diagnosis, to a more radical attempt at complete removal. Although some surgical principles universally apply, in many cases management varies from country and country, and even from centre to centre e.g. treatment of an elderly person with glioblastoma may vary from palliative care with no treatment, to maximal debulking followed by radiotherapy and chemotherapy. Some of these decisions on how aggressive one should treat the patient depend not only on surgical accessibility of the lesion but also on family views, cultural values and of course cost and availability of resources for neurosurgery. Such life-death decisions are part of the daily routine of neurosurgical practice.

Prolonging life may be less important than maximising quality of life. Sometimes the two go hand in hand, however in other circumstances, the extra time gained by surgery may result in a life of misery spent in hospital feeling sick on drugs with questionable benefit.

Glial cell	Sub-category	WHO Grade	Variants	Epidemiology
Astrocyte	Pilocytic	1		M : F, 1.2:1 0.3/100,000
	Diffusely infiltrating	2	Protoplasmic Gemistocytic Fibrillary	M : F, 1:1 0.2/100,000
		3 (anaplastic)		M : F, 1.4:1 0.5/100,000
		4 (glioblastoma multiforme)	Giant cell Gliosarcoma	M : F, 1.6:1 2.6/100,000 1-2.5% GBM 1.8-2.5% GBM
	Rarer types Subependymal giant cell astrocytoma Pleomorphic xanthoastrocytoma Desmoplastic cerebral astrocytoma of infancy	1 1 1		M > F 0.51% gliomas, M = F Rare 1st 18/12 life Rare
Oligodendrocyte	Oligodendroglioma	2		M : F, 1.3:1 0.3/100,000
	Anaplastic oligodendroglioma	3		M : F, 1.5:1 0.1/100,000
Mixed	Oligoastrocytoma	2		M : F, 1.9:1 0.1/100,000
	Anaplastic oligoastrocytoma	3		
	Other mixed			
Ependymal cell	Ependymoma	2	Cellular, papillary, clear cell, tancytic	M : F, 1.3:1 0.2/100,000
	Anaplastic ependymoma	3		
	Myxopapillary ependymoma	1		M : F, 1.6:1 0.0/100,000
	Subependymoma	1		

Table 1. Classification of gliomas, grade and incidence

2. Preoperative management

In the United Kingdom, most patients present through Accident and Emergency. There are three main ways they present: with a focal neurological deficit; seizures; or with high intracranial pressure (this is often progressive, but may be sudden onset if the tumour bleeds into itself). These presenting symptoms and signs lead to CT/MR as an emergency, followed by referral to a neurosurgery unit. If brain oedema is evident on imaging, steroids are started.

2.1 Medications

Dexamethasone is preferred due to its low mineralocorticoid activity (hence little sodium and water retention). The mechanism of action of steroids remains unclear. Dexamethasone was introduced in 1960s following Gailicich's seminal paper on its use of alleviating oedema in brain tumours, and it revolutionised the outcome of surgery for brain tumours (Gailicich et al, 1961a, 1961b). The standard dose is 4mg four times a day given orally or intravenously, following a loading dose of 10mg, and an improvement in symptoms is often seen within a few hours (Kesari et al, 2002). If a patient has had a seizure due to their tumour, an antiepileptic should be given. Phenytoin is the preferred agent in the acute setting, although Carbamazepine may be better for focal seizures. Phenytoin elimination is via zero-order kinetics near the therapeutic level and approximately 90% is protein bound. A loading dose is required (18mg/kg intravenously), which must be given slowly to reduce risk of hypotension and arrhythmias (Meek et al, 1999). The daily dosage is usually 300mg once a day, and serum levels should be measured daily until a satisfactory level is achieved. The advantages of phenytoin are the fast acting nature and cheap cost. Disadvantages include potentially reduced cognitive function, hypersensitivity, megaloblastic anaemia and cerebellar degeneration. Phenytoin is teratogenic. Toxicity (which may develop at concentrations above 20µm/ml, but more commonly above 30µm/ml) manifests with cerebellar signs, confusion and CNS depression. Carbamazepine has a half-life of 20-55 hours. A low dose should be commenced and incremented slowly, with regular checks of haematological function due to its potential for marrow suppressive effects. Its main advantages are the low risk of cognitive and dysmorphic side effects. The main disadvantages are the unavailability of parenteral form and its metabolic autoinduction (Tudur Smith et al, 2002). We will not describe the various antiepileptics here and their advantages and disadvantages in detail.

2.2 Multidisciplinary team

In most centres, tumours are discussed in a neuro-oncology multi-disciplinary meeting (MDT) to determine the best way to proceed with treatment. If patients present as an emergency however, their surgical treatment should not be delayed by the MDT. If not an immediate emergency, patients with a new diagnosis of glioma can be managed in either the inpatient or outpatient setting. A more aggressive approach would be to admit the patient directly to the neurosurgical unit from the emergency department or the referring hospital, and to plan for surgery on that admission over the following days. A less aggressive approach would be to see the patient in the outpatient clinic, especially when a "watch and wait" policy is a reasonable option. It is important to note the patient should not wait too long to be seen in this setting. Often, little or no information is given to the patient from the referring doctors, causing significant anxiety.

2.3 Conventional imaging

The practice of imaging of brain tumours has evolved over the past 20 years from a strictly morphology-based discipline to one that encompasses function, physiology as well as anatomy. Imaging not only allows determination of the location and extent of tumour but also has a key role in primary diagnosis, biopsy target selection, guiding resection margins, radiotherapy planning and delineating of tumour from functionally important neural tissue. Following treatment, imaging is used to quantify treatment response and extent of residual tumour. At follow-up or in the pre-op monitoring of inoperable low-grade glioma, imaging helps to determine tumour progression and to differentiate recurrent tumour growth from treatment-induced tissue changes, such as radiation necrosis.

In the majority of cases, plain computed tomography (CT) scans are the first brain imaging studies performed when investigating patients with suspected brain tumour. This is because CT is widely available, fast, relatively risk-free, and well tolerated. It has the advantage of being sensitive in detecting acute haemorrhage, hydrocephalus and mass effect. If an abnormality is detected on plain CT then intravenous contrast is administered which allows assessment of blood brain barrier (BBB) integrity and delineation of contrast enhancing tumour border, if present. Due to its intrinsically low soft tissue contrast, CT is not optimally suited for detecting subtle changes in brain parenchyma or patterns of tumour infiltration (Ricci, 1999), even with the addition of intravenous contrast agent. CT is inferior to MRI in its soft tissue resolution, multi-planar capability and physiology-based applications. Finally, CT involves ionizing radiation and its iodinated contrast agent can cause allergic reaction (Cha, 2009).

Magnetic resonance imaging has become the standard of imaging patients with brain tumours (Jenkinson, 2007). MR techniques can be broadly classified into 'conventional' and 'advanced'. Conventional MRI provides qualitative images of normal anatomy and pathology, whilst advanced MR techniques allow quantitative and semi-quantitative measurement of cerebral blood flow, water movement and the chemical composition of the tissue under interrogation. It is these non-invasive methods of assessing tumour physiology that are becoming increasingly important in neuro-oncology decision making. In this section we will firstly introduce the characteristic glial tumour appearances on conventional MRI studies then discuss advanced imaging modalities, focusing on diffusion MR and its potential role in tumour diagnosis, delineation and treatment planning.

2.3.1 Pilocytic astrocytomas (PA), grade I

PA are slow growing, well circumscribed tumours. Their characteristic imaging appearance is of a cystic cerebellar mass with an enhancing mural nodule. They are located in the cerebellum in 60% of cases and optic nerve/chiasm in 30% (also adjacent to the third ventricle and brainstem). On plain CT, PA form discrete cystic or solid masses with little or no surrounding oedema. They contain calcium in 20% of cases, rarely haemorrhage and frequently present with obstructive hydrocephalus. Over 95% of PA enhance, but enhancement does not indicate malignancy. On T2 weighted and FLAIR MRI scans the solid portion is hyperintense to gray matter. Cystic portions are hyperintense to CSF. On T1 studies, the solid portion is iso/hyponetense to grey matter and there is intense hetereogeneous enhancement of the solid portion. The cyst wall occasionally enhances.

2.3.2 Diffuse astrocytoma (DA), grade II

Diffuse astrocytomas are typically focal or diffuse non-enhancing white matter lesions. Two thirds of DA are located in the cerebral hemispheres (of which 1/3 in the frontal lobe, 1/3 temporal lobe) and one third are located infratentorially (50% of brainstem gliomas are low grade astrocytomas). DA are tumours of the white matter with only 20% involving deep grey matter structures (thalamus or basal ganglia). They may be variable in size and are typically homogeneous lesions causing local cortical expansion and distortion of surrounding structures. Although they may appear to have a circumscribed edge on imaging studies, studies have revealed viable tumour cells are found beyond the image margin. Plain CT studies of DA reveal ill-defined hypo or iso dense lesions. Calcification is seen in 20% of cases and rarely intra-tumoural cysts. They do not typically enhance following the administration of contrast and the presence of enhancement is likely to indicate focal anaplastic transformation. Conventional MRI studies of DA (figure 1) identify homogeneous, lesions which expand white matter and adjacent cortex. They are typically hypointense on T1 weighted MR and hyperintense on T2 weighted and fluid attenuated inversion recovery (FLAIR) studies.

2.3.3 Oligodendroglioma (ODG), grade II

ODG is a well-differentiated, diffusely infiltrating tumour which typically involves subcortical white matter and cortex. 85% of ODG are supratentorially located and are most commonly seen in the frontal lobe however may also be present in temporal, parietal and occipital lobes, posterior fossa and within the ventricle (1-10%). They may be variable size and are most commonly of mixed density of plain CT with calcification seen in 70-90% of cases and cystic degeneration in 20%. Approximately 50% enhance following contrast administration on both CT and MRI. On T1-weighted MRI studies ODG are heterogeneous and hypo or isointense to grey matter. They are cortical and subcortically located and cause surrounding cortical expansion. They are hyperintense on T2/FLAIR. Anaplastic oligodendroglioma (AO), have similar appearances as ODG however will contain foci of malignant progression which may be seen as new contrast enhancement, necrosis, cystic change or haemorrhage.

2.3.4 Anaplastic astrocytoma (AA), grade III

In common with DA, anaplastic astrocytomas are infiltrating lesions predominantly involving white matter. AA are more commonly within the cerebral hemispheres (especially temporal lobes), they may be of variable size and may appear well-circumscribed however, as in DA, tumour cells are almost always found beyond the tumour border on imaging. On CT studies, AA are low density, ill-defined mass. They rarely contain calcification and the majority do not enhance (those that do display patchy foci of enhancement). On T1 weighted MR imaging they are mixed isointense to hypointense white matter lesions. They are heterogeneously hyperintense on T2 weighted and FLAIR MR. Evidence of ring enhancement, prominent flow voids and cysts may suggest progression of AA to more malignant forms.

2.3.5 Glioblastoma multiforme (GBM), grade IV

GBM are most commonly located in supratentorial white matter within the frontal, temporal and parietal lobes however may infiltrate across white matter pathways to involve contralateral cerebral hemisphere. They may be of variable size and morphology. Most frequently they are poorly marginated, diffusely infiltrating necrotic lesions, which in rare cases are multifocal or multicentric. GBM appear as irregular, isodense or hypodense lesions with central necrotic hypodensity on plain CT. They frequently exert significant local mass effect and have peri-tumoural oedema and tumour infiltration. Of all glial tumours, GBM are the most likely to contain haemorrhage. Conventional MRI of GBM (figure 2), reveal irregular iso or hypo intense masses on T1 weighted studies and heterogeneous hyperintense masses with adjacent oedema/tumour infiltration on T2 weighted/FLAIR MRI. GBM frequently contain a necrotic core, tumoural cysts, focal haemorrhage, and flow voids secondary to tumour neovascularity. GBM most commonly have thick irregular enhancing margins surrounding central necrosis however may exhibit solid, ring or patchy enhancement on gadolinium enhanced T1 weighted MRI.

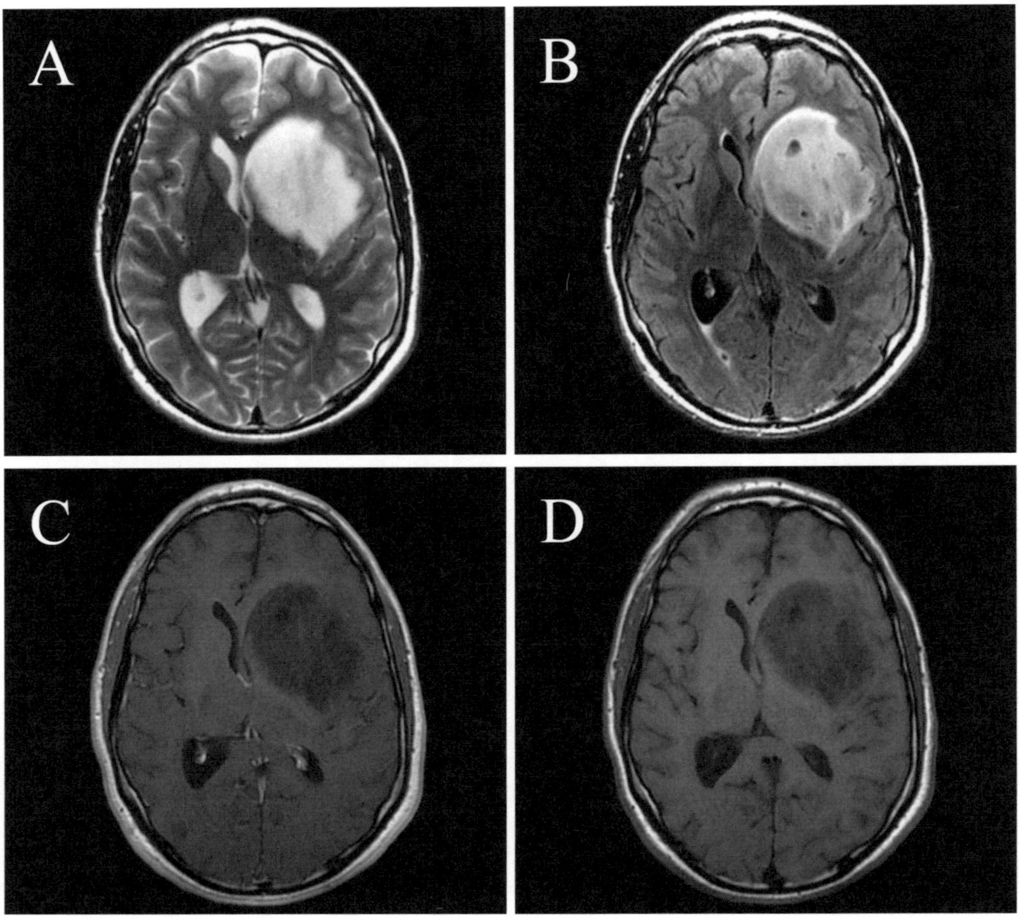

Fig. 1. MRI images of left fronto-temporal diffuse astrocytoma. A. T2-weighted image, B. Fluid attenuated inversion recovery (FLAIR) image, C. T1-weighted image following administration of 0.1 mmol/kg gadoterate meglumine, Dotarem®), D. T1-weighted image.

2.3.6 Ependymoma grade II or III

Ependymoma are slow growing tumours of ependymal cells, of which, 2 / 3 are infratentorially located (typically within the IVth ventricle) and 1 / 3 supratentorial (within periventricular white matter). They are of irregular shape, typically modelling to the shape of the ventricle or cistern. 50% of ependymomas calcify and they are heterogeneous lesions (iso or hypo inetense on T1 and T2 MRI) and display irregular degrees of enhancement.

2.3.7 Rare gliomas

Gliosarcoma (grade IV). Gliosarcomas are rare malignant neoplasms containing both glial and mesenchymal elements. Although their imaging appearances are often indistinguishable from GBM, they more commonly exhibit dural invasion and involvement of surrounding skull. In common with GBM, they infiltrate white matter and are typically supratentorially located however may have a discrete portion. They are heterogeneous masses with thick irregular enhancement on CT and share the features of GBM on conventional MRI, as a result gliosarcoma are frequently only identified following formal tumour histological analysis.

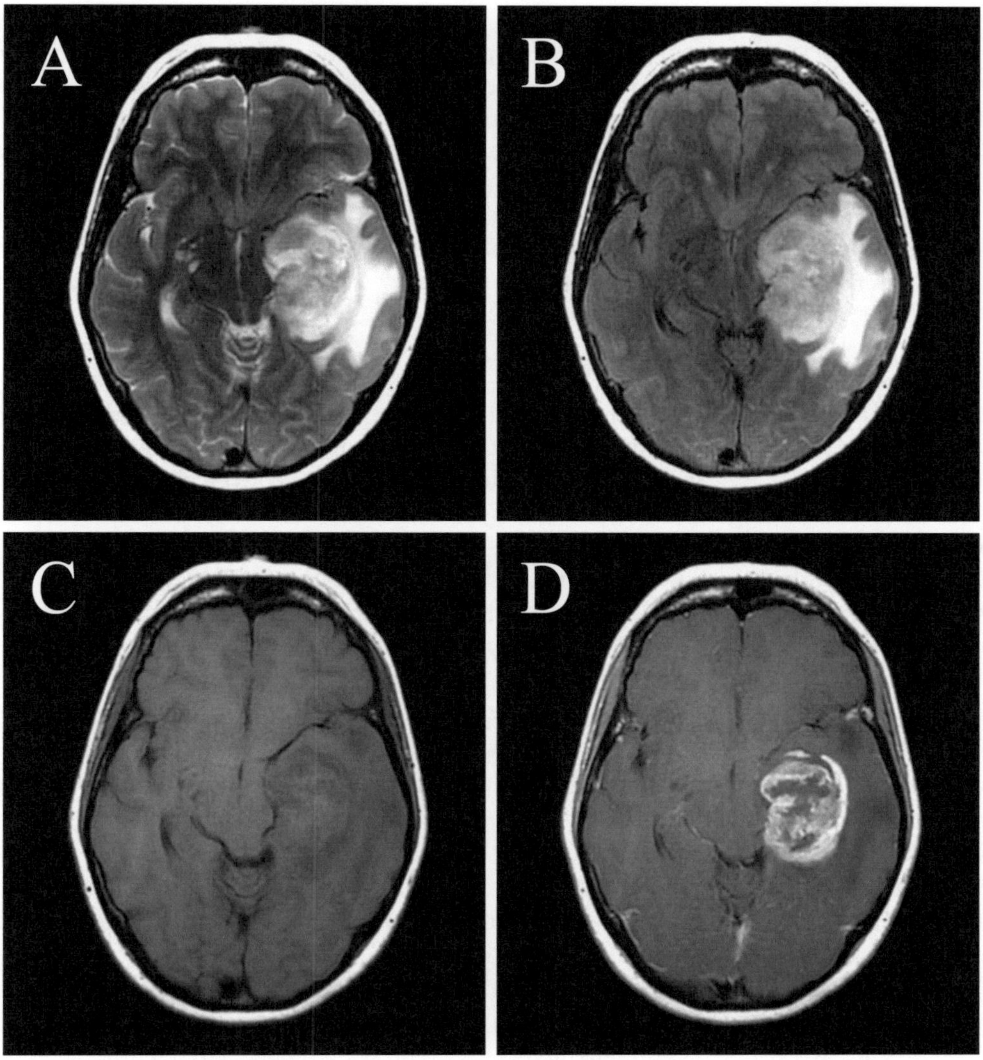

Fig. 2. MRI images of left temporal glioblastoma. A. T2-weighted image, B. Fluid attenuated inversion recovery (FLAIR) image, C. T1-weighted image, D. T1-weighted image following administration of 0.1 mmol/kg gadoterate meglumine, Dotarem®)

Gliomatosis cerebri (grade IV). Gliomatosis cerebri (GC), are diffusely infiltrating glioblastoma lesions involving two or more lobes of the brain and a frequently bilateral. Although they are typically hemispheric they may involve cortex in 19% of cases and as well as diffuse white matter may involve basal ganglia/thalami (75%), corpus callosum (50%), brainstem/spinal cord (10-15%) and cerebellum (10%). GC are infiltrative in nature, yet may preserve underlying brain architecture and cross the midline via corpus callosum or massa intermedia. GC may exhibit subtle asymmetric loss of grey-white differentiation and mild mass effect on plain CT and do not typically enhance (focal enhancement may indicate malignant progression or a focus of anaplastic change). They are iso or hypo intense on T1 weighted MR and homogenously hyperintense on T2-weighted/FLAIR MRI.

Pleomorphic xanthoastrocytoma (PXA), grade II. PXA are a distinct type of benign, supratentorial (98% of cases), astrocytoma affecting young adults. Their characteristic feature is of a cortical mass with adjacent enhancing dural 'tail' with an associated tumour cyst (50-60% of cases) and mural nodule. They are most commonly seen in the temporal lobe and may be of variable size. Despite their circumscribed appearance they often infiltrate into brain. On CT, PXAs are hypodense with a mixed density nodule, they have minimal surrounding oedema and typically avidly enhance. On T1 weighted MRI, they are hypo or isointense to surrounding grey matter and enhance following administration of gadolinium. The solid portion is hyperintense or of mixed signal intensity on T2-weight or FLAIR studies. Any cystic portions are isointense to CSF.

2.4 Advanced imaging

Despite its superb soft tissue contrast, multi-planar capability and non-invasive nature, conventional MRI is largely limited to depicting morphological abnormalities. Different disease processes can appear similar on anatomic imaging, and conversely a disease entity may have varied imaging findings. The underlying metabolic or functional integrity of brain cannot be adequately evaluated on anatomical MRI alone. To that end, several physiology-based MRI methods have been developed to improve tumour characterisation including spectroscopy, radionuclide imaging (PET and SPECT), dynamic susceptibility contrast MRI, blood oxygen level dependent (BOLD) MRI and diffusion imaging.

2.4.1 Magnetic resonance spectroscopy (MRS)

Proton MRS can be used to non-invasively evaluate the biochemical structure of tumour tissue and has been used as an adjunct to conventional MRI to diagnose 'likely' tumour grade prior to surgery, guide stereotactic biopsy, plan radiotherapy margins and differentiate radiation necrosis from tumour recurrence. Spectroscopy signals are either localised from a single selected voxel or from multiple voxels (also known as chemical shift imaging). Proton spectra reveal varying peaks at defined resonant frequencies. The commonest peaks studied in brain tumours are:

i. N-acetyl aspartate (NAA): reduced in disorders resulting in axonal loss therefore considered a surrogate marker of integrity of the neurone.
ii. Choline (cho): choline compounds involved in breakdown and manufacture of cellular membranes. Choline increases with membrane turnover.
iii. Creatine (Cr): involved in energy metabolism (ATP synthesis)
iv. Lipid: not normally seen in brain. Their presence indicates membrane breakdown and necrosis.

v. Lactate: levels increase in situations of anaerobic glycolysis

Glial tumours have a reduced NAA/Cr ratio and spectroscopic profiles such as high lactate and lipids are indicative of malignant tumour. Tumour cell density may be reflected by the magnitude of choline peak and choline:NAA ratio. MRS is useful in distinguishing neoplastic from non-neoplastic lesions however owing to the lack of reproducible 'metabolite profiles' of glial tumour subtypes, its role in routine diagnosis has yet to be elucidated.

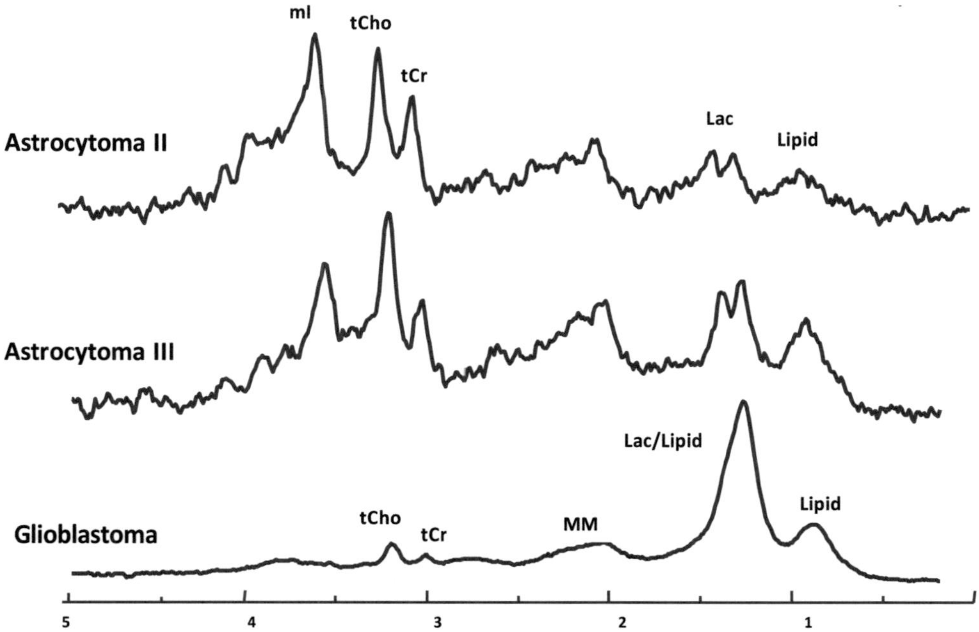

Fig. 3. Characteristic spectroscopic profiles of glial tumours. Choline (tCho) is considered a marker of tumour cell membrane proliferation and is seen to increase with tumour grade. Similarly an inverse relationship between NAA/Cr and Cho/Cr ratio and tumour grade may be used to differentiate high grade from low grade glioma. Higher lipid levels are seen in GBM, presumably a result of necrosis. Higher lactate levels with higher grades.

2.4.2 Diffusion imaging

The development of MR pulse sequences sensitised to the movement of water molecules has enabled visualisation and mathematical characterisation of the magnitude and direction of water diffusion within the brain. Diffusion weighted imaging was introduced into routine practice in the 1990s, and generation of maps of apparent diffusion coefficient (ADC) have been used to differentiate cystic lesions (arachnoid from epidermoid cysts) and abscess from tumour. Numerous studies have been performed to characterise the glial tumour environment using ADC values which are affected by both the extent of local vasogenic oedema and the degree of tumour cellularity. Despite several studies confirming a correlation between celularity and ADC, a tumour-specific DWI profile has not been identified. The underlying assumption of DWI is that water diffusion occurs in all directions (i.e. is isotropic). Investigators proposed that diffusion is likely to be restricted and directional (anisotropic) due to the influence of local intra and extra cellular structures such as white matter fibres and myelin sheaths. Mathematical determination of the resultant diffusion ellipsoid requires the use of a tensor, which contains information about the magnitude and principal directionality of diffusion on a voxel scale. This information has enabled calculation of rotationally invariant indices such as mean diffusivity (MD) and fractional anisotropy (FA) as measures of isotropic and anisotropic diffusion respectively. These metrics have been applied to a range of intracranial pathology and studies have revealed relationships between FA and tumour cell density and have attempted to characterise the peri-tumoural oedema of low and high-grade glioma yet this has yet to be used routinely in clinical practice. The most promising role for diffusion tensor imaging in glial surgery is its application in tractography. Use of this technique has allowed:

i. Definition of the anatomical relationship of a tumour to local white matter pathways, which may be incorporated on to image guidance systems to guide the surgical approach intra-operatively.
ii. Evaluation of whether there is displacement, invasion or destruction of surrounding white matter tracts by tumour.
iii. Knowledge of location of white matter tracts may assist intraoperative fibre stimulation and guide extent of resection
iv. Evidence of intact pathways following surgery may predict motor deficits and recovery.

Although the strong similarity between generated white matter structures using DTI tractography and post mortem anatomical dissection, the technique is unable to accurately define the anatomy of individual axons and may be complicated by crossing fibres thus, at present, it role is primarily for macroscopic delineation of tract configuration.

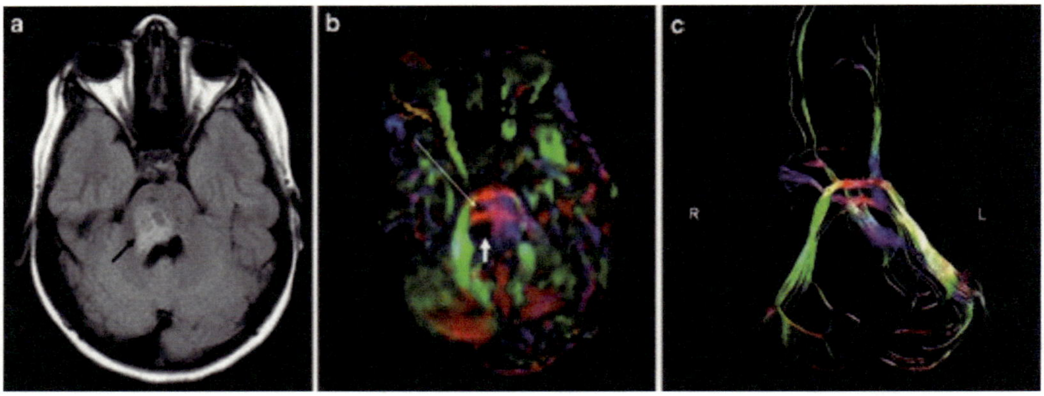

Fig. 4. A 6-year-old child with tumor arising from the brainstem. *a* Axial FLAIR image shows a tumor within the right middle cerebellar peduncle (*arrow*). *b* Axial color map shows loss of anisotropy within the right medial lemniscus resulting in lack of blue (*short arrow*). The right corticospinal tract (*long arrow*) is attenuated and has diminished anisotropy. *C* Coronal image derived from tractography shows leftward displacement of the right corticospinal tract (Rollins, 2007).

3. Common brain gliomas – surgical management

3.1 Glioblastoma multiforme (grade IV)/ anaplastic astrocytoma (grade III)

Grade III and grade IV astrocytomas are also called high-grade tumours. If the patient is young and the tumour "resectable," the primary aim is to remove as much as possible. The greater the extent of tumour removed, the better the time to tumour progression and survival (Keles et al, 1999). Surgery not only prolongs life, but also improves quality of life and the effectiveness of adjuvant therapy (Abrudan et al, 2011, Kiwit et al, 1996; Ryken et al, 2008). When considering surgery, three of the most important prognostic factors for surgeons are the patient age, the tumour grade and the patient's performance status (Karnofsky score) at presentation (Buckner, 2003; Wu et al, 2010). Each is an independent factor for survival; favouring survival is younger patient age, Karnovsky score ≥ 70 (meaning independence) and lower tumour grade. Tumour resectability predominantly refers to the tumour location and the ability to remove the tumour without leaving the patient dead or moribund. Superficial, non-eloquent lesions (e.g. non dominant frontal) are considered highly resectable. Non-resectable lesions include deep, eloquent brain e.g. brainstem gliomas. Another subset that fall under the non-resectable lesions are butterfly gliomas, so called due to their characteristic radiological appearances based around the corpus callosum, extending bifrontally. These often occur in elderly patients and treatment is usually biopsy alone. Prognosis is dismal (Agrawal, 2009).

Surgery is simple in most cases, the aim is to remove as much tumour as possible without causing damage to brain. A craniotomy is performed at the required location, followed by debulking of the tumour with suction and/ or Cavitron Ultrasonic Surgical Aspirator (CUSA). Suction pulls on surrounding brain tissue, CUSA advantageously does not. High-grade tumours are highly vascular, and may bleed substantially during surgery. It is common to encounter necrosis and thrombosed vessels intraoperatively. This is surgical evidence of a high-grade lesion. With substantial bleeding, it is important to continue resecting, as once the tumour and associated abnormal blood vessels are removed, the bleeding will stop. Do not fall into the trap of stopping every few seconds to assess and coagulate as this will take too long, will increase blood loss and will probably result in less tumour removed. The tumour often feels tougher than brain, and any cystic components have a characteristic straw coloured fluid. Surgical judgement (from feel and experience) is required to know when to stop resecting. These are diffuse tumours and therefore there is no clear margin. There is a continuum from what is all tumour to more and more percentage of brain mixed with tumour, and when to stop depends also on the eloquence of adjacent brain. At the end of the operation, haemostasis is imperative. This is achieved with a combination of coagulation, Surgicel, and woolly balls. Surgicel and woolly balls will only stop venous bleeding. We always ask the anaesthetist to increase the patient's blood pressure to normal before closing. Any arteries in spasm will then begin to bleed. It is obviously important to know this before closing, so that we coagulate rather than ignore any unaddressed bleeding to avoid postoperative haematoma! Once we are satisfied the operative field is dry, we close up and the operation is finished (Schmidek, 2005; Slacman M, 1996).

Some centres operate on high-grade tumours awake. The patient is anaesthetised for the skin incision and craniotomy parts. The patient is woken once the brain and tumour is exposed. This allows the surgeon to maximise tumour resection without causing a disabling neurological deficit. Awake surgery is not widely accepted for GBM and anaplastic astrocytoma due to their aggressive and infiltrative nature. Although there is well-documented evidence of a significant difference in outlook between a small biopsy vs. extensive resection (Arudan et al, 2011; Keles et al, 1999; Ryken et al, 2008) there is probably little to be gained in outlook between extensive resection versus achieving another small percentage resection with awake surgery.

Recently, some surgeons advocated the intraoperative use of fluorescent dye, 5-aminolevulinic acid (5-ALA), although currently this is not widely used. 5-ALA is a natural biochemical precursor of haemoglobin, which results in accumulation of porphyrins within malignant glioma tissue. Its selective intratumoural synthesis enables an accurate delineation of the tumour boundary, seen via a modified neuromicroscope. 5-ALA has been shown to improve gross total resection defined by early post operative MRI, as well as improve 6 month progression free survival (Stummer et al, 2006).

Neuronavigation (e.g. Stealth, see figure 5) is another aid to glioma surgery. This utilises preoperative CT and/or MRI images to map the patient's anatomy in a 3-dimensional configuration, calibrated using specific landmarks on the patient. It can be used to map the bone flap and to guide debulking of the abnormal tissue. The main disadvantage of this widely used technique is that the brain moves once the skull and meninges are opened, thus diminishing the accuracy of the neuronavigation (Warnick & Bath, 2002). Newer techniques include the use of intraoperative ultrasound. This allows for an updated picture on each application of the ultrasound wand, and therefore corrects for any intraoperative brain shift with almost realtime information on the tumour location and extent. The financial cost of this is high.

If a tumour is deemed unresectable but there has been an agreement to give adjuvant treatment, a biopsy is required for histological confirmation of grade. This can be performed either Stealth or stereotactic guided. The former is frameless, the latter is a frame guided system. Both yield a similar diagnostic accuracy with similar complication rates (Doward et al, 2002). Grade III glioma treatment is the same as for grade IV, including maximal resection if possible followed by radiotherapy and temozolomide. PCV chemotherapy (procarbazine, lomustine and vincristine) is used as a second line (Theeler & Groves, 2011).

3.1.1 Other considerations in high grade gliomas

Gliadel wafers. These are made by MGI pharma, Inc and contain polifeprosan 20 with carmustine implant, an alkylating agent used for brain and bone marrow tumours. Their use at the time of surgery improves survival in good performance status patients (Karnovsky $\geq$ 70) by 2.5 months compared to placebo. There is no survival benefit in recurrent high-grade glioma. The main side effects are cerebral infections, CSF leak, cerebral oedema and healing abnormalities, and this is why not everyone uses them (Hart et al, 2011).

Temozolamide. Temozolomide is used routinely as adjuvant chemotherapy for high grades. It improves survival and time to progression, without any increase in adverse events. Tumour tissue is analysed for O-6-methylguanine-DNA methyltransferase (MGMT) expression, as this enzyme diminishes the therapeutic efficacy and thus these patients receive little benefit from temozolamide (Theeler, 2011).

New treatments. *Bevacizumab* is a humanised monoclonal antibody against vascular endothelial growth factor (VEGF), necessary for tumour angiogenesis. Although there is no level 1 evidence yet, there have been impressive results of progression free survival in some cases in patients with recurrent high grade glioma (Iwamoto & Fine, 2010; Friedman et al, 2009). With the advent of new treatments beginning to improve outcome, this raises questions about reoperation for high grade gliomas. This is a controversial topic, with views across the spectrum. The advantages of reoperation are (i) it has been shown to extend survival compared with medical treatment alone and (ii) it allows for direct local delivery of chemotherapeutic agents. The disadvantages of reoperation are more time spent in hospital, and increased risk of complications, which may outweigh a potential survival benefit. (Brandes et al, 1999; Niyazi et al, 2011). Given that oncologists have more treatments to give after reoperation, perhaps we should be considering a larger role for surgery and redebulking in recurrent high-grade glioma.

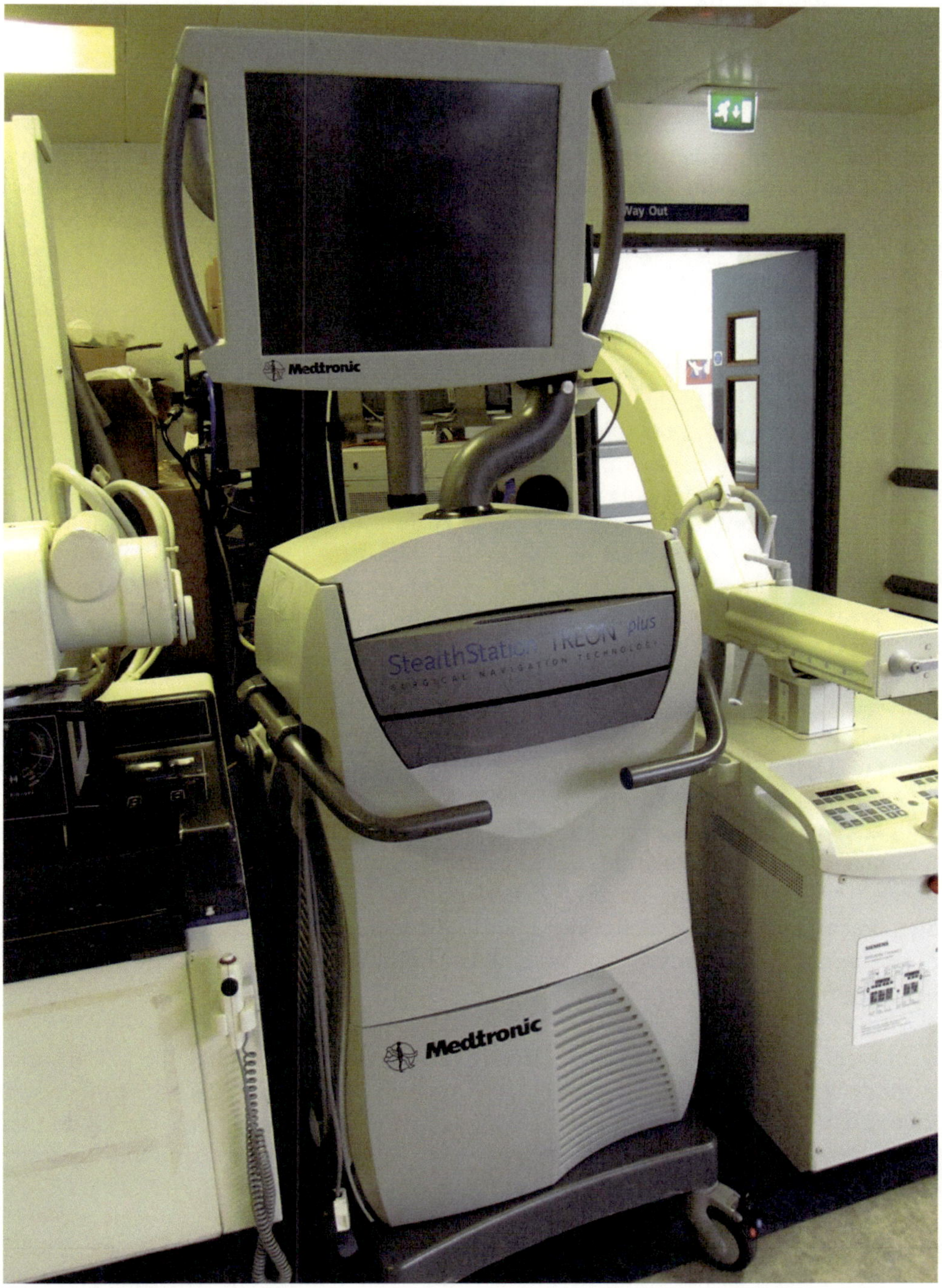

Fig. 5. Neuronavigation Stealth.

Glioblastoma subtypes. Gliosarcoma may metastasise extracranially. There are distinct gross macroscopic features described: a firm, well circumscribed lesion; and an infiltrative poorly defined lesion. Treatment and prognosis is similar as for GBM (Han et al, 2010). Giant cell GBM, another rare subtype, is treated in a similar fashion. Data suggests prognosis may be better in this subgroup compared to GBMs as a whole, especially considering long term survival (Kozak & Moody, 2009).

3.2 Grade II astrocytomas and oligoastrocytomas

There is no gold standard of treatment and management is controversial ranging from a wait and see policy with serial imaging, to biopsy, to maximal debulking. The role and timing of adjuvant radiotherapy and chemotherapy is also unclear, and is currently being investigated. There are 5 prognostic features which indicate a high risk low grade gliomas: astrocytoma histology, age over 40 years, tumours over 6cm, tumour crossing the midline, and presence of a neurological deficit. Some surgeons advocate resection followed by radiotherapy for these high risk patients (Pignatti et al, 2002; Ruiz & Lesser, 2009).
Awake surgery is well-established for low grade gliomas. The patient undergoes a general anaesthetic for the craniotomy, and is woken when the tumour is exposed. The anaesthetist runs through relevant tests of speech or motor function whilst the gyri adjacent to the tumour are stimulated to map the sensorimotor cortex. It is evident if eloquent brain is involved, as the patient may transiently become dysphasic, develop a motor weakness or experience a sensation down a limb. The surgeon is therefore able to map and avoid resection of this eloquent brain. The patient must be able to understand the procedure and tolerate surgery awake; the patient must be able to cooperate; the tumour should be close to eloquent motor or speech areas which can be tested adequately intraoperatively by stimulation and testing function; the patient must be a suitable candidate for and has consented to adjuvant treatment, as awake surgery in itself would otherwise be ineffective; at least 90% tumour resection is anticipated. There have only been two small prospective randomised controlled studies directly comparing awake versus asleep craniotomy for intrinsic brain lesions. There appears to be no difference in outcome at 3 and 6 months (Ali et al, 2009; Gupta et al, 2007). However the long term results, which are more important, are not known.
Intraoperatively low-grade tumours can look and feel almost like normal brain. A slight discolouration may indicate tumour or brain swelling and it is often difficult to differentiate between the two. Again, surgical experience is required to judge when to stop. Intraoperative MRI is a tool aimed at maximising tumour resection. Although intraoperatine MRI has been shown to improve the percentage of tumour resected, its use can be very time-consuming and there is currently no data available to show improved survival benefit (Senft et al, 2010).
The different histological subtypes of grade II gliomas are described in table 1. The variants are not prognostically important, except the gemistocytic subtype (Greek word meaning stuffed cells). These tumours behave more aggressively than their grade suggests and most oncologists will therefore treat these patients with radiotherapy and chemotherapy upfront (Krouwer et al, 1991).

3.3 Grade I pilocytic astrocytoma

These often benign lesions comprise of a cyst and solid component. The solid component often enhances, and, is the exception to the rule, in that enhancement enhancement does not mean malignancy. They are found mostly in children and occasionally in young adults, and are located most commonly in the posterior fossa. Pilocytic astrocytoma is not a diffuse tumour. Supratentorial pilocytic astrocytomas tend to be more aggressive. Pilocytic is a Greek word meaning "hairlike," so called due the appearance of the cells under a microscope. An important surgical point to note is that the cyst wall is not part of the tumour. Attempted maximal resectionof the solid component is often curative without the need for other treatment. If there is complete removal in infratentorial lesions, there is no need for long term follow up however the presence of worrying features eg supratentorial, or evidence of growth, serial MR are recommended (Fernandez et al, 2003; Krieger et al, 1997).

3.4 Rare grade I gliomas: Pleomorphic xanthoastrocytoma, desmoplastic cerebral astrocytoma of infancy and subependymal giant cell astrocytoma (SEGA)

Pleomorphic xanthoastrocytomas are most often benign tumours that tend to present in patients under the age of 30, with seizures in the majority of cases. Intraoperatively they are often well defined and in close meningeal contact (Van Rooset et al, 1996). Desmoplastic astrocytoma of infancy is a rare subtype that presents as a large hemispheric mass in infants. Radiological features are typically of a large enhancing mass with a peripheral dural based component and a central cystic component. Despite worrisome features, these tumours respond to gross total resection and prognosis is generally favourable (Serra et al, 1996; Uro-Coste et al, 2010). Subependymal giant cell astrocytomas (SEGA), part of the Tuberous Sclerosis complex, are slow growing, benign intraventricular lesions. Historically, surgical resection has been advocated however medical treatment with the mTor inhibitor Everolimus has been shown to reduce tumour size with good seizure control, and may become the hallmark of treatment for these tumours (Krueger et al, 2010; Sharma et al, 2004).

3.5 Oligodendroglioma

These WHO grade II lesions tend to be more benign, and have characteristic appearances of intralesional calcification on CT. Extensive resection followed by a watch and wait policy is an accepted treatment. 1p19q codeletion is a predictor of chemosensitivity and of improved prognosis in these tumours (Thiessen et al, 2003). Anaplastic variants should have adjuvant chemo/radiotherapy (Quon & Abdulkarim, 2008).

3.6 Ependymoma

These tumours are located predominantly in the posterior fossa and commonly present with obstructive hydrocephalus. Treatment is surgical resection followed by radiotherapy (Reni et al, 2007; Stuben et al, 1997). Subependymomas are slow-growing, benign lesions typically found in the ventricular system and may remain asymptomatic throughout life. They are well defined radiologically with little or no enhancement. Given their indolent nature, surgery should err on the side of caution i.e. on leaving tumour behind rather than causing a neurological deficit (Ragel et al, 2006).

4. Spinal cord gliomas

Primary malignant spinal cord gliomas are rare, occurring in 0.12 per 100,000 population, with an increase in ependymomas over the past three decades (Hsu et al, 2011). They usually present with progressive symptoms of numbness and tingling and loss of power.

Pain tends to be a prominent presenting feature, its nature of which is constant and poorly localised waking the patient at night, and it often precedes any neurological symptoms. Back pain that wakes the patient up at night without local tenderness is most often caused by an intrinsic tumour, ependymoma or astrocytoma. The signs are of a progressive myelopathy and may lead to a rapid quadri/paraparesis

The most common tumour type is ependymoma, followed by astrocytoma. There are characteristic MRI radiological appearances, which include an intrinsic expansive cord lesion with variable contrast enhancement, and often cystic components. Surgery is the first line treatment in ependymomas, with enbloc resection and primary dural closure if possible. CUSA is employed for resection, as well as the microscope. Gross total resection is associated with a high complication rate but good outcome and low recurrence rates. Extent of resection depends on how stuck the tumour is. Complete resection is only possible if located at the conus and not stuck, or at filum terminale. If stuck at the conus, tumour should be left behind to avoid disabling complications. Although not radiosensitive or chemosensitive, patients can go on for many years without any deterioration. Overall progression free survival is 89% and 84% at 5 and 10 years respectively (Kucia et al, 2010). Tumours are technically more difficult if higher than conus medullaris, although it still may be possible to remove completely. Intraoperative use of somatosensory evoked potentials and motor evoked potentials can help predict and even prevent post operative neurological deficit, although they may add to length of operation (Kearse et al, 1993; Kelleher et al, 2008). Low-grade astrocytomas are less curable with approximately 50% gross total resection and favourable survival outcome. Little is known about them as they are rare (Benes et al, 2009; Nakamura et al, 2008). High-grade spinal cord tumours (grade III astrocytomas and glioblastoma multiforme) carry a far worse prognosis. Given the rare nature of these tumours, actual outcome is again not known, and no centre has extensive experience. Retrospective studies have shown gross total resection is rarely possible, and most patients die of disease progression. Mean survival is quoted at 6 - 19 months for grade III and IV spinal cord gliomas. Therefore these tumours are probably just as lethal as their brain counterparts (Cohen et al, 1989; McGirt et al, 2008; Raco et al, 2010). Treatment is the same with debulking, radiotherapy and temozolomide, but often an extensive debulking as with brain GBM is not possible, and the maximum amount of targeted radiotherapy is also less than with brain GBM. For these two reasons - less debulking, less radiotherapy - the outcome of spinal cord GBM is probably worse than the outcome of brain GBM. One intriguing possibility that has yet to be explored is to remove the tumour en block with a margin of cord above and below. Obviously this would only be possible in thoracic region, and in a patient with no neurological function below the level of tumour. The theoretical advantage would be improved survival benefit. A theoretical disadvantage would be to convert a spastic paraplegia to a flaccid one.

5. Paediatric gliomas

Malignant non brain stem gliomas represent 8-10% of paediatric CNS tumours (Hargrave 2009). It is likely the molecular biology of childhood GBM is similar to that of adult GBM, however this is not as well described in the paediatric population. They are usually located supratentorially, but unlike adults, high grade gliomas are significantly less common than low grades (Pollack, 1994). As is adults, these are treated with maximal surgical resection followed by chemo/radiotherapy (Sposto et al, 1989). Diffuse intrinsic brain stem gliomas constitute 15-

20% of all CNS tumours in children, and are their main cause of death (Hargrave et al. 2006). These have characteristic radiological appearances that expand the brainstem with an epicentre situated in the pons. They do not benefit from biopsy and radical surgery is impossible. In exophytic and focal brain stem gliomas, however, surgery is the treatment of choice with radiotherapy reserved for recurrence. The prognosis is better, with 90% alive at 2 years, compared to 25% alive at 2 years in the diffuse group (Mauffrey, 2006).

6. Conclusion

In this Chapter we discussed the commonest types of brain tumour, the gliomas. Surgery is an important aspect of the management of these tumours but the extent of surgical involvement remains controversial. Unfortunately little progress has been made in this field over the last 20 years such that the outlook of patients with gliomas has not substantially improved over this period.

7. References

Abrudan C, Cocis A, Dana. (2011). Surgery of high grade gliomas - pros in favor of maximal cytoreductive surgery. *Romanian Neurosurgery*, Vol. 1, pp. 38-53.

Agrawal A. (2009). Butterfly glioma of the corpus callosum. *J Cancer Res Ther.* Vol. 5, No. 1, pp. 43-5.

Ali MZ, Fadel NA, Abouldahab HA. (2009). Awake craniotomy versus general anesthesia for managing eloquent cortex low-grade gliomas. *Neurosciences* (Riyadh). Vol. 14, No. 3, pp. 263-72.

Benes V 3rd, Barsa P, Benes V Jr, Suchomel P. (2009). Prognostic factors in intramedullary astrocytomas: a literature review. *Eur Spine J.* Vol. 18, No. 10, pp. 1397-422.

Bigner DD, Mclendon RE, Bauer JM. (Eds.). (1996). *Russell and Rubinstein Pathology of Tumors of the Nervous System.* Arnold, 9780340810071, London.

Brandes AA, Vastola F, Monfardini S. (1999). Reoperation in recurrent high-grade gliomas: literature review of prognostic factors and outcome. *Am J Clin Oncol.* Vol. 22, No. 4, pp. 387-90.

Buckner JC. (2003). Factors influencing survival in high-grade gliomas. *Semin Oncol*, Vol. 30, No. 6/19, pp. 10-4.

Cancer research UK. (2009). *Brain and central nervous system cancer survival statistics.*

http://info.cancerresearchuk.org/cancerstats/types/brain/survival/, accessed 26 April 2011.

Cohen AR, Wisoff JH, Allen JC, Epstein F. (1989). Malignant astrocytomas of the spinal cord. *J Neurosurg*, Vol. 70, pp. 50–54.

Dorward NL, Paleologos TS, Alberti O, Thomas DG. (2002). The advantages of frameless stereotactic biopsy over frame-based biopsy. *Br J Neurosurg*,Vol.16, No. 2, pp. 110-8.

Erridge SC, Hart MG, Kerr GR, Smith C, McNamara S, Grant R, Gregor A, Whittle IR. (2011). Trends in classification, referral and treatment and the effect on outcome of patients with glioma: a 20 year cohort. *J Neurooncol*. Mar 8. [Epub ahead of print]

Fernandez C, Figarella-Branger D, Girard N, Bouvier-Labit C, Gouvernet J, Paz Paredes A, Lena G. Pilocytic astrocytomas in children: prognostic factors--a retrospective study of 80 cases. (2003). *Neurosurgery*. Vol. 53, No. 3, pp. 544-53; discussion 554-5.

Friedman HS, Prados MD, Wen PY, Mikkelsen T, Schiff D, Abrey LE, Yung WK, Paleologos N, Nicholas MK, Jensen R, Vredenburgh J, Huang J, Zheng M, Cloughesy T. (2009).

Bevacizumab alone and in combination With irinotecan in recurrent glioblastoma. *J Clin Oncol*, Vol. 27 No. 28, pp. 4733–40.

Galicich JH, French LA, Melby JC. (1961). Use of dexamethasone in the treatment of cerebral edema associated with brain tumors. *J Lancet*. Vol. 81, pp. 46-53.

Galicich JH, French LA. (1961). Use of dexamethasone in the treatment of cerebral edema resulting from brain tumors and brain surgery. *Am Pract Dig Treat*. Vol. 12, pp. 169-74.

Gupta DK, Chandra PS, Ojha BK, Sharma BS, Mahapatra AK and Mehta VS. (2007). Awake craniotomy versus surgery under general anesthesia for resection of intrinsic lesions of eloquent cortex—A prospective randomised study. *Clinical Neurology and Neurosurgery*, Vol. 109, No. 4, pp. 335-343.

Han SJ, Yang I, Tihan T,Prados MD, and Parsa AT. (2010). Primary gliosarcoma: key clinical and pathologic distinctions from glioblastoma with implications as a unique oncologic entity. *Neurooncol*, Vol. 96, No.3, pp. 313-320.

Hargrave D, Bartels U, Bouffet E. (2006). Diffuse brainstem glioma in children: critical review of clinical trials. *Lancet Oncol*. Vol. 7, No. 3, pp. 241-8.

Hargrave D. Paediatric high and low grade glioma: the impact of tumour biology on current and future therapy. (2009). *Br J Neurosurg*, Vol. 23, No. 4, pp.351-363.

Hart MG, Grant R, Garside R, Rogers G, Somerville M, Stein K. (2011). Chemotherapy wafers for high grade glioma. *Cochrane Database Syst Rev*. 6;3:CD007294. Review.

Hsu S, Quattrone M, Ostrom Q, Ryken TC, Sloan AE, Barnholtz-Sloan JS. (2011). Incidence patterns for primary malignant spinal cord gliomas: a Surveillance, Epidemiology, and End Results study. *J Neurosurg Spine*. Mar 11. [Epub ahead of print]

Iwamoto FM, Fine HA. (2010). Bevacizumab for malignant gliomas. *Arch Neurol*, Vol. 67, No. 3, pp. 285–8.

Jenkinson MD, Du Plessis DG, Walker C, Smith TS. (2007). Advanced MRI in the management of adult gliomas. *Br J Neurosurg*, Vol. 21, No. 6, pp. 550-561.

Kearse LA Jr, Lopez-Bresnahan M, McPeck K, Tambe V. (1993). Loss of somatosensory evoked potentials during intramedullary spinal cord surgery predicts postoperative neurologic deficits in motor function. *J Clin Anesth*. Vol. 5, No. 5, pp. 392-8.

Keles GE, Anderson B, Brerger MS. (1999). The effect of extent of resection on time to tumour progression and survival in patients with GBM of the cerebral hemisphere. *Surg neurol*, Vol. 52, pp. 371-9.

Kelleher MO, Tan G, Sarjeant R, Fehlings MG. (2008). Predictive value of intraoperative neurophysiological monitoring during cervical spine surgery: a prospective analysis of 1055 consecutive patients. *J Neurosurg Spine*. Vol. 8, No. 3, pp. 215-21.

Kesari S, Paleologos NA, Vick NA. (2002). Corticosteroids in neurooncology. In: *Cancer neurology in clinical practice*, Schiff D, Wen PY (Eds.), pp. 47-56, Humana Press, 0896039226, New Jersey.

Kiwit JC, Floeth FW, Bock WJ. (1996). Survival in malignant glioma: analysis of prognostic factors with special regard to cytoreductive surgery. *Zentralbl Neurochir*, Vol. 57, No.2, pp. 76–88.

Kozak KR and Moody JS. (2009). Giant cell glioblastoma: A glioblastoma subtype with distinct epidemiology and superior prognosis. *Neurooncol*, Vol. 11, No.6, pp. 833–841.

Krieger MD, Gonzalez-Gomez I, Levy ML, McComb JG. (1997). Recurrence patterns and anaplastic change in a long-term study of pilocytic astrocytomas. *Pediatr Neurosurg*. Vol. 27, No. 1, pp. 1-11.

Krouwer HG, Davis RL, Silver P, Prados M. (1991). Gemistocytic astrocytomas: a reappraisal. *J Neurosurg*. Vol. 74, No. 3, pp. 399-406.

Krueger DA, Care MM, Holland K, Agricola K, Tudor C, Mangeshkar P, Wilson KA, Byars A, Sahmoud T, Franz DN. (2010). Everolimus for Subependymal Giant-Cell Astrocytomas in Tuberous Sclerosis. *N Engl J Med*, Vol. 363, pp. 1801-1811.

Kucia EJ, Bambakidis NC, Chang SW, Spetzler RF. (2010). Surgical technique and outcomes in the treatment of spinal cord ependymomas Part I. Intramedullary ependymomas. *Neurosurgery*. Vol. 68, No. 1, pp. 57-63.

Louis DN, Ohgaki H, Wiestler OD, Cavenee WK. (Eds.). (2007). *WHO Classification of tumours of the central nervous system*. IARC, 9789283224303, Lyon.

Mauffrey C. (2006). Paediatric brainstem gliomas: Prognostic factors and management *Journal of Clinical Neuroscience*, Vol. 13, No. 4, pp. 431-437

McGirt MJ, Goldstein IM, Chaichana KL, Tobias ME, Kothbauer KF, Jallo GI. (2008). Extent of surgical resection of malignant astrocytomas of the spinal cord: outcome analysis of 35 patients. *Neurosurgery*. Vol. 63, No. 1, pp. 55-60; discussion 60-1.

Meek PD, Davis SN, Collins DM, Gidal BE, Rutecki PA, Burstein AH, Fischer JH, Leppik IE, Ramsay RE. (1999). Guidelines for nonemergency use of parenteral phenytoin products: proceedings of an expert panel consensus process. Panel on Nonemergency Use of Parenteral Phenytoin Products. *Arch Intern Med*. Vol. 159, No. 22, pp. 2639-44.

Nakamura M, Ishii K, Watanabe K, Tsuji T, Takaishi H, Matsumoto M, Toyama Y, Chiba K. (2008). Surgical treatment of intramedullary spinal cord tumors: prognosis and complications. *Spinal Cord*. Vol. 46, No. 4, pp. 282-6.

Niyazi M, Siefert A, Schwarz SB, Ganswindt U, Kreth FW, Tonn JC, Belka C. (2011). Therapeutic options for recurrent malignant glioma. *Radiother Oncol*. Vol. 98, No. 1, pp. 1-14.

Office for National Statistics. (2010). *Regional Cancer Survival in England 1991 – 2006*. http://www.statistics.gov.uk/downloads/theme_health/CS-Cancer-Net-2010-data.pdf, accessed 26 April 2011.

Pignatti F, van den Bent M, Curran D, Debruyne C, Sylvester R, Therasse P, Afra D, Cornu P, Bolla M, Vecht C, Karim AB; European Organization for Research and Treatment of Cancer Brain Tumor Cooperative Group; European Organization for Research and Treatment of Cancer Radiotherapy Cooperative Group. (2002). Prognostic factors for survival in adult patients with cerebral low-grade glioma. *J Clin Oncol*. Vol. 20, No. 8, pp. 2076-84.

Pollack IF. (1994). Brain tumors in children. *N Engl J Med*, Vol. 331, pp. 1500-7.

Quon H, Abdulkarim B. (2008). Adjuvant treatment of anaplastic oligodendrogliomas and oligoastrocytomas. *Cochrane Database Syst Rev*. Apr 16;(2):CD007104.

Raco A, Piccirilli M, Landi A, Lenzi J, Delfini R, Cantore G. (2010). High-grade intramedullary astrocytomas: 30 years' experience at the Neurosurgery Department of the University of Rome "Sapienza". *J Neurosurg Spine*. Vol. 12, No. 2, pp. 144-53

Ragel BT, Osborn AG, Whang K, Townsend JJ, Jensen RL, Couldwell WT. (2006). Subependymomas: an analysis of clinical and imaging features. , Vol. 58, No. 5, pp. 881-90; discussion 881-90.

Reni M, Gatta G, Mazza E, Vecht C. Ependymoma. (2007). *Crit Rev Oncol Hematol*. Vol. 63, No. 1, pp. 81-9.

Ricci PE. (1999). Imaging of adult brain tumors. *Neuroimaging Clin N Am*, Vol. 9, No. 4, pp. 651-669.

Rollins NK. (2007). Clinical applications of diffusion tensor imaging and tractography in children. *Paediatric Radiology*, Vol. 37, No. 8, pp. 769-780.

Ruiz J, Lesser GJ. (2009). Low grade gliomas. *Curr Treat Options Oncol*. Vol. 10, No. 3-4), pp. 231-42.

Ryken TC, Frankel B, Julien T, Olson JJ. (2008). Surgical management of newly diagnosed glioblastoma in adults: role of cytoreductive surgery. *J Neurooncol*, Vol. 89, pp. 271–286.

Schmidek HH. (2005). Surgical excision of supratentorial hemispheric gliomas in adults. In: *Operative Neurosurgical Techniques. 4th ed vol 1*, Scmidek, Sweet, (Eds.), pp. 756-768. WB Saunders, 0-7216-0340-8, Philadelphia.

Senft C, Franz K, Blasel S, Oszvald A, Rathert J, Seifert V, Gasser T. (2010). Influence of iMRI-guidance on the extent of resection and survival of patients with glioblastoma multiforme. *Technol Cancer Res Treat*. Vol. 9, No. 4, pp. 339-46.

Serra A, Strain J, Ruyle S. (1996). Desmoplastic cerebral astrocytoma of infancy: report and review of the imaging characteristics. *AJR Am J Roentgenol*. Vol. 166, No. 6, pp. 1459-61.

Sharma M, Ralte A, Arora R, Santosh V, Shankar SK, Sarkar C. (2004). Subependymal giant cell astrocytoma: a clinicopathological study of 23 cases with special emphasis on proliferative markers and expression of p53 and retinoblastoma gene proteins. *Pathology*. Vol. 36, No. 2, pp. 139-44.

Slacman, M. Supratentorial gliomas: Clinical features and surgical therapy. In: *Neurosurgery 2nd ed vol 1*, Wilkins RH, Rengachary SS, (Eds). pp. 777-788. McGraw-Hill, 0070799911, New York.

Sposto R, Ertel IJ, Jenkin RD, Boesel CP, Venes JL, Ortega JA, Evans AE, Wara W, Hammond D. (1989). The effectiveness of chemotherapy for treatment of high grade astrocytoma in children: results of a randomized trial. A report from the Childrens Cancer Study Group. *J Neurooncol*, Vol. 7, pp. 165-177

Stüben G, Stuschke M, Kroll M, Havers W, Sack H. (1997). Postoperative radiotherapy of spinal and intracranial ependymomas: analysis of prognostic factors. *Radiother Oncol*. Vol. 45, No. 1, pp. 3-10.

Stummer W, Pichlmeier U, Meinel T, Wiestler OD, Zanella F, Reulen H-J and the ALA-Glioma Study Group. (2006). Fluorescence-guided surgery with 5-aminolevulinic acid for resection of malignant glioma: a randomised controlled multicentre phase III trial. *Lancet Oncol*, Vol. 7, No. 5, pp. 392-401.

Thiessen B, Maguire JA, McNeil K, Huntsman D, Martin MA, Horsman D. (2003). Loss of heterozygosity for loci on chromosome arms 1p and 10q in oligodendroglial tumors: relationship to outcome and chemosensitivity.*Neurooncol*. Vol. 64, No. 3, pp. 271-8.

Tudur Smith C, Marson AG, Clough HE, Williamson PR. (2002). Carbamazepine versus phenytoin monotherapy for epilepsy. *Cochrane Database Syst Rev 202*;(2):CD001911.

Uro-Coste E, Ssi-Yan-Kai G, Guilbeau-Frugier C, Boetto S, Bertozzi AI, Sevely A, Lolmede K, Delisle MB. (2010). Desmoplastic infantile astrocytoma with benign histological phenotype and multiple intracranial localizations at presentation. *J Neurooncol*. Vol. 98, No. 1, pp. 143-9.

van Roost D, Kristof R, Zentner J,Wolf HK, and Schramm J. (1996). Clinical, radiological, and therapeutic features of pleomorphic xanthoastrocytoma: report of three patients and review of the literature. *J Neurol Neurosurg Psychiatry*. Vol. 60, No. 6, pp. 690–692.

Warnick RE, Bath JS. (2005). Image guided neurosurgery. In: *Operative Neurosurgical Techniques. 4th ed vol 1*, Scmidek, Sweet, (Eds.), pp. 611-627. WB Saunders, 0-7216-0340-8, Philadelphia.

Wu W, Lamborn KR, Buckner JC, Novotny PJ, Chang SM, O'Fallon JR, Jaeckle KA, Prados MD. (2010). Joint NCCTG and NABTC prognostic factors analysis for high-grade recurrent glioma. *Neuro Oncol*, Vol. 12, No.2, pp. 164-72.

22

Surgical Technique for Metastatic Brain Tumors

Takeshi Okuda and Amami Kato
Department of Neurosurgery, Kinki University School of Medicine,Osaka, Japan

1. Introduction

In recent years, more effective therapies for cancer, especially systemic chemotherapy regimens, have been developed, and there has been striking improvement in the life expectancy of patients with advanced cancer. However, the benefit from systemic chemotherapy is limited in the case of brain metastases and, conversely, the recent prolongation of the life expectancy of many patients with advanced cancer has translated into a trend for an increase in brain metastases. It can thus be anticipated that there will be an even further increase in the importance of cancer therapy for brain metastases. The main treatment approaches for brain metastases are radiotherapy and surgical resection. Postoperative whole-brain irradiation is a standard therapeutic procedure for metastatic brain tumors. However, local recurrence rates of 10% to 30% have been reported even with concomitant whole-brain irradiation (Patchell et al. 1990; Schackert et al. 2001; Shinoura et al. 2002). In addition, late complications of whole-brain irradiation can greatly affect quality of life in patients (DeAngelis et al. 1989). On the other hand, with regard to surgical resection, the development of surgical devices, such as neuro-navigation systems and intraoperative monitoring, has resulted in dramatic improvements in safety and reliability (Black and Johnson 2004). However, with regard to improvement in the surgical technique itself, there has only been the recommendation for performance of "en bloc resection including a surgical margin of about 5 mm" (Modha et al. 2005), and there have been hardly any innovations, even when compared with the case of malignant glioma surgery. Thus, at first glance, it would seem that metastatic brain tumor surgery has been established. However, in fact, the local recurrence rate is high in the case of surgical resection alone, and attempts are being made to improve the local recurrence rate by performing follow-up treatments such as whole-brain irradiation, stereotactic radiosurgery on the resection cavity, or local chemotherapy (Sills 2005; Kim et al. 2006; Mathieu et al. 2006; Ewend et al. 2007; Ranasinghe and Sheehan 2007). The high local recurrence rate following surgical resection alone clearly implies the presence of residual tumor tissue (Patchell et al. 1998). On the basis of this background, we have been trying various modifications of the surgical technique for surgical resection of metastatic brain tumors to improve the resection rate and the local recurrence rate. Our modifications are explained below.

2. Surgical technique

2.1 Metastatic brain tumor surgery using fluorescein sodium

Fluorescein sodium (Alcon Japan Co., Ltd., Tokyo, Japan) is a tracer of blood-brain barrier disruption, and enhanceable tumors are stained yellow. Fluorescein sodium is extensively used in ophthalmology, and its safety has been established. The operative technique of using fluorescein sodium has a long history of use during brain tumor surgery, as reported by Moore and Murray (Moore et al. 1948; Murray 1982). A special type of filter must be provided to observe the fluorescence, but Shinoda et al. reported that observation via a normal microscope under white light without using a special type of filter was also possible by intravenously injecting a double dose (20 mg/kg) in glioma surgery (Shinoda et al. 2003). We applied this technique to metastatic brain tumor surgery (Okuda et al. 2007). After induction of general anesthesia, and the dura is opened, fluorescein sodium (20 mg/kg) is injected intravenously. Tumor resection is performed >10 minutes after injection of fluorescein sodium. A yellow-stained tumor is visible under the white light of a normal microscope without a filter. The resected tumor using fluorescein sodium and the schematic diagram are shown in Figure 1.

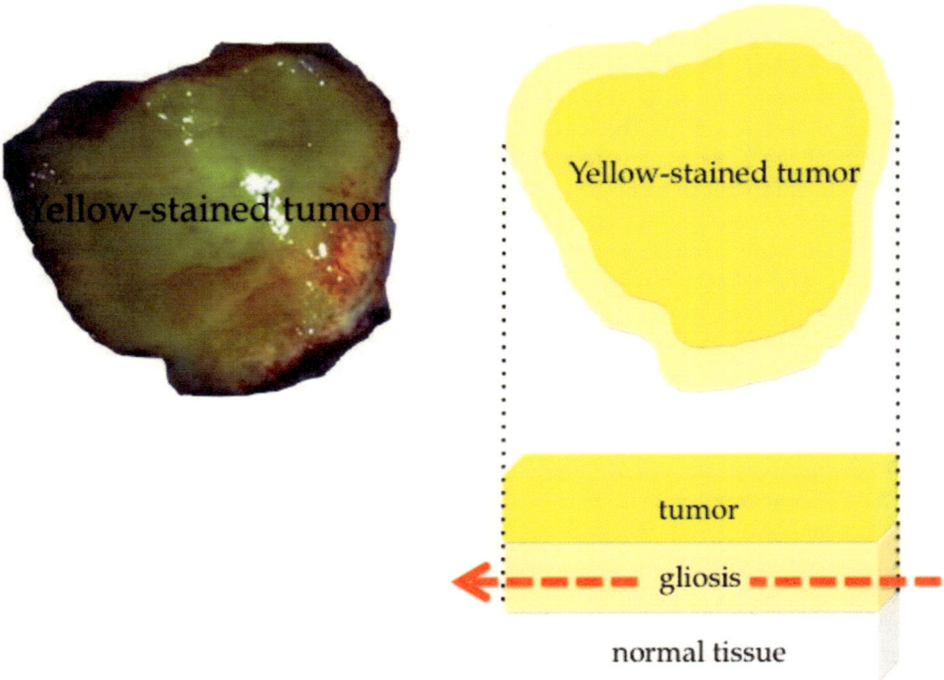

Fig. 1. Cut surface of the resected metastatic brain tumor from primary breast cancer and the schematic diagram.

The tumor parenchyma is stained, and the gliosis portion remains around the tumor. As shown in the diagram, the surrounding gliosis portion is aspirated and resected while carefully confirming the stained tumor. The edematous portion surrounding the tumor is also slightly stained, but it is easy to identify the boundary, and ideal en bloc resection can be achieved while confirming the stained tumor.

Two cases are presented below.

Case 1 was a patient with left frontal lobe metastasis from primary lung cancer (Fig. 2A). Prior to injection of fluorescein sodium (Fig. 3A), the tumor could not be distinguished from the brain surface. After injection (Fig. 3B), the yellow-stained tumor could be distinguished from the brain surface. Under magnification, the border was clearly discernable (Fig. 3C). The border of the white-colored gliosis could also be discerned (Fig. 3D), and en bloc resection was performed while performing suction and dissection (Fig. 3E). The resection cavity is shown (Fig. 3F). Postoperative MRI shows that complete resection was achieved (Fig. 2B).

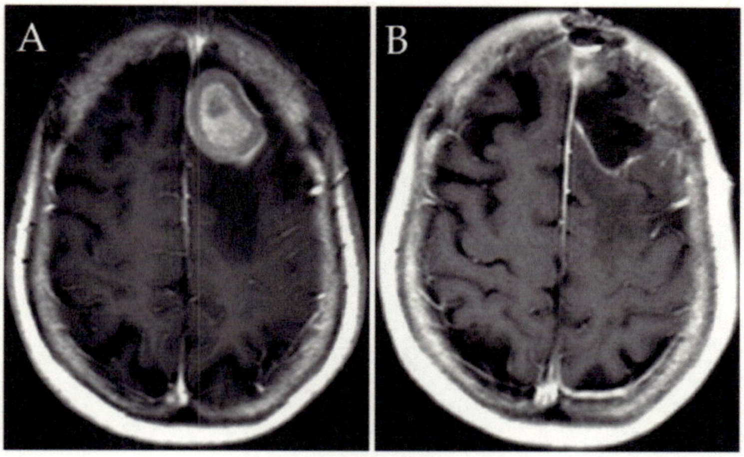

Fig. 2. MRI findings for Case 1 (A)Preoperative enhanced T1-weighted image showing a metastatic brain tumor in the left frontal lobe. (B) Enhanced T1-weighted image 1 day after surgery showing no residual tumor.

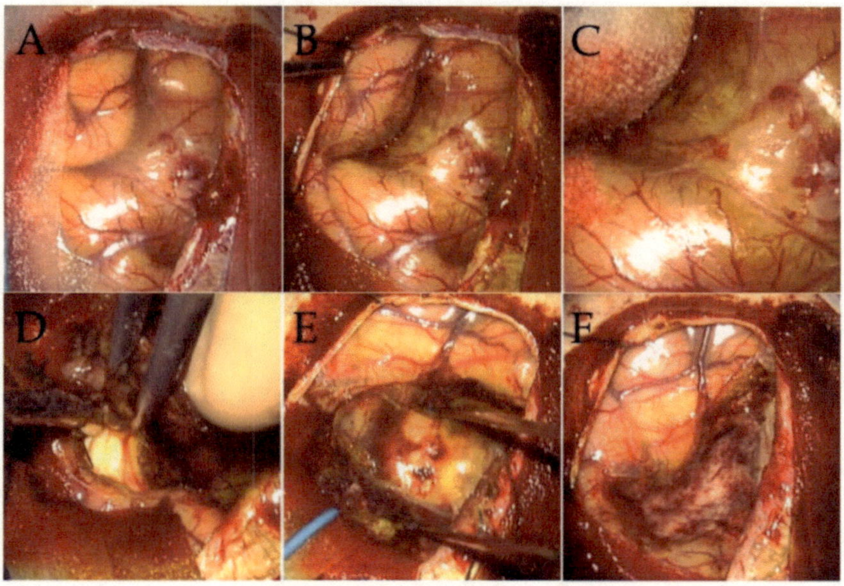

Fig. 3. Intraoperative photographs of Case 1 (A) The brain surface prior to fluorescein sodium injection. (B) The brain surface following fluorescein sodium injection. The yellow-stained tumor can be seen. (C) Magnification of B. (D) The border with the surrounding gliosis portion. (E) En bloc resection. (F) Resection cavity.

Case 2 was a patient with left frontal lobe metastasis from primary renal cell carcinoma (Fig. 4A). The tumor was located in the speech area. Fluorescein sodium was injected intravenously, the tumor was approached through minimal corticotomy, and the yellow-stained tumor surface was confirmed (Fig. 5A, B). En bloc resection was performed (Fig. 5C). Postoperatively, the aphasia symptoms improved, and MRI confirmed that complete resection had been achieved (Fig. 4B). Accordingly, even in cases of brain tumors located in eloquent areas, such as not only the speech area but also the motor area, use of fluorescein sodium makes it possible to carry out resection safely, without any special intraoperative monitoring.

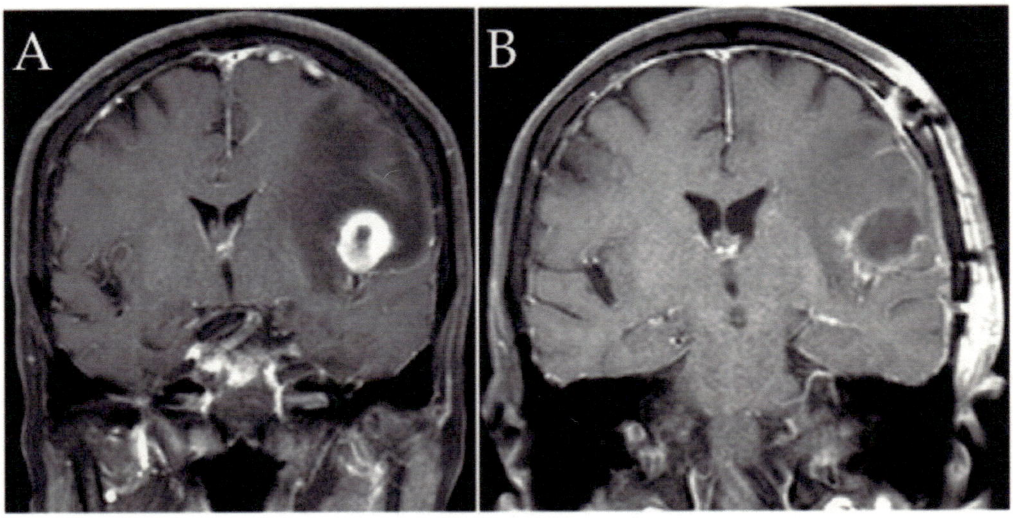

Fig. 4. MRI findings for Case 2 (A) Preoperative enhanced T1-weighted image showing a metastatic brain tumor in the left temporal lobe. (B) Enhanced T1-weighted image 1 day after surgery showing no residual tumor.

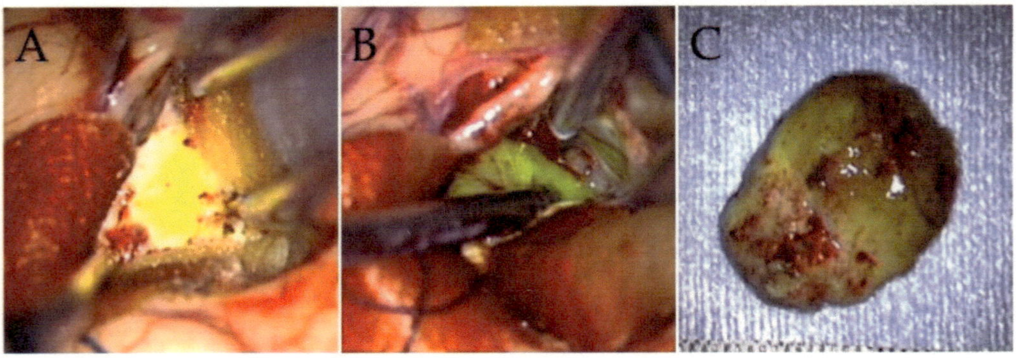

Fig. 5. Intraoperative photographs of Case 2 (A) The tumor surface has been approached, and yellow staining of the tumor by the injected fluorescein sodium is evident. (B) Dissection of the tumor. (C) The tumor was removed by en bloc resection.

To date, we have used fluorescein sodium in more than 100 patients to facilitate surgical resection of metastatic brain tumors, and there have been absolutely no instances of permanent adverse reactions. Anaphylactic shock has been reported as a serious side effect, but it is rare (Tanahashi et al. 2006) and was not observed in our study. As transient adverse events, we have seen yellow staining of the skin, mucosa, and urine, but all cases resolved within 24 hours. This technique will contribute to increasing the resection rate in metastatic brain tumor surgery. Our data also showed statistically significant improvement in the local recurrence rate. Our fluorescence-guided surgery achieved successful local control rates of metastatic brain tumors in 80% of patients without whole-brain irradiation (Okuda et al. 2010). Conversely, previous reports of conventional surgery have yielded successful local control rates of only 54% to 64% under similar conditions (Patchell et al. 1998; Schackert et al. 2001). Although these results are only a guide, based on results from very few patients, fluorescence-guided surgery might enable avoidance or postponement of subsequent whole-brain irradiation, which will not only increase quality of life for patients, but also keeps whole-brain irradiation as a therapeutic option for subsequent brain metastases. This may help to prolong survival and decrease the rate of central nervous system death. This technique is simple, inexpensive, and does not require any special equipment. We are confident that it will be recognized as an important surgical innovation for application to the field of metastatic brain tumor surgery.

2.2 Surgical technique for a cystic-type metastatic brain tumor: transformation to a solid-type tumor using hydrofiber dressing

Cystic-type metastatic brain tumors may have injury to the wall during surgery, which can in some cases result in incomplete tumor resection and dissemination of cancer cells in cyst fluid (Nakagawa et al. 1992). By transforming cystic-type tumors to solid-type tumors, we developed a surgical technique that makes it possible to carry out an ideal en bloc resection (Okuda et al. 2009). In this method, we insert a hydrofiber dressing (Aquacel; Convatec, London, UK) into a cyst, thereby transforming it to a solid-type tumor. Hydrofiber dressing is a coating agent with a high fluid-absorptive capacity that was originally used as a dressing for exudative wounds (Armstrong and Ruckley 1997). Hydrofiber dressing is a sodium carboxymethylcellulose hydrocolloid polymer with fluid-absorptive capacity equal to 25 times its own weight. This material also has a high capacity to retain absorbed water (Fig. 6).

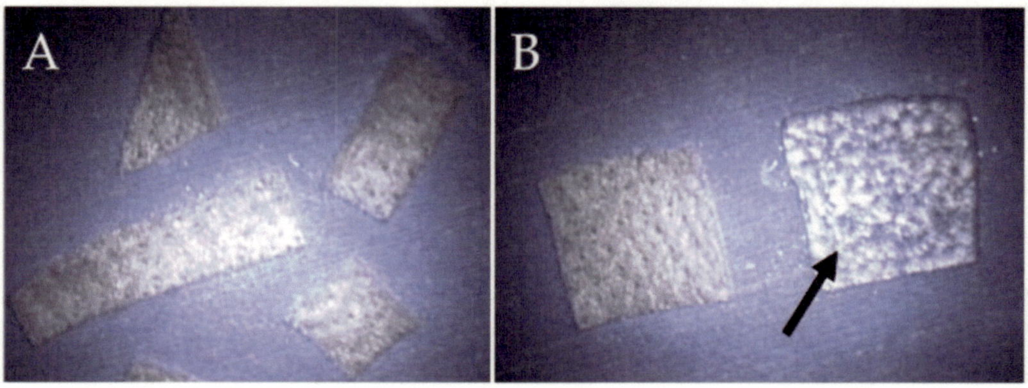

Fig. 6. Images of hydrofiber dressing (A) Hydrofiber dressing can be cut into various sizes. (B) The dotted line shows hydrofiber dressing filled with physiologic saline.

The hydrofiber dressing converts into a gel upon absorption of water, and it integrates with the tumor. As a result, the tumor becomes a soft, solid-type tumor. A flow diagram of the method for using the hydrofiber dressing during the surgical procedure is shown in Figure 7.

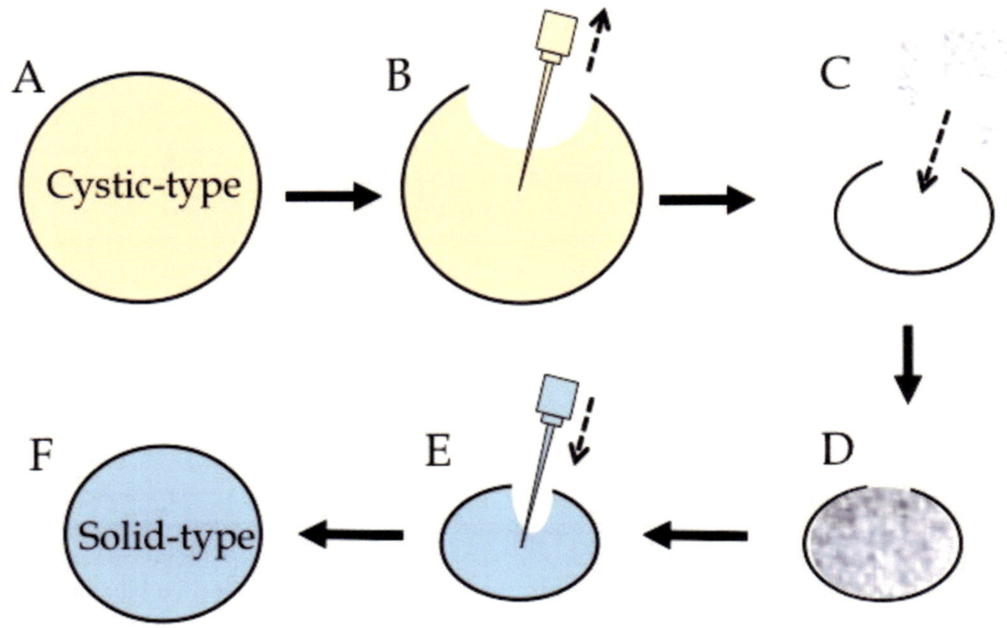

Fig. 7. Schema of cystic-type metastatic brain tumor surgery using hydrofiber dressing(A) Cystic-type tumor before use of hydrofiber dressing. (B) Suctioning of fluid in the cyst. (C, D) Hydrofiber dressing was inserted in the cyst cavity. (E) Injection of physiologic saline. F: The hydrofiber dressing absorbs the fluid in the cyst cavity and fills the cyst, thereby, transforming the tumor into a small solid-type, tumor.

This method converted the cystic-type tumor into a solid-type, small-size tumor, and ideal en bloc resection could be performed. In addition, the hydrofiber dressing absorbs the fluid contents remaining inside the cyst, and by retaining that fluid, it helps prevent tumor cell dissemination during the operation.

A case is presented below.

The patient had a right occipital lobe metastasis of a squamous cell carcinoma (Fig. 8A). First, the cyst was opened for aspiration of fluid (Fig. 9A, B). A small cut was made on the tumor surface to aspirate the fluid contents of the cyst (Fig. 9C), and then hydrofiber dressing was inserted into the cyst (Fig. 9D). Physiologic saline was then injected to fill the cyst (Fig. 9E). En bloc resection was performed (Fig. 9F), and postoperative MRI revealed no residual tumor (Fig. 8B). The tumor that was actually removed by en bloc resection is shown in Figure 10.

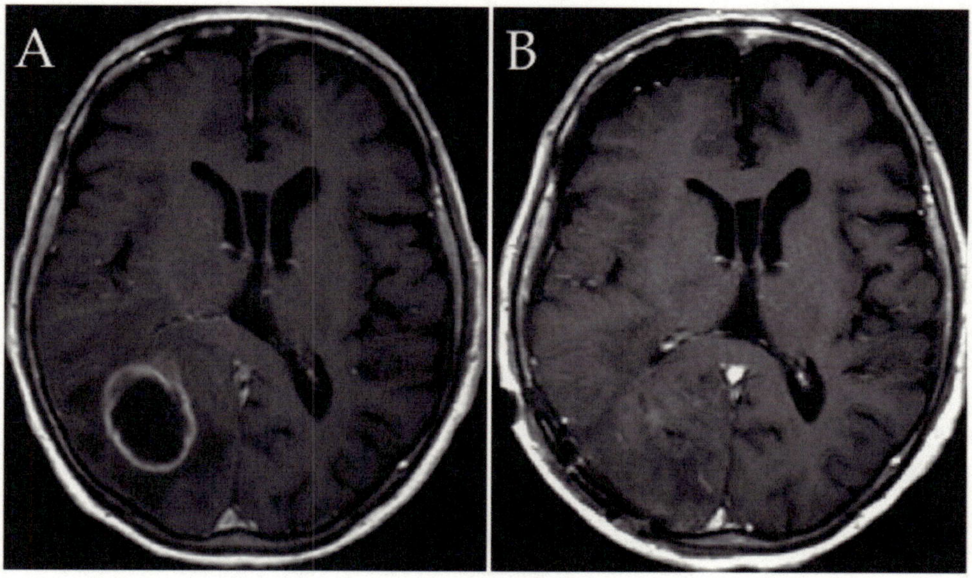

Fig. 8. MRI findings for representative case using hydrofiber dressing (A) Preoperative enhanced T1-weighted image showing a metastatic brain tumor in the right occipital lobe. (B) Enhanced T1-weighted image 1 day after surgery showing no residual tumor.

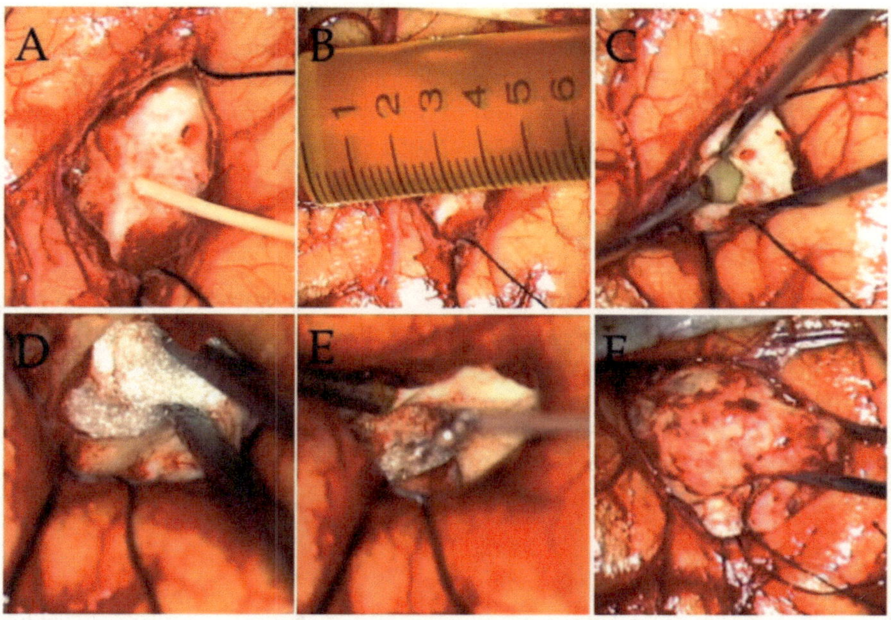

Fig. 9. Intraoperative photographs of representative case using hydrofiber dressing (A) Aspirating of the fluid contents of the cyst. (B) Fluid contents of the cyst. (C) Cyst cavity. (D) Insertion of the hydrofiber dressing. (E) Injection of physiological saline. (F) En bloc resection.

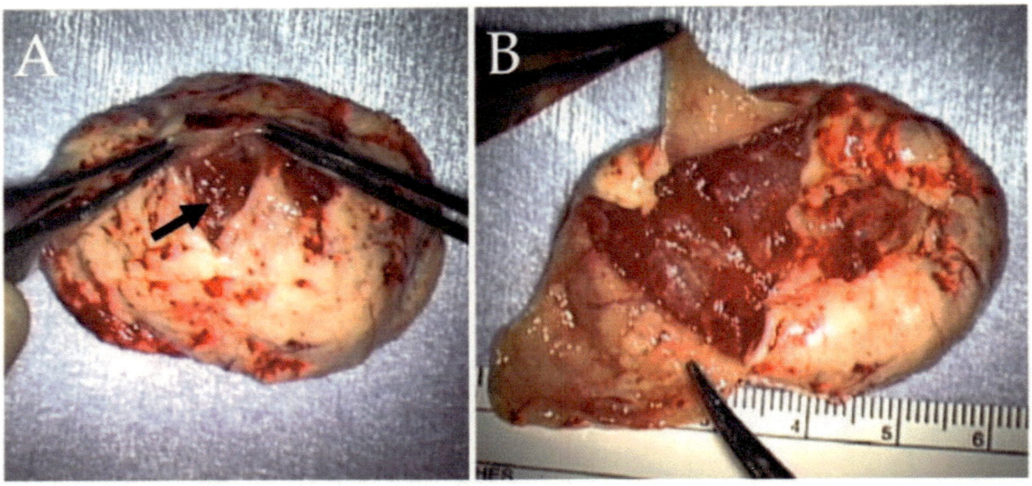

Fig. 10. The resected tumor using hydrofiber dressing (A) The black arrow indicates the opening through which the hydrofiber dressing was inserted. (B) When the cyst wall was incised, it could be seen that the hydrofiber dressing had become a gel inside the cyst.

Hydrofiber dressing is available in a blister pack that has been sterilized by irradiation. Numerous clinical trials for human wounds have confirmed the safety of hydrofiber dressing, and Hoekstra et al. observed few histologic reactions in rats in an examination of the biologic effects of hydrofiber dressing (Hoekstra et al. 2002). There were no adverse events in the 12 patients in our study, and the safety of the method we used is likely to be high, because hydrofiber dressing is used in the cyst without direct contact with brain tissue. Application of this technique to cases of cystic-type metastatic brain tumors makes it possible to perform ideal en bloc resection of the tumor. In addition, it is easy to perform and inexpensive, and we believe that it will prove similarly useful in surgical resection of other cystic brain tumors.

3. Conclusion

We have described two surgical innovations for metastatic brain tumors. Brain metastases cause serious problems in terms of the quality of life and prognosis of cancer patients. Surgery for metastatic brain tumors can have both good and bad sequelae. The surgical techniques we have described are both easy and safe, and they increase the resection rate while improving the local recurrence rate. As a result, we think that these methods will have great benefit to patients by helping avoid and/or delay radiotherapy, while also improving the clinical symptoms.

4. References

Armstrong SH, Ruckley CV. Use of a fibrous dressing in exuding leg ulcers. *J Wound Care* 6: 322-4, 1997.

Black PM, Johnson MD. Surgical resection for patients with solid brain metastases: current status. *J Neurooncol* 69: 119-24, 2004.

DeAngelis LM, Delattre JY, Posner JB. Radiation-induced dementia in patients cured of brain metastases. Neurology 39: 789-96, 1989.

Ewend MG, Brem S, Gilbert M, Goodkin R, Penar PL, Varia M, Cush S, Carey LA. Treatment of single brain metastasis with resection, intracavity carmusutine polymer wafers, and radiation therapy is safe and provides excellent local control. *Clin Cancer Res* 13: 3637-41, 2007.

Hoekstra MJ, Hermans MH, Richters CD, Dutrieux RP. A histological comparison of acte inframmatory responses with a hydrofibre or tulle gauze dressing. *J Wound Care* 11: 113-7, 2002.

Kim PK, Ellis TL, Stieber VW, McMullen KP, Shaw EG, McCoy TP, D'Agostino RB, Bourland JD, DeGuzman AF, Ekstrand KE, Raber MR, Tatter SB. Gamma knife surgery targeting the resection cavity of brain metastasis that has progressed after whole-brain radiotherapy. *J Neurosurg* 105: 75-8, 2006.

Mathieu D, Kondziolka D, Flickinger JC, Fortin D, Kenny B, Michaud K, Mongia S, Niranjan A, Lunsford LD. Tumor bed radiosurgery after resection of cerebral metastases. *Neurosurgery* 62: 817-24, 2008.

Modha A, Shepard SR, Gutin PH. Surgery of brain metastases- Is there still a place for it? *J Neurooncol* 75: 21-9, 2005.

Moore GE, Peyton WT, French LA, Walker WW. The clinical use of fluorescein in neurosurgery. The localization of brain tumors. *J Neurosurg* 5: 392–398, 1948.

Murray KJ. Improved surgical resection of human brain tumors: Part 1. A preliminary study. *Surg Neurol* 17: 316–9, 1982.

Nakagawa H, Kimura S, Kubo S, Fujita T, Tsuruzono K, Hayakawa T. Prognostic factors in patients surviving for more than 1 or 5 years after removal of metastatic brain tumors. *Neurol Med Chir (Tokyo)* 32: 947-51, 1992.

Okuda T, Kataoka K, Taneda M. Metastatic brain tumor surgery using fluorescein sodium: technical note. *Minim Invas Neurosurg* 50: 382-4, 2007.

Okuda T, Teramoto Y, Yugami H, Kataoka K, Kato A. Surgical technique for a cystic-type metastatic Brain tumor: transformation to a solid-type tumor using hydrofiber dressing. *Surg Neurol* 72: 703-6, 2009.

Okuda T, Kataoka K, Yabuuchi T, Yugami H, Kato A. Fluorescence-guided surgery of metastatic brain tumors using fluorescein sodium. *J Clin Neurosci* 17: 118-21, 2010.

Patchell RA, Tibbs PA, Walsh JW, Dempsey RJ, Maruyama Y, Kryscio RJ, Markesbery WR, Macdonald JS, Young B. A randomized trial of surgery in the treatment of single metastases to the brain. *N Engl J Med* 322: 494-500, 1990.

Patchell RA, Tibbs PA, Regine WF, Dempsey RJ, Mohiuddin M, Kryscio RJ, Markesbery WR, Foon KA, Young B. Postoperative radiotherapy in the treatment of single metastases to the brain: a randomized trial. *JAMA* 280(17): 1485-9, 1998.

Ranasinghe MG, Sheehan JM. Surgical management of brain metastases. *Neurosurg Focus* 22: E2, 2007.

Schackert G, Steinmetz A, Meier U, Sobottka SB. Surgical management of single and multiple brain metastases: results of a retrospective study. *Onkologie* 24: 246-55, 2001.

Shinoda J, Yano H, Yoshimura S, Okumura A, Kaku Y, Iwama T, Sakai N. Fluorescence-guided resection of glioblastoma multiforme by using high-dose fluorescein sodium. *J Neurosurg* 99: 597-603, 2003.

Shinoura N, Yamada R, Okamoto K, Nakamura O, Shitara N. Local recurrence of metastatic brain tumor after stereotactic radiosurgery or surgery plus radiation. *J Neurooncol* 60: 71-7, 2002.

Sills AK. Current treatment approaches to surgery for brain metastases. *Neurosurgery* 57(Suppl.): S24-32, 2005.

Tanahashi S, Lida H, Dohi S. An anaphylactoid reaction after administration of fluorescein sodium during neurosurgery. *Anesth Analg* 103: 503, 2006.

23

Stereotactic Radiosurgery for Brain Tumors

Susan C. Pannullo, Cecile Yama and A. Gabriella Wernicke
New York Presbyterian Hospital- Weill Cornell Medical College, New York USA

1. Introduction

Stereotactic Radiosurgery (SRS) is a non-invasive technique for the delivery of highly focused ionizing radiation with extreme precision. It is used in neurosurgical practice as a less invasive means of targeting benign and malignant brain tumors, vascular malformations, and functional disorders. Its ability to elicit a desired response (e.g. tumor cell death) with minimal effect on normal surrounding structures is one of the many benefits that have led to more widespread use of stereotactic radiosurgical procedures in recent years. Current standard practice involves utilizing high resolution imaging for "stereotactic" 3-dimensional (3-D) treatment planning under the guidance of a multidisciplinary team comprised of a neurosurgeon, radiation oncologist and medical physicist. To achieve the desired outcome, the SRS procedure can be performed in either a single treatment or in several applications (fractionated)[1,2].

2. Stereotactic radiosurgery: Brief history

In 1951 neurosurgeon Lars Leksell developed the first stereotactic radiosurgery technique at Karolinska Hospital in Stockholm, Sweden. Dr. Leksell pioneered the stereotactic headframe for use in noninvasive lesioning in functional neurosurgery by attaching an orthovoltage x-ray tube to a stereotactic frame in order to produce converging beams which would intersect at the treatment target[1]. In one of his first publications on the novel device he described how he could use the directed narrow beams of radiant energy in order to produce local destruction of undesirable brain tumor tissue. By adjusting the width of the beam to the size of the structure to be irradiated, and moving the beam guide transversely along the frame, the targeted radiation would meet at desired tissue site[3].

After finding his early work with the proton beam and linear accelerator radiosurgery overly cumbersome and inefficient, Dr. Leksell collaborated with Borge Larson in 1968 to design the first Gamma Knife device. This device contained 179 Cobalt 60 (Co-60) sources arranged symmetrically to irradiate a volume of brain tissue with a diameter of approximately 4, 8, or 14 mm[1]. The production and use of the Leksell Gamma Unit expanded in the late 1980s with the introduction of angiography, which enabled surgeons to delineate and therefore target arteriovenous malformations (AVMs). After getting the Food and Drug Administration (FDA) approval in 1982, the 201 Co-60 source gamma knife was used for the first time in the United States at the University of Pittsburgh, where it proved to be a therapeutically effective and economical alternative to some conventional neurosurgery practices[4].

In recent years novel imaging techniques have been developed to optimize and expand the uses of the gamma knife and other stereotactic devices. Computer tomography (CT) and magnetic resonance imaging (MRI) techniques have improved the quality of the brain image and achieved a more precise localization of abnormalities and tumors in the brain. Combining these innovative imaging technologies with high-speed workstations that rapidly calculate and display 3-D dose distributions enables more effective and productive uses of these technologies[1]. In addition, positron emission tomography (PET) scans provide images that include metabolic data and functional data and in doing so add another layer of sophistication in the treatment of more complex targets such as rapidly proliferating tumors, including gliomas and metastases. The metabolic information provided by using PET scan imaging is complementary to anatomical information derived from CT or MRI imaging and assists in more precise identification of the target in dose-planning procedures[5].

3. Stereotactic radiosurgery technologies: Gamma Knife, LINAC, CyberKnife, Proton Beam

3.1 Gamma Knife

The Gamma Knife, developed by Leksell in 1968, has been reported to have been used in 350,000 treatments by Leksell Society in 2005, at 237 centers[6]. It is made up of an 18,000 kg shield surrounding a hemispherical array of 201 sources of cobalt-60 with an average activity of 30 curie (Ci); as the cobalt-60 decays, the photons pass through various sized collimator holes in a helmet designed for the stereotactic procedure[4]. It has both fixed central and secondary beams on separate axes, with interchangeable outer collimator helmets that are used with respect to he lesion size—larger collimators are used for larger lesions, and smaller collimators for smaller diameter lesions[4]. The number of "shots" used to achieve the maximal target dose is dependent on the collimator size selected[4].

While Gamma Knife radiosurgery was originally designed to treat well-delineated lesions and targets, making it particularly useful for AVMs and benign tumors of the skull base, its uses have been expanded to include metastases, gliomas and other tumor types[5]. In addition to delineation of glial tumors, PET imaging technology has allowed for more accuracy in patients who have undergone previous surgery, which would otherwise make it difficult to define tumor recurrence accurately[5].

3.2 LINAC

The development of linear accelerators (LINAC) allowed scientists and physicians to mimic the sharply defined small volumes of radiation produced by the Gamma Knife. Presently, LINAC systems utilized for SRS represent a predominant majority of the stereotactic systems worldwide. Such treatment applications have undergone a technical evolution. Early linear accelerators developed included the use of the Talairach stereotactic coordinate system with a 10-MV photon beam in 1983, and a 4-MV linear accelerator in 1985[1]. Winston and Lutz later made use of the Brown-Roberts-Wells stereotactic frame with a floor stand in 1986 to achieve mechanical accuracy of 0.5mm, an accuracy comparable to that of the Gamma Knife[7]. In 1994 the FDA standardized commercial distribution of linear accelerator radiosurgery systems in the United States, and the expansion of such systems began[1].

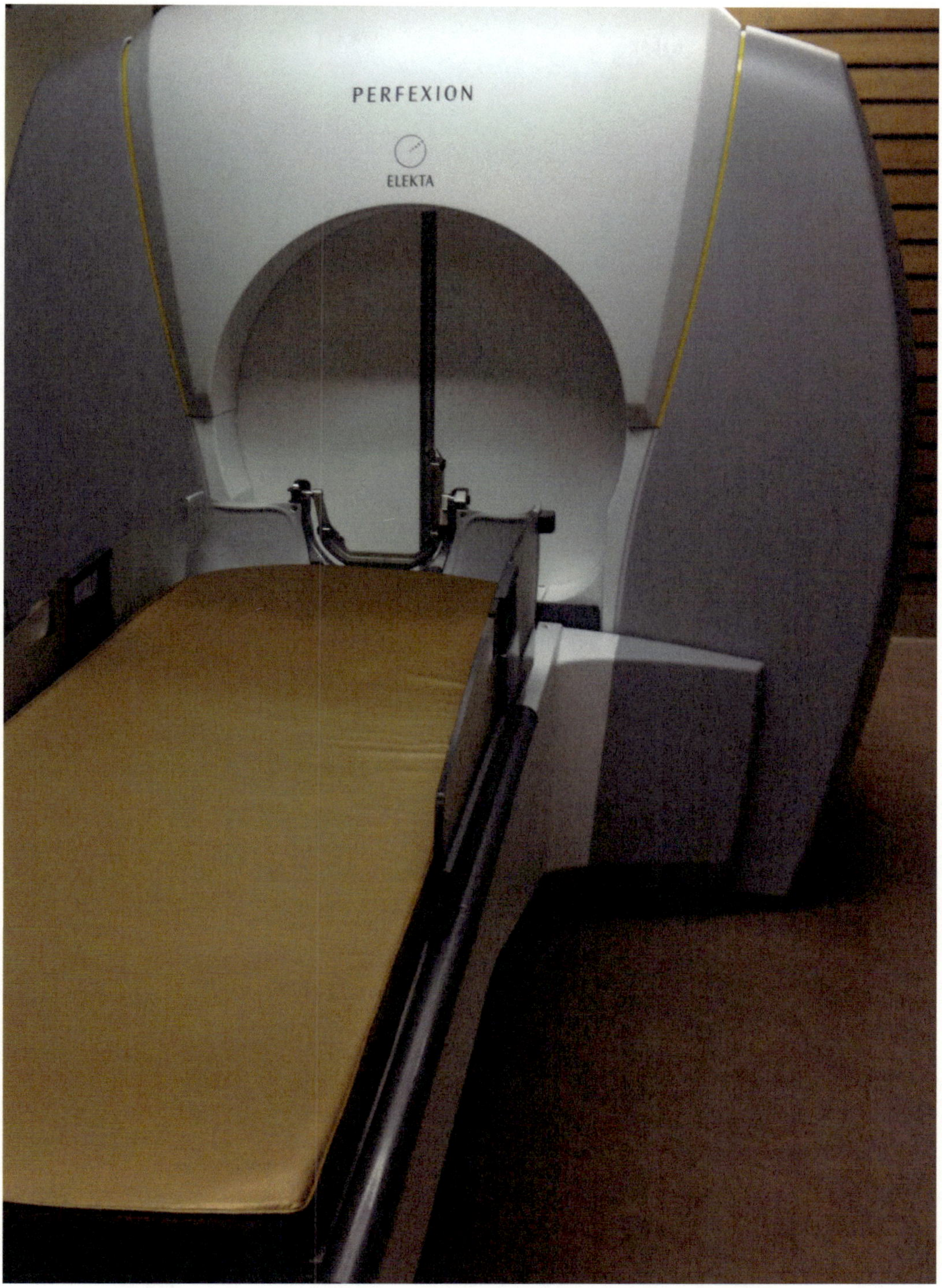

Fig. 1. Gamma Knife Perfexion Unit

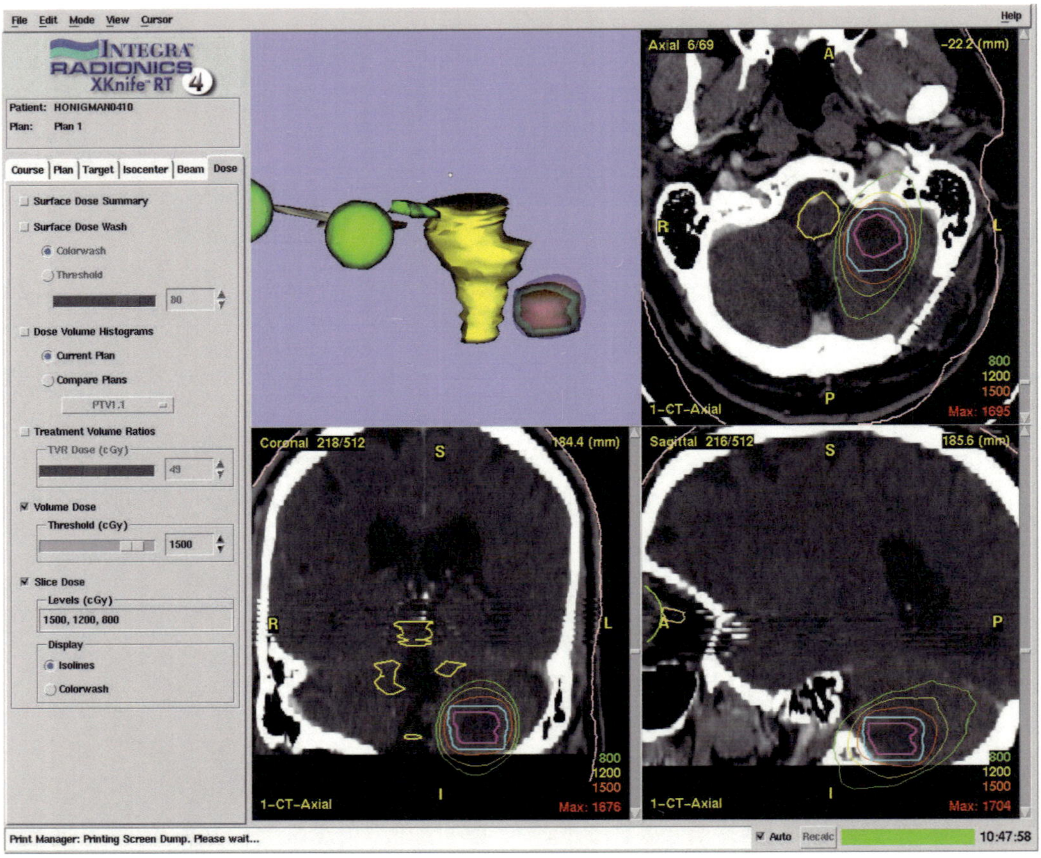

Fig. 2. LINAC Treatment Planning

The LINAC systems employ accelerated photons, much like the Gamma Knife system but rely on a different software and hardware than the Gamma Knife. It can be used with a frame or as a frameless system, and it has the advantage of being used for fractionated stereotactic radiotherapy which is for the most part not possible with Gamma Knife[1].

3.3 CyberKnife

The CyberKnife has been developed in recent years as a frameless, robotic, image-guided stereotactic radiosurgery system that manipulates an X-band linear accelerator[8]. This recent adaptation allows for a more flexible treatment both in terms of the ability to deliver the therapy without using a frame (making the experience more comfortable for the patient), increasing fractionation flexibility, as well as increasing the ability to treat extracranial lesions[8]. The CyberKnife radiosurgery system computes the dose range and quantity by using data from the robot and camera image tracking system software, along with contributions from the assembled team's treatment planning, based on CT imaging[8].

The CyberKnife enables facile stereotactic fractionation, eases patient discomfort due to lack of stereotactic frame, and does not require anesthesia in pediatric patients which is necessary with frame-based systems[8]. Additional applications of frameless radiosurgical methods include use in other organ systems and locations such as the spinal column, the mediastinum, pelvis and the retroperitoneal space[8].

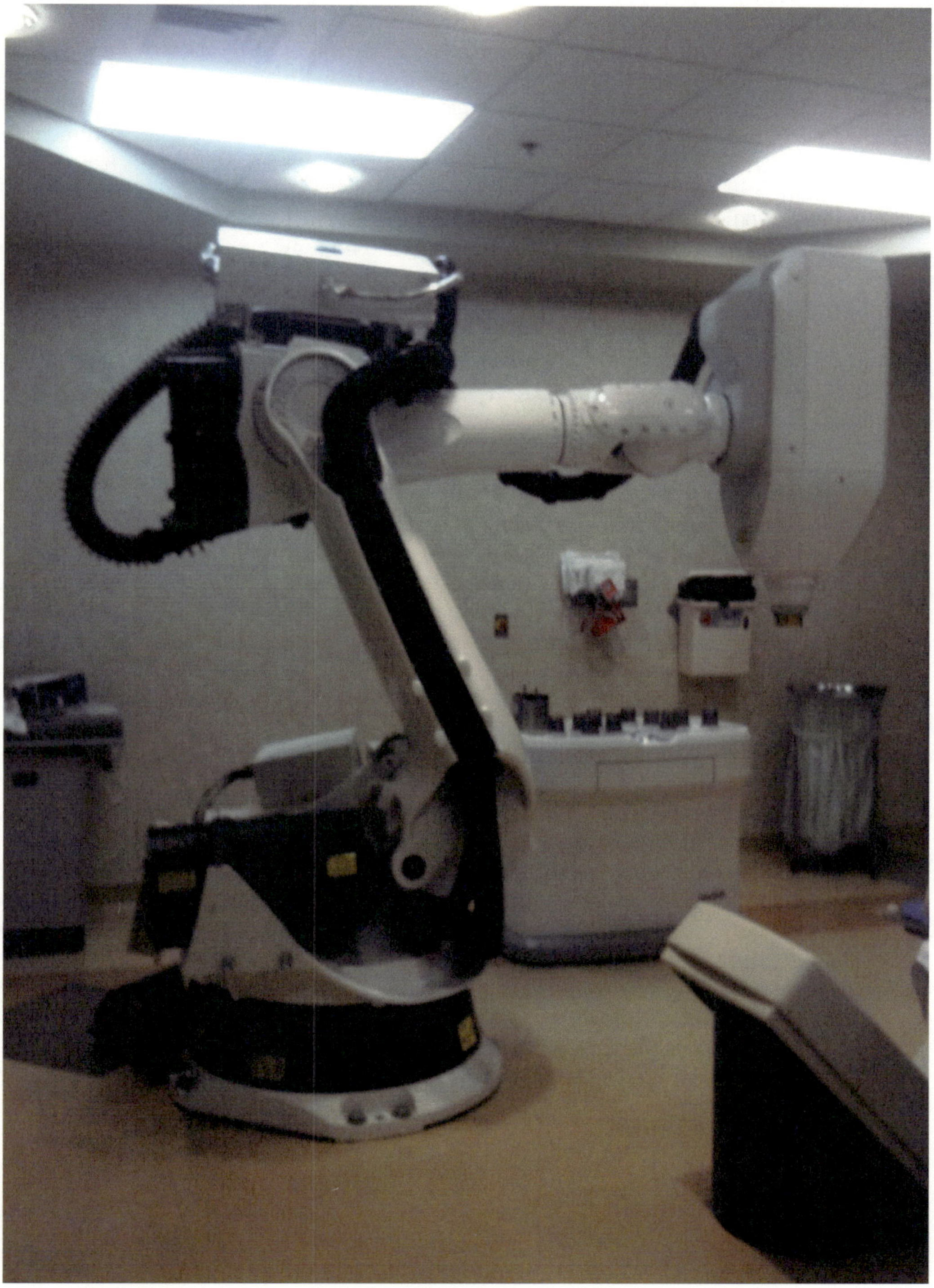

Fig. 3. CyberKnife Unit

3.4 Proton Beam

The proton beam is a significantly more costly and far less frequently used stereotactic system than the above-described applications. Due to its prohibitively high cost and special shielding, proton beam facilities are very few in the United States or worldwide. Proton beam SRS relies on generating a charged particle. Charged particle intracranial SRS was first implemented in the 1950s and 1960s when Tobias et al began to irradiate brain tumors in 1956 with high-energy, positively charged particles with a synchroclyclotron[9]. It was later used to treat intracranial lesions such as AVMs and pituitary adenomas[1]. Raju has estimated that a total of 6,500 patients had been treated with intracranial SRS using charged particle beams by 1995[10]. The beam generated can manipulate the Bragg's peak to adjust to the size of the tumor. The particular characteristics of proton radiation is a very low entry dose and a very sharp fall off dose past the Bragg peak, i.e., past the tumor. Such beam properties render proton beam application in the brain most useful for the lesions near critical structures which may produce untoward permanent damage if not spared - the optic chiasm or a brain stem - and/or special pathologies requiring very high doses of radiation (e.g., chordoma, chondrosarcoma).

4. Indications for stereotactic radiosurgery

While the first Gamma Unit using Co-60 was installed in the Sophiahemmet Hospital in Sweden in 1968 and was primarily intended for neurosurgery in deep fiber tracts or nuclei[8], its expansion to other hospitals both in Sweden and abroad allowed it to evolve in its function and use, as its capabilities were questioned and expanded. Indications for current use of stereotactic radiosurgery are multifarious, and includes certain malignant or benign tumors that meet the criteria for radiosurgical treatment as well as AVMs[11]. Radiosurgery is an especially attractive therapeutic option for brain metastases because it can be used to treat small lesions that would be otherwise inaccessible with invasive surgery due to sensitive adjacent critical structures. It presents an especially attractive alternative option to invasive surgery for patients with co-morbidities[11]. Radiosurgery continues to be constantly evaluated for its benefits, risks, and effectiveness in comparison to standard surgical, radiation and pharmacological options.

In addition to these more common uses, stereotactic radiosurgery is also used in a smaller percentage of cases for its original purpose—the treatment of functional disorders such movement disorders or intractable pain[12]. Of these functional SRS cases, the most common indication is trigeminal neuralgia, but experimental procedures for epilepsy and other psychiatric illness are also conducted in several centers under strict protocol. Ventrolateral thalamotomy is being studied as a possible radiosurgical treatment of tremor in patients with Parkinson disease or multiple sclerosis, as well as for treatment of essential tremor. A study by Friehs has shown success rates that are comparable to other treatments in older groups of patients[13].

5. Patient selection and preparation

Selecting patients for stereotactic radiosurgery involves a comprehensive account and balance of the benefits and risks of the procedure, in relation to the history of the disease, the condition of the patient, and other alternative therapies[14]. This includes thorough consideration of the demographic and medical profile of the patient as well as the nature, size, shape, and location of the lesion. Such assessment requires the expertise of several

medical professionals including neurodiagnosticians, neurosurgeons, radiationoncologists, and medical physicians[14]. Each of these medical practitioners is trained to contribute and collaborate to the procedure according to their capabilities.
Considerations with respect to the specifications of the tumor play a critical role both in deciding whether stereotactic radiosurgery is the appropriate treatment, and if so, how to approach the treatment. Radiosurgery is most often used to treat relatively small, well-circumscribed tumors or vascular malformations less than 35 mm in diameter[14,15]. Patients with larger legions are usually poor candidates. This is due to the delayed radiation-related complications from the gradual as opposed to steep fall-off of large doses of radiation as well as other adverse symptoms related to mass effect[15]. Both of these complications lead to the destruction of surrounding tissues. As a result, a neurosurgical approach is likely required for patients with larger lesions, as opposed to a radiosurgical one. In addition to the size of the lesion, the location of adjacent neural structures, such as the optic chiasm, must be considered in treatment planning as these structures often make it difficult or impossible to access the target site[13].
In terms of patient demographic, the selection of radiosurgery as opposed to other modes of treatment also involves the assessment of patient preference, the neurological hazards of open surgical resection with general anesthesia for a particular patient, and the efficacy of alternative radiation techniques[14]. Considerations such as mental and physical patient motivation and cooperation (whether they are claustrophobic or are physically able to lie flat and still for the designated amount of time of the procedure) are important in determining whether radiosurgery is the optimal choice for the patient. . It is preferable that a candidate for SRS has a Karnofsky Permonance Status (KPS) >70.

5.1 Patient preparation and frame application

Stereotactic radiosurgery is most often an outpatient single day procedure. After the patient is determined to be a good candidate for this treatment and a date has been selected, pre-operative measures must be undertaken to explain the procedure to the patient and they must also sign a form of consent. It is important that the patient understands that they will be required to lie flat and still for a prolonged period of time. Diuretics to prevent edema and anticonvulsants to prevent seizures during the procedure can be administered to the patient two weeks before the procedure.
Administration of a mild oral sedative and local anesthetic are essential for gamma-knife radiosurgery because the treatment requires rigid fixation of the patient's head in a metal head frame, which would otherwise cause discomfort. After the sedative and anesthesia is administered and allowed to take effect, the frame is then applied. Optimal frame placement is critical for frame-based radiosurgery as the placement of the frame must be precise in order to avoid cranial defects. Targets must be placed in the center of the frame so that the beams of radiation will meet properly at the planning target volume (PTV).
Accurate placement of the frame requires comprehensive imaging and treatment planning by the radiosurgical team. Essential to the placement of the frame is defining the intracranial targets in stereotactic space[16]. This is done with various combinations of cerebral angiography, CT scan and MRI technologies both before the procedure and then again once the frame has been applied, with the latter set of coordinates specifying the PTV coordinates in relationship to the frame[4]. Stereotactic localization defines the coordinates of the volume of interest within the brain in terms of the external coordinates of the frame in order to align with the radiosurgical unit[16]. A fusion of the CT scan and an MRI provides a special

orientation of the target with respect to the stereotactic coordinates. The imaging data is analyzed by dose planning system software and the radiosurgical team. In recent years, advanced technologies such as positron emission tomography (PET) have been developed and implemented as previously mentioned, which enable the possibility of more accurate determination of PTV location in complicated cases. Examples of PET uses include glial tumors which are difficult to delineate from the surrounding tissue without additional metabolic data, which differentiates malignant tumor tissue based on its proliferation, as evidenced by the uptake of the radiolabeled glucose (^{18}F)[5].

5.2 Imaging and treatment planning

Because the dosage planning for stereotactic radiosurgery is done for the most part by computer software, data including the rectilinear (x, y, z) coordinates of the target, head configuration measurements and treatment angle data must be gathered in order for the appropriate dose to be localized to the target area[4]. Stereotaxis relates the patient to a mathematic coordinate system by using the head frame's ring as a template on which the coordinate system can be applied[17]. A fiducial system attaches to the frame with imaging elements appropriate to the image modality used for treatment planning, and the data collected is inputted into a computer dose-planning system to create a stereotactic space[15]. In this way the treatment planning system identifies the coordinates of the target tissue and will administer the appropriate dosage only to that specific region.

The software used to calculate the appropriate isodose must take into account the summated isodose curves that show the cumulative effect of beam isocenter placements, collimator size, beam weighing and head angulation[15]. The system also calculates the amount of radiation that non-PTV structures are exposed to, allowing the treatment team to adjust the plan in order to minimize the effect on these surrounding structures. It is important that the software recognizes incorrect or dangerous treatment, and that the delivery system is contained in a room that protects treatment personnel as well as the public from harmful radiation[15].

Dosimetric evaluation by the clinical team often includes both qualitative and quantitative histograms, including isodose surface displays and integral dose-volume histograms[18]. Computing the appropriate dose makes up a majority of the time of the planning procedure as it requires computational algorithms in addition to clinical input in order to optimize the treatment. In computing the isocenter, small movements can alter the minimum surface dose by as much as 30%[18].

6. Selected clinical brain tumor applications of stereotactic radiosurgery

The clinical applications of stereotactic radiosurgery are numerous and include acoustic neuroma, meningioma, brain metastases, pituitary adenoma, glioblastoma multiforme, craniopharyngioma, trigeminal and other cranial nerve schwannoma, glomus jugulare tumors, hemangiopericytomas, ependymomas, and recurrent medulloblastoma. The following section will describe the specific indications for a number of these tumor types as well as the outcomes as examined by various studies. To improve treatment of many of these tumor types further research must be done in order to understand and optimize the benefits and detriments of different procedures. Contradictory data has been presented both within studies and between studies in choosing between a surgical, radiosurgical or radiation approach to tumor treatment planning.

6.1 Vestibular schwannoma / acoustic neuroma

Ideal active management for small-to-medium-sized vestibular schwannomas is still disputed and unclear, as a recent study by Pollock favored the radiosurgical over microsurgical approach, while Di Maio and Akagami showed no difference between groups of patients that were treated microsurgically, radiosurgically, or untreated with observation[19,20,21]. These studies were measured based on quality of life outcomes (QOL).

Nonetheless, stereotactic surgery is presently used to treat vestibular schwannomas with favorable disease stabilization rates upwards of 90% with some studies showing tumor control rates up to 97%[22,23]. While rates of tumor control are comparable to those of conventional microsurgery, both treatments demonstrate a preservation of hearing as well of other quality of life effects that are far from optimal. Facial weakness and facial numbness due to trigeminal and facial nerve damage during resection or radiosurgical treatment of vestibular schwannomas have presented additional challenges to current practice, but occur at a low frequency (<3%)[22]. The preservation of cochlear nerve function poses the predominant challenge to the surgical approach as well as the radiosurgical approach with a resultant preservation of useful hearing between 33-50% for small-to-medium-sized tumors, and considerably lower for larger tumors[22].

A fractionated approach has been investigated in the attempt to preserve hearing and minimize incidental cranial nerve injury[22]. Poen's study of 33 patients with vestibular schwannoma demonstrated that a 24 hour three-fraction approach allows for a preservation of useful hearing (Gardner-Robertson Class 1-2) in 77% of patients two years after the treatment procedure[22]. The fractionated SRS protocol that was designed incorporated the physical advantages of rigid stereotactic localization, the practicality of a 1-day treatment, and the potential biological advantages of an abbreviated fractionation schedule[22]. It also takes advantage of the radiobiological principles that predict that fractionated radiotherapy will allow for repair of sublethal damage in normal tissues, reoxygenation of hypoxic tumor cells and redistribution of surviving tumor cells into a more radiosensitive cell cycle phase that is more susceptible to further radiation[22].

While facial weakness and numbness is less common than hearing loss in the treatment of vestibular schwannomas, a review study by Yang has demonstrated that up to 3.8% of patients treated with Gamma Knife radiosurgery for vestibular schwannomas have poor to no facial nerve preservation after surgery[24]. As a result, facial nerve preservation is still a great concern of patients undergoing radiosurgery for vestibular schwannomas. Treatment with radiation less than 13 Gy has been shown to have better facial nerve preservation rates after Gamma Knife radiosurgery for vestibular schwannoma ($\leq$13 Gy = 98.5% vs. $\geq$13 Gy = 94.7%, $P<0.0001$)[24].

6.2 Stereotactic radiosurgery for meningiomas

Stereotactic radiosurgery is presently an alternative or adjuvant approach alongside surgical resection for treatment and management of intracranial meningiomas. Radiosurgery presents a favorable approach to microsurgery in patients with residual or recurrent small volume tumors who have had previous resection, those with high risk symptomatic primary tumors, as well as in patients with medical illness or advanced age[25]. It is not recommended for optic sheath tumors in patients with preserved vision [25]. A study by Konziolka examined the rate of tumor growth control in 972 patients with 1045 intracranial meningiomas and found the control rate to be 93% in patients with benign meningiomas and low concurrent risks[25]. In this study a mean of 7.5 isocenters were used to provide conformal radiosurgery, with a mean dose to tumor margin at 14 Gy and mean maximum delivered dose of 28 Gy[25]. Overall morbidity rate was 7.7% in patients who underwent stereotactic radiosurgical treatment for intracranial meningiomas at an average time of 11 months, and symptomatic peritumoral imaging changes were present in 4% of patients at 8 months[25].

In another study by Lee of the long-term outcomes in 176 patients who had undergone stereotactic radiosurgery for cavernous sinus meningiomas, neurological status improved in 46 patients (29%), was stabilized in 99 (62%), and worsened in 14 (9%)[26]. While microsurgical approach to skull base has become more feasible in present years to achieve rates of 22.9-100% due to technique developments, complete resection still has the likely possibility of resultant disease and death while the alternative, incomplete resection, usually fails to arrest tumor progression[26]. With a radiosurgical approach in treating cavernus sinus meningiomas, tumor volume was shown to decrease in 54 patients (34%), was stabilized in 96 (60%), and increased in nine (6%)[26]. By placing the 50% or greater isodose at the irregular tumor margin, three-dimensional conformation radiosurgery was achieved with a median maximum dose of 26 Gy, and median dose delivered to margin at 13 Gy[26]. Adverse effects of radiation occurred in 6.7% of patients where clinical or neurological deterioration occurred despite lack of tumor growth including visual deterioration, trigemnial nerve dysfunction and partial complex seizures[26].

Overall, multiple isocenter stereotactic radiosurgery allows for focused irradiation of irregular meningioma tumor margins and volumes, and prevents adjacent critical structures from injury in comparison to microsurgical techniques. Stereotactic radiosurgery is often recommended for smaller tumors, as large tumors respond poorly to due to mass effect [25,26]. Several studies have analyzed various types of intracranial meningiomas and demonstrated that tumor recurrence or progression is statistically similar in both patients who have undergone resection and those who have been treated radiosurgically, with low morbidity in small- to-moderate-sized meningiomas without the risks associated with invasive surgery[27,28].

6.3 Stereotactic radiosurgery for brain metastases

Stereotactic radiosurgery is currently being used to treat newly diagnosed metastatic tumors, recurrent brain metastases after previous whole brain radiation therapy (WBRT), and as a "boost" after WBRT. Brain metastases are the most common adult brain tumor, affecting 100,000-170,000 people annually in the United States[29]. Metastatic brain tumors have high incidence and follow a rapidly progressive course, requiring complex management which includes a combination of surgery, radiation and radiosurgery[30]. Even with the multimodal treatment, low median survival rates of around 6 months after WBRT persist, and these low survival rates have historically led the oncology community to desist from aggressive treatment of these tumors[30].

Stereotactic radiosurgery presents a non-invasive, less aggressive approach to depress the rate of growth in solitary brain metastases. Solitary metastases are especially good targets for radiosurgical treatment when they are caught in earlier stages by MRI surveillance at less than 3.5 cm, because they are usually spherical, discrete and contrast enhancing, allowing for accurate lesion delineation[30]. In addition, most metastases are uniformly sensitive to single fraction radiotherapy[30].

For multiple brain metastases, treatment becomes less effective as the number of tumors increases. A study by Pollock demonstrated that the probability of tumor control after surgery and WBRT or radiosurgery decreases from 64% for one intracranial metastasis, to 51% for two tumors, and to 41% for three³¹. Patients with fewer than four small- or medium-sized tumors can respond favorably to stereotactic radiosurgery[32]. Hypofractionated radiosurgery is the preferred option for patients that are poor surgical candidates due to co-morbidities or advanced systemic disease and it can be combined with resection for treatment of larger tumors[32]. In general, algorithms are followed to treat brain metastases through multimodal techniques that combine resection, WBRT and radiosurgery in attempt to maximize survival rates.

7. Stereotactic radiosurgery for brain tumors: Risks and benefits

7.1 Risks

The risks associated with stereotactic radiosurgery can be categorized by the time of their presentation and are determined by various factors including tumor type, size, location, prior radiation and the radiation dose given.

In a study by Warnick, complications were analyzed and categorized temporally. Acute complications occurring in the first seven days after radiosurgical treatment were rare and included nausea in 2-11% of patients within the first 24 hours, which was controlled with anti-emetics[30]. Edema was reported in 2-6% of patients, with improvement seen with corticosteroids administered pre-operatively in tumors more frequently associated with this complication[30]. Seizures were reported in 2-6% of patients within 24 hours, with greater occurrence in patients with pre-existing seizures and tumors near epileptogenic areas[33].

Subacute complications occurring within six months of the procedure, included uncommon occurrences of alopecia in 6% of patients, and the 'flare' phenomenon that presents as increased lesion volume, contrast enhancement and edema, resolving itself 9-12 months after the procedure[30]. Flare is a result of accumulation of necrotic tumor tissue. Chronic complications, referring to those persisting for longer than six months after the procedure, include radiation necrosis, which is the most severe of such side effects and is dependent on the diameter of the tumor diameter being radiated. To reduce the risk of late radiation effects on surrounding structures, WBRT is increasingly being omitted from the initial management strategy of brain metastases^{34,35}. Finally, radiation-induced secondary neoplasms have been reported infrequently in few case studies.

7.2 Potential benefits

The potential benefits of stereotactic radiosurgery are extensive, making it an attractive alternative or even replacement treatment for tumor resection. It is a safe, effective, and non-invasive procedure, and as a result is well tolerated in older patients as well as those with concurrent disease. It also allows most patients to return immediately to normal activities. Single or few treatments can produce a sustained effect in a wide variety of tumors, and multiple small tumors can be treated simultaneously while avoiding the systemic toxicity that accompanies pharmacological treatment. In addition, radiosurgery can be combined with other therapies for comprehensive, patient-specific treatment. As a result, stereotactic radiosurgery is being increasingly utilized tool in the treatment of brain tumors and its applications are bound to grow and develop in future years.

8. References

[1] Goetsch SJ. Linear accelerator and gamma knife-based stereotactic cranial radiosurgery: challenges and successes of existing quality assurance guidelines and paradigms. *International journal of radiation oncology, biology, physics*. 2008;71(1 Suppl):S118-21. Available at: http://www.ncbi.nlm.nih.gov/pubmed/18406908.

[2] Larson DA, Bova F, Eisert D, et al. Current radiosurgery practice: results of an ASTRO survey. Task Force on Stereotactic Radiosurgery, American Society for Therapeutic Radiology and Oncology. *International journal of radiation oncology, biology, physics*. 1994;28(2):523-6. Available at: http://www.ncbi.nlm.nih.gov/pubmed/8276670 [Accessed May 19, 2011].

[3] Leksell L. The stereotaxic method and radiosurgery of the brain. *Acta chirurgica Scandinavica*. 1951;102(4):316-9. Available at: http://www.ncbi.nlm.nih.gov/pubmed/14914373 [Accessed May 19, 2011].

[4] Lunsford. Stereotactic radiosurgery of the brain using the first United States 201 cobalt-60 source gamma knife. *Neurosurgery*. 1989;24(2):151. Available at: http://journals.lww.com/neurosurgery/Abstract/1989/02000/Stereotactic_Radiosurgery_of_the_Brain_Using_the.1.aspx [Accessed May 19, 2011].

[5] Levivier, M. Wikier, D. et al. Integration of the metabolic data of positron emission tomography in the dosimetry planning of radiosurgery with the Leksell gamma knife: early experience with brain tumors. *Journal of neurosurgery*. 2000; 93 (Supplement 3):233–238. Available at: http://thejns.org/doi/pdf/10.3171/jns.2000.93.supplement 3.0233 [Accessed May 19, 2011].

[6] Leksell L. Occasional Review: Stereotactic Radiosurgery. *Journal of Neurology, Neurosurgery, and Psychiatry*. 1983;46:797-803. Available at: http://jnci.oxfordjournals.org/content/87/1/34.short [Accessed May 20, 2011].

[7] Alexander E, Moriarty TM, Davis RB, et al. Stereotactic radiosurgery for the definitive, noninvasive treatment of brain metastases. *Journal of the National Cancer Institute*. 1995;87(1):34-40. Available at: http://www.ncbi.nlm.nih.gov/pubmed/7666461.

[8] Friehs GM, Park MC, Goldman M a, et al. Stereotactic radiosurgery for functional disorders. *Neurosurgical focus*. 2007;23(6):E3. Available at: http://www.ncbi.nlm.nih.gov/pubmed/18081480 [Accessed May 23, 2011].

[9] Lunsford L, Alexander E, Chapman P, Coffey R. Consensus Statement on Stereotactic Radiosurgery: Quality Improvement. *Neurosurgery*. 1994. Available at: http://scholar.google.com/scholar?hl=en&btnG=Search&q=intitle:Consensus+Statement+on+Stereotactic+Radiosurgery:+Quality+Improvement#1 [Accessed May 19, 2011].

[10] Pollock BE. *Contemporary stereotactic radiosurgery: technique and evaluation*. Wiley-Blackwell; 2002:354. Available at: http://books.google.com/books?id=yEvjyys11ugC&pg=PA1&lpg=PA1&dq=Stereotactic+radiosurgery:+evolution,+lessons+learned,+and+integration+into+neurosurgical+practice&source=bl&ots=KOApPl9wgd&sig=1wn-wXe_N5GFpMYi1Pt2KDUFwUk&hl=en&ei=Jm7VTeHkNITL0AGxpZiCDA&sa=X&oi=book_result&ct=result&resnum=1&ved=0CB4Q6AEwAA#v=onepage&q=Stereotactic radiosurgery%3A evolution%2C lessons learned%2C and integration into neurosurgical practice&f=false [Accessed May 19, 2011].

[11] Phillips MH, Stelzer KJ, Griffin TW, Mayberg MR, Winn HR. Stereotactic radiosurgery: a review and comparison of methods. *Journal of clinical oncology*. 1994;12(5):1085. Available at: http://www.jcojournal.org/content/12/5/1085.short [Accessed May 23, 2011].

[12] Buatti JM, Friedman W a, Meeks SL, Bova FJ. The radiobiology of radiosurgery and stereotactic radiotherapy. *Medical dosimetry : official journal of the American Association of Medical Dosimetrists*. 1998;23(3):201-7. Available at: http://www.ncbi.nlm.nih.gov/pubmed/9783273.

[13] Kooy HM, Nedzi LA, Loeffler JS, et al. Treatment Planning for Stereotactic Radiosurgery of Intra-Cranial Lesions. *International Journal of Radiation Oncology• Biology• Physics*. 1991;21(3):683–693. Available at: http://linkinghub.elsevier.com/retrieve/pii/036030169190687Y [Accessed June 2, 2011].

[14] Conley GS, Hirsch BE. Stereotactic radiation treatment of vestibular schwannoma: indications, limitations, and outcomes. *Current Opinion in Otolaryngology & Head and Neck Surgery*. 2010;18(5):351. Available at: http://journals.lww.com/co-otolaryngology/Abstract/2010/10000/Stereotactic_radiation_treatment_of_vestibular.2.aspx [Accessed June 2, 2011].

[15] Di Maio S, Akagami R. Prospective comparison of quality of life before and after observation, radiation, or surgery for vestibular schwannomas. *Journal of neurosurgery*. 2009;111(4):855-62. Available at: http://www.ncbi.nlm.nih.gov/pubmed/19301957 [Accessed April 17, 2011].

[16] Pollock BE. Vestibular schwannoma management: an evidence-based comparison of stereotactic radiosurgery and microsurgical resection. *Progress in neurological surgery*. 2008;21:222-7. Available at: http://www.ncbi.nlm.nih.gov/pubmed/18810223 [Accessed June 2, 2011].

[17] Poen JC, Golby a J, Forster KM, et al. Fractionated stereotactic radiosurgery and preservation of hearing in patients with vestibular schwannoma: a preliminary report. *Neurosurgery*. 1999;45(6):1299-305; discussion 1305-7. Available at: http://www.ncbi.nlm.nih.gov/pubmed/10598696.

[18] Paek SH, Chung H-T, Jeong SS, et al. Hearing preservation after gamma knife stereotactic radiosurgery of vestibular schwannoma. *Cancer*. 2005;104(3):580-90. Available at: http://www.ncbi.nlm.nih.gov/pubmed/15952200 [Accessed December 13, 2010].

[19] Yang I, Sughrue ME, Han SJ, et al. Facial nerve preservation after vestibular schwannoma Gamma Knife radiosurgery. *Journal of neuro-oncology*. 2009;93(1):41-8. Available at:

[20] Kondziolka D, Mathieu D, Lunsford LD, et al. Radiosurgery as Definitive Management for Intracranial Meningiomas. *Neurosurgery*. 2008;62(1):53. Available at: http://journals.lww.com/neurosurgery/Abstract/2008/01000/Radiosurgery_As_Definitive_Management_of.4.aspx [Accessed May 26, 2011].

[21] Lee JYK, Niranjan A, McInerney J, et al. Stereotactic radiosurgery providing long-term tumor control of cavernous sinus meningiomas. *Journal of neurosurgery*. 2002;97(1):65-72. Available at: http://www.ncbi.nlm.nih.gov/pubmed/12134934.

[22] Pollock B, Stafford S, Utter a, Giannini C, Schreiner S. Stereotactic radiosurgery provides equivalent tumor control to Simpson Grade 1 resection for patients with

small- to medium-size meningiomas. *International Journal of Radiation OncologyBiologyPhysics*. 2003;55(4):1000-1005. Available at: http://linkinghub.elsevier.com/retrieve/pii/S0360301602043560 [Accessed February 15, 2011].

[23] Duma CM, Lunsford LD, Kondziolka D, Harsh GR, Flickinger JC. Stereotactic radiosurgery of cavernous sinus meningiomas as an addition or alternative to microsurgery. *Neurosurgery*. 1993;32(5):699-704; discussion 704-5. Available at: http://www.ncbi.nlm.nih.gov/pubmed/8492844 [Accessed June 3, 2011].

[24] Nussbaum ES, Djalilian HR, Cho KH, Hall WA. Brain metastases. Histology, multiplicity, surgery, and survival. *Cancer*. 1996;78(8):1781-8. Available at: http://www.ncbi.nlm.nih.gov/pubmed/8859192 [Accessed June 3, 2011].

[25] Warnick RE, Darakchiev BJ, Breneman JC. Stereotactic radiosurgery for patients with solid brain metastases: current status. *Journal of neuro-oncology*. 2004;69(1-3):125-37. Available at: http://www.ncbi.nlm.nih.gov/pubd/15527085.

[26] Pollock B. Management of patients with multiple brain metastases. *Contemp Neurosurg 21*. 1999;21.

[27] Chang SD, Adler JR. Current treatment of patients with multiple brain metastases. *Neurosurgical focus*. 2000;9(2):e5. Available at: http://www.ncbi.nlm.nih.gov/pubmed/16836291.

[28] Aoyama H, Shirato H, Tago M, et al. Stereotactic radiosurgery plus whole-brain radiation therapy vs stereotactic radiosurgery alone for treatment of brain metastases: a randomized controlled trial. *JAMA : the journal of the American Medical Association*. 2006;295(21):2483-91. Available at: http://www.ncbi.nlm.nih.gov/pubmed/16757720.

[29] Kaido T, Hoshida T, Uranishi R, et al. Radiosurgery-induced brain tumor. Case report. *Journal of neurosurgery*. 2001;95(4):710-3. Available at: http://thejns.org/doi/abs/10.3171/jns.2001.95.4.0710 [Accessed June 3, 2011].

[30] McIver JI, Pollock BE. Radiation-induced Tumor after Stereotactic Radiosurgery and Whole Brain Radiotherapy: Case Report and Literature Review. *Journal of Neuro-Oncology*. 2004;66(3):301-305. Available at: http://www.springerlink.com/content/x7120602t456q812/ [Accessed June 3, 2011].

24

Gamma Knife Radiosurgery After Stereotactic Aspiration for Large Cystic Brain Metastases

Do Hoon Kwon and Won Hyoung Park
Department of Neurological Surgery
Asan Medical Center, College of Medicine, Univ. of Ulsan, Seoul, Korea

1. Introduction

Large cystic metastatic brain tumors can be treated with surgical resection, radiation therapy and stereotactic radiosurgery. However, single treatment modality is not effective to improve the quality of life for patients harboring these tumors. In most cases, cystic tumor can not be resected totally due to its eloquent location or patient's physical condition after chemotherapy. Radiotherapy alone is not possible due to large volume with mass effect and its effectiveness is not evaluated. Stereotactic radiosurgery alone is also dangerous due to its large volume. Therefore, in the management of large cystic metastatic brain tumors, multimodality treatment, cyst aspiration and radiosurgery with the same stereotactic frame is one option.

2. Treatment and outcome

2.1 Mechanism of cyst formation

Cystic metastatic brain tumors are common from lung cancer, and non small cell lung cancer is the most common pathology. Sometimes, even in the same pathology, multiple metastatic tumors have cystic and/or solid component.

The cause of cyst formation was not clearly established. Stem et al. suggested that the relatively large amounts of protein in cystic fluid resembled that present in inflammatory exudates, which could be the result of increased permeability of pathologic vessels and mesodermal reactive processes. Cumings et al. also suggested that formation of cystic fluid could be explained by tumor degeneration followed by transudation of fluid from blood vessels. Alternatively, Gardner et al. suggested that fluid accumulating in brain tumors is merely interstitial fluid without its normal drainage route because of the absence of lymphatics in the surrounding brain.

2.2 Surgical treatment

Conventionally, the presence of a large cystic brain tumor has been regarded as an indication for surgery. Yoshida and Morii advocated surgical treatment for patients with large cystic lesions, providing rapid relief of neurological symptoms caused by mass effect. However, if the lesions are located deep in the brain or adjacent to eloquent area, surgical procedures may result in severe neurologic deficits. In addition, surgical procedures are not possible nor effective for patients in poor general condition or those with multiple lesions.

2.3 Stereotactic radiosurgery

From the past decade, stereotactic radiosurgery, particularly with Gamma Knife, have gained increasing relevance in the treatment of cerebral metastatic tumors. The increasing use of this technique is attributable to minimal invasiveness, a substantial reduction in hospitalization time and cost with an excellent local tumor control rates even in radioresistant tumor types and a very low associated morbidity. Moreover, although there had been no direct randomized clinical comparisons of Gamma Knife Radiosurgery with other surgical-radiation protocols, the results of Gamma Knife Radiosurgery in patients with solitary lesions were similar or superior to those obtained using other methods. If the tumors are located in the eloquent areas or in the deep locations, or have large cystic component, it is difficult to remove the tumor completely. Also, large cystic brain metastases do not appear suitable for radiosurgery, because the volume of the lesion is the limiting factor for radiosurgery given that it correlates with radiation induced complication.

Pan et al. reported that tumors with large cystic components (> 10 cc) were not effectively controlled by Gamma Knife Radiosurgery alone.

2.4 Cyst aspiration and stereotactic radiosurgery

In large cystic tumors, Gamma Knife Radiosurgery after stereotactic cyst aspiration could be the better treatment modality than surgical resection or Gamma Knife Radiosurgery alone.

Stereotactic cyst aspiration is a safe and effective procedure. Stereotactic cyst aspiration reduced tumor volume in most of our cases and relieved the neurologic symptom rapidly. The mean volume reduction after aspiration was about 76% compared to the preradiosurgical tumor volume in our results and we could increase the prescription dose to the tumor margin.

The high viscosity of cystic contents can make aspiration difficult. But even in the case of intratumoral hemorrhage which was noted in MR images before radiosurgery, aspiration was not difficult because hemorrhage was mixed with cystic fluid.

Collapsed cystic tumor after aspiration became smaller than initial tumor volume, but remained as a irregular shape. These irregular shaped mass made dose planning difficult in the radiosurgical procedure and needed multiple small isocenters.

This treatment method is composed of two stereotactic procedures with a single frame application. Stereotactic cyst aspiration and Gamma Knife Radiosurgery are performed with a single frame application on the same day with pre and post operative MR guidance. When large cystic tumors were multiple or even septated, aspiration is relatively easy and not difficult to perform under MR guidance. As we experienced several cases of cystic fluid reaccumation in the follow-up period after radiosurgery, Ommaya reservoir was applied after cyst aspiration.

Combined methods, aspiration and radiosurgery were performed in the same day if patient's condition was permitted. But in some cases, the two procedure time was too long, when the patient had have multiple brain metastases or patient's condition was unable to have frame fixation for several hours. In that case, we performed stereotactic cyst aspiration and Ommaya insertion first and delayed Gamma Knife Radiosurgery several days later. The time period of

Ommaya insertion and Gamma Knife Radiosurgery was usually within 7 days, because some cases had have rapid tumor progression or reaccumulation of the cystic fluid.
Applying Ommaya reservoir can make repeated aspiration without difficulty during and after radiosurgery.

2.5 Treatment result

The result of cyst aspiration combined with radiosurgey was rarely reported in the literature. Franzin et al. reported that preoperative tumor volume (mean volume 21.8 cc) was decreased about 46% postoperatively(mean volume 10.1 cc) and he could irradiate above 18 Gy to the tumor margin. He also reported that 92.3% of tumor control rates, overall median survival time was 15 months, the acturarial survival rates at 1 and 2 years was 54.7% and 34.2%, respectively and 26.3% of patients died from neurological progression.
In our study, preoperative tumor volume(mean 24.2cc) decreased about 76% postoperatively(mean 5.6cc), irradiated 20 Gy to the tumor margin. Our results showed that the tumor control rates were 50%, the overall median survival was 17.6 months and 11.1% of the patient died from progression of the brain metastases after treatment (Table 1, 2), (Fig 1, 2).

Characteristics	Number of patients (%)
Age	
<65 years	26 (76.0)
>65 years	8(24.0)
Sex	
Male	17 (50.0)
Female	17 (50.0)
Tumor volume, mean	pre 24.2cc post 5.6cc
Marginal dose, mean	20 (13-25) Gy
Primary tumor	
Non small cell lung cancer	17 (50.0)
Small cell lung cancer	2 (5.9)
Breast cancer	7 (20.1)
Ovarian cancer	2 (5.9)
Colorectal cancer	2 (5.9)
Endometrial carcinoma	2 (5.9)
Hepatocellular carcinoma	1 (2.9)
Malignant melanoma	1 (2.9)
Number of metastases	
1	20 (55.6)
2	8 (22.2)
3	1 (2.9)
>4	5 (14.7)
RPA Classification	
Class I	18 (52.9)
Class II	11 (32.4)
Class III	5 (14.7)

RPA: Recursive partitioning analysis

Table 1. Clinical characteristics of the 34 study patients.

Outcome	Number of patients (%)
Tumor control	17 (50.0)
Local tumor progression	8 (23.5)
Remote tumor progression	9 (26.5)
Death	27(50.0)
Brain metastasis progression	3 (11.1)
Unrelated illness	14 (51.9)
Primary cancer progression	10 (37)

Table 2. Outcomes of the 34 study patients.

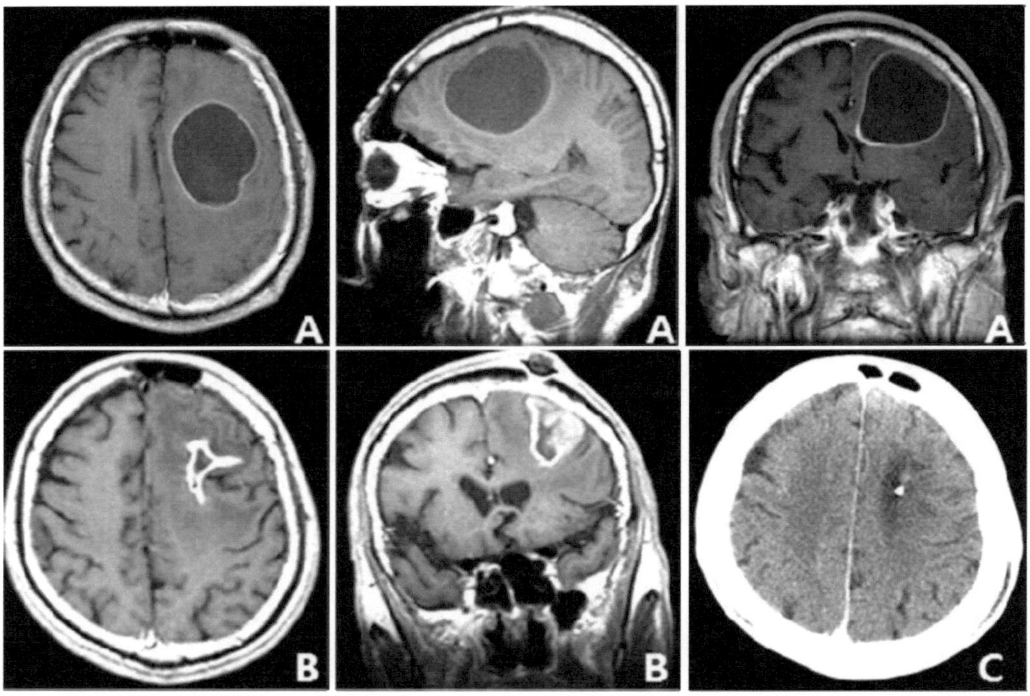

Fig. 1. Gadolinium-enhanced T1-weighted MR image of a 63-year-old man with a large cystic brain metastasis developing from non small cell lung cancer. A : Before aspiration : initial cyst volume, 36.0 cc. B : After cyst aspiration, volume, 8.0 cc. The prescription dose was 20 Gy. C : Enhanced CT scan obtained 6 months postradiosurgery showing no definite enhancing tumor.

Tendulkar et al. reported that median survival was reported to be 8.7 months after subtotal resection for single brain metastasis and 10.6 months after gross total resection of a single brain metastasis. Although it is difficult to directly compare these findings, the results of Gamma Knife Radiosurgery after stereotactic cyst aspiration of large cystic metastases were as good as that of gross total surgical resection of single brain metastasis.
The results of combined treatment modality, median survival and tumor control rates are nearly the same as the results of radiosurgery for solid metastatic brain tumors as reported in Coffey, Flickinger et al., Lutterbach et al. and Sansur et al.

Patient's prognosis is related to numerous parameters, such as KPS score, RPA class, age, location, number of cerebral lesions, character of primary tumor. Among them, RPA class is known as the most important prognostic factor.

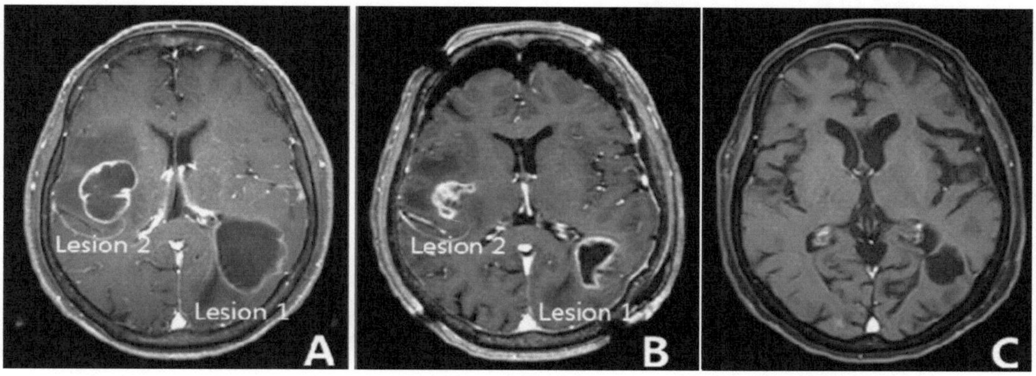

Fig. 2. Axial gadolinium-enhanced T1-weighted MR image of a 70-year-old woman with two large cystic brain metastases developing from breast cancer. A : Before aspiration : initial cyst volume of lesion 1, 34.7 cc; of lesion 2, 11.0 cc. B : After cyst aspiration : cyst volume of lesion 1, 8.0 cc ; of lesion 2, 0.9 cc. The prescription dose was 23 Gy for lesion 1 and 25 Gy for lesion 2. C : Image obtained 12 months postradiosurgery showing no definite enhancing tumors.

Tendulkar et al. reported that patients with unresectable brain metastases classified into RPA class I, II, and III, the median survival time was 7.1 months, 4.2 months and 2.3 months respectively. Lutterbach et al. reported median survival time as 13.4, 9.3 and 1.5 months in RPA class I, II and III, respectively. We observed median survival of 17.8 months, 10.9 months, and 6.1 months in RPA classes I, II and III, respectively. These data and our results confirmed that RPA class is an important tool to predict the patient prognosis in metastatic brain tumors. Moreover, some patients in RPA class III were too weak to permit general anesthesia. But, this combined treatment modality does not require general anesthesia. These findings further reinforce the efficacy of Gamma Knife Radiosurgery after stereotactic cyst aspiration for unresectable cystic brain metastases.

Perfoming Ommaya insertion and cyst aspiration just before Gamma Knife Radiosurgery is the most recommended procedure when the metastatic tumors have a large cyst even patient 's condition is not good after chemotherapy or poor general condition.

2.6 Complications

Ommaya reservoir insertion carries risks such as infection, leptomeningeal dissemination or tumor recurrence along the tube site. We have one case of this complication, tumor recurrence along the tube site, but there was no procedure related mortality nor morbidity.

Another possible complications include hemorrhage, neurosurgical deficits and seizures. The mortality rate in several large series has been less than 1%, and complication rates vary from 0% to 7%.

The complications of stereotactic radiosurgery are related to the effects of radiation on the brain and structures in proximity to the lesions. Significant early complications include

seizures and worsening neurological deficits, but they are very rare. Approximately one-third of patients experiences mild transient symptoms, including headache, nausea and dizziness. Late complications occur 6 to 9 months after the procedure and can include neurologic symptoms according to the tumor location. Patients may become symptomatic from radiation necrosis or local brain edema in the follow-up periods.
Franzin et al. reported that there was no acute complication and 7.6% of the patients experienced radionecrosis after stereotactic aspiration and Gamma Knife Radiosurgery of cystic brain metastases.

3. Conclusion

Cyst aspiration and stereotactic radiosurgery with a same stereotactic frame reduced tumor volume, relieving acute symptoms, permitting decrease in radiation dose to the brain, increasing tumor control rates, increasing median survival, decreasing the associated risks of radiation necrosis and post-radiation complications. Our results support the usefulness and safety of stereotactic radiosurgery after cyst aspiration for large cystic metastatic brain tumors.

4. Acknowledgement

The authors report no conflict of interest concerning the materials or methods used in this study or the findings specified in this chapter.

5. References

Andrews DW, Scott CB, Sperduto PW, et al (2004). Whole brain radiation therapy with or without stereotactic radiosurgery boost for patients with one to three brain metastases : phase III results of the RTGO 9585 randomized trial. Lancet 363 : 1665-1672

Arnold SM, Patchell RA (2001). Diagnosis and management of brain metastases. Hemato Oncol Clin North Am 15 : 1085-1107

Bernstein M, Parrent A (1994). Complication of CT guided stereotactic biopsy of intra-axial brain lesions. J Neurosurg 81 : 165-168

Borgelt B, Gelber R, Kramer S, et al (1980). The palliation of brain metastases : final results of the first two studies by the Radiation Therapy Oncology Group. Int J Radiat Oncol Bio Phys 6 : 1-9

Coffey RJ (1995). Stereotactic radiosurgical treatment of brain metastases in Cohen AR, Haines SJ (Ed) : Minimally invasive Techniques in Neurosurgery. Baltimore : Williams & Wilkins, 1995, pp139-143

Cumings JN (1950). The chemistry of cerebral cysts. Brain 73 : 244-250, 1950

Diener-West M, Dobbins TW, Phillips TL, Nelson DF (1989). Identification of an optimal subgroup for treatment evaluation of patients with brain metastases using RTGO study 7916. Int J Radiat Oncol Bio Phys 16 : 669-673

Flickiner JC (2001). Radiotherapy and radiosurgical management of brain metastases. Curr Oncol Rep 3 : 484-489

Franzin A, Vimercati A, Picozzi P, et al (2008). Stereotactic drainage and Gamma Knife radiosurgery of cystic brain metastasis. J Neurosurg 109 : 259-267

Gardner WJ, Collis JS, Lewis LA (1963). Cystic brain tumors and the blood-brain barrier. Comparision of protein fractions in cyst fluids and sera. Arch Neurol 8 : 291-298

Kim MS, Lee SL, Sim SH (1999). Brain tumors with cyst treated with Gamma Knife Radiosurgery : Is Microsurgery Indicated? Stereotact Funct Neurosurg 72 (Suppl 1) : 38-44

Kondziolka D, Firlik AD, Lunsford LD (1998). Complications of stereotactic brain surgery. Neurol Clin 16 : 35-54

Lohr F, Pirzkall A, Hof H, Fleckenstein K, Debus J (2001). Adjuvant treatment of brain metastases. Semin Surg Oncol 20 : 50-56

Lunsford LD, Martines AJ (1984). Streotactic exploration of the brain in the era of computed tomography. Surg Neurol 22 : 222-230

Lutterbach J, Cyron D, Henne K, Ostertag CB (2003). Radiosurgery followed by planned observation in patients with one to three brain metastases. Neurosurgery 52 : 1066-1074

Mandell L, Hilaris B, Sullvian M, Sundaresan N, Nori D, Kim JH, (1986). The treatment of single brain metastasis from non-oat cell lung carcinoma : surgery and radiation versus radiation therapy alone. Cancer 58 : 641-649

Mingione V, Oliveira M, Prasar D, Steiner M, Steiner L (2002). Gamma surgery for melanoma metastases in the brain. J Neurosurg 96 : 544-551

Muacevic A, Kreth FW, Horstmann GA, et al (1999). Surgery and radiotherapy compared with gamma knife radiosurgery in the treatment of solitary cerebral metastases of small diameter. J Neurosurg 91 : 35-43

Pan HC, Sheehan J, Stroila M, Steiner M, Steiner L (2005). Gamma knife radiosurgery for brain metastases from lung cancer. J Neurosurg 102: 128-133

Park WH, Jang IS, Kwon DH, et al (2009). Gamma Knife radiosurgery after stereotactic aspiration for large cystic brain metastases. J Korean Neurosurg Soc 46: 360-364

Patchell RA, Tibbs PA, Walsh JW, et al (1990). A randomized trial of surgery in the treatment of single metastases to the brain. N England J Med 322 : 494-500

Pullicino P, Thompson EJ, Moseley IF, Zilkha E, Shortman RC(1979). Cystic intracranial tumors. Cyst fluid, biochemical changes and computerized tomographic findings. J Neurol Sci 44 : 77-85

Tendulkar RD, Liu SW, Barnett GH, et al (2006). RPA classification has prognostic significance for surgically resected single brain metastasis. Int J Radiat Oncol Biol Phys 66 :810-817

Sansur CA, Chin LS, Ames JW, et al (2000). Gamma knife radiosurgery for the treatment of brain metastases. Stereotact Funct Neurosurg 74 : 37-51

Stem K (1939). Chemical study of fluids obtained from cerebral cysts : report on 56 cases. Brain 62 : 88

Weissman DE (1988): Glucocorticoid treatment for brain metastases and epidural spinal cord compression : a review. J Clin Oncol 6 : 543-551

Werner-Wasik M, Rudoler S, Preston PE, et al (1999). Immediate side effects of stereotactic radiotherapy and radiosurgery. Int J Radiat Oncol Biol Phys 43 : 299-304

Yoshida S, Morii K (2004). The role of surgery in the treatment of brain metastasis : a retrospective review. Acta Neurochir (Wien) 146 : 767-770

25

Management of Brain Tumors in Eloquent Areas

José Manuel González - Darder and Pablo González - López
Department of Neurosurgery, Hospital Clínico Universitario Valencia
Spain

1. Introduction

Brain tumours in eloquent areas represent a great challenge for Neurosurgeons due to its surgical resection complexity. The main goal of this chapter is the comprehensive study of perioperative work-up, diagnostic and preoperative functional techniques, microsurgical skills and intraoperative monitoring for the management of brain tumours located in eloquent areas.

Integral management of brain tumors in eloquent areas involves different but related disciplines. So to reach a correct diagnosis, localization, treatment and prognosis, it is necessary to follow neuroclinical, neuroanatomical, neuroradiological, neurophysiological and neuropathological protocols. A complete resection is thought to be the best initial treatment for glial - type tumors, although there is no scientific evidence that a greater extent of resection is associated with a better prognosis (Berger et al., 1994; Keles et al., 2001, 2006; Pesudo et al., 2001; Sanai & Berger, 2008; Shaw et al., 2008).

The infiltrative growth pattern of the neuropil by glial tumors is the reason for surgical treatment not being curative (Claes et al., 2007) and therefore the majority of patients will suffer a relapse or local progression of the disease some time after surgery. The known molecular mechanisms that drive this pattern of cellular migration have been deeply studied (Giese et al., 1995, 1996, 2003; Hwang et al., 2008). Although until new treatments for glial tumors are developed, the cytoreduction provided by surgery will maintain its value, because it offers material for diagnosis and research, alleviates both the focal and clinical symptoms of intracranial hypertension, and contributes to a greater efficacy of oncological treatments. Following this line of reasoning, there is a large number of modern series supporting the idea of resecting the largest possible volume of tumor (Giese et al., 2003; McGirt et al., 2008, 2009; Sanai & Berger 2008). The price to pay for radical resection may be an increase in morbidity, fact that takes a special challenge in case of highly eloquent areas. In this sense, a great number of imaging, neurophysiological, neurochemical, and even surgical techniques have recently been developed and incorporated into the management of these tumors, with the ultimate objective being to optimize the resection limits; to extend them to the maximum while minimizing the eventual associated morbidity (Price et al., 2006; Provenzale et al., 2004; Stummer et al., 1998; Tanaka et al., 2009).

The final objective of this approach is to resect the lesion identified as tumoral based on the imaging techniques, as well as the neighboring brain tissue that is normal in appearance during surgery, but that is suspected of being invaded by tumor cells, or with cells already affected by the molecular disorder that would convert them into tumor cells. In this way, the tumoral resection limit would be taken to the point where there may be deterioration of any neurological function considered important (functional resection limit). This concept of functional resection limit extremes in case of brain tumors in eloquent areas due to the high eloquence of the surrounding brain tissue.

2. Neuroanatomy of eloquent areas

An accurate knowledge of function distribution over the human brain is necessary for the preoperatory planification development. The functional cortical and subcortical structures can be identified during tumor resection in different ways. In the same way, preoperative localization of intra-axial tumors and functional areas can be performed using multiple non-invasive imaging techniques.

2.1 Motor function

Most of brain areas related with motor function are located in the frontal lobe (Fig.1). The classical primary motor area is anatomically located in the precentral gyrus just anterior to the boundary between the frontal and parietal lobe, the central sulcus. In 1870, Gustav Fritsch and Eduard Hitzig published a paper entitled 'On the Electrical Excitability of the Cerebrum', which experimentally demonstrated that cortical stimulation of certain brain areas induced tonic muscle contractions in the contralateral body side. These areas have been largely studied since then, and the primary motor area has been demonstrated to be the area with a lower threshold for induction of movements after electrical stimulation. However there are other cortical areas related with the planning and control of movement. In this sense the Premotor and Supplementary Motor Area stand out. Both the premotor area and the supplementary motor area are included in the superior frontal gyrus, on its lateral and mesial side, right in front of the precentral sulcus. Other brain area related with the movement control remains located in the Primary Somatosensitive Area in the Parietal Lobe. This area is supposed to process and incorporate the nociceptive inputs to the motion generation. Some regions in the insular lobe have also been related with the motor control.

All these brain cortical regions receive and send inputs and outputs to the corticospinal fiber tract in order to build coordinate movements. The corona radiata is a white matter region composed by these fibers, which come and go to different structures as the corpus callosum and especially to the internal capsule. The internal capsule can be subdivided in anterior and posterior limbs, and genu. The genu and posterior limb mainly contain motor and sensitive information. The motor fiber pathways get into the cerebral peduncles at the level of the diencephalo - mesencephalic junction, and finally decussate just before reaching the spinal cord.

2.2 Sensitive function

The path followed by the sensitive information is opposite to the motor system. It comes from the spinal cord through the medial lemniscus at the level of the mesencephalon. These fibers and the trigeminothalamic fiber tract join together and enter in the ventroposterior lateral nucleus of thalamus, where after synapsing are launched to the sensitive cortex through the superior thalamic peduncle, which joins to the posterior limb of the internal capsule at the level of the caudate body in the lateral wall of lateral ventricles. This sensitive information mainly travels to the Primary Somatosensitive Area located in the Postcentral Gyrus, posterior to the central sulcus in the Parietal Lobe.

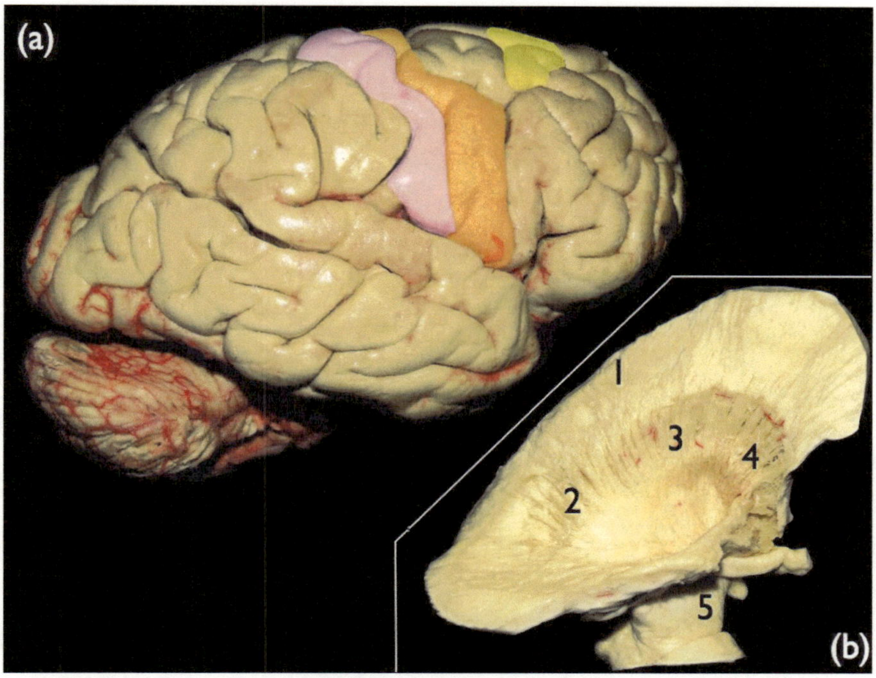

Fig. 1. (a) Right lateral view of the brain and cerebellar hemisphere in a cadaveric specimen after removing the arachnoid and vessels of the supratentorial cortex, where it is possible to appreciate the primary motor area in orange, the primary somatosensitive area in pink, and part of the supplementary motor area in yellow color; (b) right lateral view of the internal capsule where it is possible to appreciate the corona radiata (1), genu (3), anterior (4) and posterior (2) limbs of internal capsule, and caudally the cerebral peduncle (5)

2.3 Speech

In the XIX century, Paul Broca first described the language area after studying brain specimens of patients suffering aphasia. This area, nowadays known as Broca´s Area, is anatomically located in the Inferior Frontal Gyrus of the dominant Frontal Lobe, filling the pars triangularis and opercularis (Fig.2). This area is essential in producing fluent speech. A lesion of Broca's area results in a non-fluent aphasia. Patients emit few words, both spoken and written, and understanding is maintained. The nondominant inferior frontal gyrus is involved in controlling the rhythm, intonation and emotion of verbal content, which is known as prosody. Therefore, any injury on that region will produce aprosodia, which is the lack of emotion in words. Both the premotor and supplementary motor area of the dominant hemisphere, are also involved in speech production. Speech also seems to consist of different areas located in the cortex of the temporoparietal and insular dominant hemispheres, as well as scattered groups of neurons that are activated parallely. The anterior commissure is a white fiber bundle that connects both temporal lobes and is supposed to be integrated in the speech circuit. However the main fiber tract involved in language comprehension and production is the superior longitudinal fasciculus, which connects the frontal, parietal, occipital and temporal lobes. This fasciculus is the longest of the association fiber bundles. It remains superior to the lentiform nucleus and lateral to the insula.

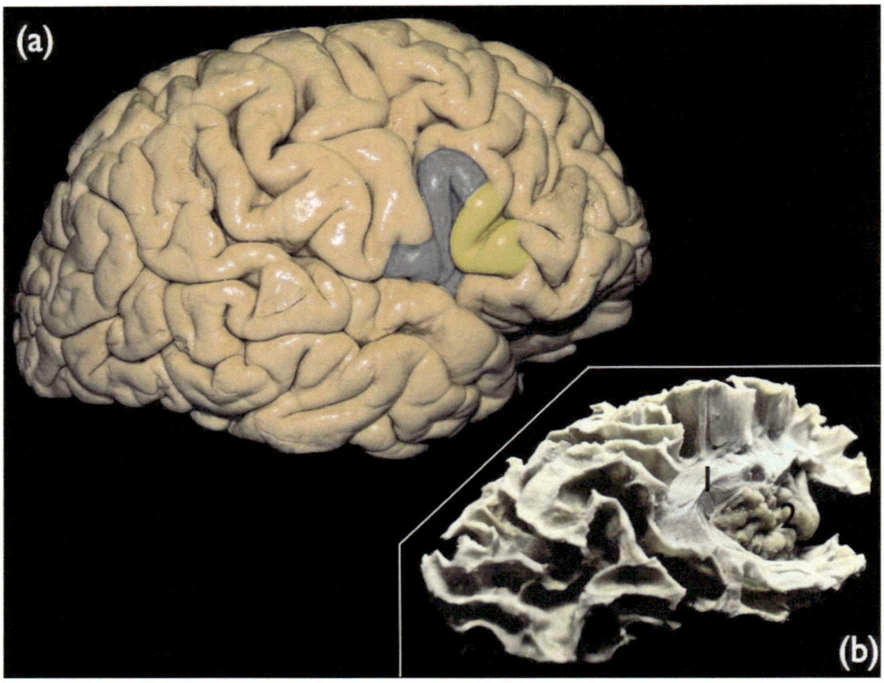

Fig. 2. (a) Right lateral see of the brain where it is possible to view in blue the pars opercularis and in yellow the pars triangularis; (b) posterolateral view of the superior longitudinal fasciculus (1) surrounding the insular lobe (2)

2.4 Vision and eyes movement

The Primary Visual Area, also known as striate cortex, is located in the Occipital Lobe, surrounding the calcarine sulcus. The visual information travels from the optic nerves and tracts till reaching the lateral geniculate bodies, from where after synapsing, the electrical impulse is transmitted to the striate cortex through the optic radiations, which remain located in the deep inferior temporal gyrus surrounding the temporal horn of lateral ventricles, is integrated in the posterior thalamic radiations and sagittal stratum at the level of the corona radiata, and finally ends in the occipital lobe surface.

Related with the process of vision it is important to highlight the Frontal Eye Field, which is ahead of the representation of the face and hand in the primary motor cortex, just behind the middle frontal gyrus and precentral sulcus. This area is responsible for saccadic eye movements, and their stimulation causes horizontal conjugate eye movements or oblique to the contralateral side. An injury of the frontal eye area can cause inability to turn its gaze on a voluntary basis to the contralateral visual field. Its main outputs or frontopontine projections travel together within the anterior limb of the internal capsule.

2.5 Memory and learning

A region highly implicated in learning and memory is located in the prefrontal cortex, receiving outputs from associative somatosensitive, visual and auditive areas. This area is responsible of the commonly known as working memory, related with planning and problem - solving and attention span. The orbital and medial prefrontal cortex receives connections from limbic structures like the amygdala. The mesial structures of the temporal lobe and the limbic circuit are also important structures in memory and learning ability. The limbic circuit is integrated by important mesial structures as the cingulum, amygdala, hippocampus, parahippocampal gyrus, fornix, mammillary body, mammillothalamic tract and some thalamic nuclei, among others.

2.6 Reading

J. Jules Dejerine in the XIX century first described different syndromes related to reading disability. The reading ability is known to be located mainly in the Gyrus Angularis in the Parietal Lobe, and posterior part of the Superior (Wernicke´s Area) and Inferior Temporal Gyri in the Temporal Lobe, both in the dominant hemisphere.

2.7 Hearing

The auditory pathways are quite complex and include different white matter fiber tracts and nuclei in different levels of the encephalon. The main structures related with the audition are the vestibulocochlear nerve, cochlear nucleus, superior olive, inferior colliculus, medial geniculate body of thalamus, and finally the auditory cortex. The Primary Auditory Area is composed of the Transverse Gyrus of Heschl deep to the Superior Temporal Gyrus in the Sylvian Fissure, which crosses the upper surface and posterior Temporal Lobe.

3. History and physical examination

Physical examination remains of great interest in neurological diseases, but this fact takes on special significance when dealing with intrinsic brain tumors in Eloquent Areas.
Prior to modern neuroimaging, neurological treatment decisions were based on findings obtained from patient history and clinical examination. Despite the great information given by new imaging techniques, the clinical exam of associated neurological disturbances can be very helpful in order to identify intracranial tumors in the clinical practice (Maranhao et al., 2010). History and clinical exam offer important information to diagnose brain tumors and their location. Actually a detailed physical examination and a complete imaging analysis, is often enough as a perioperative assessment.
Clinical presentation of brain tumors commonly appears as irritative symptoms like seizures (almost 80% of intrinsic brain tumors; presenting and also once diagnosed). Although its high frequency, irritative symptoms do not clearly orient to the tumor location.
Neurological deficit is also a classic event referred in cases of brain tumors in eloquent areas, and the kind of neurological disturbance can help to clarify the tumor location. Tumors affecting the frontal lobe can show clinical findings like hemiparesis, conjugate deviation of eyes, fluent speech deficits or difficulty with word finding in case of dominant hemisphere and memory and learning difficulties. Patients diagnosed of brain intrinsic tumors affecting the Parietal Lobe can present hemiparesis, paresthesias and dysesthesias, and aphasia and symptoms as reading and hearing disturbances when affecting the dominant hemisphere. Parietal lobe tumors can even present hemianopia and spatial disorientation. Temporal Lobe tumors usually present a large variety and even mixed symptoms. The most common symptoms are temporal seizures. Lesions in the dominant hemisphere can show different degrees and varieties of speech, hearing and reading abnormalities. Memory and learning disabilities are also symptoms frequently found in this kind of tumors. Quadrantanopia is also a frequent symptom present after an ophthalmologic revision in temporal lobe tumors.

Patients affected by Occipital Lobe intrinsic brain tumors can notice visual problems as contralateral hemianopia, although these findings can be misinterpreted, fact that makes necessary a specific visual examination. Insular lobe connects the limbic system and cortical areas, taking part in many superior functions, so tumors located in this deep area can affect sensitive, motor, speech and auditive tasks. Lesions affecting the limbic circuit usually present as cognitive disorders or memory disabilities. Subcortical lesions infiltrating or displacing important white matter fiber bundles can cause hemiparesis, sensitive and eyes movement disturbances in case of the internal capsule, memory and cognitive disorders in case of the uncinate fascicle, speech problems when affecting the superior longitudinal fascicle and of course visual problems in case of lesions damaging the optic radiations.

Lobe affected	Symptomatology
Frontal	Personality and gait disturbances, expressive aphasia, hemipharesis, conjugate deviation of eyes, seizures
Parietal	Sensory disturbances, receptive aphasia, hemianopia, spatial disorientation
Temporal	Behaviour disturbances, hearing loss, comprehension inabilities, symptoms of autism, memory loss, quadrantanopia
Occipital	Hemianopia
Insular	Comprehension and expression disturbances, hemiparesis, personality changes, memory problems

Table 1. Focal Neurologic Signs and Symptoms of Primary Brain Tumors

Brain tumors can also show different degrees of cognitive disabilities. These symptoms can be difficult to interpret because of the inability of most of these patients to perceive changes in memory and personality, and even to relate a comprehensive history. In this sense a close family member can help to uncove some clinical findings.

Moreover the type of symptoms, it is also really helpful exploring the timing. Evolutive and progressive changes orient to a tumor diagnosis. In this sense it remains of great interest to perform specific questions with the aim of remarking symptoms that could have been misinterpreted by the patient. Slow progression of symptomatology focuses to a low - grade tumor, while a rapid progression focuses the study to a high - grade tumor. The duration of symptoms varies greatly, due to the fact that some patients have harbored lower grade gliomas that have undergone malignant transformation, leading to longer histories than those high - grade gliomas that arise de novo.

4. Medical management

Initial medical treatment is almost always the first step in managing brain tumors. In addition to provide a definitive treatment, an important role of neurosurgeons taking care of patients recently diagnosed of brain tumors is to alleviate the most common appearing symptoms as increased intracranial pressure due to peritumoral edema, headache, medication side effects, pain, symptomatic seizures, venous thromboembolism, fatigue and cognitive dysfunction. Effective medical management results in decreased morbidity and mortality and improved quality of life for affected patients. Although there are relatively few studies addressing these issues (Wen et al., 2006), guidelines can be offered to maximize quality of life and minimize hospital admissions.

4.1 Initial medical treatment

4.1.1 Peritumoral edema

Tumor - associated vasogenic edema is due to increased capillary permeability in the blood - brain barrier. This vasogenic edema surrounding brain tumors contributes significantly to the morbidity experienced by patients, resulting in headache with emesis and even seizures exacerbation (Papadopoulos et al., 2001); when severe, this edema can result in herniation and death. Corticosteroids are routinely employed when treating patients affected of brain tumors with symptomatic mass effect and cerebral edema, resulting in an essential early part of brain tumor therapy (Kaal & Vecht, 2004).

In selected cases, when a fast depletive treatment is required, other measures as elevation of the head of the bed, diuretics, or fluid restriction, can be chosen till the steroid therapy becomes effective. Although the mechanism is not well known yet, steroids are thought to reduce the permeability of tumor capillaries.

The empirical initial dose of steroids is an intravenous bolus of 10 mg of dexamethasone, followed by a maintenance dose of 4 mg every 6 hours in patients with significant symptomatic edema. Complete absorption from gastrointestinal tract is quite fast, and oral therapy should be used as soon as possible. Higher doses to these proposed can be employed in patients who do not respond to the usual initial dose. Response to steroids must be measured in terms of neurological deficits improvement during the first 48 hours. The dose may be increased up to 100 mg/day when necessary (Vick & Wilson, 1985). For asymptomatic patients with peritumoral edema on neuroimaging studies, corticosteroids are usually unnecessary.

Unfortunately corticosteroids are associated with a number of side effects, and the benefit should be balanced with the appearing of common side effects. The most common and important to notice complications in patients with brain tumors during steroid treatment are gastrointestinal disturbances, insomnia, manic behavior and hyperglycemia. Most of these side effects are solved after withdrawal of therapy (Wen et al., 2006). Patients with diabetes should be daily monitored in order to control their glycemic values to modify insulin dosage when necessary.

4.1.2 Seizures

Seizures are the presenting symptom of a brain tumor in up to 40% of patients and occur during the course of the illness in more than 60% of patients with tumors in the cerebral hemispheres (Moots et al., 1995). A cortical location of tumor is particularly common in patients with tumor - related epilepsy, with white matter and deep gray nuclei less common. Although the pathogenesis is poorly understood, some factors may be involved, as altered peritumoral amino acids, alteration and distribution of glutamate receptors, pH, neuronal and glial enzyme and protein expression (Schaller & Ruegg, 2003).

Antiepileptic drug treatment is universally accepted when a recognized seizure has appeared. However, there is strong evidence against the prophylactic use of antiepileptic drugs in patients just diagnosed brain tumors and free of seizures (Glantz et al., 2000).

The treatment should be performed with standard antiepileptic drugs. The selection of drugs usually depends on the surgeon´s preferences. Phenytoin is the most commonly used antiepileptic when treating and preventing seizures in neurosurgery. Its pharmacokinetics remains quite variable among different patients, so its blood levels must be monitored until reaching the clinically effective serum level (10-20 mcg/mL). A loading dose must be employed at the beginning, inyecting 15-18 mg/kg/24h spread in three doses: half a dose initially, a quarter after 8 hours, and the last quarter after 16 hours. The maintenance dose ranges between 5-7 mg/kg/24h spread in three doses (once each 8 hours again). Once effective serum levels have been achieved, the dosage usually ranges between 300-500 mg/d in three doses. With recommended dosage, a period of 7-10 days may be required to achieve a steady state. Sodium valproate is also commonly employed in case of epileptogenic brain tumors. As other antiepileptic drugs, serum levels are difficult to be reached at the beginning. The usually employed intravenous loading dose remains in 15 mg/kg spread in 10-20 minutes, continuing after half an hour with a continuous perfusion of 1 mg/kg/h. The optimum dose must be balanced attending to the clinical efficacy. The plasmatic efficient levels range between 50-125 mcg/mL. Oral administration must be used as soon as possible, dealing 20-30 mg/kg between 2 and 3 doses a day. Carbamazepine is usually administered with a gradual increase of dosage. The optimal dosage is 800-1200 a day. Although its antiquity, phenobarbital is still used in cases of refractory symptomatic seizure disorders in patients affected by intrinsic brain tumors.

The unnecessary use of antiepileptic agents can alter the metabolism of many other drugs as steroids, chemotherapeutic agents and other antiepileptic, after inducing hepatic P450 enzymes (phenytoin, carbamazepine, phenobarbital). Actually there are a large number of agents free of inducing hepatic enzymes, with relatively few drug interactions (French et al., 2004).

Although infrequent, patients with brain tumors comprise 4-12 % of patients developing status epilepticus (Wen et al., 2006). Intravenous administration of antiepileptic agents is necessary in these cases.

4.1.3 Reduced mobility

Venous thromboembolism is a common cause of morbidity and mortality among patients with brain tumors of all types, particularly during the perioperative period (Rosenfeld & Pruitt, 2007). This fact takes on special significance when dealing with brain tumors in eloquent areas, specially in motor areas, due to the reduced mobility from paretic limbs, which increase the risk for deep vein thrombosis and subsequent pulmonary emboli. An interesting study estimated the rate of symptomatic deep vein thrombosis to be 24% over the 17 months beyond the first 6 postoperative weeks. Although the pathogenesis is not completely understood yet, several risk factors have been identified: venous stasis in paretic limbs, age > 60, larger tumor size, prolonged surgery, chemotherapy, high - dose steroid therapy and hormonal therapy (Marras et al., 2000).

Most neurosurgeons prefer the use of low - dose heparin (3500-5000 U subcutaneously/day), with which postoperative bleeding is uncommon.

4.2 Preoperative medical treatment

Preoperative medical protocols for surgery of brain tumors in eloquent areas differ from other brain tumors due to the special intraoperative techniques and anaesthesic management employed.

General medical guidelines include steroid therapy, anticonvulsant agents and prophylaxis of venous thromboembolism in patients undergoing surgery for brain tumors. The effectiveness of prophylactic antiepileptic agents in patients who have undergone craniotomy is unclear. Different studies have showed no differences in risk of postoperative seizures between groups treated and no treated with anticonvulsant prophylaxis. However others have shown that prophylactic antiepileptic agents reduced the frequency of post - operative seizures during the first week after a supratentorial surgery (North et al., 1983). In cases of awake or slept but non - relaxed surgery for brain tumors, the use of anticonvulsant drugs remains necessary and serum levels should be achieved days before surgery. The morning of surgery, antiepileptic dosage should be doubled (10 mg/kg followed by 5 mg/kg/day postoperative in case of phenytoin). However the dosage could depend on the tumor location, and definitive studies should be designed in order to adjust all the variables implicated. Preoperative steroids are used when peritumoral edema is obvious before surgery. As mentioned before, the effect of dexamethasone begins effective 24-48 h after its introduction. In case of preoperative treatment an initial bolus of 10 mg followed by 10 mg/6h 24h before surgery should be enough.

4.3 Postperative medical treatment

General medical management after a craniotomy performed to treat a brain tumor primary implies control of intracranial pressure due to cerebral edema, seizures due to cortex irritation, analgesia and deep vein thrombosis due to immobilization. Dexamethasone can be progressively reduced after surgery, but higher dosages are recommended during the first 24-48 h (6-8 mg/6h). Serum levels of antiepileptic drugs must be ranged between their clinical effective values. However, the most frequent systemic complication after craniotomy is deep vein thrombosis, reaching values of 1-10% of patients during the first month (Brandes et al., 1997). Multimodality venous thrombosis prophylaxis should begin at the time of the original surgery, taking patients out of bed and mobilized as soon as possible after surgery, using external leg compression until the patient is ambulatory and introducing anticoagulation with 5000 U of heparin or low molecular weight heparin subcutaneously 24 hours after the craniotomy. However, it must not be forgotten the risk of bleeding (7/1000 intracranial hemorrhage and 28/1000 minor bleedings) (Hamilton et al., 2011).

Patients with primary brain tumors suffer a high risk of being affected by postoperative medical and surgical complications. The most accepted classification about postoperative complications after a craniotomy was performed in 1998 dividing them into three major groups: neurological, regional and systemic complications (Sawaya et al., 1998). Main neurologic postoperative deficits are motor, sensory, language and visual disturbances. When dealing with regional complications, we mean wound infections, CSF fistula, hydrocephalus, seizure, brain abscess, cerebritis and meningitis. Infectious processes require antibiotic drugs that cross the blood - brain barrier, and sometimes delayed surgeries. Other regional complications as hydrocephalus and CSF fistula usually require individualized mixed treatments. Seizures must be treated through antiepileptic drugs when there are not image findings, which justify them. Systemic complications include deep vein thrombosis, pulmonary embolus, myocardial infarction, urinary tract infection, pneumonia and sepsis. Each one of these entities requires individual treatments, but most of them, as neurological and regional complications, can be prevented through a careful preoperative planning, meticulous surgical technique, and attentive postoperative care.

Complication		Treatment
NEUROLOGICAL		
	Motor/Sensory disability	Depending on the cause (retraction, ischemic, compression, bleeding, mass effect)
	Aphasia	
	Visual disturbances	
REGIONAL		
	Seizures	Antiepileptic drugs
	Hematoma	Depending on the location and clinical symptomatology
	Hydrocephalus	External ventricular drainage ± Definitive shunt
	Pneumocephalus	Observation vs. Revision depending on the clinical symptomatology
	Cerebrospinal fluid leak	Medical treatment and/or wound revisión
	Wound infection	Surgical revisión and Antibiotics
	Meningitis	Antibiotics
SYSTEMIC		
	Pulmonary, urinary tract, central line infections and sepsis	Antibiotics
	Deep vein thrombosis	Anticoagulation therapy

Table 2. Postoperative complications in patients after craniotomies (Sawaya et al., 1998)

5. Imaging

Dealing with brain tumors has been dramatically changed since the improvement of diagnostic imaging techniques. Neuroimaging with either magnetic resonance imaging or computed tomography improves the accuracy of diagnosis and remains indispensable for surgical planning.

Nowadays, modern imaging techniques are necessary to detect or confirm a structural abnormality, localize and assess the abnormality, characterize the abnormality, plan the surgical approach and extension, predict the possible postoperative neurological deficits, orient to the metabolism and metabolites composition of the tumor and surroundings, understand the 3D anatomical relation of the tumor with brain eloquent areas (cortical and subcortical) through functional and anatomical sequences, as well as to rate the surgical extent of resection intra and postoperatively.

5.1 Diagnostic techniques

5.1.1 Computed tomography

Computed tomography is a great screening method and almost always the most commonly used image modality for the initial patient evaluation, mainly in cases of supratentorial abnormalities, due to its accuracy and availability.

CT scanners provide enough specific information for the initial management of brain tumors. Once detected a lesion it is also important to try to characterize it, due to the immediate management differences between neoplasms and non - neoplastic processes. This is the main reason to perform a CT with the aid of contrast agents. This modality differentiates between intrinsic and extrinsic tumors, and is also helpful to delimitate the edema from necrotic or cystic areas.

Brain tumors may be hypodense, isodense or hyperdense on a noncontrast CT scan, depending on tumor location and histology. Isodense or small tumors with few peritumoral edema and mass effect can be difficult to be visualized on noncontrast CT, but highlight after contrast injection. Extra - axial brain tumors show a good resolution with CT and usually enhance after contrast administration, while low - grade gliomas and epidermoid tumors do not enhance. Although MRI is preferable for tumor definitive evaluation, CT is preferred to detect calcifications, intratumoral hemorrhage or bone abnormalities as destruction, erosion, infiltration and hyperostosis.

5.1.2 Magnetic resonance imaging

Despite initial CT scanners, MRI is nowadays the imaging method of choice in the pre - therapeutical evaluation of brain tumors.

Usual MRI sequences let visualizing both normal anatomy and pathological findings. They are used in the clinical set for lesion detection, localization, characterization, determination of tumor extension, planning and guiding tumor biopsy and therapeutical actions, and monitoring of treatment response. Advanced MRI sequences allow semi-quantitative and quantitative measurements of several entities, such as movement of water molecules, cerebral blood volume and flow or chemical tissue composition (Cha, 2006).

5.1.2.1 Anatomic imaging

Brain tumors localization and relations with their surroundings reach the highest interest in cases of tumors in eloquent areas. Once diagnosed a brain tumor, the next point on its evaluation remains in the fact of its anatomic location. Some MRI techniques are recommended for this purpose: T1- and T2-weighted sequences, including FLAIR, after gadolinium T1-weighted sequences with at least one spin-echo sequence, and an additional T1-weighted 3D sequence. In order to achieve a good localization of tumors in the different eloquent areas, it is recommended to perform at least the T1- and T2-weighted sequences in the axial, coronal and sagittal planes of the space.

The goal of anatomic imaging sequences in case of brain tumors in eloquent areas is centered on identifying some cortical areas as the supplementary motor area, premotor area, primary motor area in case of motor function; primary somatosensitive area in case of sensory; frontal aye field and primary visual or striate cortex in case of visual function; primary auditive cortex or transverse gyrus of Heschl in case of auditive function; and Broca´s and Wernicke´s area in case of language and comprehension.

As known by anatomy the supplementary motor, premotor area and frontal eye field are located respectively along the most medial, posterior and lateral portion of the superior frontal and immediately facing the precentral gyrus, seen in axial and sagittal T2-weighted slices. The central sulcus of Rolando and therefore the primary motor area (precentral gyrus), and primary somatosensitive area (postcentral gyrus) located just in front and behind it can be easily located by selecting the most rostral axial T2-weighted slices.

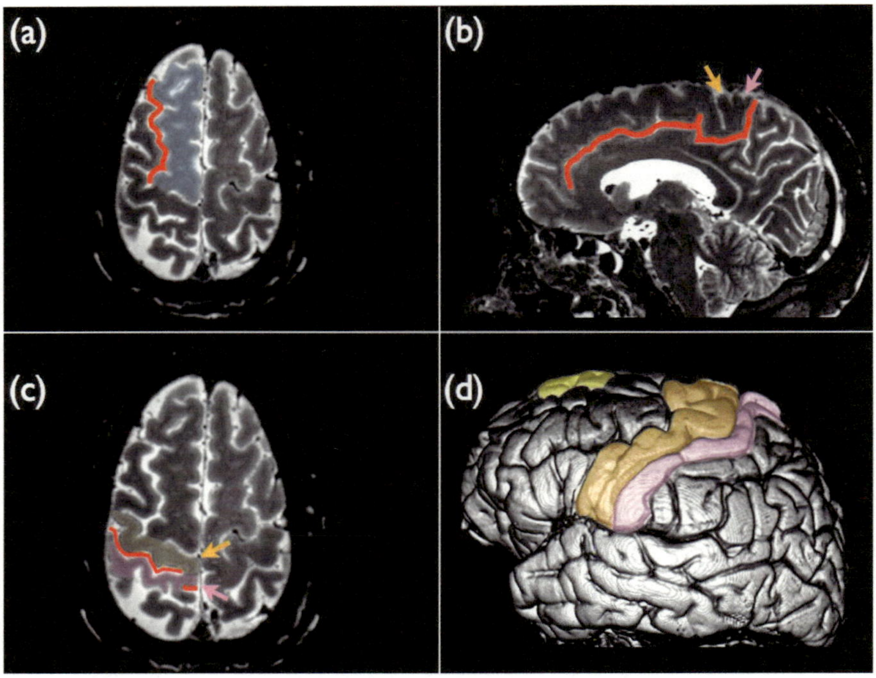

Fig. 3. (a) Axial T2 - weighted MRI slice where the superior frontal gyrus and superior frontal sulcus are marked in blue and red respectively; (b) midline sagittal T2 - weighted slice with the cingulate sulcus marked in red, showing the primary motor and somatosensitive areas through orange and pink arrows; (c) Axial T2 - weighted MRI slice where the primary motor and somatosensitive areas are marked in orange and pink, and the central sulcus in red; (d) 3D reconstruction from a T2 - weighted multislice study, with the supplementary motor, primary motor and somatosensitive areas in yellow, orange and pink respectively

The central sulcus is a good reference for the location of the motor homunculus, since despite the mass effect is always present and allows the preoperative study of the motor areas. In a parafalcian sagittal section, the Rolandic cortex (motor and somatosensory areas) is easily identifiable by following the superior cingulate gyrus and then to its end point (ascendent or marginal gyrus). The rolandic cortex is just anterior to this groove. In more lateral sagittal images, drawing a perpendicular line upward from the posterior corner of the insular triangle can easily identify the precentral sulcus (Fig.3).

Broca´s area is located in the dominant hemisphere in the opercular and triangular parts of the inferior frontal gyrus, which can be easily visualized in a lateral sagittal slice (Gallucci, 2007; Ribas, 2010). This area is visible on coronal sections of the brain, when this section, perpendicular to the commissural plane, is located within 15 or 20 mm in front of the anterior commissure.

In the same sagittal slice, Wernicke Area is located over the reverse C - shaped convolution constituted by the connection of the supramarginal and superior temporal gyri that encircles the posterior end of the sylvian fissure (Fig. 4).
The primary auditive cortex is located in the transverse gyrus of Heschl, which can be located using the sylvian fissure and superior temporal sulcus as the main landmarks. In a coronal slice at a point where the body of the lateral ventricles becomes into the atrium, the transverse gyrus shows a typical convex image between the superior temporal and lateral sulcus (Fig.5).
The main landmarks to locate the primary visual area are the calcarine and parieto - occipital fissures, and remain well outlined on a midline sagittal section of the brain.
Despite all these landmarks and reference points to locate the brain eloquent areas, in the clinical practice this fact can be more difficult due to the peritumoral edema and mass effect, which usually distorts the normal brain anatomy. In this sense other imaging techniques have appeared to solve this problem.

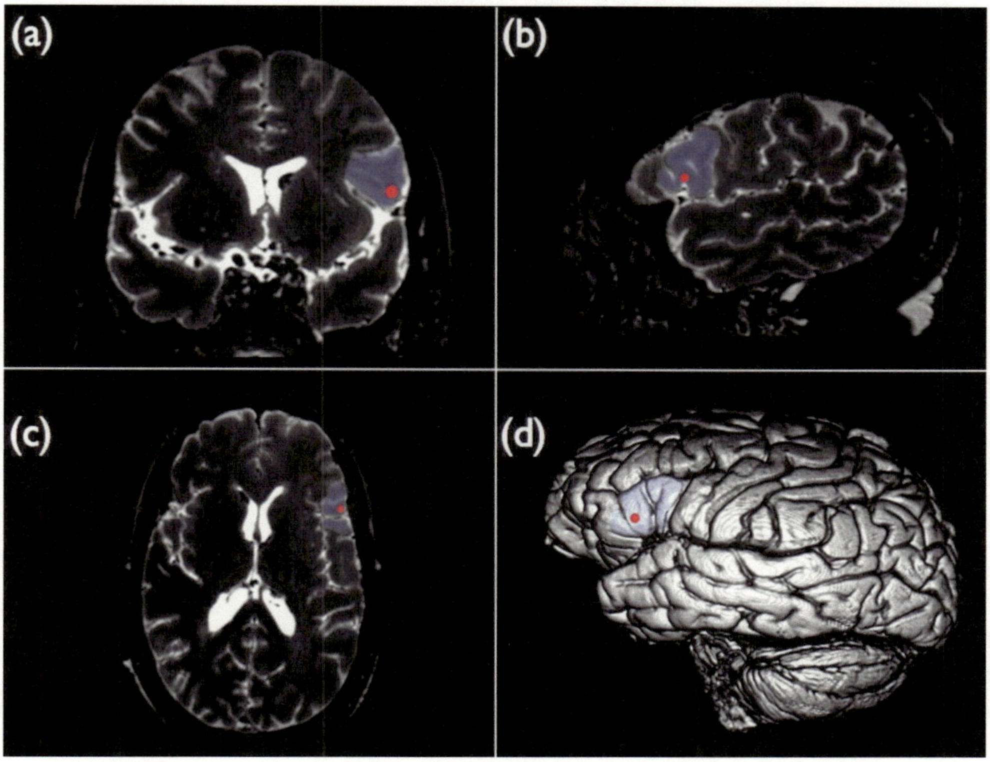

Fig. 4. (a) Coronal T2 - weighted MRI slice 15 mm rostral from the anterior commissure with the pars opercularis in blue and a red dot as reference for the next slices; (b) sagittal T2 - weighted MRI slice from the red dot of the coronal slice and part of pars triangularis and pars opercularis in blue; (c) axial T2 - weighted MRI slice with Broca´s area in blue; (d) 3D reconstruction from a T2 - weighted multislice study, where Broca´s area can be identified in blue

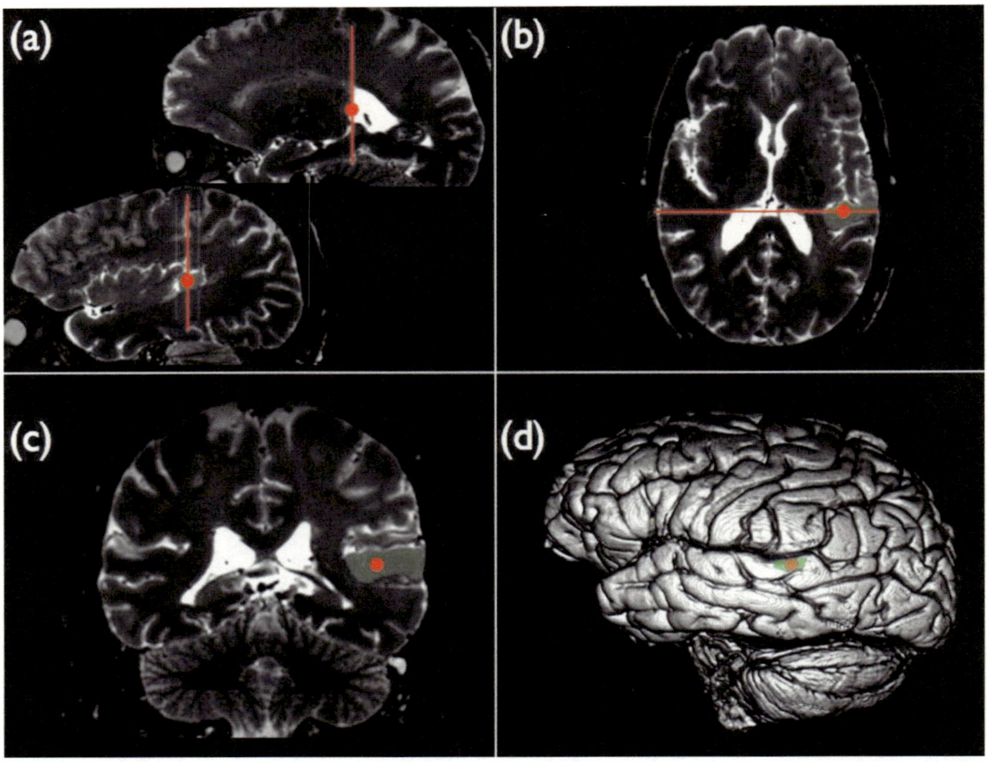

Fig. 5. (a) Sagittal T2 - weighted MRI slice at a point where the body of the lateral ventricles becomes into the atrium and its lateral translation till reaching the transverse gyrus of Heschl in green; (b) axial T2 - weighted MRI slice with transverse gyrus of Heschl in green; (c) coronal T2 - weighted MRI slice at a point where the body of the lateral ventricles becomes into the atrium and the transverse gyrus of Heschl can be easily located in green; (d) 3D reconstruction from a T2 - weighted multislice study, where primary auditive cortex can be identified in green

5.1.2.2 Metabolic imaging

These modern imaging modalities have been developed with the aim of offering information about metabolic changes in the core of the tumor and also in the supposed infiltrated surrounding gray and white matter. This information is extremely helpful in cases of tumors in eloquent areas due to the planning for extent of resection.

Classical anatomic MRI sequences are highly sensitive but nonspecific, cannot differentiate tumor and treatment effect, are unable to assess early therapy failure and predict clinical outcome. In this sense, neuroimaging should improve in characterizing brain tumor biology and assessing therapeutic response. Advances in neuroimaging have allowed a transition from anatomy to biology through physiology. Two new imaging modalities are being reviewed: perfusion - weighted imaging and proton MR spectroscopy.

5.1.2.2.1 Perfusion – weighted Imaging

This imaging modality offers a relative measure of blood volume and an indirect degree of angiogenesis inside a tumor (Fig.6). Perfusion MR provides additional information to standard gadolinium enhanced sequences. Gadolinium enhancement in standard contrast sequences shows blood-brain barrier breakdown, while in case of perfusion MR, it offers information about tumor tissue perfusion through its microvasculature (Kim & Zee, 2007). When a patient with a brain tumor receives an injection of gadolinium, a T2 - weighted image is used to measure the decrease in signal intensity of the perfused tissue volume, and different perfusion parameters as time to peak, mean transit time, relative cerebral blood volume (rCBV), and regional cerebral blood flow (rCBF) can be calculated (Kim & Zee, 2007; Ostergaard, 2005). The rCBV reveals significantly lower values in low - grade gliomas than in high grade gliomas, in fact, several studies have found a significant correlation between the rCBV inside a tumor and glioma grading. However, it can not differentiate yet between grade I and II, grade II and III or grade III and IV neoplasms.

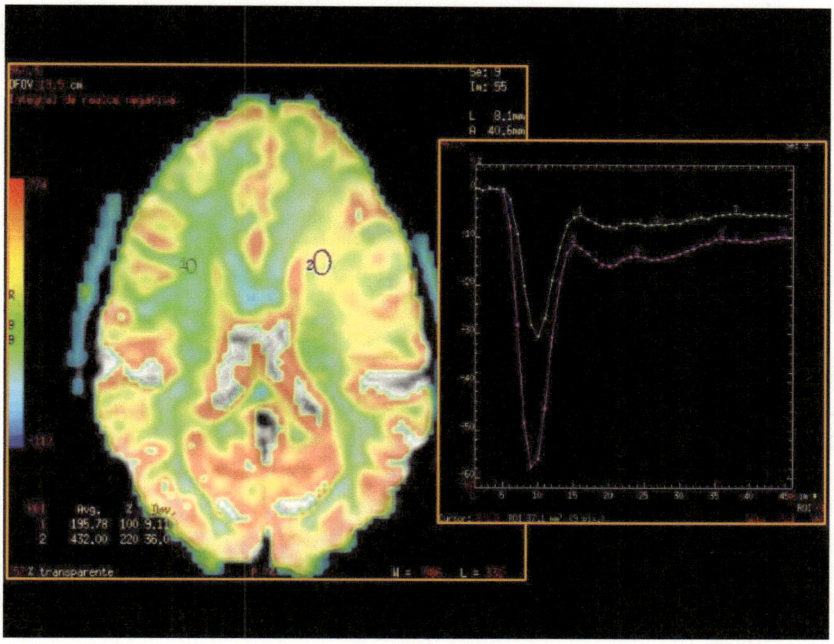

Fig. 6. MRI sequence showing the color map from the perfusion analysis and the increase of perfusion in a point of left centrum semiovale

Despite the general information offered by this imaging modality, one of the main interest in surgical planning, is the fact that rCBV values can be found significative higher in areas surrounding the contrast enhanced mass, where other imaging modalities do not show alterations due to the artifact of the edema.

5.1.2.2.2 Proton MR Spectroscopy

Spectroscopy allows the detection of heterogeneous metabolic areas within a tumor, which may be present beyond the margins that show classic MRI sequences. This technique detects increases of choline (Cho) in glial lesions, which represents cell proliferation, decreased concentrations of N - acetylaspartate (NAA) denoting loss of neurons as tumor cells replace them, and especially in high-grade gliomas increase of lactate (marker of necrosis) and increase of mobile lipids (Fig.7).

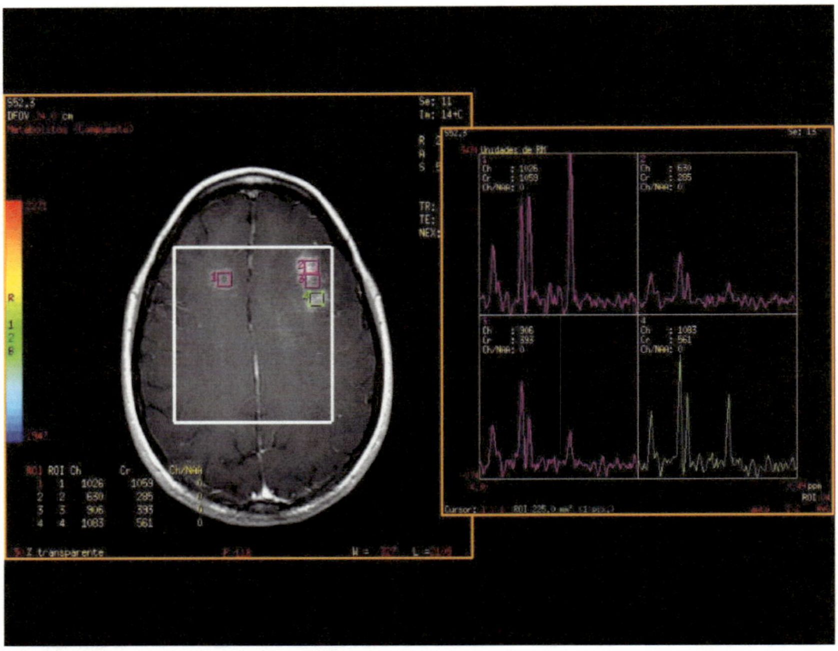

Fig. 7. Proton MR spectroscopy analysis of four different voxels. The numbers 2, 3 and 4 are compared with number 1, a control in the healthy side

5.2 Preoperative study

The classic, anatomic and metabolic MR modalities are really helpful in diagnosing, localizing and characterizing a brain tumor. However, for surgical planning of a brain tumor in a highly functional area, the most important point is to perform a 3D reconstruction of the brain where the surgeon can easily recognize the tumor volume, the involved gyri and the subcortical white matter tracts displaced and/or affected. For this purpose some imaging modalities have been developed: Functional MRI, DTI - based tractography and 3D anatomic sequences.

5.2.1 Functional imaging

Its main goal is the preoperative localization of eloquent areas prior to tumor resection to minimize intraoperative damage to these brain areas and thereby to reduce postoperative morbidity.

Functional MRI (fMRI) looks at changes in cerebral blood flow, and more specifically, in the balance of oxy and deoxyhemoglobin in the capillary circulation, and it can be viewed dynamically as a result of stimulation and performing tasks that are marked. Neuronal activation is measured indirectly through changes in blood oxygenation - dependent signal (BOLD). There is wide evidence that the location of motor and language areas by this technique is really helpful for preoperative planning in addition to being a noninvasive technique. A concept we should not forget is that it remains a technique that without the ability to distinguish between the various components of any specific functional response, and therefore may overlap different functional areas of brain processes, magnifying certain eloquent regions.

In surgical routine the cortical regions mainly mapped through fMRI are speech, comprehension, motor, sensitive, visual and memory areas (Fig.8). In order to detect changes in blood oxygenation in speech areas, the patient is asked to pronounce different words or phrases. The chosen task in case of comprehension mapping consists on asking the patient to listen to and think about different phrases. If the chosen task is for motor mapping, patients are asked to move different parts of their bodies repeating the movements at least during 50 or 60 seconds in order to try to become these movements in a routine with the aim of avoiding blood oxygenation changes in prefrontal areas, cerebellum and basal ganglia. When the desired mapping is for sensory areas, the task will consist on pressing different parts of the body of the patient through a mechanic system. Memory mapping is performed through the task called "walking in my city", asking the patient to mentally remember all the details in a walk between two chosen points in his city.

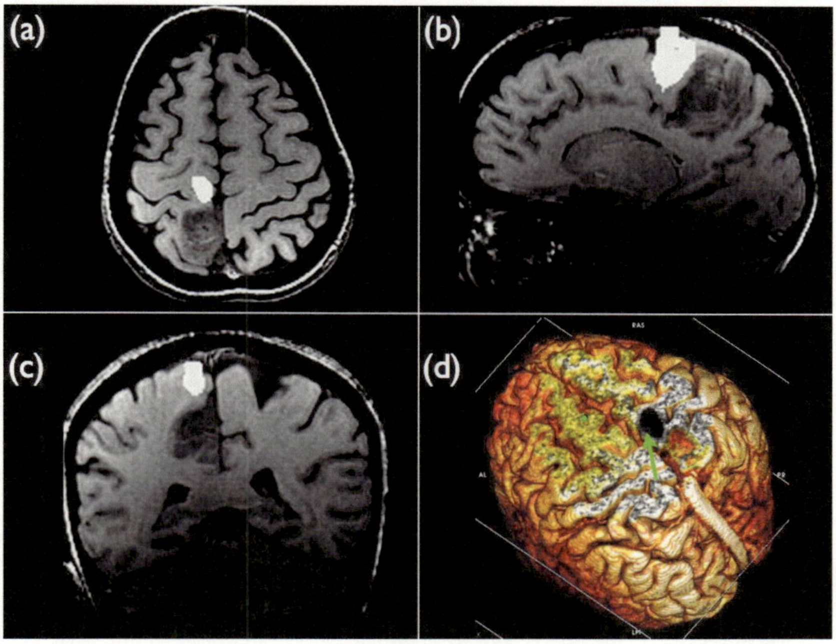

Fig. 8. Axial, sagittal and coronal T2 - weighted MRI slices (a), (b), (c), where a intrinsic tumor is located in the postcentral area and the activation from the fMRI for the leg (white stain) is located just anterior to the tumor; (d) 3D reconstruction from a T1 - weighted multislice study, where the three - dimensional relation between the activated area and the tumor are easily recognized

5.2.2 DTI – based tractography

Diffusion tensor imaging (DTI) is able to detect the characteristics of water diffusion in tissue distribution and display particular dimensional Brownian motion. The diffusion of water particles is facilitated by the ordered distribution of neural fibers through the membranes covering the axons. This imaging modality allows displaying the white matter fiber tracts by selecting a place where they can be easily visualized and then performing a three - dimensional reconstruction of them. DTI allows the visualization of bundles of axons in the human brain, by selecting regions with the same values of Fractional Anisotropy as "seed" for the start of production of tracts in the three - dimensional space (Berger & Hadjipanayis, 2007).

Craniocaudal direction fascicles contain not only motor tracts, but also consist on somatosensory tracts that will be visible depending on where the seed is placed. The motor and somatosensory fascicles are located differently in the brainstem, at cerebral peduncle the first, and medial lemniscus the second. Following this reasoning, tractography can become a great tool for locating the primary motor area using the same regions with fractional anisotropy values when deciding where to place the seed.

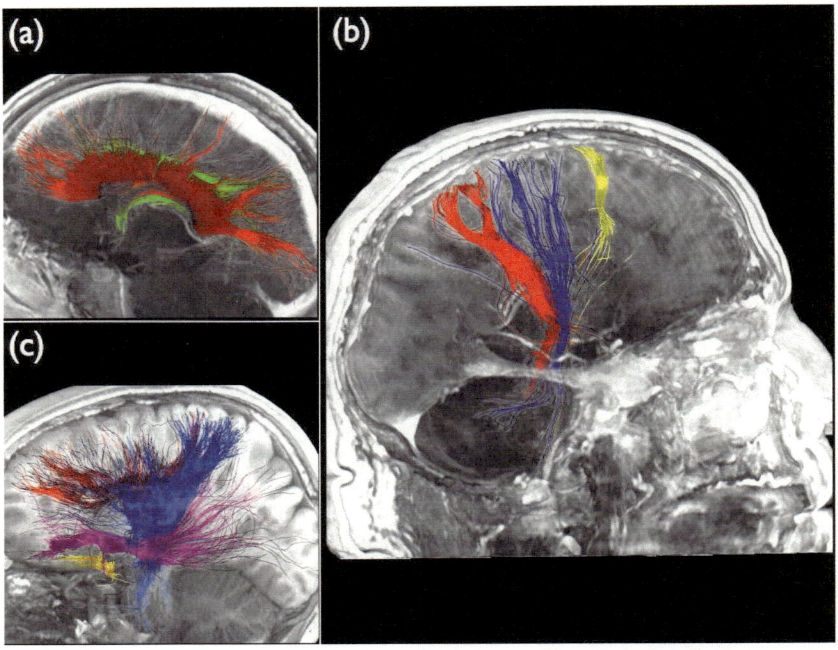

Fig. 9. (a) DTI - based tractography of the corpus callosum, cingulum and fornix in red and green; (b) DTI - based tractography showing the somatosensitive, motor and frontopontine fiber bundles of the internal capsule in red, blue and yellow respectively; (c) DTI - based tractography of uncinate, occipitofrontal, internal capsule and corpus callosum in yellow, purple, blue and red respectively

Tractography provides information about the normal course, the displacement or disruption of white matter tracts around the tumor, as well as damage to these tracts due to vasogenic edema or tumor infiltration. In Neurosurgery tractography is starting being used not only to understand the subcortical relation between the tumor and clinically relevant white matter fiber tracts, but also with the intention of localizing the motor and association pathways starting from their corresponding cortical areas, which are the neurons that leave these axons (Fig.9). In this sense DTI - based tractography can result of great help in cases in which fMRI cannot be easily performed. One of the biggest problems in functional MRI is the large number of variations of the venous circulation and the variety of hemodynamic responses that a brain in pathological conditions presents. Moreover, in patients with focal deficits or cognitive processing of tasks requiring fMRI is often very laborious and can not be done in many cases due to the inability of the patient (Basser, 2000). In these cases DTI is a really helpful tool to distinguish different cortical areas. It is important to have in mind that tractography is also limited in areas where tracts cross tumors or peritumoral vasogenic edema, so this fact should be noticed when deciding the place for the seed.

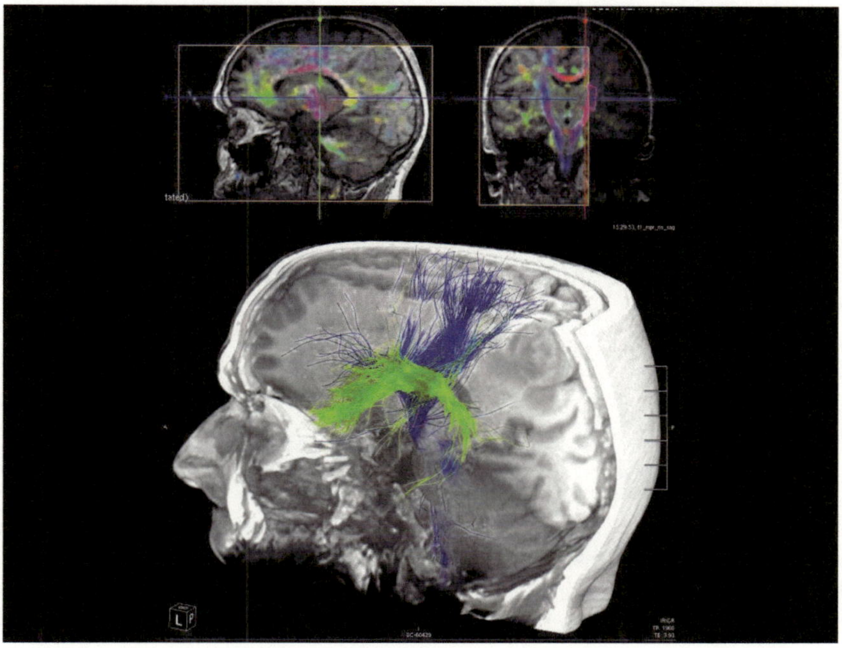

Fig. 10. Tensor preparation and seed placement of the internal capsule (pink boxes in sagittal and coronal slices in the color map), and 3D reconstruction showing the superior longitudinal fasciculus and internal capsule in green and blue

A great number of fascicles can be visualizes through DTI - based tractography, but in the neurosurgical practice the main studied fiber bundles are the corticospinal tract that contain motor and somatosensory fibers from the central lobe, passing through the corona radiate to join the internal capsule where the sensory part incorporates from the thalamic nuclei, and the motor fibers will lead to the cerebral peduncle; the superior longitudinal fascicle contains the arcuate fasciculus, which joins Broca´s and Wernicke´s area, resulting of great interest in cases of tumors located in the surroundings of the inferior frontal, angular and superior temporal gyri; and the optic radiations are also of great interest dealing with tumors not only in the occipital lobe, but also deep in temporal and parietal lobes (Fig.10).

5.2.3 Three – dimensional anatomic sequences

Once localized the tumor, marked the eloquent cortical areas and fiber tracked the subcortical white matter related to the tumor, next step consists on integrating all these data over a 3D anatomic sequence. The best sequence to perform this step is the one known as Three Dimensional Magnetization Prepared Rapid Acquisition Gradient Echo (3D MP-RAGE). A 3D T2 - weighted image can be also helpful in some cases because it also offers a great accuracy of sulci and gyri (Fig.11).

These sequences offer the chance of performing a 3D reconstruction of the brain, being very helpful to plan the surgical approach and transulcal microsurgical technique.

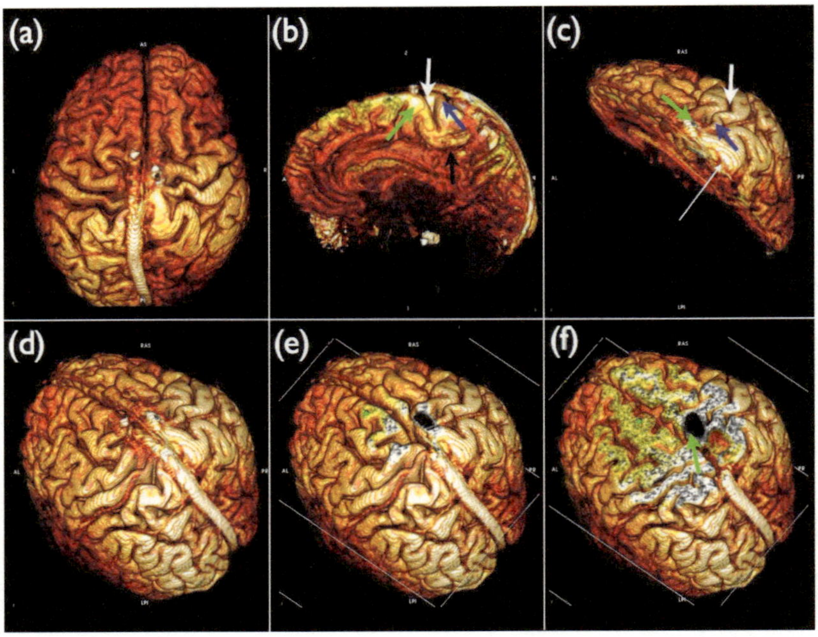

Fig. 11. Different views of a 3D reconstruction from a T1 - weighted multislice study showing the relation of a postcentral tumor (swollen gyrus marked with a thin white arrow in (c)), the precentral gyrus marked with a green arrow in (b) and (c), postcentral gyrus marked through a blue arrow in (c), and the fMRI activation for the left leg showed through a grey stain in (f)

5.3 Intraoperative neuronavigation

A neuronavigator is a passive intraoperative position-sensing system. Its main task is to encode the six-dimensional position of a surgical tool, to register the coordinate frame of the position sensor with some preoperative three-dimensional medical images using anatomic landmarks or fiducials, and thus to display in real time the location of the surgical tool on preoperative images. To establish a relation between a coordinate in physical space and its corresponding coordinate in image space a computer workstation calculates a transformation matrix (Vahala et al., 2001).

This technology allows the surgeon implementing all the chosen imaging modalities over a system of brain navigation, having stereotactic frameless control of the theoric extent of resection, and the relative location of different brain structures, of course including the tumor.

Image-assisted surgery is continuously being developed to help neurosurgeons to practice surgery on brain tumors more safely and effectively. Neuronavigation allows surgeons to locate intra-axial brain tumors more accurately choosing the best path to the lesion. All intraoperative navigation systems are fed with imaging studies, either a CT or MRI. The choice of appropriate images is really important, as for example, low-grade gliomas are best defined by T2-weighted sequences, whereas high-grade primary tumors are best seen on a T1 contrast (Berger & Hadjipanayis, 2007).

The competency to combine functional studies of the diffusion tensor is a tool that provides relevant data when intraoperative planning surgical approach.

Integration of preoperative functional data extracted from fMRI, known as functional neuronavigation, has become a routine practice in surgery of lesions adjacent to eloquent areas of the human brain, in order to avoid postoperative deficits (Fig.12). But in addition to eloquent cortical areas, deep structures, as are the bundles of white matter fibers connecting these areas should also be respected during surgery. The images produced by the tractography help the surgeon to understand the connections and the location of the tracts during surgery, and their relationship with cortical anatomy and brain disorders.
These new additions to the surgical planning are a major consumer of time spent on analysis and data processing. The accuracy of the information provided by tractography depends largely on the experience of the individual processing. Since the introduction of these technologies in the routine surgical procedure for brain tumors, the extent of resection avoiding surgical morbidity has improved exponentially.

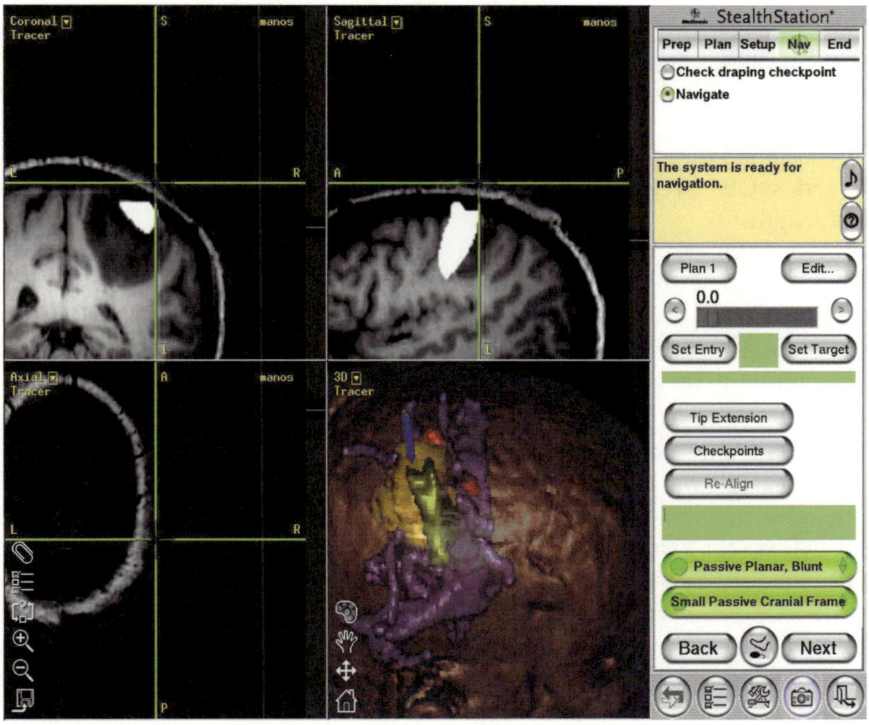

Fig. 12. Screenshot from the intraoperative neuronavigator showing the three orthogonal slices showing the white stain from the arm activation of fMRI and its relation with the tumor in precentral gyrus, and the 3D reconstruction where it is easy to visualize the tumor, arm and leg activations and internal capsule motor projections, in yellow, green, red and blue respectively

5.4 Intraoperative imaging modalities

The role of radical surgery in the management of glial - type brain tumors is still controversial. In fact, there is no scientific evidence that a greater extent of resection is associated with a better prognosis. Class II data show that the extent of resection for malignant gliomas improves survival and in case of low - grade gliomas, improves survival and time to tumor recurrence (Keles et al., 2001). This is the main reason why until new treatments for glial tumors are developed, the cytoreductive treatment provided by surgery will maintain its value. The price to pay for radical resection may be an increase in morbidity. In this sense, different intraoperative imaging modalities have been incorporated to the clinical practice with the ultimate objective being to optimize the resection limits; to extend them to the maximum while minimizing the eventual associated morbidity (Gonzalez-Darder et al., 2010).

The main limitation of neuronavigation is its reliance on preoperative images. Upon opening the skull and dura mater, movements inevitably occur, making data derived from these images unreliable and then loosing accuracy. Only intraoperative imaging is able to offer the updated information needed to maintain accurate navigation during the surgical procedure. These images are useful to confirm that tumor resection has been completed, a fact often not verifiable under the surgical microscope vision (Schulder & Carmel, 2003).

5.4.1 Intraoperative magnetic resonance

Intraoperative magnetic resonance imaging (iMRI) is a technology not largely employed yet due to its high cost and its special needs in the operating room (OR). An OR must be previously designed to host an iMRI. The complexity of the OR setup is greater for the use of iMRI, and safety as well as equipment details increase proportionally to the field magnetic strength.

How iMRI may influence quality of life and survival remains to be studied yet, but it seems that selected patients with low and high - grade gliomas will clearly benefit from the use of intraoperative imaging techniques as iMRI, due to the ability of them to offer in real time a direct control of the extent of resection, the relative location of the cortical and subcortical eloquent regions with the tumor (Nimsky et al., 2005).

5.4.2 Intraoperative ultrasound

Intraoperative MRI technical pitfalls have let to the development of intraoperative ultrasonography in many centers. Ideally all brain tumors are at least partially hyper echogenic. Diffuse calcifications inside lesions produces stronger echo patterns, while cysts or areas of necrosis are hypo echogenic. The local invasion of gliomas tends to appear as intermediate echogenicity. The edema can also be distinguished from the surrounding healthy parenchyma.

The main limitation of ultrasound is image resolution and the correlation of preoperative MRI scans and intraoperative ultrasonography images. This problem has been partially solved with the aim of modern neuronavigation systems, which allow overlapping of real - time ultrasound images with preoperative MRI data (Berger & Hadjipanayis, 2007).

5.4.3 Fluorescence guided resection with 5 – aminolevulinic acid

This technique allows the visualization of malignant tissue during surgery for malignant glioma (grades III and IV WHO). Tumor resection guided by fluorescence involves giving the patient a natural precursor, 5-aminolevulinic acid (5-ALA HCl), which is taken up by cells of malignant gliomas and, when summed, becomes a fluorescent substance. Thus, by applying a special light during surgery, the malignant cells are stained red offering the surgeon a clear distinction between the healthy and which are not, letting increasing the extent of tumor resection, minimizing brain damage (Stummer at al., 2006)(Fig.13).

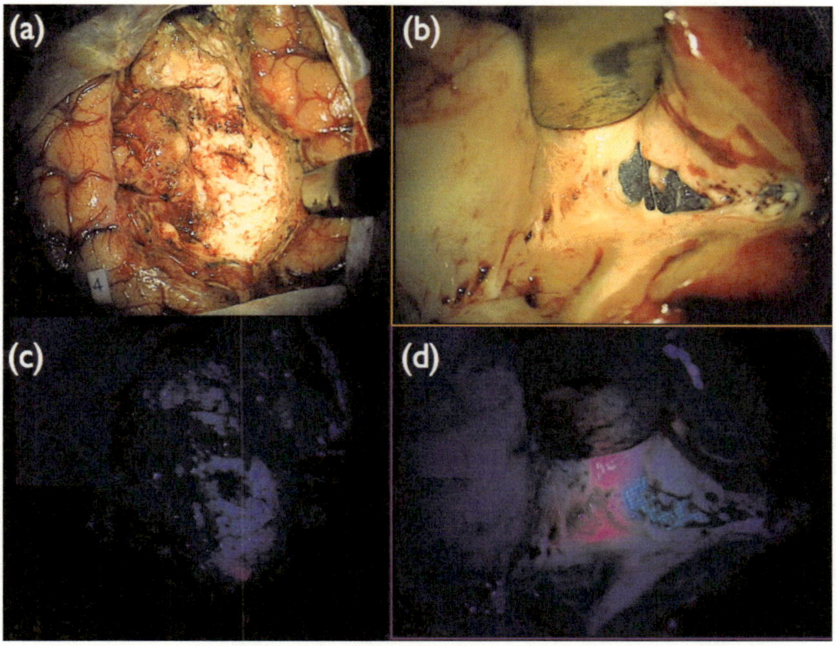

Fig. 13. Intraoperative views from brain tumor resection cavity and tumoral piece resected under the white light of the microscope (a) and (b); views of the same pieces under fluorescence special light where it is possible to appreciate pink areas which show the invasion by tumoral cells

5.5 Postoperative follow – up

Obviously the best imaging technique to evaluate the surgical resection of a brain tumor is MRI. The time between imaging controls to update the evolution of a brain tumor after surgery will depend on the initial extent of resection and the tumor grade. The sequences employed will be the same used preoperatively, as T1 - weighted with contrast and T2 - weighted imaging, flair, perfusion - weighted imaging and spectroscopy.

An important point in gliomas follow - up is to perform an early postoperative image control, in order to use it as the starting point to evaluate possible future complications and tumor recurrences, and also to evaluate tumoral remains. In this sense, although the contrast enhanced T1 - weighted imaging, the diffusion - weighted has emerged as a really helpful sequence. This early image control should be performed in the first 48 hours after the surgical procedure.

Acute cellular damage in the surrounding parenchyma after brain tumor resection occurs due to direct surgical trauma, retraction and vascular injury, and devascularization of tumor. This cellular damage results in acute intracellular swelling and decrease in the surrounding extracellular space can lead to reduced diffusion in the brain. This fact remains really important in the evaluation of an early postoperative MRI. These areas of immediate postoperative diffusion abnormality invariably undergo a phase of contrast enhancement on routine anatomic images that can be easily misinterpreted as tumor recurrence. This is the reason why an early detection (24-48 h post - surgery) of these areas let the surgeon differentiate a tumor rest from a resection ischemic damage.

6. Functional mapping

The goal of neurophysiological techniques in the identification of eloquent areas before and during brain tumor surgery is to achieve a better definition of eloquent areas in order to increase tumor resection with greater safety in avoiding damaging structures and potential functional irreversible neurological sequelae.

Locating eloquent areas is very useful considering the large interindividual anatomical variability, which is more pronounced in case of patients with space - occupying lesions that cause a distortion and displacement of anatomical structures, infiltrate functional areas and suffer neuronal plasticity phenomena.

There are several functional mapping techniques, which can be subdivided in two major groups depending when they are performed: preoperative and intraoperative techniques.

6.1 Preoperative mapping

6.1.1 Navigated transcranial magnetic stimulation

Transcranial Magnetic Stimulation (TMS) is based on the stimulation or inhibition of neuronal activity through a magnetic field centered over the skin. This technique was born as the evolution of Transcranial Electric Stimulation, improving the procedure due to the accuracy when applying the electrical flow.

The physical basis consists on a current discharged into an electromagnetic coil resting on the scalp, creating a magnetic field that induces a perpendicular electric field. The field produces an electric stimulus in the cortex. TMS may be used to map the motor, sensitive or language cortex. One of the best advantages of TMS is that it is the only noninvasive inhibition technique. Disadvantages include the risk of repetitive TMS causing seizures.

The main advantage of TMS over other non-invasive brain functional imaging techniques is that when a physiological response is evoked by stimulation of a cortical area, that specific area can be assumed to be directly responsible of evoking that response. With other imaging methods, it is only possible to detect and map a brain area that takes part in a previously decided task (Ruohonen & Karhu, 2010). This fact assumes that TMS is much more selective in order to map the tumor surroundings, so as to avoid damaging them during surgery.

Although there has been relatively little reported use of TMS in surgical planning, recent technical advantages have introduced this technique in some neuronavigation systems, allowing neurosurgeons preoperatively mapping the desired cortex of their patients, and then introducing the data over a 3D brain anatomic reconstruction with the aim of improving the surgical planning (Tharin & Golby, 2007). Neuronavigation of TMS enables the localization of eloquent cortex in patients with distorted anatomy as it is often found in brain tumors. Some advantages are present comparing with fMRI, as they are the fact that some tasks are difficult to be performed by patients with a brain tumor near the motor cortex, it avoids the artifacts given by fMRI and it can be monitored by neurosurgeons, allowing them to choose the cortex to be mapped (Forster, 2011).

6.1.2 Somatosensory evoked potentials

The SEP consist on the distal stimulation of afferent pathways with the aim of identifying short latency responses evoked from specific cortical areas (Fig.14). When stimulating the sciatic nerve distally, the response is detected on its specific area of the contralateral postcentral gyrus devoted to the representation of the lower extremity, while stimulation of the upper extremity will elicit a similar response from a different portion of the contralateral postcentral gyrus. With this approach, it is possible to elaborate a functional map of the somatosensory projection cortex in the postcentral gyrus.

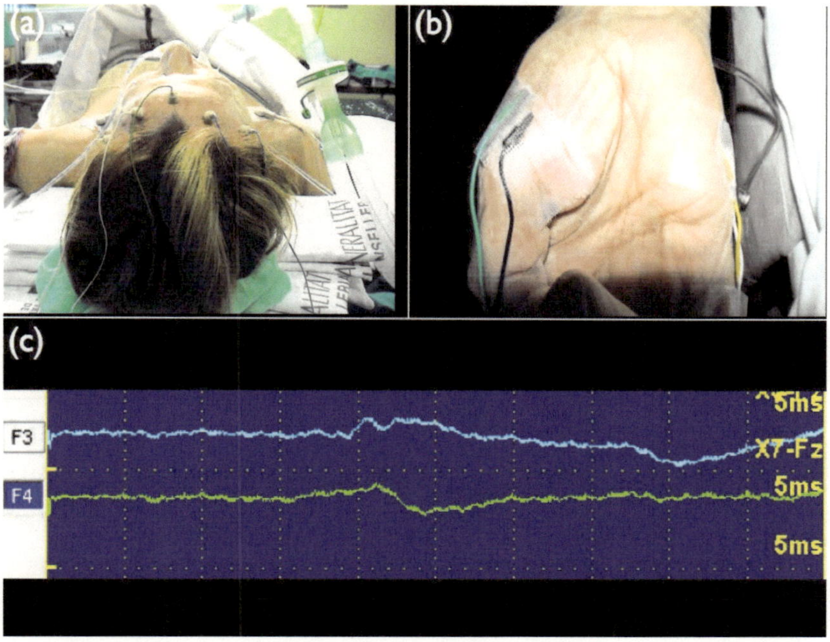

Fig. 14. (a) Scalp distribution of electrodes to receive the signal from the (b) median nerve stimulation in order to detect the (c) somatosensory evoked potentials register

The evoked potential method has been subsequently developed as a practical noninvasive clinical method to study conduction in the visual, auditory, and somatosensory systems. In the clinical practice this technique is used to check the somatosensory pathway integrity before, during and after surgery. Its preoperative status is of great importance in order to have a control to fastly detect any changes during surgery.

6.2 Intraoperative mapping

6.2.1 General considerations for intraoperative brain mapping

Different intraoperative mapping techniques have improved the results when resecting brain tumors near eloquent areas. Some of these techniques require the patient´s collaboration in order to detect for example a speech arrest during Broca´s Area stimulation.

Asleep craniotomy for brain tumors surgery is a useful technique in selected cases. When the tumor affects the area of language, the surgical procedure is performed under conscious sedation, in which the patient actively participates (object naming, counting and reading numbers) in much of the procedure. Therefore they must understand exactly the technique, the objectives, limitations and complications of the method. In these cases the aim consists on achieving conscious sedation, which means that the patient is asleep but responds to verbal commands. This sedation is objectified through an anesthetic depth monitor (Bispectral Index whose values should be between 70-80). With this level of sedation achieved good cooperation of the patient.

If the patient's cooperation is not needed, there will be a total intravenous anesthesia preferably with appropriate depth level (BIS 40-50). Using propofol with remifentanil both in continuous intravenous infusion. The use of drugs that reduce or alter the potential such as neuromuscular relaxants, volatile anesthetics and benzodiazepines should be avoided.

However neuromuscular relaxants can be used to obtain a partial blockage, in such a way as to reduce an important part of the movement and to facilitate the surgical procedure, being able to obtain adequate monitoring (with an appropriate lock), except during the mapping.

One of the possible complications of this method is the appearance of post-discharges associated with stimulation, such as to trigger a seizure. If a post-discharge appears over 30 sec, it suggests the use of midazolam 2 mg or lorazepam 2 mg, or low intravenous dose of barbiturates. It is also recommended the use of serum ringer at a lower temperature than ambient directly over the exposed cortex.

Other factors that influence the monitoring are: an adequate blood flow, intracranial pressure, optimal hematocrit, adequate ventilation and oxygenation and temperature of the patient.

6.2.2 Somatosensory evoked potentials

The somatosensory evoked potentials technique has exactly the same purpose intra than preoperatively, and has just been commented in the preoperative mapping section. Its main goal consists on monitoring the somatosensory pathways during surgery.

6.2.3 Phase reversal of somatosensory evoked potentials technique: N20/P30 wave

When dealing with cortico - subcortical tumors near the central sulcus, the fact of identifying this anatomical structure when opening the dura mater may result really complex due to the anatomical distortion caused by the tumor. For this purpose the N20 wave technique has been developed. SEP can identify primary areas of sensory and motor control (precentral and postcentral grooves).

The reverse phase of SEP is based on changes in the polarity of the dipole field generated by the cortical afferent pathway. The stimulus applied to a peripheral nerve generates an electric dipole on the postcentral gyrus. The polarity of this dipole changes on the adjacent precentral gyrus. Thus, a SEP (N20/P30) can register from the postcentral gyrus and a reverse image from the turn precentral (P'20 / N'30).

Once performed the craniotomy and opened the dura, a strip of silicone that have set a variable number of electrodes (4 or 6) of platinum of 1-1.5 mm in diameter aligned in rows, with an interval of 0.5-1 cm, will be placed over the cortex (Fig.15). The strip of electrodes should be placed across the alleged central sulcus, covering the area of the hand or foot at the sensorimotor gyri, with an angle of 15 ° to the sagittal direction. For the SEP of the median nerve, the electrode should be placed in a cortical area between 3 and 8 cm from the midline. For the tibial nerve, the cortical area is limited to 0-3 cm from the midline.

In tumors affecting the central area close to the interhemispheric fissure, the posterior tibial nerve stimulation is used. This technique is more difficult to obtain, but very useful in these cases.

An electrical stimulator current of constant voltage will be employed for this purposes. Intensity should be gradually increased until a motor response in the first finger (median nerve) or the big toe (tibial nerve) appears. Once obtained the wave, it is easy to locate the central sulcus between the electrodes in which the phase reversal is given.

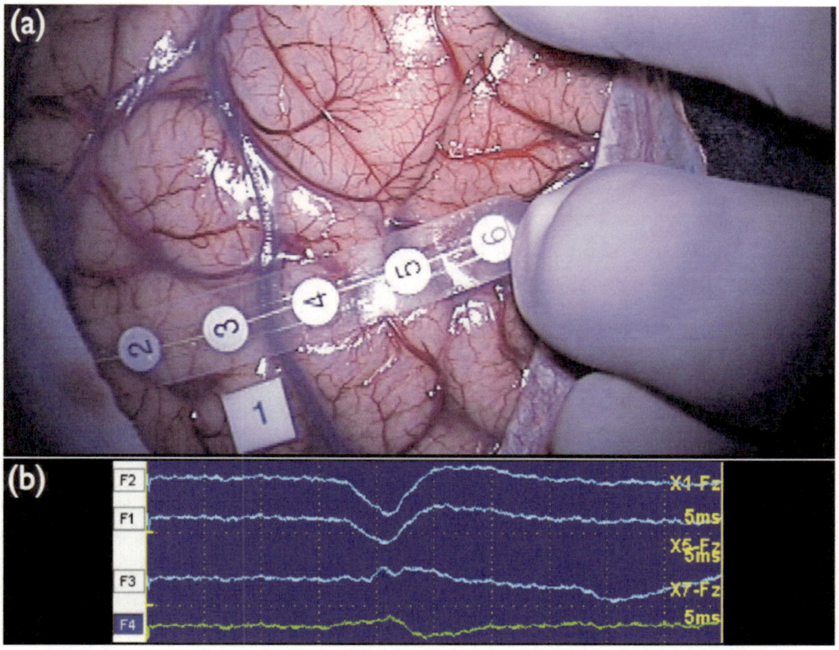

Fig. 15. (a) Flat strip over the brain surface to locate the central sulcus and the register (b) given after the stimulation where it is possible to appreciate the wave inversion between number 4 and 5 poles

6.2.4 Direct cortical stimulation: looking for the functional gray mater

This neurophysiological technique allows the surgeon localizing the functional areas with awake (language areas) or non - relaxed (motor areas) patients, through direct brain stimulation.

The technique of mapping by direct cortical electrical stimulation allows the realization of a functional map of the cerebral cortex exposed, both to identify areas that are functionally significant as areas that are not.

The neurosurgeon places the electrode at a small region of cortical area of the brain, and the stimulator from the computer applies a train of stimuli, which can result in neurological changes as patient movement or numbness or inhibit neurological function as speech arrest. When stimulation of a focal brain region produces any of the above symptoms not accompanied by a crisis or post-discharge, it is confirmed that the stimulated cortex region is important for brain function. The criteria for considering an area as eloquent, involves that a functional response occurs for at least three separate stimuli into a single cortical region (Pouratian, 2004).

The most employed technique for direct cortical stimulation is the repetitive bipolar cortical stimulation or Penfield technique (Fig.16). Bipolar stimulation technique of Penfield is based on the activation of the cortical circuit applying electrical pulses repeatedly.

For the stimulation is commonly used a bipolar electrode with carbon tips 5 mm apart, with a cable connected to an external stimulator that acts as a generator of continuous electrical power trains of biphasic pulse. To assess motor or sensory function, applying a train of 2-3 seconds long is enough, while assessing language function requires longer durations of 5-7 seconds. Stimuli should not be encouraged two consecutive times in order to prevent post - discharges and seizures. Three positive tests in the same location are enough to ensure that it is essential for language. Occasionally it is necessary to extend the duration of the train to 7-10 seconds to map the language, due to the complexity of questions and answers to the questions.

It is recommended to begin with a current of 1mA from 2 mA to increase to the minimum intensity that produces a sensorimotor response (not higher than 8-10 mA). The procedure finishes by marking with sterile labels the cortex with positive response using the legend chosen by each surgeon, in order to avoid damaging these eloquent areas.

6.2.4.1 Motor areas

Registration can be done with the patient awake, determining the evoked movement by direct visualization or with the patient asleep using as control a continuous electromyographic recording.

Recording electrodes should be placed when the patient is anesthetized. The needle electrodes are subcutaneous monopolar and disposable (12 mm or 20 mm in length, placed 2 separate needles 5-10 mm between them) and are placed in the muscle groups that correspond to the stimulated brain area (right / left, contralateral to the lesion; or bilateral, depending on the location of the tumor), for example, it is possible to monitor facial muscles (orbicularis oris) upper limb muscles (deltoid, biceps, extensor digitorum and short Abductor) and lower limb (femoral adductor, quadriceps, tibialis anterior and abductor). Best when it is possible to monitor the entire side of the body, with impedances below 5 K Ω.

The stimulus causes muscle jerking or tonic contractions that can start immediately to stimulation or after several seconds. In other regions the stimulation can cause inhibition of movement (when an awake patient is told to move his fingers, stimulation can slow or halt the movement), as supplementary motor cortex stimulation and other regions that can assume an integrative role in motor function.

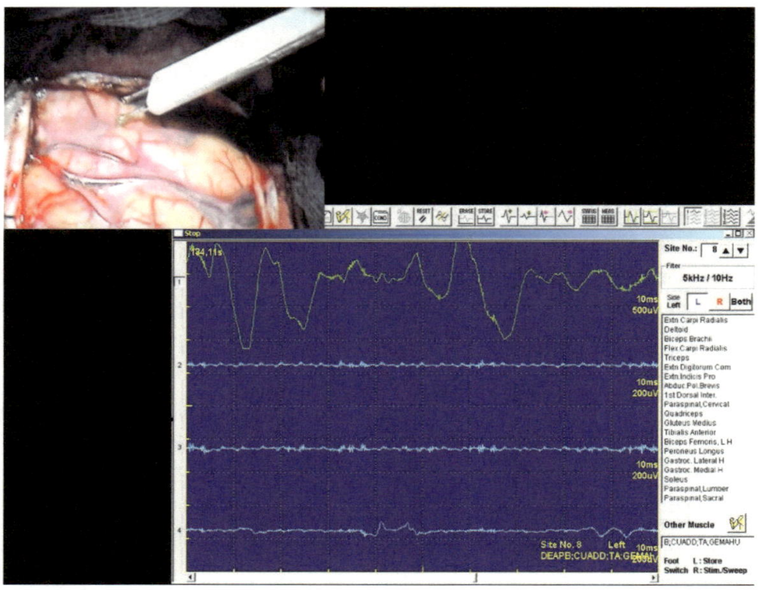

Fig. 16. Direct cortical stimulation and its register showing activation in the left cuadriceps

6.2.4.2 Sensitive areas

It is performed with the patient awake and requires of his/her cooperation. The presence of sensory impairment is assessed by the patient, paresthesias in the contralateral regions of the body and occasionally on both sides of tongue or face, or both sides of the neck.

6.2.4.3 Visual areas

Visual areas are not usually intraoperatively mapped, but when performed, the patient must be awake and his cooperation is needed. It values the appearance in the contralateral visual field: lights, colors, shadows (when stimulated primary visual cortex). Stimulation in the visual association cortex may cause hallucinations.

In the event that a craniotomy is large enough, placing a blanket of subdural electrodes allows identifying and monitoring the bioelectric response of the visual region throughout the procedure, using visual stimuli from special glasses with LEDs. This technology facilitates the surgical procedure and avoids keeping the patient awake. This same methodology can be used to identify the primary auditory area.

6.2.4.4 Language areas

It is performed with the patient awake and requires their collaboration. The administration of drugs must be stopped at least 15 minutes before beginning the cortical stimulation.

It is desirable the involvement of a neuropsychologist for interpretation of different language errors caused by the stimulation. There should be a preoperative training about the tasks to be performed intraoperatively, and stop the monitoring in case the patient in a basal situation fails more than 25% of the tasks presented.

In a first step the sensorimotor response should be mapped to confirm a positive response. After confirming the response, next steps are:

a. Mapping cortical areas
b. Language sites whose answers after stimuli are known are mapped and produce the same inhibition (speech arrest, dysarthria or anomia).

   A good beginning is naming and counting tasks (expressive language): asking the patient to count (1 to 10, again and again) or name objects presented visually (different test can be used, selected according to different variables such as frequency, familiarity, age of acquisition, and education). It helps to choose pictures of items that the patient can name quickly and easily in the test.

   Phonetic Association: asking the patient to tell as many names beginning with the letters F, P and L (one minute for each letter).

   Semantic association: the patient is asked to read the largest number of cars, fruits or animals.

   Nomination of famous faces: showing the patient 50 pictures from famous people and 50 non - famous.

   Object Naming.

   Calculations simple: multiplication or subtraction.
c. Failures are coded and responsible areas are registered again with sterile labels:

   Aphasia (loss of the ability to produce and / or comprehend language).

   Phonemic paraphasias (changes in the articulation of one or more phonemes).

   Semantic paraphasias (changes in the phonology of the word, weakness with the onset of the alterations).

   Anomia (difficulty in retrieving words when speaking)

   Perseverance (repeat previous items as the following items were submitted)

   Speech arrest.

6.2.5 Electrocorticography

The electrocorticography is a technique that involves recording cerebral bioelectrical activity through a strip of subdural electrodes. The procedure is more useful when is associated with direct cortical stimulation.

This neurophysiological procedure has the ability to detect both tumoral and irritative regions. It is often possible to identify directly the peri - rolandic region by the presence of a typical spindle shape of mu rolandic rhythm. It also allows detecting the stimulus artifact while stimulating the cortex, which verifies that cortex is being stimulated and electrocorticography is recorded.

The maximum stimulus intensity can be defined, and the incidence of post-discharges and seizures induced by electrical stimulation can be detected. The incidence of post-discharges or seizures following a train of stimuli during direct cortical stimulation, increases the possibility that the physiological effect of the train should be not localized due to the spread to a wider cortical region, fact that could cause a misinterpretation by the surgeon in case of not using the electrocorticography.

This technique is necessary when the intraoperative brain functional mapping is supposed to be longer than usual.

6.2.6 Direct subcortical stimulation: extent of resection in the white matter

Subcortical stimulation is a novel technique that has reached as importance as cortical mapping in brain tumor surgery. Its main indication remains when dealing with tumors with a subcortical extension in the surroundings or inside important white matter fiber bundles. The technical details and the tools employed are the same explained in the section about direct cortical stimulation.

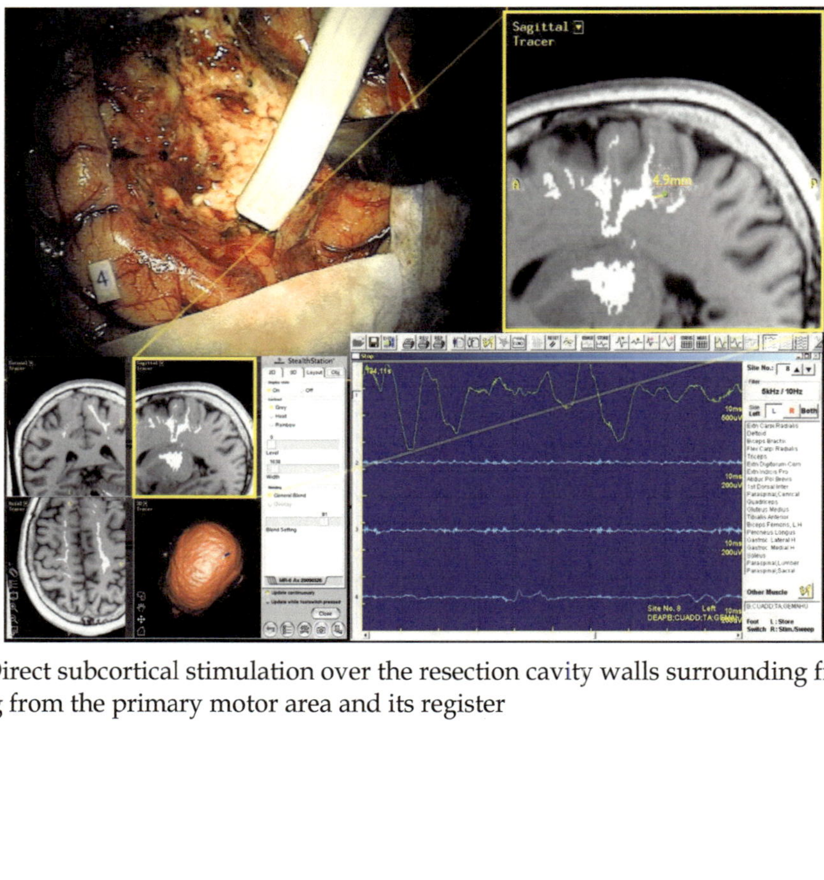

Fig. 17. Direct subcortical stimulation over the resection cavity walls surrounding fibers emerging from the primary motor area and its register

Once removed the main tumor volume, the oncologic surgical concept forces to resect as much relative healthy tissue as possible, in order to complete a total macroscopic resection. This fact is easier when the tumor involves not functional fiber bundles, but in cases of highly eloquent white matter fiber tracts, the prize to pay by a total resection may be too high.
In this sense the direct subcortical stimulation appears as a great tool. The most accepted approach consists on stimulating the walls of the resection cavity each 3 or 4 mm, using a bipolar stimulator during 2 - 4 sec, with intensities between 2 and 10 mA for the motor and sensitive pathways (Fig.17).
In cases of language areas, during tumor resection, the functional pathway mapping will follow outlining the eloquent cortical sites at depth. The patient should be nominating and counting in different phases until the end of tumor resection.

7. Microsurgical treatment

7.1 Surgical approaches and patient´s position

Surgical position and approach is the result of a careful and concise preoperative surgical planning, and probably, one of the most important points to consider during the surgical procedure. Generally, it is assumed that a good position and surgical approach is performed when the venous return is facilitated, the patient´s limbs are not forced, the surgeon has an optimal angle and vision of the field and all the neurosurgical team has space enough to develop their functions.
The preoperative imaging and functional tests can resemble very helpful to decide the surgical approach, however, the anatomic knowledge is basic to decide the patient´s position in the operating room table. The patient´s neck must not be forced to facilitate the venous return, so when necessary, different mechanisms will be used to elevate different parts of the body in order to get a free neck position. It is also a general recommendation to keep the head elevated between 6 and 10 cm from the level of the heart, fact that improves the venous return.
When the surgery is going to be performed with the patient awake, the position will be the same if possible, but the surgeon will employ all care with the aim that the patient is as comfortable as possible.
Patients undergoing craniotomies for intrinsic brain lesions are generally positioned in such a way that the lesion is highest in the field. However, the position and surgical approach in cases of tumors near eloquent areas will follow some general rules, depending on the location of the lesion (Fig.18).

7.1.1 Precentral and postcentral areas at the sagittal level of the superior and middle frontal gyri. Anterior midline lesions in the cingulate gyrus

In cases of tumors surrounding the paracentral lobe, it will be necessary to expose the rolandic cortex in order to facilitate stimulation and visual control of this area. The patient´s head must be positioned straight up with a slightly flexion of the neck or 5 - 10º turned to the contralateral side after fixation with the cephalostat device, in order to expose the field perpendicular to the surgeon´s hands. The incision is usually performed in a horseshoe - shape centered in the lesion and including the motor cortex. When the tumor remains located in the anterior cingulate gyrus or in the mesial side of the paracentral lobe, the incision must be highly extended to the contralateral side, in order to facilitate a crossing - midline craniotomy.

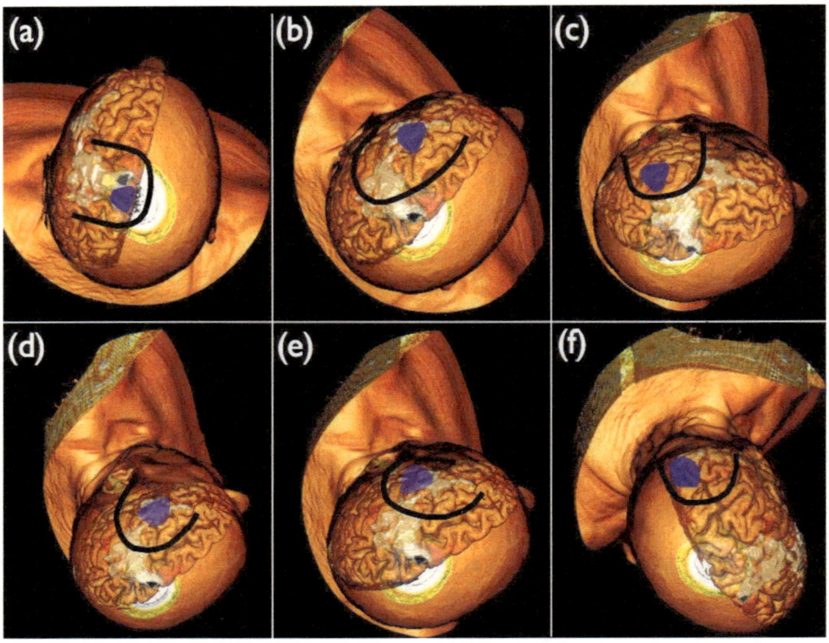

Fig. 18. Patient´s position and skin incision for intrinsic brain tumors located in medial paracentral lobe (a), lateral paracentral lobe and Broca´s area (b), angular and supramarginal gyrus and Wernicke´s area (c), superior edge of insular lobe (d), inferior edge of insular lobe (e) and occipital lobe (f)

7.1.2 Precentral and postcentral areas at the sagittal level of the inferior frontal gyrus. Pars triangularis and opercularis of the inferior frontal gyrus (Broca´s Area)

In these cases the approach philosophy is exactly the same than in more medial tumors of this area, so the rolandic cortex should be exposed, the tumor centered on the craniotomy and the field perpendicular to the surgeon´s hand. To get these facts, positioning can be facilitated by turning the head between 45 - 60° toward the contralateral side, elevating the ipsilateral shoulder to avoid forcing the ipsilateral side of the neck, improving with this maneuver the venous return. The skin incision can be performed in a horseshoe - shape not crossing the midline, or if preferred by the surgeon it can be traced as a C - shaped incision emerging above the zygomatic root, curving posteriorly enough to expose the lateral rolandic cortex and again curving anteriorly including the tumor till reaching the hair implantation line. This last skin incision is supposed to better respect the blood flow on the wound, making easier the healing process.

7.1.3 Superior frontal gyrus (premotor area, supplementary motor area and frontal aye field)

In cases of tumors affecting different parts of the superior frontal gyrus, the head position and skin incision is really similar to the midline rolandic lesions. The head is usually fixed in a central neutral position, not flexed and 8-10 cm elevated from the level of the heart. It is not necessary to expose the paracentral lobe, in fact it should be avoided, so the incision remains quite more anterior. The incision requires usually crossing the midline, so many times a posterior bicoronal incision replaces the typical horseshoe - shaped one.

7.1.4 Angular, supramarginal and posterior part of superior temporal gyri (Wernicke´s area). Transverse gyrus of Heschl (primary auditive area)

For approaching these tumors, the head is turned nearly 90° to the contralateral side, elevating the shoulder as far as possible to get a free of tension neck, turning the head as far as getting it almost parallel to the floor. The incision is began at the root of zygoma, extending superiorly and then posteriorly to end well behind the pinna of the ear in a horseshoe - shaped (Berger & Hadjipanayis, 2007), exactly the same as for a subtemporal approach. When the lesion affects the angular and supramarginal gyri, the incision can be moved quite more posterior and superior, even leaving the ear free. These incisions can be centered with the help of a neuronavigator system.

7.1.5 Insular tumors

Although the skin incision and craniotomy will always be the same (a extended pterional approach), the patient´s position will highly depend on the relative location of the tumor inside the insula. The insula is hidden under the frontal, temporal and parietal opercula, so retraction is needed to approach this region. Avoiding retraction as much as possible is the reason to the different positions of the head, taking advantage from the force of gravity. When dealing with lesions affecting the superior aspect of insula (frontal part of the sulcus circularis insulae), the head will be turned 60-75° to the contralateral side and extended at least 15°, to obtain a frontal lobe anatomical retraction when opening the sylvian fissure (Berger & Hadjipanayis, 2007). In cases of tumors affecting the inferior part or temporal sulcus, and the limen insulae, the philosophy will be opposite, flexing the head 10-20° in order to get a direct angle with minimal retraction.

7.1.6 Lateral occipital lobe (primary visual area)

In cases in which the tumor affects the occipital lobe the chosen position is the known as three - quarter prone position or park - bench. With this approach, the head is midly flexed and turned following the contralateral shoulder direction so that the nose points to the floor. This locates the occipital lobe in a nondependent fashion, avoiding pressure on the abdomen, although it is extremely difficult to be performed when dealing with obese patients. A sling supports the ipsilateral arm with a roll under the armpit to prevent brachial plexopathy, and the ipsilateral shoulder is taped to minimize its profile. A horseshoe - shaped incision is then performed centered in the tumor.

7.2 Surgical technique

The development of neuroimaging, intraoperative functional mapping technologies and especially the incorporation of microneurosurgery skills to the intrinsic brain tumors surgery, has largely improved the extent of resection of these tumors with a great clinical impact over the postoperative morbidity and mortality.

7.2.1 Transulcal microsurgical approach

Understanding the gyral and sulcal anatomy is the first step in all neurosurgical procedures. Glial tumors grow in a completely different way from the rest of the human body neoplasms. They do not behave as a mass, but they present a special growing pattern, extending away the origin of the neoplasms using as corridors the vessels external walls and overall the white matter substance. In a given gyrus, there are at least two kinds of white matter fiber bundles, the arcuate or U - shaped fibers that join adjacent gyri at the deep of the sulci, and long fiber bundles, which can be commissural or associative pathways. Modern neuroimaging has developed techniques, which offer a high definition about which gyri and white matter tracts are infiltrated, so the classical way to define a brain tumor location is nowadays dramatically changing. Thanks to these imaging modalities a brain tumor can be said to affect the pars opercularis of the inferior frontal gyrus and the frontal portion of the arcuate fascicle of the superior longitudinal fascicle in the left side, avoiding the classical nomenclature, which would have named it as a left frontal tumor.

All these information is needed to plan a surgical approach, and to reach a macroscopic complete resection of a given tumor. In this sense the surgical excision must be performed following the anatomical concepts offered by neuroimaging, so once localized the eloquent areas surrounding the tumor, and the affected gyri, the dissection will begin following the natural corridors of the brain, also known as sulci. Once completely deeply dissected the involved sulci and having respected the functional regions, a gross resection of the main tumor volume must be done.

The transulcal microsurgical resection remains of great interest, and brings the concept of oncologic resection to the field of brain tumors.

7.2.2 Ultrasonic aspiration

This technology was first introduced in the neurosurgical procedures 25 years ago, and actually has become an indispensable tool in the neurosurgical armamentarium for the resection of intracranial tumors.

The ultrasonic aspirator presents two effects over the tissue interface. The first effect supposes a suction that brings the surrounding tissue to the tip of the aspirator and forces it to vibrate, accelerate, and decelerate with the tip, fragmenting it away from harder tissues as vessels. The second important effect consists on a rapidly oscillating tip that produces localized pressure waves, which cause vapor pockets around cells in tissues with high water contents; the collapse of these pockets causes the tissue cells to rupture. The speed of fragmentation depends on the amplitude setting of the system (Jallo, 2001).

The use of this technology remains of great interest when dealing with intrinsic brain tumors, especially when these tumors are close to eloquent areas. Classical resection of intrinsic brain tumors is performed through an electric coagulating bipolar system to destroy tissue and a conventional suction system to aspirate it. This procedure can result as effective as ultrasonic aspiration, but there is a great difference. Bipolar coagulation systems increase the local temperature of the surrounding tissue and it has been demonstrated to be responsible of damaging neighbor areas to the resected tissue. On the contrary, the ultrasonic aspirator is at least as effective removing infiltrated tissue, but shows the advantage of not damaging the healthy surrounding healthy and sometimes functional tissue.

The use of ultrasonic aspirators can increase the extent of resection, respecting vessels and healthy surrounding tissue, and then improving the functional result.

7.2.3 Subcortical resection

A precise subcortical resection usually marks the difference between a good and an excellent brain tumor resection. Different procedures as intraoperative imaging modalities, neuronavigation systems, fluorescence - guidance and direct electrical stimulation, can help neurosurgeons on decision making about when to stop the tumor resection.

Once performed the transulcal approach and the main tumor volume removal, the main challenge appears about when to stop the subcortical deep resection. This fact takes especial consideration in cases of adjacent white matter functional fiber bundles. To optimize this purpose the neurosurgeon´s main armamentarium is based on different technical procedures.

Intraoperative imaging modalities as iMRI and intraoperative ultrasonography show in real - time the extent of resection, and in some cases they can offer the visualization of important fiber bundles near the walls of the resection cavity (Nimsky et al., 2005).

Other modalities as fluoresecence guided - resection, offer the ability of visualizing infiltrated tissue under a special wavelength, which could not be visualized under the usual white microscope light.

All these imaging and metabolic techniques are of great interest when resecting the tumoral mass, but in case of functional subcortical areas, the gold standard remains being the direct subcortical electric stimulation in order to localize the function and stop the resection to avoid postoperative morbidity. Different studies have been performed to study the optimal distance between the location of fiber tracts on the navigated DTI and the positive response to the subcortical electrical stimulation (Gonzalez-Darder et al., 2010; Nimsky et al., 2005), proposing a safety margin of 5 - 8 mm. A positive response is accepted as to directly stimulate the involved fiber tract, when applying a stimulus of 2-8 mA during at least 2 seconds. The appearing of a positive response under these parameters must make the surgeon to stop the resection in that area.

8. Conclusions

The integration of pre- and intraoperative anatomical, imaging and functional studies allows for a functional resection that significantly widens the extent of resection in lesions in relevant eloquent areas. Navigation allows neurosurgeons to integrate and understand the correlation between the preoperative data and the intraoperative findings. The cortical functional areas are anatomically and functionally defined in the preoperative period by using MR and fMR imaging studies, as well as other non-invasive techniques as the Transcranial Magnetic Stimulation, and the subcortical functional areas are defined by DTI - based tractography, whereas intraoperative confirmation is achieved using CS and the N20 wave inversion study for the cortical areas and sCS for the subcortical areas. Microsurgical treatment supported by intraoperative imaging techniques and fluorescence, guided by navigation and with the aid of the studies described above, allows great tumor resections in lesions located in cortical and subcortical eloquent motor areas, with a relatively high neurological morbidity in the immediate postoperative period, which is significantly reduced both quantitatively and qualitatively during the first postoperative weeks. The ongoing studies should define safety margins for functional resection that take the brain shift into consideration. Finally, the benefit of these protocols for disease-free interval, recurrence, or ultimate patient survival remains to be defined in future.

9. Acknowledgements

The authors would like to thank the collaboration of all medical and nonmedical members of the Services Neurosurgery, Neurophysiology and Anesthesiology from Hospital Clinico Universitario, Valencia; of ERESA (Exploraciones Radiológicas SA), and of the Department of Basic Psychology, and Clinical Psychobiology from UJI (Universitat Jaume I). Also thank to Medtronic by their technical support. This work was supported in part by the grant 2008/005 Foundation ERESA Group for Development and Research Medical Area (Neurology).

10. References

Basser P.J., Pajevic S., Pierpaoli C., Duda J. & Aldroubi A. (2000). In vivo fiber tractography using DT-MRI data. *Magnetic Resonance Medicine,* Vol.44, pp625–632

Berger M.S., Deliganis A.V., Dobbins J. & Keles G.E. (1994). The effect of extent of resection on recurrence in patients with low grade cerebral hemisphere gliomas. *Cancer,* Vol.74, pp1784–1791

Berger M.S. & Hadjipanayis C.G. (2007). Surgery of intrinsic cerebral tumors. *Neurosurgery,* Vol.61: pp279-305

Brandes A.A., Scelzi E., Salmistraro G., Ermani M., Carollo C., Berti F., Zampieri P., Baiocchi C. & Fiorentino M.V. (1997). Incidence of risk of thromboembolism during treatment of high - grade gliomas: a prospective study. *European Journal of Cancer,* Vol.33, pp-1592-1596

Cha S. (2006). Update on brain tumor imaging: from anatomy to physiology. *American Journal of Neuroradiology,* Vol.27, pp475-487

Claes A., Idema A.J. & Wesseling P. (2007). Diffuse glioma growth: a guerilla war. *Acta Neuropathologica,* Vol.114, pp443–458

Forster M.T., Hattingen E., Senft C., Gasser T., Seifert V. & Szelényi A. (2011). Navigated Transcranial Magnetic Stimulation and functional Magnetic Resonance Imaging - advanced adjuncts in preoperative planning for central region tumors. *Neurosurgery,* 2011 Jan 26. [Epub ahead of print]

French J.A., Kanner A.M., Bautista J., Abou-Khalil B., Browne T., Harden C.L., Theodore W.H., Bazil C., Stern J., Schachter S.C., Bergen D., Hirtz D., Montouris G.D., Nespeca M., Gidal B., Marks W.J., Turk W.R., Fischer J.H., Bourgeois B., Wilner A., Faught R.E., Sachdeo R.C., Beydoun A. & Glauser T.A. (2004). Efficacy and tolerability of the new antiepileptic drugs I: treatment of new onset epilepsy: report of the therapeutics and technology assessment subcommittee of the American Academy of Neurology and the American Epilepsy Society. *Neurology,* Vol.62, pp1252-1260

Gallucci M., Capoccia S. & Catalucci A. (2007). Functional Systems, In: *Radiographic atlas of skull and brain anatomy,* Heilmann U., Stoeck M. & Steinen-Bro F. (ed.), pp208-262, Springer-Verlag, ISBN-10 3-540-34190-0, New York.

Giese A., Loo M.A., Rief M.D., Tran N. & Berens M.E. (1995). Substrates for astrocytoma invasion. *Neurosurgery,* Vol.37, pp294–302

Giese A., Kluwe L., Laube B., Meissner H., Berens M.E. & Westphal M. (1996). Migration of human glioma cells on myelin. *Neurosurgery,* Vol.38, pp755–764

Giese A., Bjerkvig R., Berens M.E. & Westphal M. (2003). Cost of migration: invasion of malignant gliomas and implications for treatment. *Journal of Clinical Oncology,* Vol.21, pp1624–1636

Glantz M.J., Cole B.F., Forsyth PA, Recht L.D., Wen P.Y., Chamberlain M.C., Grossman S.A. & Cairncross J.G. (2000). Practice parameter: anticonvulsant prophylaxis in patients with newly diagnosed brain tumors. Report of the quality standards subcommittee of the American Academy of Neurology. *Neurology,* Vol.54, pp1886-1893

González-Darder J.M., González-López P., Talamantes F., Quilis V., Cortés V., García-March G. & Roldán P. (2010). Multimodal navigation in the functional microsurgical resection of intrinsic brain tumors located in eloquent motor areas: role of tractography. *Neurosurgical Focus*, Vol.28(2), ppE5

Hamilton M.G., Yee W.H., Hull R.D. & Ghali W.A. (2011). Venous thromboembolism prophylaxis in patients undergoing cranial neurosurgery: a systematic review and meta - analysis. *Neurosurgery*, Vol.68, pp571-581

Hwang J.H., Smith C.A., Salhia B. & Rutka J.T. (2008). The role of fascin in the migration and invasiveness of malignant glioma cells. *Neoplasia*, Vol.10, pp149–159

Jallo G.I. (2001). CUSA EXcel Ultrasonic Aspiration System. *Neurosurgery* Vol.48, pp695-697

Kaal E.C. & Vecht C.J. (2004). The management of brain edema in brain tumors. *Current Opinion in Oncology*, Vol.16(6), 593-600

Keles G.E., Lamborn K.R. & Berger M.S. (2001). Low - grade hemispheric gliomas in adults: a critical review of extent of resection as a factor influencing outcome. *Journal of Neurosurgery*, Vol.95, pp735-745

Keles G.E., Chang E.F., Lamborn K.R., Tihan T., Chang C.J., Chang S.M. & Berger M.S. (2006). Volumetric extent of resection and residual contrast enhancement on initial surgery as predictors of outcome in adult patients with hemispheric anaplastic astrocytoma. *Journal of Neurosurgery*, Vol.105, pp34–40

Kim P.E. & Zee C.S. (2007). Imaging of the cerebrum. *Neurosurgery*, Vol.61, ppSHC-123–SHC-146

Maranhao E.T., Maranhao-Filho P., Lima M.A. & Vincent M.B. (2010). Can clinical tests detect early signs of monohemispheric brain tumors? *Journal of Neurologic Physical Therapy*, Vol.34, pp145-149

Marras L.C., Geerts W.H., & Perry J.R. (2000). The risk of venous thromboembolism is increased throughout the course of malignant glioma: an evidence - based review. *Cancer*, Vol.89, pp640-646

McGirt M.J., Chaichana K.L., Attenello F.J., Weingart J.D., Than K., Burger P.C., Olivi A., Brem H. & Quinoñes-Hinojosa A.R. (2008). Extent of surgical resection is independently associated with survival in patients with hemispheric infiltrating low-grade gliomas. *Neurosurgery*, Vol.63, pp700–708

McGirt M.J., Chaichana K.L., Gathinji M., Attenello F.J., Than K., Olivi A., Weingart J.D., Brem H. & Quinoñes-Hinojosa A.R. (2009). Independent association of extent of resection with survival in patients with malignant brain astrocytoma. *Journal of Neurosurgery*, Vol.110, pp156–162

Moots P.L., Maciunas R.J., Eisert D.R., Parker R.A., Laporte K. & Abou-Khalil B. (1995). The course of seizure disorders in patients with malignant gliomas. *Archives of Neurology*, Vol.52, pp717-724

Nimsky C., Ganslandt O., Hastreiter P., Wang R., Benner T., Sorensen A.G. & Fahlbusch R. (2005). Preoperative and intraoperative diffusion tensor imaging based fiber tracking in glioma surgery. *Neurosurgery*, Vol.56, pp130 –137

North J.B., Penhall R.K., Hanieh A., Frewin D.B. & Taylor W.B. (1983). Phenytoin and postoperative epilepsy. *Journal of Neurosurgery* Vol.58, pp672-677

Ostergaard L. (2005): Principles of cerebral perfusion imaging by bolus tracking. *Journal of Magnetic Resonance Imaging*, Vol.22, pp710–717

Papadopoulos M.C., Saadoun S., Davies D.C. & Bell B.A.: Emerging molecular mechanisms of brain tumor oedema. *British Journal of Neurosurgery*, Vol.15, pp101-108

Pesudo J.V., González-Darder J.M., Feliu R., Belloch V., Vera J. & Gil J.L. (2001). Assessment of the degree of resection of high grade supratentorial gliomas with early postoperative magnetic resonance. *Neurocirugia* Vol.12, pp43–50

Pouratian N., Cannestra A.F., Bookheimer S.Y., Martin N.A. & Toga A.W. (2004). Variability of intraoperative electrocortical stimulation mapping parameters across and whithin individuals. *Journal of Neurosurgery*, Vol.101, pp458-466

Price S.J., Jena R., Burnet N.G., Hutchinson P.J., Dean A.F., Peña A., Pickard J.D., Carpenter T.A & Gillard J.H. (2006). Improved delineation of glioma margins and regions of infiltration with the use of diffusion tensor imaging: an image-guided biopsy study. *American Journal of Neuroradiology*, Vol.27, pp1969–1974

Provenzale J.M., McGraw P., Mhatre P., Guo A.C. & Delong D. (2004). Peritumoral brain regions in gliomas and meningiomas: investigation with isotropic diffusion-weighted MR imaging and diffusion-tensor MR imaging. *Radiology*, Vol.232, pp451–460

Ribas G.C. (2010). The cerebral sulci and gyri. *Neurosurgical Focus*, Vol.28(2), ppE2

Rosenfeld M.R. & Pruitt A.A. (2007). Managing medical complications in patients with brain tumors. *Community Oncology*, Vol.4, pp411-416

Ruohonen J. & Karhu J. (2010). Navigated transcranial magnetic stimulation. La stimulation magnétique transcrânienne. *Clinical Neurophysiology*, Vol.40, pp7-17

Sanai N. & Berger M.S. (2008). Glioma extent of resection and its impact on patient outcome. *Neurosurgery*, Vol.62, pp753–766

Sawaya R., Hammoud M., Schoppa D., Hess K.R., Wu S.Z., Shi W.M. & Wildrick D.M. (1998). Neurosurgical outcomes in a modern series of 400 craniotomies for treatment of parenchymal tumors. *Neurosurgery*, Vol.42(5), pp1044-1055

Schaller B. & Ruegg S.J. (2003). Brain tumor and seizures: pathophysiology and its implications for treatment revisited. *Epilepsia*, Vol.44(9), pp1223-1232

Schulder M. & Carmel P.W. (2003). Intraoperative magnetic resonance imaging: impact on brain tumor surgery. *Cancer Control Journal*, Vol.10, pp115–124

Shaw E.G., Berkey B., Coons S.W., Bullard D., Brachman D., Buckner J.C., Stelzer K.J., Barger G.R., Brown P.D., Gilbert M.R. & Mehta M. (2008). Recurrence following neurosurgeon-determined gross-total resection of adult supratentorial low-grade glioma: results of a prospective clinical trial. *Journal of Neurosurgery*, Vol.109, pp835–841

Stummer W., Stocker S., Wagner S., Stepp H., Fritsch C., Goetz C., Goetz A.E., Kiefmann R. & Reulen H.J. (1998). Intraoperative detection of malignant gliomas by 5-aminolevulinic acid-induced porphyrin fluorescence. *Neurosurgery*, Vol.42, pp518–526

Stummer W., Pichlmeier U., Meinel T., Wiestler O.D., Zanella F. & Reulen H.J. (2006). Fluorescence-guided surgery with 5-aminolevulinic acid for resection of malignant glioma: a randomised controlled multicentre phase III trial. *The Lancet Oncology*, Vol.7(5), pp392-401

Tanaka Y., Nariai T., Momose T., Aoyagi M., Maehara T., Tomori T., Yoshino Y., Nagaoka T., Ishiwata K., Ishii K. & Ohno K. (2009). Glioma surgery using a multimodal navigation system with integrated metabolic images. *Journal of Neurosurgery*, Vol.110, pp163–172

Tharin S. & Golby A. (2007). Functional brain mapping and its applications to neurosurgery. *Neurosurgery*, Vol.60, ppONS-185–ONS-202

Vahala E., Ylihautala M., Tuominen J., Schiffbauer H., Katisko J., Yrjänä S., Vaara T., Ehnholm G. & Koivukangas J. (2001). Registration in interventional procedures with optical navigator. *Journal of Magnetic Resonance Imaging*, Vol.13(1), pp93-98

Vick N.A. & Wilson C.B. (1985). Total care of the patient with a brain tumor. *Neurologic Clinics*, Vol.3, pp705-710

Wen P.Y., Schiff D., Kesari S., Drappatz J., Gigas D.C. & Doherty L. (2006). Medical management of patients with brain tumors. *Journal of Neurooncology*, Vol.80, pp313-332

26

Therapeutic Embolization of Cranial Tumors

Antonin Krajina, Tomas Cesak, Kamil Zelenak and Svatopluk Rehak
University Hospital, Hradec Kralove
University Hospital, Martin
Czech Republic,
Slovakia

1. Introduction

The aim of embolization is to devascularize the tumor bed by filling intratumoral vascularization as deep as possible into the precapillary level to initiate tumor necrosis, decrease blood loss during surgery and thus make it easier and possibly, more radical, and in tumor of nasal cavity to stop epistaxis (Berenstein, 2004, Valavanis, 2002, Gupta, 2006, Smith, 2006). The procedure is angiographically guided. Embolization of a tumor is performed by either an intraarterial catheterization approach or direct puncture of the tumor artery. Selection of one of these approaches depends of the location, and number of arterial feeders of the tumor. Result of devascularization is verified by contrast enhanced CT or MR imaging.

Endovascular therapy is not only limited to devascularization procedures for head and neck tumors. Central nervous system lymphomas can be treated with intraarterial chemotherapy infusions after blood brain barrier disruption (Neuwelt, 1991), and squamous cell carcinomas of the skull base and neck are treated with selective infusions of high dose chemotherapy (Simunek, 1993). In this review, we will discuss the endovascular approach to induce tumor ischemia and necrosis of central nervous system and skull base tumors. In spite of the fact that methods of preoperative devascularization of hypervascularized tumors of the head have been established for many years, the number of patients treated endovascularly using this technique is relatively low. This is mainly due to a small proportion of the head and neck tumors suitable for this therapy and controversies in terms of its risk-benefit ratio (Latchaw, 1993).

2. Indications

There are basically three main indications for head and neck vascularized tumor embolization: presurgical embolization, palliative treatment, and to stop epistaxis. Presurgical embolization is believed to reduce blood loss, shorten the operative procedure time and potentially increase the chances of radical surgical resection as well as decrease the incidence of tumor recurrence. Palliative treatment may led to a decrease in tumor mass with improvement of neurological symptoms due to intracranial expansion. In some cases, shrinkage of tumor may alleviate intractable pain.

The most common skull base hypervascular tumors treated with embolization are meningiomas, paragangliomas, hemangiopericytomas, juvenile nasopharyngeal angiofibromas. The most frequent intraaxially located tumors indicated for embolotherapy are hemangioblastomas, hypervascularized metastases and ependymomas (table 1).

Cranial tumors that are treated with endovascular embolization
1. Meningiomas
2. Paragangliomas
3. Juvenile nasopharyngeal angiofibromas
4. Hemangioblastomas
5. Intracranial and extracranial mestastases
6. Hemangiopericytomas

Table 1. The list of the most common hypervascularized tumors in which embolization may be benefitial.

3. Embolization technique

3.1 Functional Angiography

Selective internal, external carotid and vertebral angiograms are followed by selective catheterizations of feeding arteries to analyze arterial supply of the tumor.
Complex vascular anatomy of the skull base requires meticulous digital subtraction angiograms to reveal dangerous anastomoses from external carotid artery branches to internal carotid or vertebral arteries (Russell, 1986, Geibprasert, 2009). These arterial connections should be checked during embolization since they might open up as the occlusion of target artery progresses (Berenstein, 2004, Russell, 1986).
For complex procedures, meticulous angiograms without motion artifacts are required, and simple intravenous sedation may be inadequate. In such procedures general anesthesia will often be appropriate. Arteficial ventilation is stopped during selective injections to avoid any movement artefacts. High-quality biplanar imaging is generally recommended at the skull base and around the eye arterial network studies.
Depending on tumor size and extension, unilateral or bilateral internal and external carotid and vertebral angiograms are performed using 5F catheter system as the first step of embolization procedure. Then selective studies are accomplished via various types and diameters of microcatheters. Their selection depends on diameter of the target artery and also on the operator´s experience. Care should always be exercised to avoid proximal vasospasms which may preclude flow directed embolization. Vasospasms occurrence varies from patient to patient and should be minimized by careful catheterization techniques and administration of vasodilators (Kurata, 1996).
The feeding pedicles should be tested for supply to cranial nerves before infusion of embolic agents. Awake patient can be evaluated for appropriate cranial nerve or visual deficits after selective injection of 1-2 ml of local anesthetic before embolization starts. In the sleeping patient we have to rely on anatomical angiographic studies and thorough knowledge of anatomy.
Ideally the capillary bed of the tumor is slowly saturated with embolic microparticles or liquid agent. This is accomplished under fluoroscopic guidance to assess blood flow velocity in the artery and potential backflow and reflux of embolic agent is observed. During embolization the operator should perform selective angiograms, the quality of which

enables not only to assess progress in occlusion, but to reveal potential filling of collaterals. Some neuroradiologists say: "When you see collaterals, it is always too late."

3.2 Special techniques

For tumors in cavernous region supplied by dural feeders coming off the internal carotid artery the non-detachable balloon is inflated above the feeding arteries origin to protect the ophthalmic artery and all pial networks (Théron, 1986, Gonzales, 1990, Tymianski, 1994, Jungreis, 1991). The microparticles can be safely injected nonselectively into these feeders. Repeated flushing and aspiration should be performed before the balloon is deflated to minimize distal embolization.

Usually, it is most important to embolize surgically inaccessible arterial feeders. Then depending on risk-benefit ratio and compartmental supply of some tumors, second-order size feeders are closed as well. Finally, we prefer to embolize the largest feeders.

The blood flow in the magistral arteries with potentially dangerous collaterals can be modified by temporal balloon occlusion. Distal arterial beds can be protected by microcoil placement to avoid penetration of embolic agent into normal tissue and minimize risk of the skin necrosis or delayed healing of the future surgical wound.

Direct percutaneous puncture of some hypervascular tumors is performed with a system of coaxial needles (Casasco, 1994, Chaloupka, 1999, Abud, 2004, Lonser, 1998, Casasco, 1999). This has to be done under general anesthesia and simultaneous angiographic control. Liquid agents are most used in this technique (Lonser, 1998). Complications from intratumoral anastomoses to surrounding neurovascular structures are observed with this technique, similar to those of transarterial embolization (Casasco, 1999).

3.3 Embolic agents

The operator´s selection of embolic agent is directed by a balance between risk and efficacy. Smaller particles (45-150 μm) (Wakhloo, 1993) and liquid embolic agents (bucrylate, ethanol, ethylenevinylalcohol) penetrate tumor better and achieve a higher degree of necrosis. However, these agents definitely carry a higher risk of collateral tissue ischemia of the vasa nervorum. The critical size of microparticles is generally considered to be above 150 μm (table 2).

The most frequent causes of neurologic deficit after embolization of cranial base tumors
1. selection of inappropriate embolic material
2. reflux of emboli (vasospasm, nonselective injection, too many particles injected too fast)
3. failure to recognize dangerous anastomoses (incomplete angiogram, inadequate analysis)

Table 2. The list of frequent causes of ischemic neurological deficit after embolization in the skull base (Lasjaunias, 1980).

4. Results of embolization

Comparisons between groups of patients with surgical therapy of meningiomas with and without preoperative embolization revealed that embolization reduces blood loss and the number of transfusions needed during operation. This effect is higher in large tumors than small, and when a high degree of obliteration was achieved. These facts can be generalized to other vascularized tumors of the skull base and brain which are much less frequent than meningeomas. The authors will discusse embolization in specific lesions as meningeomas, paragangliomas, juvenile angiofibromas and some of intraaxial tumors.

4.1 Meningiomas

Meningiomas are the most common extraaxial intracranial tumors in adults. They are derived from meningothelial cells concentrated in the arachnoid villi. The most frequent sites of origin of these tumors are where the arachnoid villi are the most numerous, i.e. the major dural sinuses, veins, and along the root sleeves of the exiting cranial and spinal nerves. However, ectopic meningiomas may arise from ectopic arachnoid cell inclusions (Black, 1993).

The grade of vascularization varies on histological type of meningioma (Toktas, 2010, Ketter, 2008). The World Heath Organization grade II and III, which are labeled as atypical and anaplastic, as well as angioblastic and syncytial types tend to be more vascular then grade I, and fibroblastic type which are considered benign.

For practical reasons three types of this diseases are classified in the literature. The most common is the globular meningioma. It presents with compact rounded mass with invagination of brain. The tumor is flat at base, and originates in at basal or convexity dura, tentorium or falx. The second type is meningioma en plaque, which induces hyperostosis of underlying bone. This type is not indicated for angiography or embolization. The third type is multicentric meningioma. It might be associated with neurofibromatosis type II.

Preoperative angiography is indicated only for purposes of devascularization in potentially highly vascularized tumors evaluated by CT or MR. These are predominantly large in size and located at skull base (Nelson, 1994).

Angiography demonstrates early opacification of tumoral blush which stays late into the venous phase, so called "mother-in-law" phenomenon. The early draining vein sign is rare, and may be seen in angioblastic meningiomas. Tumorous vascularization has a characteristic "sunburst" pattern. Meningiomas in certain locations have particular arterial feeders. The degree of their pial supply varies.

Hypervascularized meningiomas involving the skull base are the most frequently embolized (Macpherson, 1991, Rosen, 2002). Meningiomas originating from the anterior fossa (the olfactory groove, planum sphenoidale) may receive their dural blood supply from the ethmoidal arteries of the ophthalmic artery (Figure 1). Meningiomas of the cavernous sinus and clinoid region are fed by the inferolateral and meningohypophyseal trunks of the internal carotid artery and by the cavernous branch of the middle meningeal artery, recurrent meningeal branch of the ophthalmic artery and the accessory meningeal artery (Valavanis, 2002).

Meningiomas of the middle fossa and sphenoid wing are supplied by the sphenoidal branch of the middle meningeal artery. In general, meningiomas of the lateral third of the sphenoid wing are supplied by external feeders, and tumors of the medial third are supplied off internal carotid artery feeders. Meningiomas located in the tentorium and posterior fossa receive their supply from the internal carotid artery via the marginal tentorial artery, the lateral clival branch, and tentorial branch of the middle meningeal artery. Infratentorial meningeal supply is through the posterior meningeal artery and posterior falx artery which arise from the vertebral artery. Petroclival and cerebellopontine angle meningiomas are supplied by branches of the internal carotid artery, middle meningeal artery, mastoid artery and ascending pharyngeal artery (Valavanis, 2002, Natarajan, 2007).

Convexity meningiomas receive their dural supply from the middle menigeal artery. There may be bilateral feeders when these lesions are located close to the midline. Meningiomas, invading into the bone may receive transosseous supply from scalp arteries.

Angiography is expected to evaluate relationship of convexity meningiomas to the dural sinuses. If a meningioma has obliterated the sinus, it is easier for the neurosurgeon to remove than if it has compressed the sinus. In this case, preservation of the sinus is necessary (Raza, 2010).

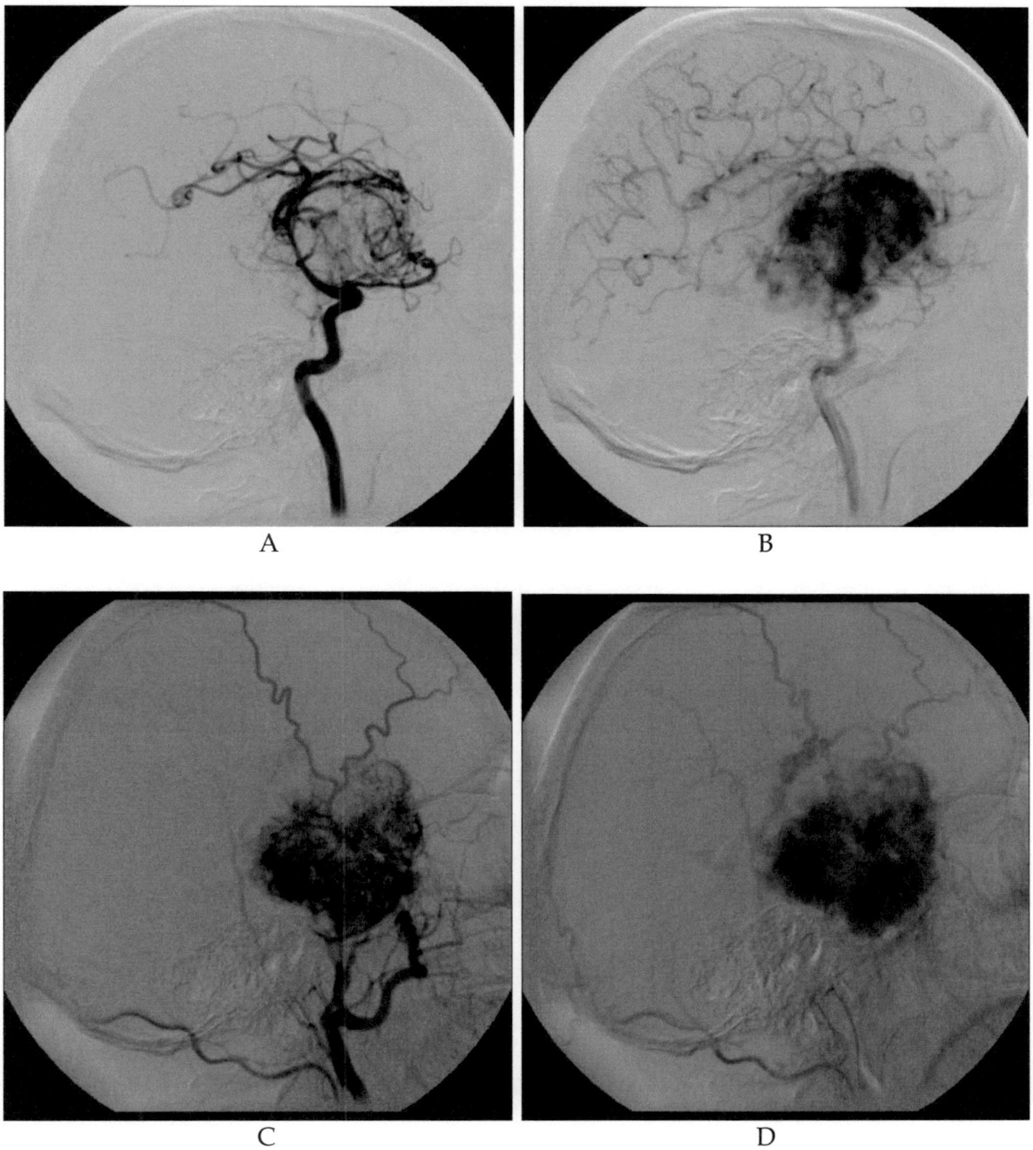

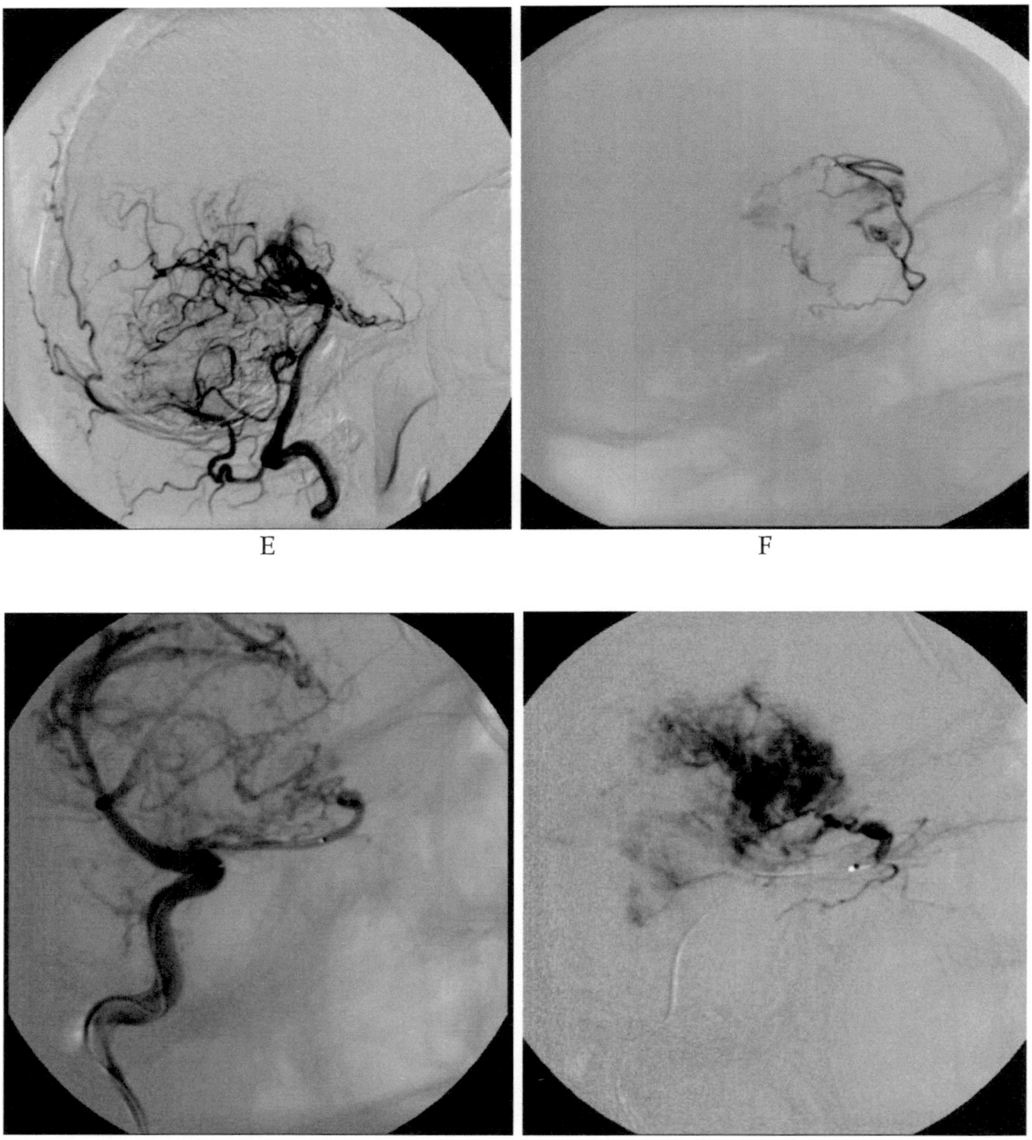

E F

G H

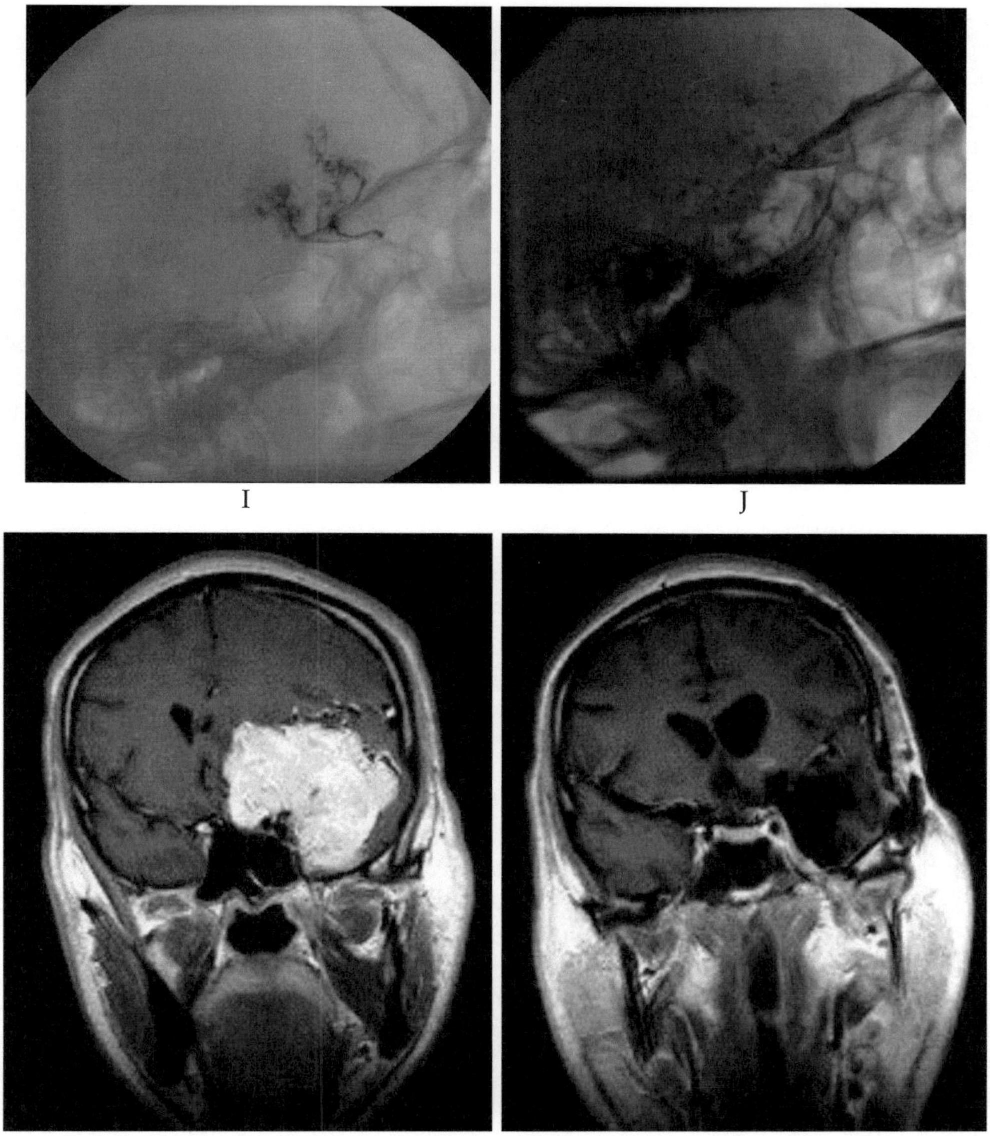

Fig. 1. A 48-year-old male with large meningioma of the sphenoid wing. **A, B.** Selective internal carotid angiogram shows hypervascularized tumor. **C, D.** The external carotid angiogram demonstrates rich vascularization fed from the middle and accessory meningeal arteries. **E.** The posterior part of the tumor is supplied by pial feeders arising from posterior circulation. **F.** Embolization of the tumor was started from hypertrophied pial feeders. **G-I.** After embolization of the external carotid artery branches (not shown), the opththalmic artery feeder was catheterized and embolized. **J.** The lateral view of the skull reveales penetration of radiopaque acrylic glue into the tumor. **K.** Preoperative MR image of the tumor. **L.** Postoperative MR image demonstrated total tumor removal inspite of the fact that preoperative embolization was estimated to be only 50 %. The patient suffered from ipsilateral oculomotor palsy after surgery which improved with time.

4.1.1 Results

In last two decades several comparative studies to prove whether embolization really reduces operative blood loss have been published, including whether it justifies the potential risk.

In 1994 Dean et al. selected 18 matched pairs of meningiomas (size, location, angioblastic versus nonangioblastic) out of 33 embolized and 193 nonembolized meningiomas to compare both groups for blood loss during operation, surgical resection time, cost and complications. Embolization was revealed to be beneficial since the estimated blood loss was significantly lower (533 ml versus 836 ml), number of transfusions was significantly lower (0.39 units versus 1.56 units), surgical resection time was shorter (305.8 minutes versus 337.5 minutes) and length of hospitalization was shorter (10.6 days versus 15.0 days). The mean cost was lower for the embolized group. There were zero major and ten minor complications in embolized group and three major and nine minor complications in the non-embolized group (Dean, 1994).

In 1998 Oka et al. analysed a group of 12 patients with meningiomas larger than 4 cm in diameter which were embolized prior surgery after the year 1990. The control group included 8 patients who were operated without embolization between 1980-1989. The results showed that in tumors smaller than 6 cm, the average blood lost was significantly lower in the embolized group (1.1. units versus 12.8 units).

Differences in the number of blood units required during surgery for patients with meningiomas over 6 cm in size did not reach statistical significance. This paradox was explained by a tendency of larger meningiomas in recruiting blood vessels that were unsuitable for preoperative embolization. The authors did not find a difference in the lenght of the operation between the two groups and the embolized group tended to show a better clinical outcome than the non-embolized group (Oka, 1998).

In 2000 Bendszus et al. compared 30 patients who were preoperatively embolized for meningiomas at one center with another 30 patients at a second center who were not. Both protocols were considered to be routine at each neurosurgical center. The mean tumor sizes were 29.6 cm^3 in embolized group versus 29.9 cm^3 in non-embolized group. There were no effect on blood loss (636 ml in embolized group versus 646 ml in non-embolized group) except when there was more than 90 % tumor devascularization as assessed by postembolization MR imaging. The observations of the neurosurgeons regarding hemostasis, tumor consistency, and intratumoral necrosis did not differ significantly. There was one permanent neurological deficit (3%) caused by embolization. The rates of surgical morbidity with permanent neurological worsening were 16 % in a center where embolization was used, and 20 % in a center without preoperative embolization (Bendszus, 2000).

The efficacy of preoperative meningiomas embolization was studied retrospectively in numerous monocentric studies. Investigators analysed embolic agent, methods of tumor necrosis verification, proportion of the feeders from the external and internal carotid artery, timing of surgery after embolization and complications.

4.1.2 Embolic agents

In 1993 Wakhloo et al. compared group of 14 patients whose meningiomas were embolized with polyvinylalcohol particles of 150 to 300 μm in size, with a group of 20 patients where smaller (50 to 150 μm) particles were used. The patients were evaluated by CT, MR, MR spectroscopy and MR volumetry of their tumors. Angiography after embolization demonstrated the total elimination of tumor blush in all patients. Contrast-enhanced MR after larger particles embolization proved a reduction of tumor enhancement in only 14 %. While after smaller particles necrosis ranged from 30 to 95 % was proved in 60 % with some volume reduction in 20 %. The appearance of the tumor at surgery, and histopathologic examination of different parts of the tumor confirmed MR finding of necrosis. The authors concluded that extended embolization with 50 to 150 μm microparticles improved the surgical treatment of meningiomas, as compared with larger particles embolization. They suggested to use this technique in palliative embolization in patients who are not candidates for surgery (Wakhloo, 1993).

Small particles penetrated deep into the tumorous vasculature, while larger particles produced proximal occlusion of feeding arteries. This proximal occlusion results in clot formation which, over time, can be recanalized and such embolization is less efficient. On the other hand, the operator has to balance the use of the aggressive embolization techniques in a particular vascular territory against possible complications. Another study which compared a historically new embolic agent with polyvinylalcohol microparticles was published in 2000 (Bendszus, 2000). The new embolic microparticles were much more sophisticated. They are trisacryl gelatin microspheres non absorbable collagen-coated, precisely calibrated microspheres (Embospheres, Guerbet). The study included 60 patients and revealed that use of the trisacrylmicrospheres in size 150 to 300 μm were significantly more efficient than embolization with polyvinylalcohol microparticles of both sizes of 45 to 150 μm or 150 to 300 μm regarding blood loss at surgery. The result was explained by deeper arterial penetration of the trisacryl microspheres (Wakhloo, 1993).

In some anatomical territories or if the tip of microcatheter is positioned inside tumoral vasculature, successful embolization using liquid agents have been reported. The use of n-butyl-2-cyanoacrylate (Histoacryl, B. Braun) is recommended in presence of intratumoral arteriovenous shunts. This liquid agent is diluted by oily contrast medium which delays rapidity of its solidification.

Use of highly concentrated ethanol for skull base meningiomas was reported in a series of seven patients at cavernous region. The cavernous part of the internal carotid artery was occluded with a non detachable balloon and from 1 to 12 ml of ethanol was injected during 5-40 minutes. In 2 patients (30 %) permanent cranial nerve palsies developed (Jungreis, 1991).

Another liquid embolic agent is composed of ethylenevinylalcohol copolymer suspended in dimethylsulfoxide with tantalum added for radioopacity (Onyx, ev3). This agent is increasingly used either for transcatheter of direct needle puncture embolization of tumors. The technique of its injection is quite different than on previous agents. The injection is slow and penetration of the agent can be clearly seen on fluoroscopy (Gemmete. 2010) (Figure 2).

4.1.3 Tumor necrosis verification

Angiography performed at the end of embolization is considered not to be valid proof of effective embolization even if the tumor blush disappears completely (Valavanis, 2002, Benszus, 2000). This could be either due to arterial spasms or proximal extratumoral occlusion of feeders. Gadolinium enhanced MR provides more valuable imaging of tumor necrosis. MR spectroscopy has been studied, but is not used routinely (Bendszus, 2000). In our practice - contrast enhanced CT scanning is most likely equal to MR for evaluating those meningiomas that have not been operated and for their remmants (Figure 3).

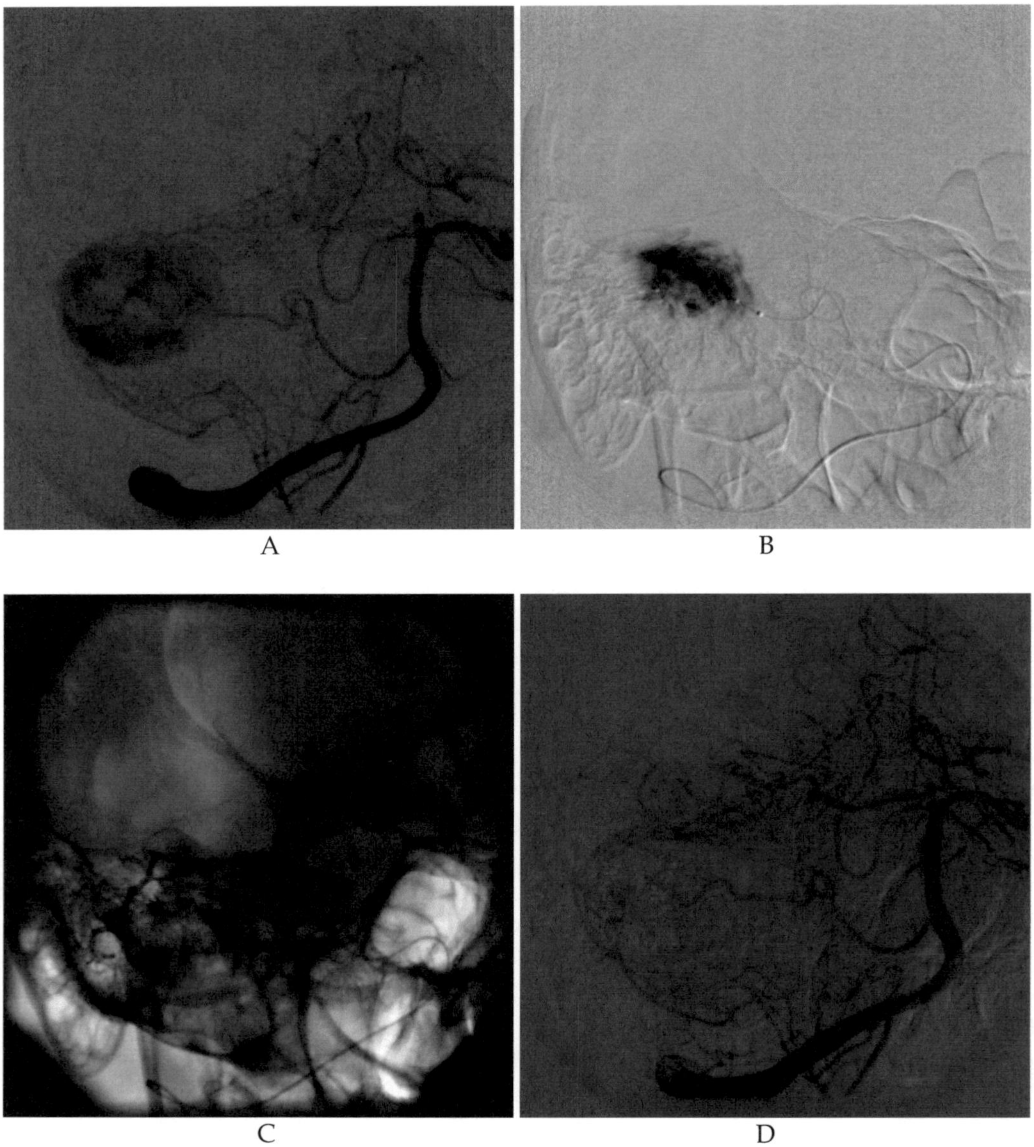

Fig. 2. **A.** A 42-year-old man with intraaxial hypervascularized hemangioblastoma supplyied mainly by the anterior inferior cerebellar artery. **B.** Selective injection through the Sonic 1,5F microcatheter (Balt). **C.** The tumor was embolized with 0.4 ml of ethylenevinylalcohol (Onyx 18, ev3). Filling of the tumorous arteries with radiopaque liquid can be seen. **D.** Postembolization arteriogram depicting the lack of tumor blush with preservation of the anterior inferior cerebellar artery. The patient was operated.

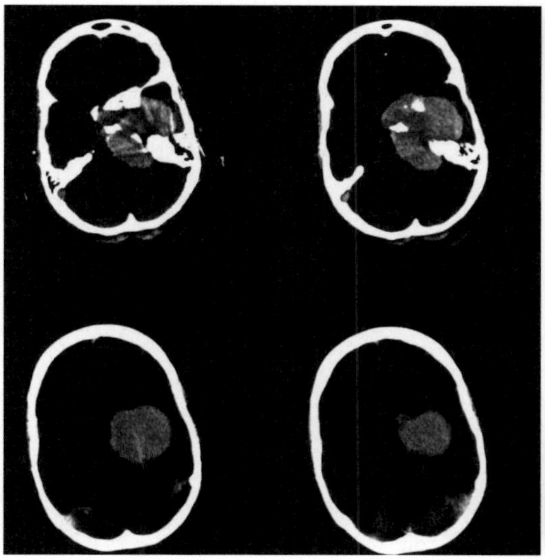

A

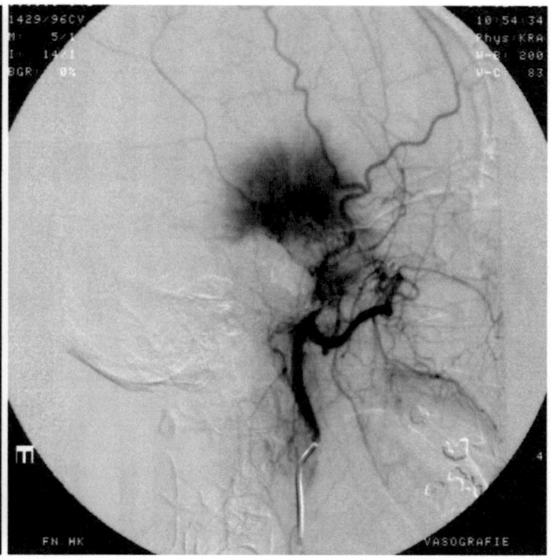
1429/96CV
10:54:34
Phys KRA
FN HK
VASOGRAFIE

B

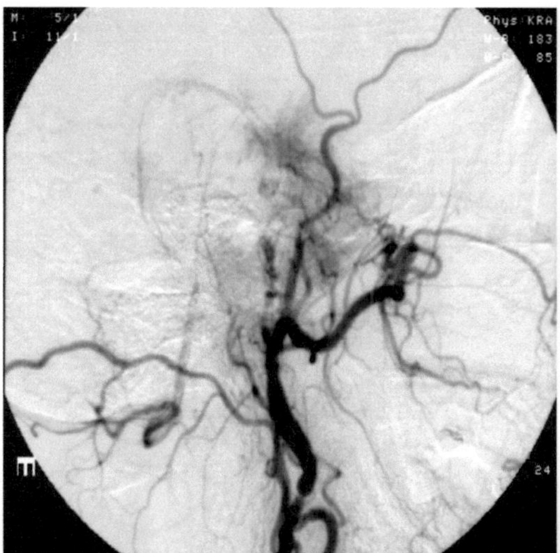
Phys KRA
FN HK
VASOGRAFIE

C

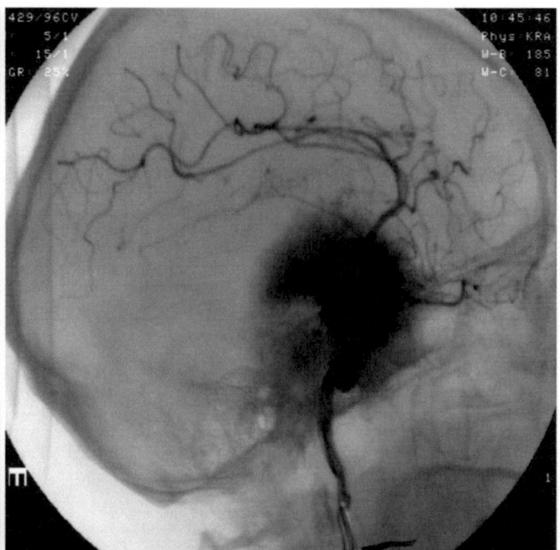
429/96CV
10:45:46
Phys KRA
FN HK
VASOGRAFIE

D

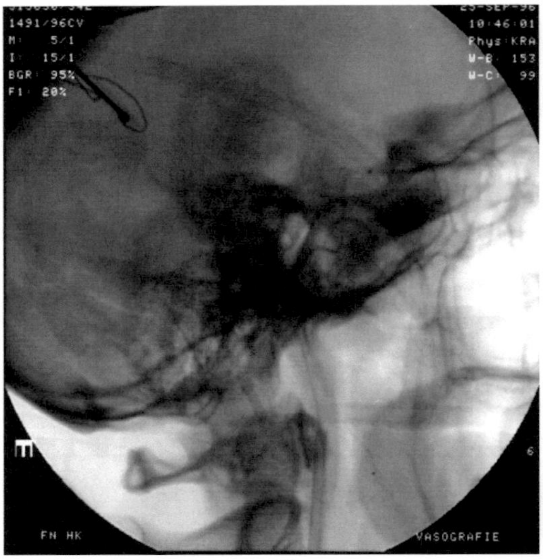
1491/96CV
M: 5/1
I: 15/1
BGR: 95%
F1: 20%
10:46:01
Phys:KRA
W-B: 153
W-C: 99
6
FN HK
VASOGRAFIE

E

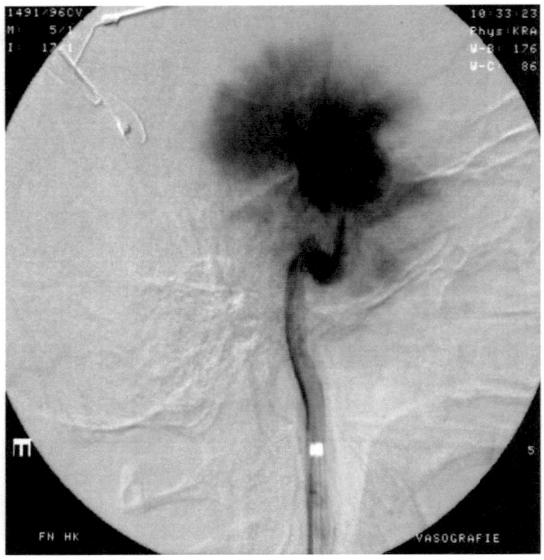
1491/96CV
10:33:23
Phys:KRA
176
86
5
FN HK
VASOGRAFIE

F

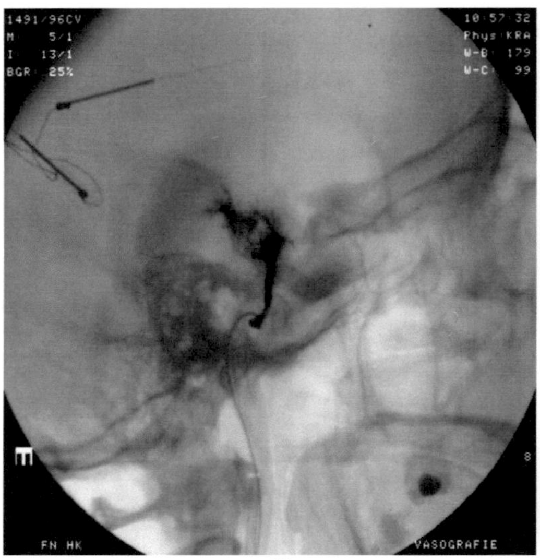
1491/96CV
M: 5/1
I: 13/1
BGR: 25%
10:57:32
Phys:KRA
W-B: 179
W-C: 99
8
FN HK
VASOGRAFIE

G

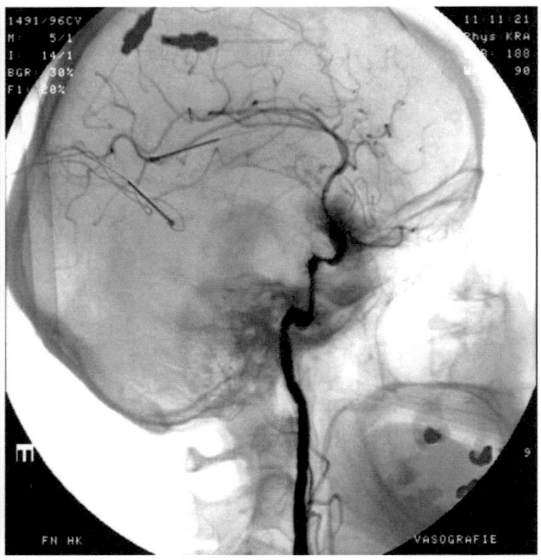
1491/96CV
11:11:21
9
FN HK
VASOGRAFIE

H

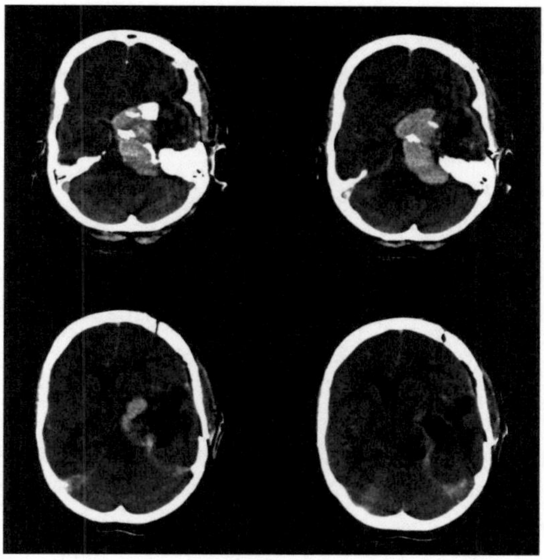

I

Fig. 3. **A.** A 45-year-old woman with large hypervascular meningioma which occupies the middle fossa. **B.** The external carotid angiogram reveals typical sunburst pattern of meningioma. **C.** There is minimal residual blush after embolization of the middle and accessory meningeal arteries. **D.** The majority of the tumor is fed from the internal carotid artery branches. **E.** The guiding catheter was placed into the internal carotid artery and nondetachable balloon was inflated below the level of the ophthalmic artery origin. The second parallel microcatheter was placed below the balloon for injection of microparticles (polyvinylalcohol 150-300 μm). **F.** The internal carotid artery angiogram with balloon inflated above the tumor feeders. **G.** The internal carotid artery angiogram after embolization demonstrates some filling of intratumoral arteries. The blood from the internal carotid artery was aspirated before the balloon was deflated. **H.** The internal carotid artery angiogram revealed significant tumorous blush reduction. **I.** The contrast enhanced CT performed after surgery revealed persistent midline portion of the tumor. The tumor remnant was treated by stereotactic radiosurgery.

4.1.4 Embolization of the internal carotid artery feeders

This point is of importance for skull base meningiomas. Some of the internal carotid branches are not accessible at the beginning of surgery, but their embolization presents a much higher risk for the patient than standard embolization of the external carotid artery branches. But if we look closer at the distribution of permanent neurological deficit after embolization, the artery with the highest risk is the ascending pharyngeal artery followed by the meningohypophyseal trunk, accessory meningeal artery, middle meningeal artery and ophthalmic artery. In this study, which included 167 meningiomas with 280 feeders the most frequently embolized artery was the middle meningeal artery followed by meningohypophyseal trunk and ascending pharyngeal artery. The rate of permanent deficit was 9 % (Rosen, 2002) (table 3).

In the other study, which included, 119 meningiomas with embolization of 18 % of the internal carotid artery feeders, permanent complication rate was 2.5 %. None of them was not in relation to the internal carotid artery feeder embolization (Waldron, 2011).

Most frequent permanent neurological deficit after cranial base meningiomas embolization. Distribution according embolized arteries
1. ascending pharyngeal artery 2. meningohypophyseal trunk 3. accessory meningeal artery 4. middle meningeal artery 5. ophthalmic artery

Table 3. The list of the arteries with the most frequent permanent neurological deficit after cranial base meningiomas embolization (Rosen, 2002).

4.1.5 Timing of surgery after embolization

It is general practice to schedule meningioma surgery within 24 hours after embolization, especially to prevent revascularization and avoid problems due to tumor swelling in some cases.

Two interesting studies have been performed. The first proved no difference in operative blood loss in delayed surgery and the greatest degree of tumor softening at surgery was found between 7th and 9th day after embolization (Kai, 2002).

The second study compared two groups of patients. In the first group of 28 patients surgery was done within 24 hours, while in the second group the meningioma was resected later (2-7 days). There was found to be significantly decreased in operative blood loss in the delayed surgery group (Chun, 2002).

4.1.6 Neurologic complications

Causes of neurologic complications after meningiomas embolization include brain or cranial nerve ischemia, hemorrhage, and tumoral swelling (Yu, 2004).

Depending on aggressiveness of the operator the rate of ischemic complications is reported from 0 % to 9 %. Bendzus et al reported on 185 consecutive cases undergoing microspheres embolization of meningiomas, 12 (7 %) complications related to the procedure. Six of them were ischemic (hemiparesis and amaurosis) and another six hemorrhagic. The authors concluded that microspheres embolization of meningiomas is associated with substantial risk of ischemic and hemorrhage events. The individual risk-to-benefit ratio of embolization should be thoroughly considered (Bendszus, 2005).

Kallmes et al. reviewed literature in 1997 and found only seven cases of hemorrhage of a meningioma after embolotherapy at that time. All those meningiomas were large (> 6 cm) and highly vascular (Kallmes, 1997). In the report of Bendzus et al. (Bendszus, 2005) were observed 6 cases of postembolization meningioma hemorrhage occurred in a series of 185 cases. One of them was fatal and the others necessitated urgent surgical tumor removal, but resulted in no persistent neurological deficit. The atypical meningiomas, and tumors with previous hemorrhage, with cystic changes within tumor were positive predictors of hemorrhage. Worsening of mass effects after embolization of meningiomas with significant edema should be prevented by pretreatment with steroids (Gilad, 2009).

4.2 Paragangliomas

Paragangliomas are derived from paragangliomic chemoreceptor cells of neural crest origin. These neoplasms are locally aggressive with a low metastatic potential (Gerosa, 2006). The

most common location in the head and neck region for these tumors is along the temporal bone (almost 50 %) involving the tympanic plexus or jugular fossa, followed by the carotid bifurcation and vagal nerve. Detailed description of last two entities is beyond the scope of this chapter. Multicentricity is observed in 22 %, especially in patients with a positive family history. Secretory catecholamines activity occurs in 1 % (Berenstein, 2004, Valavanis, 2002).
Definitive treatment for these tumor is surgical excision. Preoperative arterial embolization has been accepted for selected cases of head and neck paragangliomas. A ten year survival of only in 29 % in untreated temporal paragangliomas justifies aggressive treatment of these patients (Valavanis, 2002, Valavanis, 1986, Tikkakoski, 1997, Persky, 2002).

4.2.1 Glomus tympanicum tumor

Glomus tympanicum tumor is the most common tumor in the middle ear, which presents with hearing loss and pulsatile tinnitus. It originates from the tympanic plexus on cochlear promontory of the middle ear. The extent of bone involvement can be demonstrated on CT using bone algorithm protocol. Local spread may cause invasion of the carotid canal, jugular foramen, facial and hypoglossal nerves canals, cerebellopontine angle and mastoid process. MRI provides typical "salt and pepper" appearance of hypervascular soft tissue tumor and relationship to the carotid artery (Valavanis, 2002, Van den Berg, 2002).

4.2.2 Glomus jugulare tumor

This is the most common tumor in the jugular fossa with intracranial extension. It arises from the adventitia of the jugular vein and shows similarity to tympanicum tumor with hearing loss and tinnitus. CT may reveal destruction of the posteroinferior petrous pyramid (Ramina, 2005).

4.2.3 Preoperative and preembolization angiography

Paragangliomas are hypervascularized with enlarged arterial feeders. Catheterization angiography should include separate internal and external carotid artery studies with venous phase imaging.
The ascending pharyngeal artery is the most important feeder of paragangliomas in all four regions and therefore has been called "the artery of the paraganglioma" (Lasjaunias, 1976, Lasjaunias, 1978, Cavalcanti, 2009). While the tympanic paraganglioma is sometimes difficult to visualize because of its small size, the jugular paraganglioma is usually seen as a hypervascular mass with persistent homogeneous reticular stain. On the basis of the compartmental theory, temporal paragangliomas supplied by both neuromeningeal and tympanic branches of the ascending pharyngeal artery may represent two separate tumors appearing as one mass. The compartmental arrangement of paragangliomas has been described in which one artery supplies a single area with a specific venous drainage. More than one compartment occurs in 85 % cases. This type of tumor compartmentalization is explained by its encapsulation, which restricts recruitment of feeders from adjacent territories (Moret, 1982).
The presence of other arterial supply can be a sign of intracranial extension of skull base paraganglioma. These feeders are recruited from meningeal arteries of both external and internal carotid arteries. True intradural tumor ingrowth is proved if there is supply from the anterior inferior and posterior inferior cerebellar arteries.

Patency of the internal jugular vein may be impossible to prove due to washout from arteriovenous shunting of the tumor. It is recommended to evaluate jugular vein on postembolization angiography (Valavanis, 2002).

Preoperative or intraoperative occlusion of the internal carotid artery should be considered when CT shows extensive destruction of the horizontal portion of the carotid canal or the tumor spreads to foramen lacerum and cavernous sinus. In such instances, the balloon test occlusion is useful as a part of angiographic work up.

Similarly to meningiomas, there is controversy as to whether embolization is useful before surgical resection. Tikkakoski et al. compared blood loss between paragangliomas embolized before surgery with that of non embolized paragangliomas and revealed a significantly

($p < 0.04$) lower amount of blood loss in the embolized group (588 ml versus 1374 ml) (Tikkakoski, 1997).

The diameter of arteries supplying paragangliomas is about 90 μm proximally and enlarges deep within the tumor. In the central part of the tumor arteries may reach a diameter of 300-600 μm. The most frequently used embolic agent are microparticles and in order to reach central part of the tumor, their diameter should be less than 90 μm then. The presence of arteriovenous shunting in some paragangliomas warrants the use of n-butyl-2-cyanoacrylate (Figure 4) or ethylenevinylalcohol (Valavanis, 2002).

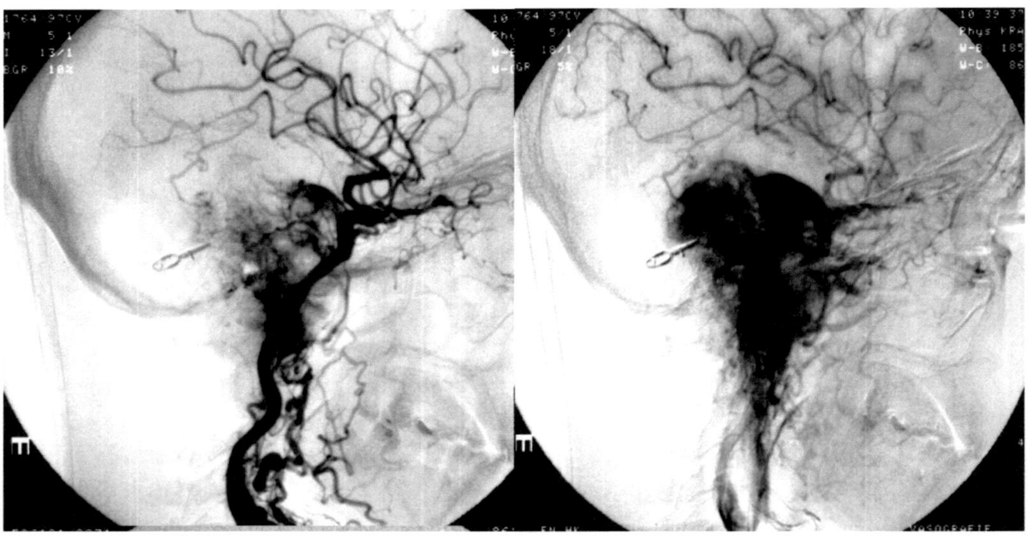

A B

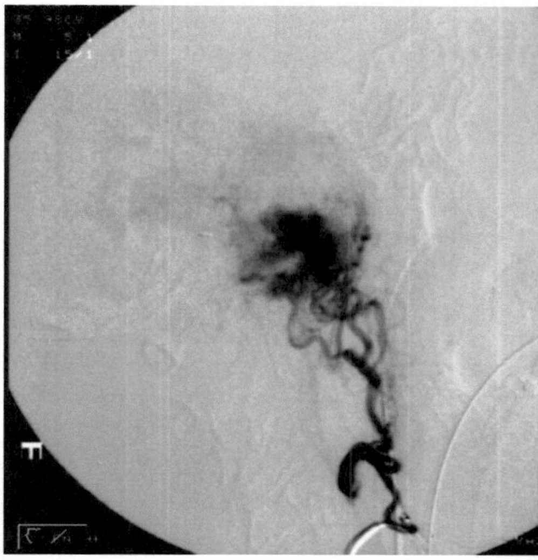

C

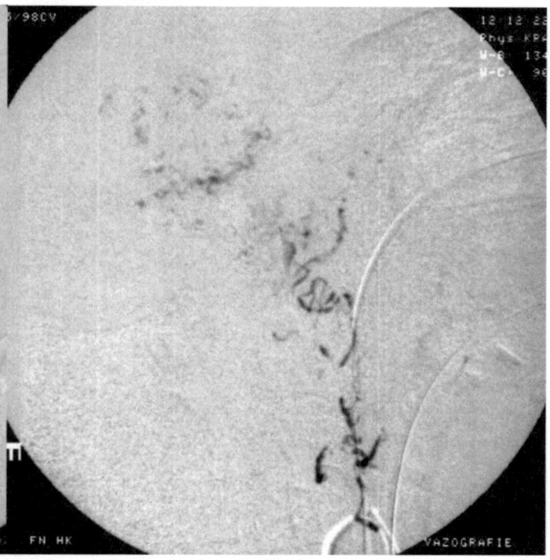

D

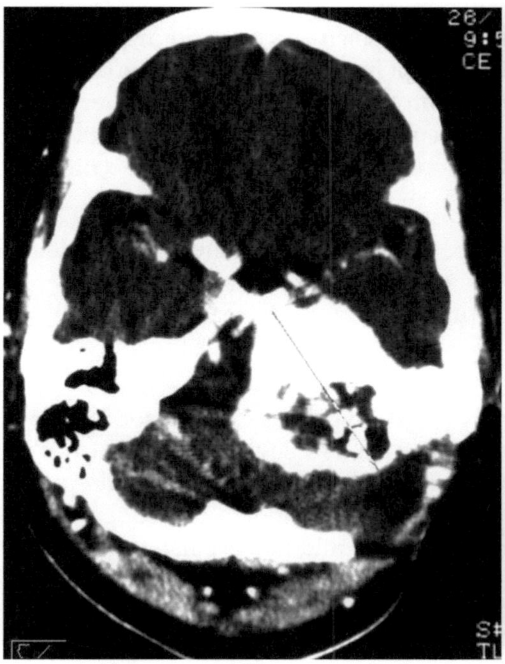

E

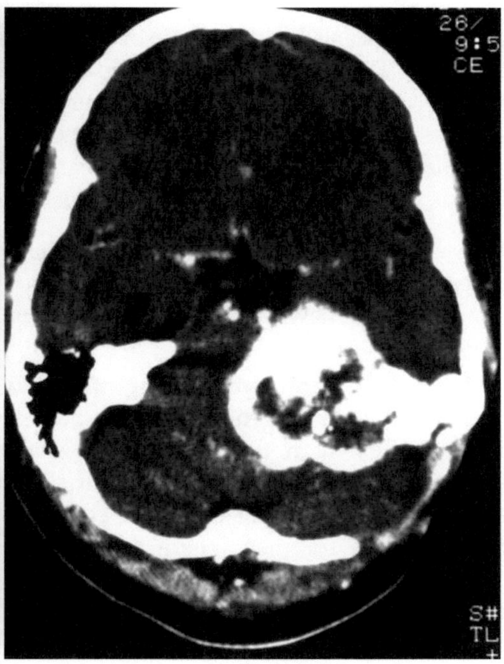

F

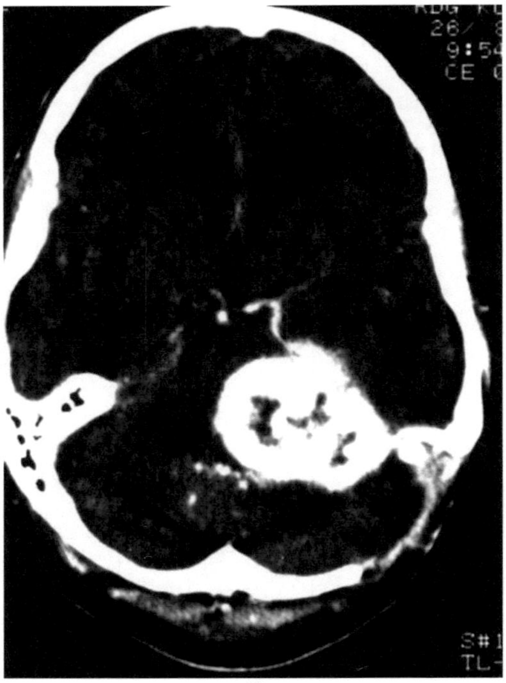

G

Fig. 4. A 48-year-old woman with large paraganglioma. **A.** The left common carotid angiogram reveals ligation of the external carotid artery which was done during previous surgery. **B.** The late arterial phase shows opacification of hypervascularized tumor. **C.** The external carotid was reached via collateral branch from the superior thyreoidal artery. **D.** The substracted image demonstrates injection and penetration of the acrylic glue into the vascular bed of the tumor. **E-G.** Follow-up contrast enhanced CT scans revealed central necrosis with radiopaque glue deposit inside it.

The use of percutaneous, direct puncture therapeutic embolization is relatively new technique. Successful devascularization with direct percutaneous injection of n-butyl-2-cyanoacrylate ethanol or ethylenevinylalcohol has been reported (Casasco, 1994, Gemmete, 2010).

4.3 Juvenile nasopharyngeal angiofibroma

Juvenile nasopharyngeal angiofibroma is a benign hypervascular tumor. Although histologically benign, they behave in a locally invasive manner having a propensity to thin and erode bone and displace adjacent structures. The lesion originates from the postero-lateral wall of the nasal cavity in close proximity to the superior aspect of the middle sphenopalatine foramen where the posterior part of the middle turbinate attaches. The tumor later occupies the nasopharynx and posterior nasal cavity, sphenoid sinus, middle cranial fossa, maxillary sinus, oropharynx infratemporal fossa, orbit, and parapharyngeal space (Berenstein, 2004).

Symptoms are related to size and direction of spread. They may include repeat epistaxis (in 59 %), which may be life threatening, obstruction of paranasal sinuses and auditory canal, anosmia, decreased hearing and typical nasal speech due to nasal obstruction. It may be difficult to differentiate paranasal tumor invasion from purulent sinusitis. Sarcomatous transformation has been reported after radiation therapy. Juvenile nasopharyngeal angiofibroma occurs in young males between 8 and 23 years of age. Tumors decrease in size with exogenous estrogen administration, and increase in size with testosterone (Johns, 1980).

CT and MR can preoperatively reveal bone involvement and extent of the tumor (Chagnaud, 1998, Kania, 2005). Since the introduction of preoperative embolization, both the blood loss and operative time have decreased (Garcia-Cervigon, 1988, Moulin, 1995). More recent transnasal endoscopic surgical techniques may be applied to many of these tumors and tend to rely on preoperative devascularization to decrease blood loss, enhancing the chances for complete tumor resection (Scholtz, 2001, Douglas, 2006). Polyvinylalcohol microparticles are used by most of operators.

A systematic angiographic protocol of juvenile nasopharyngeal angiofibromas begins with injection of the contralateral common carotid artery followed by the ipsilateral common and internal carotid arteries injections. Then the ipsilateral external carotid angiography for evaluation of the maxillary and ascending pharyngeal arteries is performed. The maxillary, accessory meningeal, ascending pharyngeal, and ascending palatine arteries are the most often embolized. If the tumor crosses the midline embolization of appropriate contralateral feeders is done.

In cases with extensive tumorous spread, the supply from the internal carotid artery branches may be embolized if possible, especially if the internal carotid artery needs to be sacrificed prior to surgery. Neurologic deficit is the most feared complication of preoperative embolization. Particularly blindness is of major concern as a result of ethmoidal supply (Lasjaunias, 1980).

Since the introduction of embolization of juvenile nasopharyngeal angiofibroma by Roberson in 1972 (Roberson, 1972) there have been several studies proving benefit of preoperative embolization by decreasing blood loss and operative times. One of the most recent proved, that additional supply from the internal carotid artery in high-grade tumors correlated with recurrences and if only the external carotid artery feeders were embolized, such preoperative embolization did not significantly decrease intraoperative blood loss (Liu,2000, Petruson, 2002).

The majority of studies are 10 to 20 years old and many reports do not even describe embolization techniques at the time (McCombe, 1990). Tumor recurrence after surgery may correlate with preoperative embolization. This fact could be due to tumor postsurgical remnants which are more probable after previous embolization (Petruson, 2002).

4.4 Hemangioblastomas

Hemangioblastomas are highly vascular benign tumors which occur predominantly in the cerebellum and spinal cord. Although 10 % to 20 % are associated with von Hippel-Lindau disease, most occur sporadically. Von Hippel-Lindau disease is a autosomal dominantly inherited disorder with incomplete penetrance and expression (Tampieri, 1993, Gläsker, 2005).

Hemangioblastomas become symptomatic by progressive growth either of the hemangioblastic nodule or an associated cyst or, more acutely, by spontaneous hemorrhage. The role of angiography is to demonstrate vascular supply. Cerebellar hemangioblastomas are opacified from cerebellar arteries, but additional feeders from meningeal tentorial and vertebral feeders have been reported. However, angiography and preoperative embolization are done only if the tumor is larger than 1,5 cm since such small hemangiomas are not associated with significant risk of pre-, intra- or postoperative hemorrhage (Gläsker, 2005, Gerlach, 2002).

Preoperative embolization of larger tumors may be performed without additional neurologic deficit even if the tumor is fed by more than one pedicle (Tampieri, 1993, Eskridge, 1996).

However, there have been reports of worsening of preexisting hydrocephalus within 12 hours of embolization (Cornelius, 2007), and intratumoral hemorrhages after small microparticles embolization. The authors hypothesized that 45-150 μm could initiated processes which led to fatal hemorrhage. The authors conclusion is, that if preoperative embolization of cerebellar hemangioblastomas appears absolutely necessary, proximal glue embolization or larger microparticles could be safer (Limaye, 2000, Cornelius, 2007).

4.5 Other hypervascularized tumors

Among other hypervascularized cranial tumors, which have been reported to be embolized, are hemangiopericytomas (Craven, 1992), chorioid plexus papillomas (Oten, 2006), metastases, schwannomas, hemangiomas, neurinomas, esthesioneuroblastomas (Berenstein, 2004). The embolization techniques follows that of meningiomas which are by far the most common tumors in this area.

5. Conclusion

We have rewieved embolization therapy of the cranial tumors. Pre-surgical embolotherapy for hypervascularized tumors is a well-established method. First of all, familiarity with the arterial anatomy of this region is fundamental for safe and successful treatment. Appropriate imaging work up and periprocedural detailed angiographic studies as well as careful selection of embolic agents help to decrease the ischemic complications.

6. References

Abud DG, Mounayer CH, Benndorf G, Piotin M, Spelle L, Moret J. (2004). Intratumoral Injection of Cyanoacrylate Glue in Head and Neck Paragangliomas. *Am J Neuroradiol*, Vol. 25, pp. 1457- 1462.

Bendszus M, Klein R, Burger R, Warmoth-Metz M, Hofmann E, Solymosi L. (2000). Efficacy of Trisacryl Gelatin Microspheres Versus Polyvinyl Alcohol Particles in the Preoperative Embolization of Meningiomas. *Am J Neuroradiol,* Vol. 21, pp. 255-261.

Bendszus M, Martin-Schrader I, Warmuth-Metz M, Hofmann E, Solymosi L. (2000). MR Imaging- and MR Spectroscopy-Revealed Changes in Meningiomas for which Embolization was Performed without Subsequent Surgery. *Am J Neuroradiol, Vol.* 21, pp. 666-669.

Bendszus M, Rao G, Burger R, et al. (2000). Is there a Benefit of Preoperative Meningioma Embolization? *Neurosurgery,* Vol. 47, No. 6, pp. 1306-1312.

Bendszus M, Monoranu CM, Schütz A, Nölte I, Vince GH, Solymosi L. (2005). Neurologic Complications after Particle Embolization of Intracranial Meningiomas. *Am J Neuroradiol,* Vol. 26, pp. 1413-1419.

Black PM. (1993). Meningiomas. *Neurosurgery,* Vol. 32, No. 4, pp. 643-657.

Berenstein A, Lasjaunias P, TerBrugge KG. (2004). Dural and Bony Tumors, Nasopharyngeal Tumors, Paragangliomas. In: Berenstein A, Lasjaunias P, TerBrugge KG, *Surgical Neuroangiography 2.1, Second edition, Springer,* pp. 154-276, ISBN 3-540-41668-4, Berlin.

Chagnaud CH, Petit P, Bartoli JM, Champsaur P, Gaubert JY, Dessi P, Zanaret M, Cannoni M, Moulin G. (1998). Postoperative Follow-Up of Juvenile Nasopharyngeal Angiofibromas: Assessment by CT Scan and MR Imaging. *Eur Radiol* , Vol. 8, pp. 756-764.

Chaloupka JC, Mangla S, Huddle DC, Roth TC, Mitra S, Ross DA, Sasaki CT. (1999). Evolving Experience with Direct Puncture Therapeutic Embolization for Adjunctive and Palliative Management of Head and Neck Hypervascular Neoplasms. *Laryngoscope,* Vol. 109, No.11, pp. 1864-1872.

Chun JY, McDermott MW, Lamborn KR, Wilson CB, Higashida R, Berger MS. (2002) Delayed Surgical Resection Reduces Intraoperative Blood Loss for Embolized Meningiomas. *Neurosurgery,* Vol. 50, No.6. pp. 1231-1237.

Casasco A, Herbreteau D, Houdart E, et al. (1994). Devascularization of Craniofacial Tumour by Percutaneous Tumour Puncture. *Am J Neuroradiol,* Vol. 15, pp. 1233-1239.

Casasco A. (1999). Major Complications of Percutaneous Embolization of Skull Base Tumors. *Am J Neuroradiol,* Vol. 20, pp. 179-181.

Cavalcanti DD, Reis CVC, Hanel R, Safavi-Abbasi S, Deshmukh P, Spetzler RF, Preul MC. (2009). The Ascending Pharyngeal Artery and its Relevance for Neurosurgical and Endovascular Procedures. *Neurosurgery,* Vol. 65, No. 1, pp. ONS114-ONS120.

Cornelius JF, Saint-Maurice JP, Bresson D, George B, Houdart E. (2007). Hemorrhage after Particle Embolization of Hemangioblastomas: Comparison of Outcomes in Spinal Cerebellar Lesions. *J Neurosurg,* Vol. 106, pp. 994-998.

Craven JP. Quigley TM, Bolen JW, Raker EJ. (1992). Current Management of Clinical Outcome of Hemangiopericytomas. *Amer J Surg,* Vol. 163, pp. 490-493.

Dean BL, Flom RA, Wallace RC, et al. (1994). Efficacy of Endovascular Treatment of Meningiomas: Evaluation with Matched Samples. *Am J Neuroradiol,* Vol. 15, pp. 1675-1680.

Douglas R, Wormand PJ. (2006). Endoscopic Surgery for Juvenile Nasopharyngeal Angiofibroma: Where are the Limits? *Curr Opin Otolaryngol Head Neck Surg,* Vol. 14, pp. 1-5.

Eskridge JM, McAuliffe W, Harris B, Kim DK, Scott J, Winn HR. (1996). Preoperative Endovascular Embolization of Craniospinal Hemangioblastomas. *Am J Neuroradiol,* Vol. 17, pp. 525-531.

Garcia-Cervigon E, Bien S, Rüfenacht D, Thurel C, Reizine D, Huy PTB, Merland JJ. (1988). Pre-operative Embolization of Nasopharyngeal Angiofibromas. *Neuroradiology,* Vol. 30, p. 556- 560.

Geibprasert S, Pongpech S, Armstrong D, Krings T. (2009). Dangerous Extracranial-Intracranial Anastomoses and Supply to the Cranial Nerves: Vessels the Neurointerventionalist Needs to Know. *Am J Neuroradiol,* Vol. 30, pp. 1459-1468.

Gemmete JJ, Chaudhary N, Pandey A, Gandhi D, Sullivan SE, Marentette LJ, Chepeha DB, Ansari SA. (2010). Usefulness of Percutaneously Injected Ethylenevinyl Alcohol Copolymer in Conjunction with Standard Endovascular Embolization Techniques for Preoperative Devascularization of Hypervascular Head and Neck Tumors:

Technique, Initial Experience, and Corelation with Surgical Observations. *Am J Neuroradiol,* Vol. 31, pp. 961-966.

Gerlach R, Marquardt G, Wissing H, Scharrer I, Raabe A, Seifert V. (2002). Application of Recombinant Activated Factor VII During Surgery for a Giant Skull Base Hemangiopericytoma to Achieve Safe Hemostasis. *J Neurosurg,* Vol. 96, pp. 946-948.

Gerosa M, Visca A, Rizzo P, Foroni R, Nicolato A, Bricolo A. (2006). Glomus Jugulare Tumors: the Option of Gama Knife Radiosurgery. *Neurosurgery,* Vol. 59, No. 3, pp. 561-569.

Gilad R, Fatterpekar GM, Gandhi CD, Win HR, Johnson DM, Patel AB, Bederson JB, Naidich TP (2009). Intracranial Tumors: Cisternal Angle as a Measure of Midbrain Compression for Assessing Risk of Postembolization Clinical Deterioration. *Radiology,* Vol. 251, No. 3, pp. 892-900.

Gläsker S, Van Velhtoven V. (2005). Risk of Hemorrhage in Hemangioblastomas of the Central Nervous System. *Neurosurgery,* Vol. 57, No. 1, pp. 71-76.

Gonzales CF, Moret J. (1990). Balloon Occlusion of the Carotid Artery Prior to Surgery for Neck Tumors. *Am J Neuroradiol,* Vol. 11, pp. 649-652.

Gupta R, Thomas AJ, Horowitz M. (2006). Intracranial Head and Neck Tumors: Endovascular Considerations, Present and Future. *Neurosurgery,* Vol. 59, No. 5, pp. S3-251-S3-260.

Johns ME, McLeod RM, Cantrell RW. (1980). Estrogen Receptors in Nasopharyngeal Angiofibromas.*Laryngoscope,* Vol. 90, pp. 630-634.

Jungreis CHA. (1991). Skull-base Tumors: Ethanol Embolization of the Cavernous Carotid Artery. *Radiology,* Vol. 181, pp. 741-743.

Kai Y, Hamada JI, Morioka M, Yano S, Todaka T, Ushio Y. (2002). Appropriate Interval Between Embolization and Surgery in Patients with Meningioma. *Am J Neuroradiol,* Vol. 23, pp. 139- 142.

Kallmes DF, Evans AJ, Kaptain GJ, Mathis JM, Jensen ME, Jane JA, Dion JE. (1997). Hemorrhagic Complications in Embolization of a Meningioma: Case Report and Review of the Literature. *Neuroradiology,* Vol. 39, pp. 877-880.

Kania RE, Sauvaget E, Guichard JP, Chapot R, Tran Ba Huy P, Herman P. (2005). Early Postopertive CT Scanning for Juvenile Nasopharyngeal Angiofibroma: Detection of Residual Disease. *Am J Neuroradiol,* Vol. 26, pp. 82-88.

Ketter R, Rahnenführer J, Henn W, Kim YJ, Feiden W, Steudel WI, Zang KD, Urbschat S. (2008). Correspondence of Tumor Localization with Tumor Recurrence and Cytogenetic Progression in Meningiomas. *Neurosurgery,* Vol. 62, No. 1, pp. 61-70.

Kurata A, Miyasaka Y, Tanaka C, Tokiwa K, Saegusa H, Fujii K, Kan S. (1996). Prevention of Complications During Endovascular Surgery on the External Carotid Arteries, with Special Reference to Use of Nitropaste and the Lidocaine Test. Intervent Neuroradiol, Vol. 2, pp. 193-200.

Lasjaunias P, Moret J. (1976). The Ascending Pharyngeal Artery: Normal and Pathological Radioanatomy. *Neuroradiology,* Vol. 11, pp. 77-82.

Lasjaunias P, Doyon D. (1978). The Ascending Pharyngeal Artery and the Blood Supply of the Lower Cranial Nerves. *J Neuroradiol,* Vol. 5, pp. 287-301.

Lasjaunias P. (1980). Nasopharyngeal Angiofibromas: Hazards of Embolization. *Radiology,* Vol. 136, pp. 119-123.

Latchaw RE. (1993). Preoperative Intracranial Meningioma Embolisation: Technical Consideration Affecting the Risk-to-Benefit Ratio. *Am J Neuroradiol,* Vol. 14, pp. 583-586.

Limaye U, Siddhartha W, Shrivastava M, Parmar H. (2000). Posterior Fossa Hypervascular Tumor Embolization. An Unusual Complication. *Riv Neuroradiol,* Vol. 13, pp. 593-598.

Liu L, Wang R, Huang D, Han D, Ferguson EJ, Shi H, Yang. (2002). Analysis of Intra-Operative Bleeding and Recurrence of Juvenile Nasopharyngeal Angiofibromas. *Clin Otolaryngol,* Vol. 27, pp. 536-540.

Lonser RR, Heiss JD, Oldfield EH. (1998). Tumour Devascularization by Intratumoral Ethanol Injection During Surgery. *J Neurosurg,* Vol. 88, pp. 923-924.

Macpherson P. (1991). The Value of Pre-operative Embolisation of Meningioma Estimated Subjectively and Objectively. *Neuroradiology,* Vol. 33, pp. 334-337.

McCombe A, Lund VJ, Howard DJ. (1990). Recurrence in Juvenile Angiofibroma. *Rhinology,* Vol. 28, pp. 97-102.

Moret J, Delvert C, Lasjaunias P. (1982). Vascular Architecture of Tympanojugular Glomus Tumours: its Application Regarding Therapeutic Angiography. *J Neuroradiol,* Vol. 9, pp. 237-260.

Moulin G, Chagnaud Ch, Gras R, et al. (1995). Juvenile Angiofibroma: Comparison of Blood Loss During Removal in Embolized Group versus Nonembolized Group. *Cardiovasc Intervent Radiol,* Vol. 18, pp. 158-161.

Natarajan SK, Sekhar LN, Schessel D, Morita A. (2007). Petroclival Meningiomas: Multimodality Treatment and Outcomes at Long-Term Follow-Up. *Neurosurgery,* Vol. 60, No. 6, pp. 965-981.

Nelson PK, Setton A, Choi IS, Ransohoff J, Berenstein A (1994). Current Status of Interventional Neuroradiology in the Management of Meningiomas. *Neurosurgery Clinics of North America,* Vol. 5, No. 2, pp. 235-259.

Neuwelt EA, Goldman DL, Dahlborg SA, Crossen J, Ramsey F, Roman-Goldstein S, Braziel R, Dana B. (1991). Primary Central Nervous System Lymphoma Treated with Osmotic Blood-brain Barrier Disruption: Prolonged Survival and Preservation of Cognitive Function. *J Clin Oncol,* Vol. 9, pp. 1580-1590.

Oka H. (1998). Preoperative Superselective Embolization of Skull Base Meningiomas: Indications and Limitations. *J Neuro-Oncology,* Vol. 40, pp. 67-71.

Oten ML, Riina HA, Gobin YP, Souweidane MM. (2006). Preoperative Embolization in the Treatment of Chorioid Plexus Papilloma in an Infant. *J Neurosurg,* Vol. 104, pp. 419-421.

Persky MS, Setton A, Niimi Y, Hartman J, Frank D, Berenstein A. (2002). Combined Endovascular and

Surgical Treatment of Head and Neck Paragangliomas - a Team Approach. *Head Neck,* Vol. 24, pp. 423-431.

Petruson K, Rodriguez-Catarino M, Petruson B et al. (2002). Juvenile Nasopharyngeal Angiofibroma: Long-term Results in Preoperative Embolized and Non-embolized Patients. *Acta Otolaryngol,* Vol. 122, pp. 96-100.

Ramina R, Maniglia JJ, Fernandes YB, Paschoal JR, Nizan L, Neto MC. (2005). Tumors of the Jugular Foramen: Diagnosis and Management. *Neurosurgery,* Vol. 57, No. 1, pp. ONS59-ONS68.

Raza SM, Gallia GL, Brem H, Weingart JD, Long DM, Olivi A. (2010). Perioperative and Long-term Outcomes from the Management of Parasagittal Meningiomas Invading the Superior sagittal sinus. *Neurosurgery,* Vol. 67, No. 4, pp. 885-893.

Roberson GH, Biller H, Sessions DG et al. (1972). Presurgical Internal Maxillary Artery Embolization in Juvenile Angiofibroma. *Laryngoscope,* Vol. 82, pp. 1524-1532.

Rosen CL, Ammerman JM, Sekhar LN, Bank WO. (2002). Outcome Analysis of Preoperative Embolization in Cranial Base Surgery. *Acta Neurochir,* Vol. 144, pp. 1157-1164.

Russell EJ. (1986). Functional Angiography of the Head and Neck. *Am J Neuroradiol,* Vol. 7, pp. 927-936.

Scholtz AW, Appenroth E, Kammen-Jolly K et al. (2001). Juvenile Nasopharyngeal Angiofibroma: Management and Therapy. *Laryngoscope,* Vol. 111, pp. 681-687.

Simunek A, Krajina A, Hlava A. (1993). Selective Intraarterial Chemotherapy of Tumors in the Lingual Artery Territory by a New Approach. *Cardiovasc Intervent Radiol,* Vol. 16, pp. 392-395.

Smith TP. (2006). Embolization in the External Carotid Artery. *J Vasc Interv Radiol,* Vol. 17, pp. 1897-1913.

Tampieri D, Leblanc R, TerBrugge K. (1993). Preoperative Embolization of Brain and Spinal Hemangioblastomas. *Neurosurgery ,* Vol. 33, No. 3, pp. 502-505.

Théron J, Cosgrove R, Melanson D, Ethier R. (1986). Embolization with Temporary Balloon Occlusion of the Internal Carotid or Vertebral Arteries. *Neuroradiology,* Vol. 28, pp. 246-253.

Tikkakoski T, Luotonen J, Leinonen S, Siniluoto T, Heikkilä O, Päivänsälo M, Hyrynkangas K. (1997). Preoperative Embolization in the Management of Neck Paragangliomas. *Laryngoscope,* Vol. 107, No. 6, pp. 821-826.

Toktas ZO, Akgun E, Ozkan A, Bozkurt SU, Bekiroglu N, Seker A, Konya D, Kilic T. (2010). Relationship of Angiogenic Potential with Clinical Features in Cranial Meningiomas: a Corneal Angiogenesis Study. *Neurosurgery,* Vol. 67, No. 6, pp. 1724-1732.

Tymianski M, Willinsky RA, Tator CH, Mikulis D, TerBrugge KG, Markson L. (1994). Embolization with Temporary Balloon Occlusion of the Internal Carotid Artery and in Vivo Proton Spectroscopy Improves Radical Removal of Petrous-Tentorial Meningioma. *Neurosurgery,* Vol. 35, No. 5, pp. 974-977.

Van den Berg R, Rodesch G, Lasjaunias P. (2002). Management of Paragangliomas. Clinical and Angiographic Aspects. *Intervent Neuroradiol,* Vol. 8, pp. 127-134.

Valavanis A. (1986). Preoperative Embolization of the Head and Neck: Indications, Patient Selection, Goals, and Precautions. *Am J Neuroradiol,* Vol. 7, pp. 943-952.

Valavanis A, Christoforidis G. (2002). Tumours of the Head and Neck. In: J Byrne *Interventional Neuroradiology. Theory and Practice.* Oxford University Press, pp. 213-238. ISBN 0-19-263154-3, Oxford

Wakhloo Ak, Juengling FD, Van Velthoven V, et al. (1993). Extended Preoperative Polyvinylalcohol Microembolization of Intracranial Meningeomas: Assessment of two Embolization Techniques. *Am J Neuroradiol,* Vol. 14, pp. 571-582.

Waldron JS, Sughrue ME, Hetts SW, Willson SP, Mills SA, McDermott MW, Dowd CF, Parsa AT. (2011). Embolization of Skull Base Meningiomas and Feeding Vessels Arising from the Internal Carotid Circulation. *Neurosurgery,* Vol. 68, No. 1, pp. 162-169.

Yu SCH, Boet R, Wong GKC, Lam WWM, Poon WS. (2004). Postembolization Hemorrhage of a Large and Necrotic Meningioma. Am J Neuroradiol, Vol. 25, pp. 506-508.

27

Advanced Surgical Management of Gliomas: Technological Requirements, Concept of Information-Guided Resection, and Clinical Results

Yoshihiro Muragaki et al.*
Department of Neurosurgery and
Faculty of Advanced Techno-Surgery
Tokyo Women's Medical University, Tokyo
Japan

1. Introduction

Contemporary technological developments revolutionized surgical management of intracranial gliomas. In fact, decades of the previous clinical experience clearly demonstrated that in such cases routine surgical technique usually does not permit to perform aggressive resection of the lesion without significant risk of the permanent postoperative neurological morbidity. The main associated surgical problem is evident. Arising from the cerebral tissue itself the majority of these tumors has a propensity for invasive growth, therefore their boarders could not be clearly distinguished and precisely differentiated from the adjacent functionally important brain structures, which may preserve their function even in presence of tumor infiltration. It typically led to incomplete resection of the neoplasm, which, however, may have significant negative impact on prognosis.

Nowadays, the availability of the intraoperative MRI (iMRI) and related updated neuronavigation permits for neurosurgeons to perform resection of glioma under precise anatomical guidance. Moreover, the efficacy and safety of surgery is further enhanced by use of comprehensive neurophysiological monitoring, cortical and subcortical brain mapping, particularly performed during awake craniotomy, neurochemical navigation with 5-aminolevulinic acid (5-ALA), and regular histopathological characterization of the resected tissue. Combined application of these techniques provides an opportunity for aggressive removal of the intraaxial brain lesions with minimal risk of neurological complications. Surgery performed under such conditions can be designated as "information-guided procedure" (Iseki et al., 2008; Muragaki et al., 2011).

---

*Hiroshi Iseki, Takashi Maruyama, Mikhail Chernov, Takashi Suzuki, Kitaro Yoshimitsu, Manabu Tamura, Soko Ikuta, Masayuki Nitta Taiichi Saito, Jun Okamoto and Kintomo Takakura
Department of Neurosurgery and Faculty of Advanced Techno-Surgery
Tokyo Women's Medical University, Tokyo, Japan

The present chapter summarizes the experience with resection of the intracranial gliomas gained in the Tokyo Women's Medical University (TWMU) from 2000 till 2011 with an emphasis on applied intraoperative technology, treatment concept, and clinical results.

2. Rationale for aggressive resection of intracranial gliomas

The well-known benefits of resective surgery in cases of glioma include relief of compression of the tumor bulk on the surrounding brain (important for neurological improvement), reduction of the volume of the neoplasm (can render postoperative radiochemotherapy more effective), and establishment of the precise histopathological diagnosis, which is important for choice of the adjuvant therapy, optimal follow-up, and prediction of prognosis. Additionally, extensive removal of the tumor may positively influence patients' survival. While the latter does not formally proved up to date (Proescholdt et al., 2005) there is a growing agreement, that total resection of glioma is associated with better long-term outcome, even in cases of malignancies.

Stummer et al. (2008) adjusted biases of age and eloquent area location in the dataset of randomized study on use of neurochemical navigation with 5-ALA during resection of glioblastoma multiforme (GBM), and found that median overall survival after complete removal of the contrast-enhanced lesion was significantly longer compared to cases with its incomplete resection (17 months vs. 12 months). In concordance, in the report on EORTC 26951 randomized trial of combined chemotherapy for anaplastic gliomas, the overall survival was better after complete tumor removal compared to partial ones or to biopsy (van den Bent et al., 2006). It was demonstrated that 98% or more resection of GBM is associated with significant improvement of the long-term outcome (Lacroix et al., 2001), whereas recently the same trend was revealed even at 78% resection rate (Sanai et al, 2011). The similar results were marked by The Committee of Brain Tumor Registry of Japan (2003): analysis of 6400 cases of WHO grade III and IV gliomas showed that more than 90% tumor removal is associated with survival advantage, while such resection rate was attained in 6%-to-10% of cases only.

It is still questionable what should be defined as total removal of glioma. In our practice such resection rate is considered if postoperative MRI performed within first week after surgery confirms elimination of more than 95% of the mass lesion with regard to signal hyperintensity on T_2-weighted images in cases of low-grade neoplasms, or contrast-enhanced area on postgadolinium T_1-weighted images in cases of high-grade ones.

It should be specifically emphasized that complete surgical resection is highly desirable, but not ultimate goal of surgery for glioma, therefore it should not be performed if can cause major permanent postoperative neurological morbidity or lead to significant decline of the quality of life.

3. Surgical strategy for intracranial gliomas

Selection of the optimal surgical strategy for intracranial gliomas is based on the detailed preoperative clinical and radiological evaluation of the patient. The main details of the typical clinical protocol, which is used in our clinic, are following.

Before surgery the history of the disease, general condition and neurological status of the patient are carefully assessed. The Karnofsky Performance Scale (KPS) score and Medical Research Council (MRC) Neurological Scale grade are defined. Of note, in our practice age of the patient has limited influence on the choice of the treatment strategy, but presence of co-morbidities definitely plays an important role. Risk of surgery is estimated by anesthesiologist according to American Society of Anesthesiologists (ASA) grading system.

Preoperative neuroimaging protocol includes volumetric MRI (T_1-weighted images in axial, coronal, and sagittal projections without and with single-dose gadoteridol, and T_2-weighted images), Fluid Attenuation Inversion Recovery (FLAIR) images, diffusion-weighted imaging (DWI), susceptibility-weighted imaging (SWI), perfusion-weighted imaging (PWI), single- and multivoxel proton magnetic resonance spectroscopy (^{1}H-MRS). For this purpose at present we use 3 Tesla MR scanner due to its advantages in image acquirement and resolution. Additionally, positron emission tomography (PET) with ^{11}C-methionine, [^{18}F] Fluorodeoxyglucose, and ^{11}C-Choline is performed (Kato et al, 2008). At present cerebral angiography in patients with gliomas is usually omitted, whereas interrelationships between the tumor and vascular structures are evaluated on MR angiography and SWI. Based on results of these investigations tumor size, location, and mass-effect are evaluated, and histopathological type and grade of the neoplasm are predicted.

The functional grade of the tumor is assigned according to its location (Sawaya et al., 1998). If the neoplasm is located in close vicinity to the pyramidal tract diffusion-tensor imaging (DTI) is attained for evaluation of its interrelationships with the lesion and estimation of the possible shift in location. In cases of cortical gliomas functional MRI is performed for identification of the motor and language areas and their correspondence to the tumor location. If according to functional MRI glioma occupies the language area Wada test is performed.

Preoperative invasive cortical or subcortical brain mapping with implanted subdural grid or stereotactic electrodes is used occasionally, particularly in cases with symptomatic epilepsy.

3.1 Indications for stereotactic biopsy

Image-guided stereotactic biopsy represents a standard neurosurgical technique, routinely used in cases of parenchymal brain lesions. Tissue sampling from the area, which looks the most abnormal on MRI, results in high rate of positive histopathological findings. Nevertheless, heterogeneity of the lesion, frequently observed in gliomas, limits the diagnostic accuracy of the procedure, and not infrequently leads to erroneous tumor typing and/or grading. Moreover, the stereotactic tissue sampling does not seem justified if further resection of the lesion is planned.

Since we advocate aggressive surgical management of gliomas, not more than 10% of patients with parenchymal brain lesions undergoing stereotactic biopsy in our clinic (Muragaki et al, 2008; Chernov et al., 2009). The indications for this procedure are limited to following:

- clarification of the histopathological diagnosis, which can not be established based on clinical and radiological investigations, particularly for differentiation of neoplastic and non-neoplastic lesions;
- histopathological confirmation of the diagnosis of the tumor, for which treatment with chemotherapy and/or irradiation is planned (for example, malignant lymphoma);
- stereotactic implantation of electrodes for preoperative brain mapping in cases of gliomas (simultaneous tissue sampling is usually performed);
- extremely extensive or diffuse lesions, which are not amenable even for subtotal resection (such as gliomatosis cerebri).

For guidance of stereotactic brain biopsy combined use of structural MRI and metabolic imaging (^{1}H-MRS and/or PET) is reasonable, especially in recurrent cases or highly vascular lesions (Chernov et al., 2009).

3.2 Strategy for glioma resection

Optimal strategy of glioma resection is mainly determined by 3 interrelated factors: tumor size, histopathological grade, and functional grade. The goal of surgery should be attainment of the maximal possible removal of the neoplasm, defined as radiologically total, or as subtotal leaving the residual lesion within the functioning eloquent brain structures identified with neurophysiological monitoring and/or brain mapping.

In general, the best result of surgery is maximal possible removal of the whole area of the hyperintense signal detected on preoperative T_2-weighted or FLAIR images. It can be frequently achieved in cases of low-grade neoplasms, but rarely attained in high-grade lesions surrounded by prominent peritumoral edema. In latter cases surgery is usually directed on the maximal possible resection of the contrast-enchanced area.

In rare occasions resection of extensive tumors affecting functioning eloquent brain structures can be directed on the most metabolically active part of the neoplasm detected according to ^{11}C-methionine uptake on PET.

4. Intelligent operating theater of the Tokyo Women's Medical University

Intelligent operating theater was established in TWMU in 2000. Its internal organization is presented below.

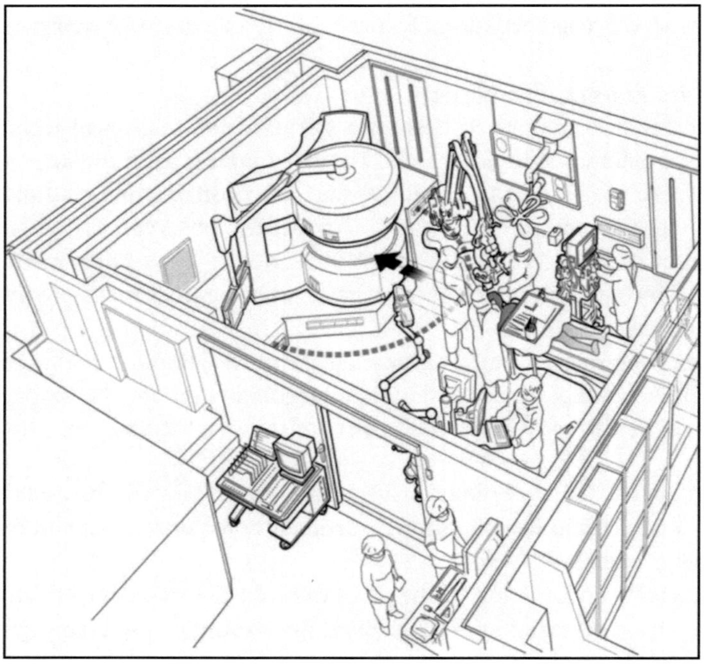

Fig. 1. Internal organization of the intelligent operating theater in TWMU. Arrow indicates direction of the operating table movement during iMRI investigation. Dots correspond to 5-gauss line.

4.1 Intraoperative MRI

First iMRI systems were introduced in neurosurgery at the end of 1990`s. Since then, such devices have been used for real-time observation of surgical manipulations, for assessment of the extent of tumor resection, and evaluation of the intraoperative complications. While real-time guidance of the surgical manipulations with iMRI is theoretically presumed to be the most effective, such systems usually provide relatively narrow working space and necessitate all surgical devices to be composed of non-ferromagnetic materials (Iseki et al., 2005). By contrast, if iMRI investigations are performed at some temporary break points during surgical procedure, it can provide a higher degree of freedom for the surgeon and permit to use standard (not MRI-compatible) neurosurgical instrumentarium. It should be noted that any type of iMRI system increases the operation time, because MR imaging by itself is a time-consuming process.

During the last decade there is a trend for introduction of iMRI scanners with high magnetic field strength of 1.5 and 3 Tesla. Their advantages include high image quality, possibility to attain diffusion tensor and spectroscopic images, as well as short scanning time. Increase of magnetic field strength, however, is associated with greater possibility of image distortion artifacts. The risk of the latter is 5 times greater in 1.5 Tesla MR scanner compared to 0.2 Tesla one (Fransson et al., 2001). Additionally, the maintenance costs of high-field-strength iMRI scanners is significant.

Intelligent operating theater of the TWMU is equipped with a low-field-strength (0.3 Tesla) open iMRI scanner (AIRIS II™; Hitachi Medical Co., Chiba, Japan). It has a hamburger-like shape with a 43 cm gantry gap and a disc-shaped permanent magnet producing vertical magnetic field with resonance frequency of 12.7 MHz. This scanner does not require a cooling system, which significantly reduce its operating cost by approximately 10.000 Japanese yen (around 100 US $) per month. Low magnetic field strength creates narrow 5-gauss line, extending 2 meters from both sides, 2.2 meters in front, 1.8 meters backwards, and 2.5 meters upwards, which permits for the surgeon to use some conventional surgical instruments in the working space outside of it (for example, high-speed drill). Nevertheless, all surgical devices that are used within the 5-gauss line, such as operating table (MOT2000-MRI; Mizuho Ltd., Tokyo, Japan) and operating microscope (MRI-30; Mitaka Co., Tokyo, Japan) are constructed from non-ferromagnetic material to prevent accidents and avoid image artifacts.

Originally developed radiofrequency receiver coil integrated with Sugita head-holder (Head-holder coil; Mizuho Ltd., Tokyo, Japan) significantly improved the quality of the intraoperative images (Ozawa et al., 2008a, 2008b). Positioning of the coil in close vicinity to the visualized region provides one an opportunity to perform MRI investigations with minimal distortion artifacts and maximum structure contrasting in any plane irrespectively to orientation of the object. It means, that fixation of the patient head can be done in the most desirable position for tumor removal, therefore use of any required surgical approach, including retrosigmoid and transtentorial, is possible. In fact, the quality of the intraoperative images in our practice is comparable to those ones obtained on scanners with higher magnetic field strength.

After induction of the general anesthesia the patient`s head is firmly fixed with titanium pins in the modified Sugita head-holder, representing the lower arch of the Head-holder coil. It is connected to the operating table with a special supporting arm, which provides easy adjustment of the head position according to the surgical needs. Before iMRI investigation several fiducial markers are fixed to the skull on the periphery of the surgical field, and an additional one is inserted into the surgical wound and located in the vicinity to the target. Both semicircular arches of the Head-holder coil are connected. A wide transparent sterile drape is used to cover the whole body of the patient including the head, and the operating table is moved into the gap of the iMR scanner.

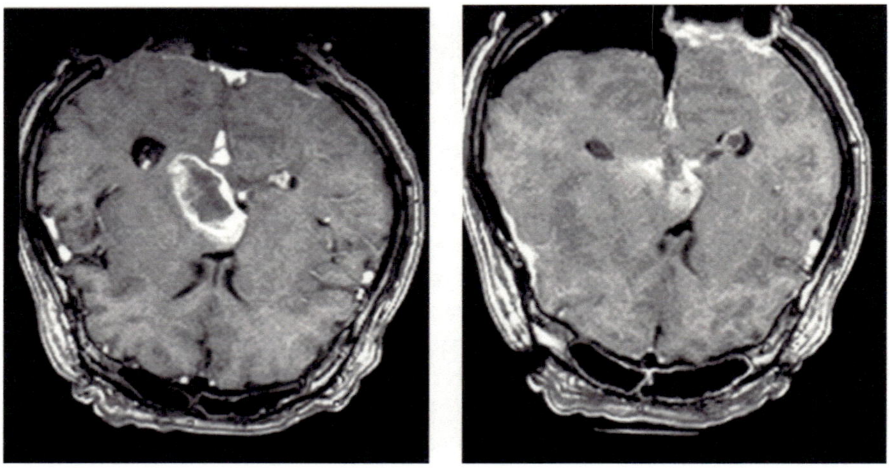

Fig. 2. Intraoperative images obtained using 0.3 Tesla MR scanner before (*left*) and after (*right*) 85% resection of the of GBM of the left thalamus via occipital-transtentorial approach in prone position of the patient.

Integration of the Head-holder coil with modified Komai stereotactic frame permits to perform stereotactically guided surgical procedures under the control of iMRI (Taniguchi et al., 2006).

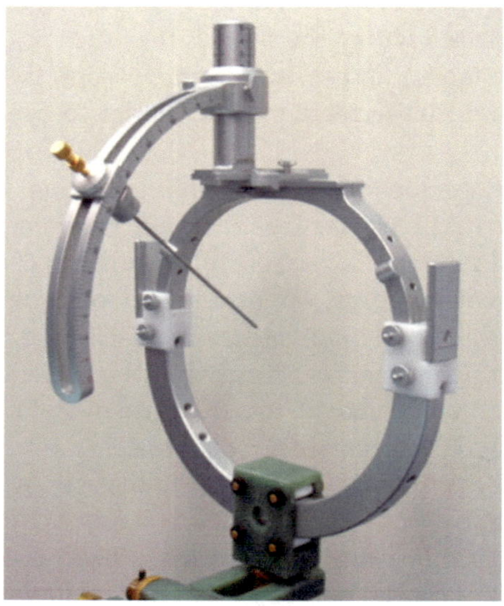

Fig. 3. Head-holder coil integrated with modified Komai stereotactic frame for stereotactically guided surgical procedures under the control of intraoperative MRI.

4.1.1 Intraoperative diffusion-weighted imaging

Use of Head-holder coil permits for us to acquire intraoperatively not only volumetric MR images, but to perform MR angiography, functional investigations (Gasser et al., 2011), and DWI. The latter is of particular importance, because it provides nearly real-time information on spatial interrelationships between the pyramidal tract, the lesion, and position of the surgical instruments, including the electrical stimulator for subcortical functional mapping, which can be effectively used for prevention of the inadvertent injury of the pyramidal tract and corresponding avoidance of the postoperative deterioration of the motor function.
The estimated positional accuracy of iDWI in our practice is within 5 mm, which corresponds to the conducting depth of the electrical stimulation during subcortical brain mapping (Ozawa et al., 2009a). It should be marked, however, that diffusion anisotropy of the white matter tracts may be reduced by presence of the tumor or peritumoral edema, which may occasionally lead to poor visualization of the pyramidal tract on the affected side (Ozawa et al., 2008b).

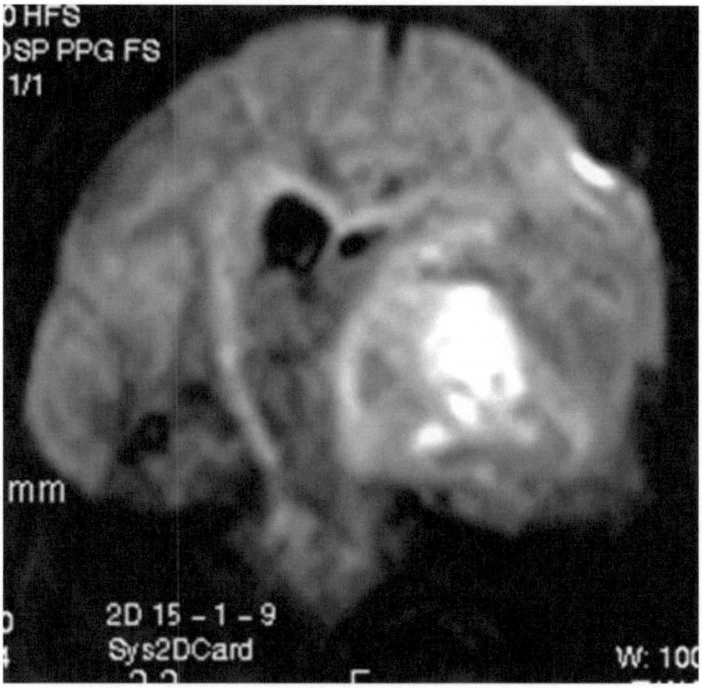

Fig. 4. Intraoperative DWI obtained on MRI scanner with magnetic field strength of 0.3 Tesla: both pyramidal tracts are clearly seen and its shift on the affected side can be easily evaluated.

4.2 Updated intraoperative neuronavigation

Simultaneous to installation of iMRI in the intelligent operating theater of TWMU, the special system for updated neuronavigation based on the intraoperative neuroimaging has been developed in 2000. Its main advantage is avoidance of the adverse effects caused by brain shift and deformation, which allows precise identification of the tumor position and its interrelationships with surrounding brain structures.

For facilitation of the tumor removal and detection of the neoplastic remnants we use previously developed navigator for photon radiosurgery system (PRS navigator; Toshiba Medical Co. Ltd., Tokyo, Japan), which allows fast and easy updating of the information obtained with iMRI. The mislocalization errors of the device constitute 0.8 mm in average, 1.5 mm at maximum, and 0.5 mm at minimum, and typically do not exceed 1 mm (Iseki et al., 2008). The system permits co-registration, fusion and three-dimensional reconstruction of the various images, and provides easy-to-understand information. The different areas of the perilesional brain can be color-coded according to the safety of manipulations and probable risk of complications. Additionally, the device may be integrated with special sound alarm, which is automatically activated if surgical instruments are coming in close proximity to the high-risk area.

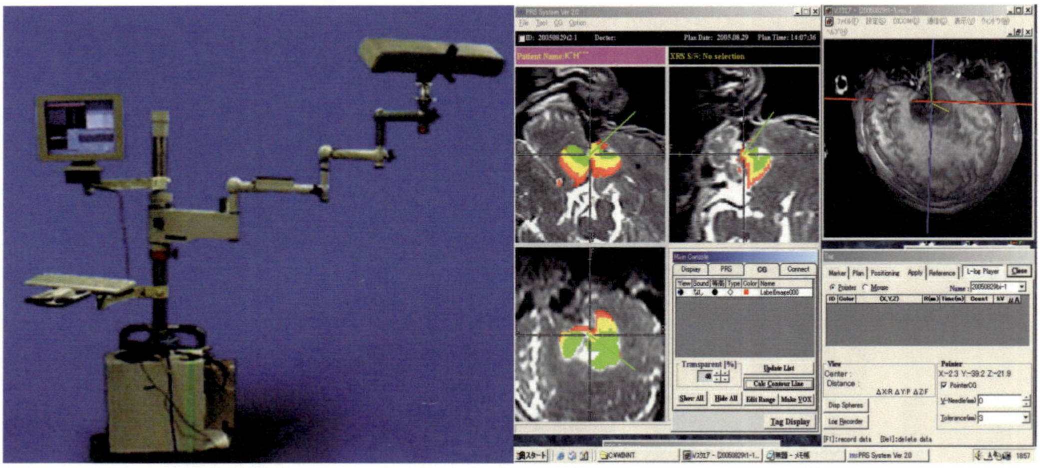

Fig. 5. Intraoperative neuronavigation system (PRS navigator; Toshiba Medical Co. Ltd., Tokyo, Japan) used in intelligent operating theater of TWMU (*left*) and its screen with color-coded safety areas of the tumor resection (*right*), showing areas located less than 5 mm, between 5 and 10 mm, and more than 10 mm to the pyramidal tract, which are demarcated, respectively, as red, yellow, and green.

4.3 Intraoperative neurophysiological monitoring, brain mapping, and awake craniotomy

During surgical procedures in the intelligent operating theater of TWMU comprehensive intraoperative neurophysiological monitoring is used routinely. The depth of anesthesia, which may interfere with results of such examinations is constantly monitored with bispectral index (BIS) monitor.

Somatosensory evoked potentials (SEP) are recorded with stimulation of the median nerve. The values of the latencies and amplitudes obtained after craniotomy just before the dural incision are considered as an individual baseline. The central sulcus is localized based on the polarity inversion of the N20 component of SEP.

Motor evoked potentials (MEP) are monitored using transcranial electrodes and measurement of the electromyograms at the thenar, quadriceps femoris, anterior tibial, and gastrocnemius muscles on both sides. Direct cortical mapping of the primary motor area is also performed. The parameters of stimulation depend on the various surgical conditions, but as a rule low-frequency current is used initially for prevention of seizures (Otani et al., 2005; Mikuni & Miyamoto, 2010).

The main indication for awake craniotomy in our practice is location of glioma in the vicinity to the language centers. During examination speech production, repetition, object naming, verb generation, and reading tasks are used with simultaneous stimulation of the different language areas. Meanwhile, several problems may arise with identification of the cortical speech centers using brain mapping. Particularly, elimination of anarthria produced by positive motor response of the tongue and face or from the negative motor response of the tongue during cortical stimulation is of paramount importance for precise evaluation of the language function (Mikuni & Miyamoto, 2010).

4.3.1 Intraoperative examination monitor for awake surgery (IEMAS)

To facilitate the process of brain mapping our group had developed dedicated Intraoperative Examination Monitor for Awake Surgery (IEMAS). It is an information-sharing device, which provides ones an opportunity for simultaneous real-time visualization of the wide spectrum of co-registered intraoperative data (Iseki & Nambu, 2005; Iseki et al., 2008; Sakurai et al., 2011). For example, the patient's mimic and face movements during answering on the specific test questions, type of the examination test, position of the surgical instruments and cortical stimulator in the surgical field, parameters of BIS monitor, and general view of the surgical field through the operating microscope, can be presented compactly in one screen with several displays. From 2010 wireless modification of the device became available (Yoshimitsu et al., 2010).

4.4 Neurochemical navigation with 5-ALA and intraoperative histopathological diagnosis

Neurochemical navigation with 5-ALA during resection of gliomas is based on the effect of its accumulation in the tumor cells and areas with impaired blood-brain barrier (BBB) and further conversion into protoporphyrin IX, which fluorescence is visible under ultraviolet light (Ando et al., 2011). This method can be effectively used for identification of the neoplastic tissue and its differentiation from the brain itself, which may be particularly important at the periphery of the neoplasm.

It should be noted, however, that erroneous results of neurochemical navigation with 5-ALA are possible. False negative cases may be met in low-grade gliomas due to relative preservation of the BBB, or be caused by presence of the adherent blood on the tissue surface since erythrocytes can absorb ultraviolet light, which in such case does not reach protoporphyrin IX in the pathological tissue (Ando et al., 2011). Contrary, false positive fluorescence may be observed in the areas with high vascularisation, reactive astrocytosis, or BBB impairment in the absence of the neoplastic elements.

Regular intraoperative histopathological investigation of the resected tissue on the frozen sections effectively complement neurochemical navigation and may be efficiently used for guidance of the tumor resection, identification of the neoplastic remnants, and confirmation of completeness of the lesion removal.

4.5 Management of the intraoperative information and surgical information strategy desk

Appropriate management of the intraoperative medical information may have a significant impact on the clinical decision-making, and, therefore, may influence the outcome. During neurosurgical procedure a wide spectrum of data, such as various pre- and intraoperative images, details of the intraoperative neuronavigation, parameters of the neurophysiological monitoring, nuances of the cortical mapping, and main characteristics of the current patient condition, should be provided. Moreover, those data have to be constantly updated, presented in a real-time regime, and widely distributed between members of the surgical team. At optimal, the scientific information from evidence-based sources, integrated using probability assessment technique, should be also available upon request. It is evident, that for a purpose of high quality surgery all information should be not only precise and proved, but presented in a most compact, comfortable and friendly way for optimal visualization, easy understanding, and effective use.

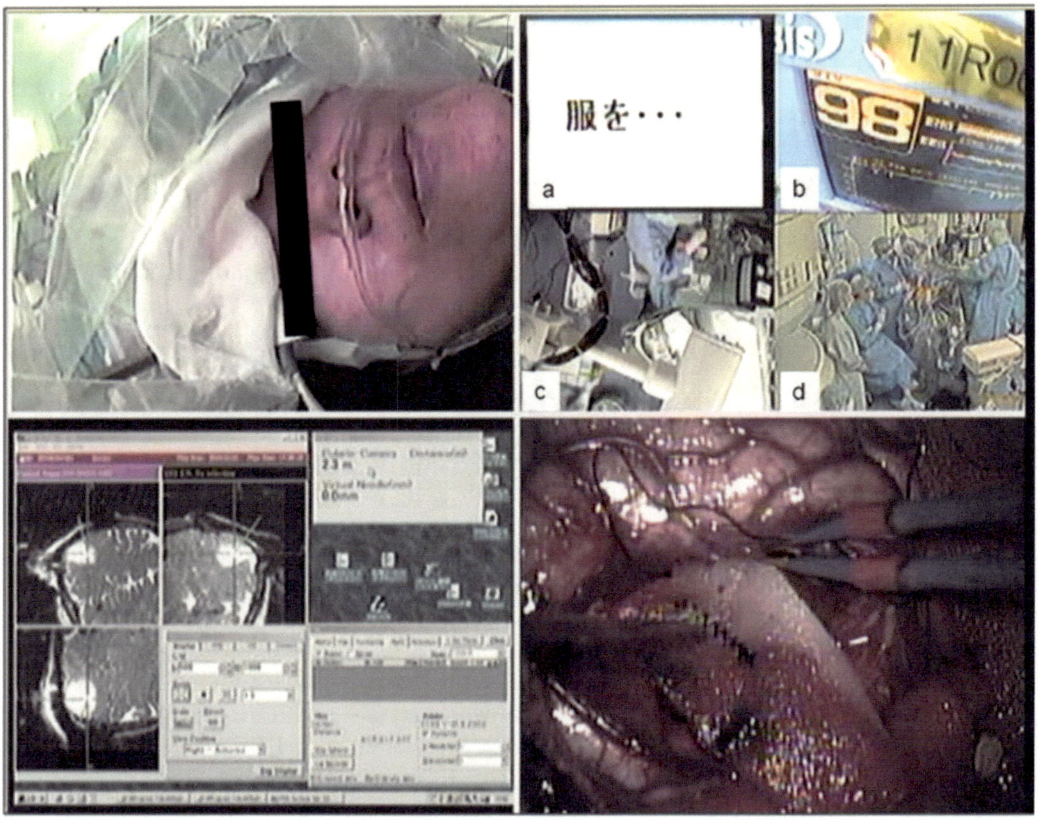

Fig. 6. Integration of the multiple intraoperative data on the screen of IEMAS. On the upper left display, the patient's face can be seen to facilitate checking of the consciousness status and mimics during response to test questions. On the lower left display, the anatomical data from the real-time updated neuronavigation system is shown, which allows localization of the exact position of the cortical stimulator. On the lower right display the view of the surgical field through the operative microscope is seen, which can be helpful for precise identification of the timing of stimulation. On the upper right display, 4 different types of information are presented: the test question provided for a patient (a), parameters of the BIS monitor reflecting the patient's awakening state (b), and general view of the operating theater (c and d).

Intelligent operating theater of TWMU has several in-room liquid crystal display (LCD) monitors, therefore integrated real-time information can be easily distributed and quickly analyzed by all members of the surgical team, practically without interruption of the surgical manipulations. Additionally, a special surgical information strategy desk has been designed to facilitate search of an optimal solution in a constantly changing surgical situation. It provides for a surgeon the whole spectrum of the integrated information about situation in the surgical field, chemical neuronavigation, neurophysiological monitoring, intraoperative images, histopathological investigation etc. All data are presented in a real time regime and their visualization can be easily changed or combined in a different way just by a click of the network switch. The system makes possible transfer of the information into the distant areas, therefore, urgent consulting service with the specialists, located outside the operating theater, can be provided.

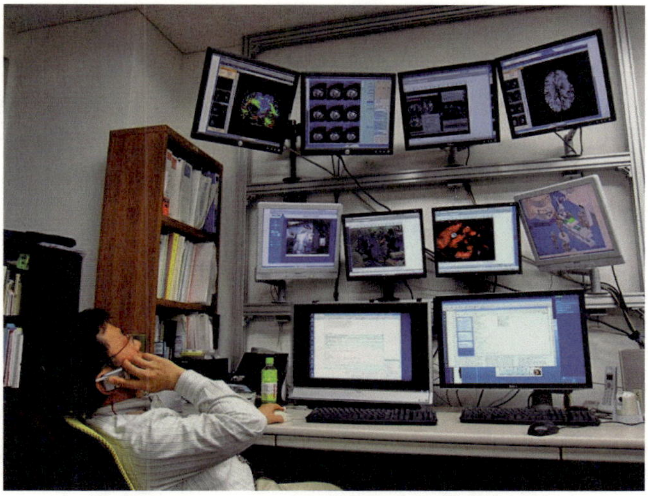

Fig. 7. Senior neurosurgeon supervising removal of glioma from the neurosurgical office using surgical information strategy desk.

5. Concept of the information-guided tumor resection

The concept of the information-guided surgical management of gliomas is based on the integration of the various intraoperative anatomical, functional, and histopathological data with a purpose to attain maximal surgical resection of the tumor with minimal risk of postoperative neurological morbidity.

In our usual practice the initial iMRI investigation with subsequent installation of data into the neuronavigation system is performed after craniotomy and completion of the approach to the tumor. After removal of the neoplasm, the investigation is repeated for assessment of the completeness of resection, identification of the residual lesion or possible adverse effects such as hemorrhage. If residual glioma is identified and considered suitable for additional resection, the newly obtained iMRI data are installed into neuronavigation device and further removal of the neoplasm is performed using this updated information (Muragaki et al., 2006, 2011). After completion of such additional resection iMRI is repeated once again.

It should be clear, however, that anatomical data alone, even if obtained with iMRI, are not sufficient enough for guidance of the tumor resection. Location of the eloquent brain structures has known individual variability and may be displaced during growth of the neoplasm, which necessitates use of comprehensive neurophysiological monitoring and intraoperative cortical and subcortical brain mapping with or without awake craniotomy, and further integration of the neurophysiological and anatomical data within the updated neuronavigation system. In any occasion the first priority in surgical decision-making should be given to such functional information (Senft et al., 2010).

Additionally, resection of the residual part of the neoplasm after removal of its main bulk should be guided by neurochemical navigation with 5-ALA and regular intaoperative histopathological investigations of the walls of the surgical cavity (Muragaki et al., 2011).

Certainly, effectiveness of the information-guided tumor resection is strongly depended on the quality of the related information (Iseki et al., 2008).

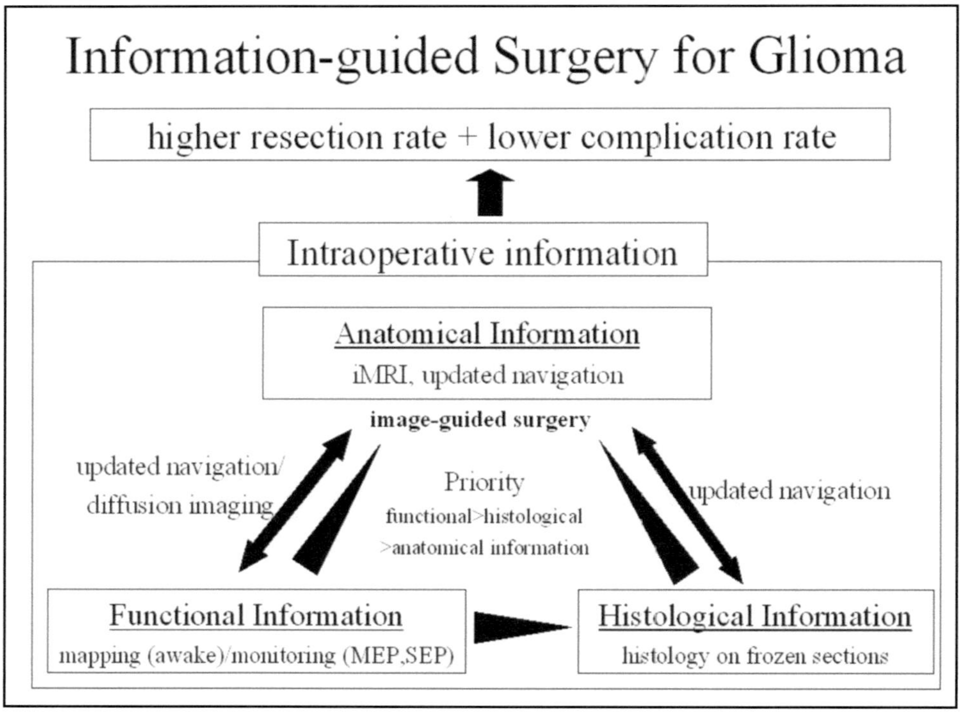

Fig. 8. Main principles of the information-guided surgery for glioma (iMRI, intraoperative MRI; MEP, motor evoked potentials; SEP, somatosensory evoked potentials).

6. Surgical experience and outcome

From March 2000 till January 2011, 939 neurosurgical interventions directed on resection of the intracranial gliomas, including 220 awake craniotomies, were performed in the intelligent operating theatre of the TWMU.

6.1 Resection rate

Maximal possible resection of glioma was attained in 99% of cases. Mean resection rate was 92%. It did not depend on histopathological grade and constituted, in median, 91%, 93%, and 92% for WHO grade II, III, and IV tumors, respectively.

Median residual tumor volume was 0.17 cc. In general, it was greater in neoplasms of higher histopathological and functional grade, but such trends did not reach statistical significance. Radiologically total tumor removal was achieved in 46% of cases.

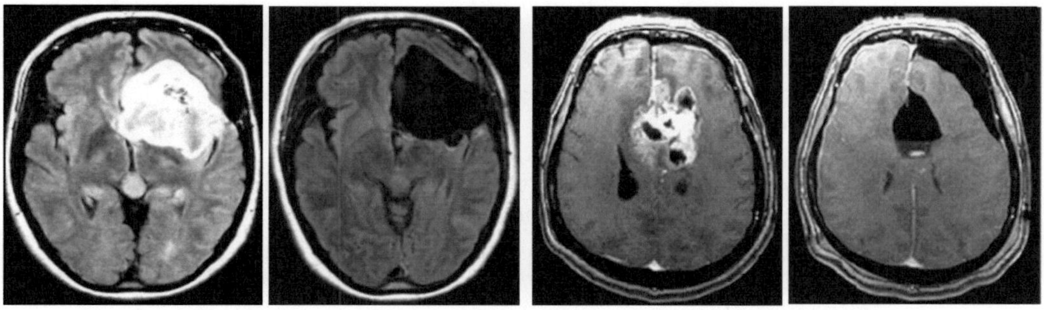

Fig. 9. Examples of the total surgical resection of the low-grade (*left*) and high-grade (*right*) gliomas.

6.1.1 Effectiveness of iMRI

Low-field-strength iMRI showed high sensitivity for detection of the residual glioma, which was confirmed by postoperative high-field-strength MRI investigations. In no one case of our series unexpected residual tumor was disclosed.

6.2 Technical failures and complications

In 0.3% of cases technical troubles with iMRI did not permit to perform aggressive surgery. In 2% of awake craniotomies tumor resection was not completed as planned due to lost of cooperation with the operated patient.

Immediately after surgery more or less prominent neurological deterioration was marked in 34% of patients. It should be noted, however, that in more than half of these cases, the symptoms regressed at least up to preoperative level within 3 subsequent months. The risk of such temporary postoperative neurological deterioration was found to be higher in cases with greater resection rate.

Wound infection after tumor removal was met in 2% of cases. Hemorrhage complicated stereotactic brain biopsy in 1% of cases.

6.2.1 Learning curve

Gradual gaining of experience of surgical management of gliomas in the intelligent operating theater resulted in statistically significant increase of tumor resection rate, and decrease of the volume of residual neoplasm, especially in cases of histopathological WHO grade IV and Sawaya functional grade III tumors.

Nevertheless, in our latest series of patients with WHO grade II and III gliomas the resection rate was intentionally decreased (in median up to 84-88%) for avoidance of postoperative neurological deterioration and providing optimal quality of life.

6.2.2 Diagnostic accuracy of stereotactic biopsy

In overall the diagnostic yield of stereotactic biopsy in our practice constituted 94%, while attained 100% in ^{1}H-MRS-supported procedures (Chernov et al., 2009). However, comparison of the histopathological diagnoses after stereotactic biopsy and subsequent surgical resection of the lesion revealed complete diagnostic agreement in 35% of cases only, whereas minor disagreement was noted in 38%, and major one in 27%. Among the latter undergrading of non-enhancing WHO grade III gliomas was the most common (Muragaki et al., 2008; Chernov et al., 2009).

6.3 Neurological outcome after glioma resection

In 13% of patients pre-existing signs and symptoms improved after surgery, whereas in 12% of patients permanent neurological deterioration was marked. After intentional decrease of resection rate in our latest series of patients with WHO grade II and III gliomas, the risk of permanent postoperative neurological deterioration reduced to 9%.

6.4 Long-term survival

In patients with available long-term follow-up the prognosis was significantly worse for WHO grade IV gliomas, but did not reach statistically significant differences between WHO grade II and III tumors (Shinohara et al., 2008). Among patients who were followed more than 2 years after surgery (46% of the total number of cases) with WHO grade II, III, and IV gliomas the corresponding actuarial 5-year survival rates were 87%, 69%, and 19%, respectively. For comparison, according to The Committee of Brain Tumor Registry of Japan (2003) the same rates in general neurosurgical practice, constitute 75%, 40%, and 7%, respectively (Muragaki et al., 2011).

In patients with low-grade glioma the extent of tumor resection was significantly associated with prolonged overall survival, progression-free survival, and malignant-progression-free survival.

7. Further perspectives

Use of iMRI and real-time updated neuronavigation has proved their great efficacy in the neurosurgical management of parenchymal brain tumors. Anyway, several problems still require solution, and necessity of further technological improvements is evident.

7.1 Computer-based system for correction of distortion artifacts

In fact, the intraoperative neuronavigation system, which is used in our practice, is not "real-time", but nearly "real-time". It means that the risk of some mislocalization errors, particularly caused by brain deformation and its movements due to surgical manipulations, is still preserved. It may be of critical importance if the lesion is located in the nearest vicinity to the eloquent brain structures. For example, the magnitude of pyramidal tract displacement due to removal of the neoplasm varies on the affected side from 0.5 to 8.7 mm (Ozawa et al., 2009b). Therefore, development of the special computer-based system for constant real-time estimation and correction of the mislocalization errors is required.

7.2 Overcoming the shortages of the low-magnetic-field iMRI

While use of low-field-strength iMRI has definite practical advantages, it also has some shortages compared to the high-field-strength devices. It is evident, that despite any technological achievements the spatial resolution of 3 Tesla MR scanner is much better. Additionally, some specific investigations, such as ^{1}H-MRS, can not be effectively attained with 0.3 Tesla iMRI. To overcome these limitations the special computer-based program for fusion of the preoperative images obtained at high-field-strength MRI or PET, with intraoperative images of low-field-strength iMRI is highly desirable, since it can potentially provide highly informative anatomic and metabolic data adjusted to intraoperative brain shift and deformation.

7.3 Robotic neurosurgery

Incorporation of the robotic systems into neurosurgical practice may provide extremely high preciseness (up to 10 µm), and may potentially reduce the risk of neurological deficit if surgery is performed in highly vulnerable brain areas. Other potential advantages of the robotics include opportunity to perform manipulations in extremely limited working space, as well as possibility of initial computer-aided modeling and simulation of the planned surgical actions.

7.4 Information-guided treatment simulation and pre-emptive risk management

In order to improve safety and effectiveness of the neurosurgical procedures their precise planning is absolutely necessary. Therefore, it is important to develop special computer-aided modalities and tools for neurosurgical simulation based both on the previous clinical experience and available scientific data. To attain such a purpose just installation of the surgical records and video into databases is not sufficient, but special system for their automatic analysis with possible immediate extraction of the very particular information important for intraoperative decision-making should be created. Such a system should permit prediction of the possible risks and inform the surgeon about their probability. The possible consequences of the various surgical manipulations have to be analyzed and the optimal solution "what to do" in constantly changing surgical situation should be offered. Moreover, at optimal such a system should simulate not only the surgical procedure, but the whole clinical course of the particular patient with comparison of the different treatment options, evaluation of the various risks, and scientifically-based choice of the optimal treatment strategy for attainment of the best possible outcome (Iseki et al, 2008, 2010).

7.5 Development of effective adjunctive treatment options

It is evident, that despite further development of the intraoperative technology, significant proportion of the intracranial gliomas will not undergo total resection due to safety concerns. It necessitates continuous search for effective adjuvant treatment modalities. Seemingly, radiosurgery may be successful in some low-grade gliomas. In cases of high-grade neoplasms addition of tumor vaccine therapy to the standard treatment protocol may provide some benefits for the patients. Individually-based choice of the chemotherapeutic drugs based on the genetic profile of the tumor also requires further investigation.

8. Conclusion

Information-guided surgical management of intracranial gliomas based on the intraoperative integration of the various anatomical, neurophysiological, and histopathological data permits to perform aggressive tumor resection with minimal risk of permanent postoperative neurological morbidity, and may result in meaningful prolongation of the patients' survival. Particularly, survival advantage in patients with WHO grade III neoplasms seems to be of special clinical significance, since may render their long-term prognosis similar to cases of low-grade tumors. It can be expected, that further development of the intraoperative technologies will permit to increase the rate of glioma resection. Nevertheless, due to safety reasons total removal seemingly will not be possible in significant proportion of these tumors, which necessitates continuous search for effective adjuvant treatment modalities.

9. Acknowledgements

The authors wish to express their gratitude to the members and technical stuff of the Departments of Neurosurgery and Anesthesiology, Surgical Facility Unit, and Faculty of Advanced Techno-Surgery of the Tokyo Women`s Medical University, as well as to maintenance team of the Hitachi Medical Corporation, for long-term friendly and fruitful collaboration during clinical work both inside and outside of the Intelligent Operating Theater, which allows for us to provide the best possible care for the patients with brain tumors. Special thanks are devoted to prof. Yoshikazu Okada, prof. Tomokatsu Hori, and Dr. Masahiko Tanaka for their constant support of our clinical and research activities.

10. References

Ando, T.; Kobayashi, E.; Liao, H.; Maruyama, T.; Muragaki, Y.; Iseki, H.; Kubo, O. & Sakuma, I. (2011). Precise comparison of protoporphyrin IX fluorescence spectra with pathological results for brain tumor tissue identification. *Brain Tumor Pathology*, Vol. 28, No. 1, (February 2011), pp. 43-51, ISSN 1433-7398

Chernov, M.F.; Muragaki, Y.; Ochiai, T.; Taira, T.; Ono, Y.; Usukura, M.; Maruyama, T.; Nakaya, K.; Nakamura, R.; Iseki, H.; Kubo, O.; Hori, T. & Takakura, K. (2009). Spectroscopy-supported frame-based image-guided stereotactic biopsy of parenchymal brain lesions: comparative evaluation of diagnostic yield and diagnostic accuracy. *Clinical Neurology and Neurosurgery*, Vol. 111, No. 6, (July 2009), pp. 527-535, ISSN 0303-8467

Fransson, A.; Andreo, P. & Potter, R. (2001). Aspects of MR image distortions in radiotherapy treatment planning. *Strahlentherapie und Onkologie*, Vol. 177, No. 2, (February 2001), pp. 59-73, ISSN 0179-7158

Gasser, T.; Szelenyi, A.; Senft, C.; Muragaki, Y.; Sandalcioglu, I.E.; Sure, U.; Nimsky, C. & Seifert, V. (2011). Intraoperative MRI and functional mapping. *Acta Neurochirurgica Supplementum*, Vol. 109, pp. 61-65, ISSN 0065-1419

Iseki, H.; Muragaki, Y.; Nakamura, R.; Ozawa, N.; Taniguchi, H.; Hori, T. & Takakura, K. (2005). Intelligent operating theater using intraoperative open-MRI. *Magnetic Resonance in Medical Sciences*, Vol. 4, No. 3, (February 2006), pp. 129–136, ISSN 1347-3182

Iseki, H. & Nambu, K. (2005). Intraoperative Examination Monitoring for Awake Surgery (IEMAS). *No Shinkei Geka*, Vol. 33, No. 10, (October 2005), pp. 1028–1031, ISSN 0301-2603

Iseki, H.; Nakamura, R.; Muragaki, Y.; Suzuku, T.; Chernov, M.; Hori, T. & Takakura K. (2008). Advanced computer-aided intraoperative technologies for information-guided surgical management of gliomas: Tokyo Women's Medical University experience. *Minimally Invasive Neurosurgery*, Vol. 51, No. 5, (October 2008), pp. 285-291, ISSN 0946-7211

Iseki, H.; Muragaki, Y.; Maruyama, T.; Chernov, M.; Suzuki, T.; Yoshimitsu, K.; Ikuta, S. & Tamura, M. (2010). Neurosurgical workflow in TWIns,. Proceedings of the 6th Asian

Conference on Computer Aided Surgery (ACCAS 2010), pp. 31-32, Busan, Korea, November 26-27, 2010

Kato, T.; Shinoda, J.; Nakayama, N.; Miwa, K.; Okumura, A.; Yano, H.; Yoshimura, S.; Maruyama, T.; Muragaki, Y. & Iwama T. (2008). Metabolic assessment of gliomas using 11C-methionine, [18F] fluorodeoxyglucose, and 11C-choline positron-emission tomography. *AJNR Am J Neuroradiol*, Vol. 29, No. 6, (June 2008), pp. 1176-1182, ISSN 0195-6108

Lacroix, M.; Abi-Said, D.; Fourney, D.R.; Gokaslan, Z.L.; Shi, W.; DeMonte, F.; Lang, F.F.; McCutcheon, I.E.; Hassenbusch, S.J.; Holland, E.; Hess, K.; Michael, C.; Miller, D. & Sawaya R. (2001). A multivariate analysis of 416 patients with glioblastoma multiforme: prognosis, extent of resection, and survival. *Journal of Neurosurgery*, Vol. 95, No. 2, (August 2001), pp. 190–198, ISSN 0022-3085

Mikuni, N. & Miyamoto, S. (2010). Surgical treatment of glioma: extent of resection applying functional neurosurgery. *Neurologia Medico-Chirurgica*, Vol. 50, No. 9, (September 2010), pp. 720-726, ISSN 0470-8105

Muragaki, Y.; Iseki, H.; Maruyama, T.; Kawamata, T.; Yamane, F.; Nakamura, R.; Kubo, O.; Takakura, K. & Hori, T. (2006). Usefulness of intraoperative magnetic resonance imaging for glioma surgery. *Acta Neurochirurgica Supplementum*, Vol. 98, pp. 67-75, ISSN 0065-1419

Muragaki, Y.; Chernov, M.; Maruyama, T.; Ochiai, T.; Taira, T.; Kubo, O.; Nakamura, R.; Iseki, H.; Hori, T. & Takakura K. (2008). Low-grade glioma on stereotactic biopsy: how often is the diagnosis accurate? *Minimally Invasive Neurosurgery*, Vol. 51, No. 5, (October 2008), pp. 275-279, ISSN 0946-7211

Muragaki, Y.; Iseki, H.; Maruyama, T.; Tanaka, M.; Shinohara, C.; Suzuku, T.; Yoshimitsu, K.; Ikuta, S.; Hayashi, M.; Chernov, M.; Hori, T.; Okada, Y. & Takakura, K. (2011). Information-guided surgical management of gliomas using low-field-strength intraoperative MRI. *Acta Neurochirurgica Supplementum*, Vol. 109, pp. 67-72, ISSN 0065-1419

Otani, N.; Bjeljac, M.; Muroi, C.; Weniger, D.; Khan, N.; Wieser H.G.; Curcic, M. & Yonekawa, Y. (2005). Awake surgery for glioma resection in eloquent areas: Zurich's experience and review. *Neurologia Medico-Chirurgica*, Vol. 45, No. 10, (October 2005), pp. 501-511, ISSN 0470-8105

Ozawa, N.; Muragaki, Y.; Nakamura, R. & Iseki, H. (2008a). Intraoperative diffusion-weighted imaging for visualization of the pyramidal tracts. Part I: Pre-clinical validation of the scanning protocol. *Minimally Invasive Neurosurgery*, Vol. 51, No. 2, (April 2008), pp. 63-66, ISSN 0946-7211

Ozawa, N.; Muragaki, Y.; Nakamura, R. & Iseki, H. (2008b). Intraoperative diffusion-weighted imaging for visualization of the pyramidal tracts. Part II: Clinical study of usefulness and efficacy. *Minimally Invasive Neurosurgery*, Vol. 51, No. 2, (April 2008), pp. 67-71, ISSN 0946-7211

Ozawa, N.; Muragaki, Y.; Nakamura, R. & Iseki, H. (2009a). Identification of the pyramidal tract by neuronavigation based on intraoperative diffusion-weighted imaging combined with subcortical stimulation. *Stereotactic and Functional Neurosurgery*, Vol. 87, No. 1, (February 2009), pp. 18-24, ISSN 1423-0372

Ozawa, N.; Muragaki, Y.; Nakamura R.; Hori, T. & Iseki, H. (2009b). Shift of the pyramidal tract during resection of the intraaxial brain tumors estimated by intraoperative diffusion-weighted imaging. *Neurologia Medico-Chirurgica*, Vol. 49, No. 2, (February 2009), pp. 51-56, ISSN 0470-8105

Proescholdt, M.A.; Macher, C.; Woertgen, C. & Brawanski A. (2005). Level of evidence in the literature concerning brain tumor resection. *Clinical Neurology and Neurosurgery*, Vol. 107, No. 2, (February 2005), pp. 95-98, ISSN 0303-8467

Sakurai, Y.; Muragaki, Y.; Okada, Y.; Nambu, K. & Iseki, H. (2011). The development and application of the device for intraoperative examination monitor for awake surgery. *Journal of Tokyo Women's Medical University*, Vol. 81, No. 1, (February 2011), pp. 32-40, ISSN 0040-9022

Sanai, N.; Polley, M.Y.; McDermott, M.W.; Parsa, A.T & Berger M.S. (2011). An extent of resection threshold for newly diagnosed glioblastomas. *Journal of Neurosurgery*, (in press), ISSN 0022-3085

Sawaya, R.; Hammoud, M.; Schoppa, D.; Hess, K.R.; Wu, S.Z.; Shi, W.M. & Wildrick, D.M. (1998). Neurosurgical outcomes in a modern series of 400 craniotomies for treatment of parenchymal tumors. *Neurosurgery*, Vol. 42, No. 5, (May 1998), pp. 1044-1056, ISSN 0148-396X

Senft, C.; Franz, K.; Ulrich, C.T.; Bink, A.; Szelenyi, A.; Gasser, T. & Seifert. V. (2010). Low field intraoperative MRI-guided surgery of gliomas: a single center experience. *Clinical Neurology and Neurosurgery*, Vol. 112, No. 3, (April 2010), pp. 237-243, ISSN 0303-8467

Shinohara, C.; Muragaki, Y.; Maruyama, T.; Shimizu, S.; Tanaka, M.; Kubota, Y.; Oikawa, M.; Nakamura, R.; Iseki, H.; Kubo, O.; Takakura, K. & Hori. T. (2008). Long-term prognostic assessment of 185 newly diagnosed gliomas: Grade III glioma showed prognosis comparable to that of Grade II glioma. *Japanese Journal of Clinical Oncology*, Vol. 38, No. 11, (November 2008), pp. 730-733, ISSN 0368-2811

Stummer, W.; Reulen, H.J.; Meinel, T.; Pichlmeier, U.; Schumacher, W.; Tonn, J.C.; Rohde, V.; Oppel, F.; Turowski, B.; Woiciechowsky, C.; Franz, K.; Pietsch, T. & ALA-Glioma study group. (2008). Extent of resection and survival in glioblastoma multiforme: identification of and adjustment for bias. *Neurosurgery*, Vol. 62, No. 3, (March 2008), pp. 564-576, ISSN 0148-396X

Taniguchi, H.; Muragaki, Y.; Iseki, H.; Nakamura, R. & Taira, T. (2006). New radiofrequency coil integrated with a stereotactic frame for intraoperative MRI-controlled stereotactically guided brain surgery. *Stereotactic and Functional Neurosurgery*, Vol. 84, No. 4, (September 2006), pp. 136-141, ISSN 1423-0372

The Committee of Brain Tumor Registry of Japan. (2003). Report of brain tumor registry of Japan (1969-1996), 11th edition. *Neurologia Medico-Chirurgica*, Vol. 43, Supplement, (September 2003), pp. 1-111, ISSN 0470-8105

van den Bent, M.J.; Carpentier, A.F.; Brandes, A.A.; Sanson, M.; Taphoorn, M.J.; Bernsen, H.J.; Frenay, M.; Tijssen, C.C.; Grisold, W.; Sipos, L.; Haaxma-Reiche, H.; Kros, J.M.; van Kouwenhoven, M.C.; Vecht, C.J.; Allqeier, A.; Lacombe, D. & Gorlia, T. (2006). Adjuvant procarbasine, lomustine, and vincristine improves progression-free survival but not overall survival in newly diagnosed anaplastic oligodendrogliomas and oligoastrocytomas: a randomized European Organisation for Research and Treatment of Cancer phase III trial. *Journal of Clinical Oncology*, Vol. 24, No. 18, (June 2006), pp. 2715-2722, ISSN 0732-183X

Yoshimitsu, K.; Suzuki, T.; Muragaki, Y.; Chernov, M. & Iseki H. (2010). Development of modified Intraoperative Examination Monitor for Awake Surgery (IEMAS) system for awake craniotomy during brain tumor resection, *Proceedings of the 32nd Annual International Conference of the IEEE Engineering in Medicine and Biology Society*, pp. 6050-6053, ISBN 978-1-4244-4123-5, Buenos Aires, Argentina, August 31- September 4, 2010